Arrhythmia – A Guide to Clinical Electrocardiology

Foreword by
Ronald Campbell

Arrhythmia – A Guide to Clinical Electrocardiology

Erik Sandøe
Bjarne Sigurd

Foreword by
Ronald Campbell

Publishing Partners Verlags GmbH

The authors and publisher have made every effort to ensure that drug selection and dosage outlined in this text comply with current recommendations and clinical application at the time of publication. However, in the light of ongoing research and the voluminous inflow of information concerning drug therapy as well as the outside possibility of typographical inconsistencies, the reader is urged to check any dosage carefully also against package insert for any change in indications and dosage and for added warnings and precautions. This becomes increasingly important with any new and/ or infrequently employed drug.

Publishing Partners Verlags GmbH
Ockenheimer Chaussee 5
D-6530 Bingen

ISBN-Nr. 3-927925-02-0

Lay-out and art work of all ECGs:
STUDIO Z
Corporate Communication
Ockenheimer Chaussee 5
D-6530 Bingen

Drawings: Figs. 1.7, 1.11–1.16, 1.20–1.23, 1.25, 1.31 and 3.6: Peter Skanning

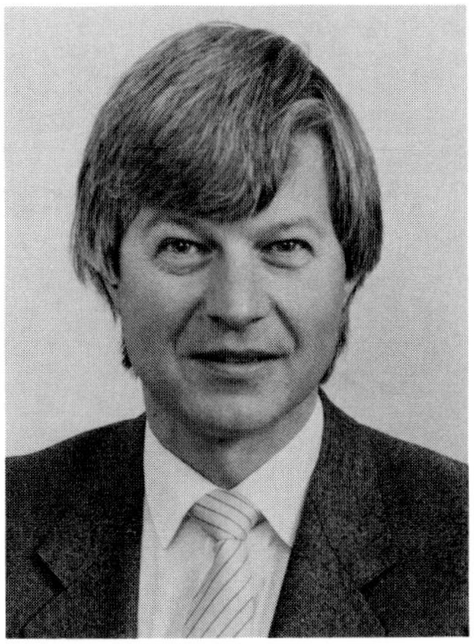

Ronald Campbell

Professor Campbell, born 1946, is a Cardiologist with a special interest in arrhythmias, electrophysiology and electrosurgery. He graduated from Edinburgh in 1969 and worked at Duke University Medical Centre before returning to the U.K. to work in Newcastle upon Tyne. In 1986 he was appointed chief of the Academic Department of Cardiology. His Department, supported by the British Heart Foundation, has an international reputation for arrhythmia management and electrophysiological research.

Foreword

Over the years there have been many great textbooks devoted to electrocardiography: Lewis *"The Mechanisms and Graphic Registration of the Heart Beat"* 1925; Korth *"Klinische Elektrokardiographie"* 1941; Katz *"Electrocardiography"* 1941; Lepeschkin *"Modern Electrocardiography"* 1951; Marriott *"Practical Electrocardiography"* 1952; Graybiel et al *"Electrocardiography in Practice"* 1952; Scherf and Boyd *"Clinical Electrocardiography"* 1953; Scherf and Schott *"Extrasystoles and Allied Arrhythmias"* 1953; Goldman *"Principles of Clinical Electrocardiography"* 1956; Sodi Pallares and Calder *"New Basis of Electrocardiography"* 1956; Katz and Pick *"Clinical Electrocardiography"* 1956; Grant *"Clinical Electrocardiography"* 1957; Latour and Puech *"Electrocardiographie endocavitaire"* 1957; Massie and Welsh *"Clinical Vectorcardiography and Electrocardiography"* 1960; Hoffman and Cranefield *"Electrocardiography of the Heart"* 1960; Wolff *"Electrocardiography. Fundamentals and Clinical Applications"* 1962; Bellet *"Clinical Disorders of the Heart Beat"* 1963; Hoffman *"Sudden Cardiac Death"* 1964; Langendorf and Pick *"Mechanisms and Therapy of Cardiac Arrhythmias"* 1966; Rosenbaum *"Los Hemibloques"* 1968; Stock *"Diagnosis and Treatment of Cardiac Arrhythmias"* 1969; Schamroth *"The Disorders of Cardiac Rhythm"* 1971; Bayes and Cosin *"Diagnosis and Treatment of Cardiac Arrhythmias"* 1980.

As the dates attest, the pace has slowed. Have time and research revealed the final mysteries of the surface ECG? Experience tells otherwise. The surface ECG pattern of ischaemia and infarction are well recognised but their cellular basis is not understood. Considerable precision in arrhythmia diagnosis is possible from the surface ECG but the fundamental mechanisms of the arrhythmia are rarely exposed. In an era of aggressive intervention for ischaemia, infarction and arrhythmias, these deficiencies are not merely of academic interest. The surface ECG is a fragile tool. It offers a simple non-invasive "average" view of cardiac electrical events but cellular phenomena are not exposed, rather they are inferred from clinical experience and from basic research results. There have been dramatic advances in cellular cardiac electrophysiological research. The ionic fluxes and control mechanisms responsible for electrical events are now relatively well established and in the isolated heart or in tissue bath preparations, the fundamental mechanisms of arrhythmia production have been studied and analysed, stripped of confounding and confusing external factors. The advent of invasive electrophysiological examinations in man in 1969 was heralded as the bridge between basic research and clinical practice but those expectations have been satisfied only in part. Invasive electrophysiology has helped understand some specific arrhythmias although disappointingly, arrhythmia management remains empirical and unscientific. Interpreting the surface electrocardiogram still owes as much to art as it does to science. The clinician must allow for underlying autonomic influences and the effects of destabilising disease, yet remarkably, from this volatile representation of the heart's electrical activity, clinical diagnosis and management of cardiac electrical events and arrhythmias has reached its present day sophistication.

It is a major challenge to communicate the art and science of electrocardiography. This book is a unique and worthy addition to the library of electrocardiography. It combines the experience and wisdom of traditionalist grand masters of cardiology with modern knowledge of cellular cardiac electrophysiology. Here are spectacular high quality examples of cardiac arrhythmias – common and uncommon. Here are explanations that involve basic science and clinical invasive electrophysiology. Here are up-to-date key references for every aspect of electrocardiography and of arrhythmias and their management. Here are treatment suggestions that acknowledge our ever increasing armamentarium for the management of arrhythmias and include the new non-pharmacological procedures of ablation, antitachycardia pacing, implantable defibrillators and surgery. Here is a good common sense. As a reference text, as a teaching source or as a primer in clinical electrocardiography, there is something in this fine book for everyone.

Newcastle upon Tyne, October 1990

Ronald W.F. Campbell

Preface

This textbook aims to present current knowledge about cardiac arrhythmias in a clinical context for a wide medical audience from the general practitioner to the internist and clinical cardiologist, and also including the nurse in the Coronary Care Unit. Information is set out in guideline form to make it useful for dealing with cardiac arrhythmias as they are encountered in the day-to-day life in the clinic. The principles of arrhythmia mechanisms and antiarrhythmic interventions are outlined in the simplest of terms in an attempt to render the text understandable for the reader without specific background in physics or electronics.

The book is illustrated with a number of ECG recordings reproduced on a scale of 1:1. The legend of each figure explains the characteristics of the ECG tracing in some detail so that the book can be used as an ECG atlas with a comprehensive representation of common arrhythmias and a reasonable selection of the rare and often serious arrhythmias which may endanger the life of the patient.

To avoid misunderstandings stemming from inconsistent or nonspecific terminology we have adhered strictly to recommendations of the Task Force assigned by the World Health Organization (WHO) and the International Society and Federation of Cardiology (ISFC) to define and classify cardiac arrhythmias (see WHO/ISFC Task Force. Definitions of terms related to cardiac rhythm. Eur J Cardiol 1978, 8: 127-44).

The many ECG illustrations presented in the book are almost all from Medical Department B, Rigshospitalet, University Hospital of Copenhagen. Special thanks are in order to the nursing staff of the Coronary Care Unit who assisted in the assembling of the ECG examples.

Acknowledgement and expression of our gratitude is extended to Professor R.W.F. Campbell, Freeman Hospital, Newcastle upon Tyne without whose astute reading of the manuscript and eloquent language editing of the text this volume would not have been the one it has become.

The publication of the book was made possible by a generous educational grant from Boehringer Ingelheim. We wish to express our gratitude to this pharmaceutical company for its understanding and cooperation in meeting our needs during our work with the book.

Erik Sandøe Bjarne Sigurd

Contents

Contents

Chapter 1
Fundamentals of electrocardiography

The myocardial cell [1, 2]

Cardiac muscle cells are striated muscle cells containing both myosin and actin filaments. The processes of adjacent cells are joined end-to-end by structures known as intercalated disks (Fig. 1.1). These disks are, in fact, cell membranes, but they have a very low electrical impedance (resistance) which facilitates impulse propagation from one cell to the next. Thus the atria and ventricles function as a coherent network of cells, a functional syncytium. When the first cell in the network is activated, it will fire off the next and so on until the whole atrial or ventricular myocardium has been activated.

The conduction system of the heart [1, 2]

The *conduction system of the heart* comprises collections of specialized cells with particular electrophysiological properties for conduction and impulse formation (pacemaker activity). The system is composed of (Fig. 1.2): The *sinoatrial (SA) node,* the *atrioventricular (AV)* node, *the His bundle,* the *right bundle branch,* the *left bundle* branch and its two fascicles, the slender *left anterior fascicle* and the broad *left posterior fascicle,* and the *Purkinje fibres.*

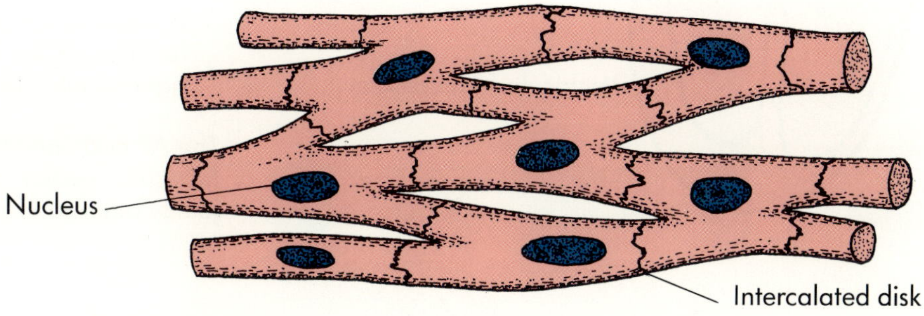

Fig. 1.1
A section of the myocardium seen under the microscope. The striated muscle cells are delimited and at the same time attached end-to-end by modified cell membranes, the intercalated disks, facilitating impulse propagation from cell to cell.

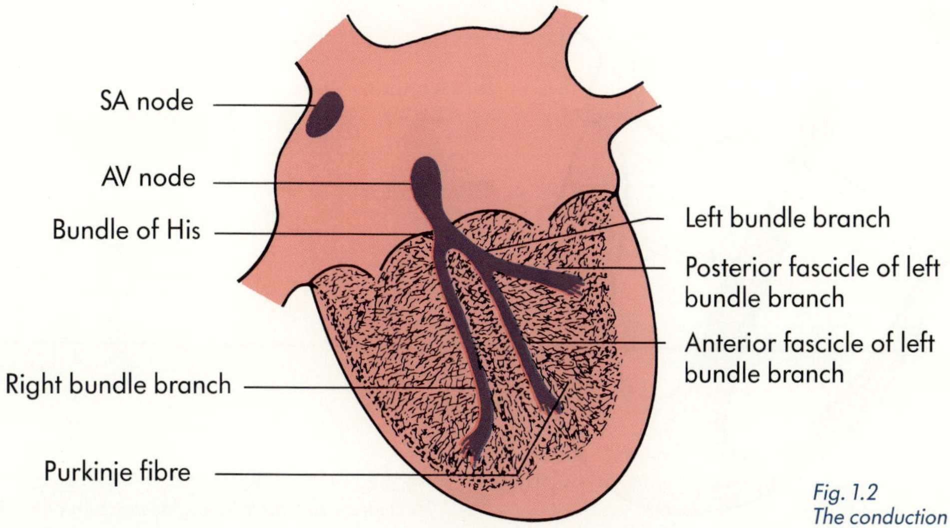

Fig. 1.2
The conduction system of the heart

The two-chambered heart [2, 3]

Electrophysiologically the heart is "two-chambered" (Fig. 1.3) with the atrial and ventricular myocardium separated from each other by the fibrous tissue of the atrioventricular rings. The only link between the two "chambers" of the atria and the ventricles, is a thin muscular bridge, the AV conduction system.

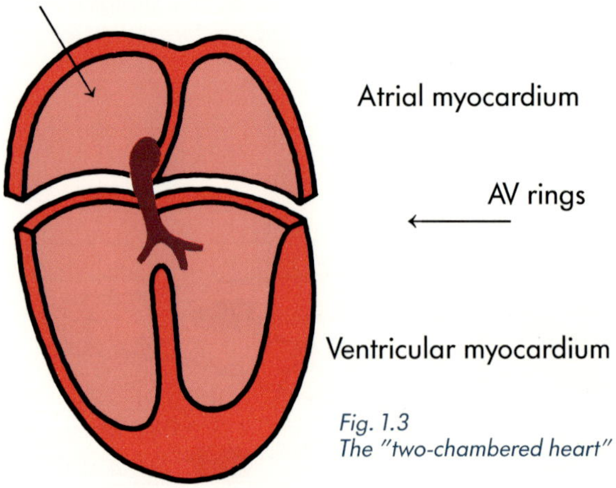

Fig. 1.3
The "two-chambered heart"

AV conduction system [2, 4–8]

The muscular link between the atria and the ventricles, the AV conduction system is composed of (Fig.1.4):

1 A monofascicular pathway: The AV node and its continuation, the bundle of His.

2 A bifascicular pathway: The left bundle branch and, parallel with it, the first part of the right bundle branch.

3 A trifascicular pathway: The anterior and posterior fascicles of the left bundle branch parallel with the right bundle branch.

The AV node and the bundle of His (forming the monofascicular section of the AV conduction pathway) are jointly referred to as the AV junction.

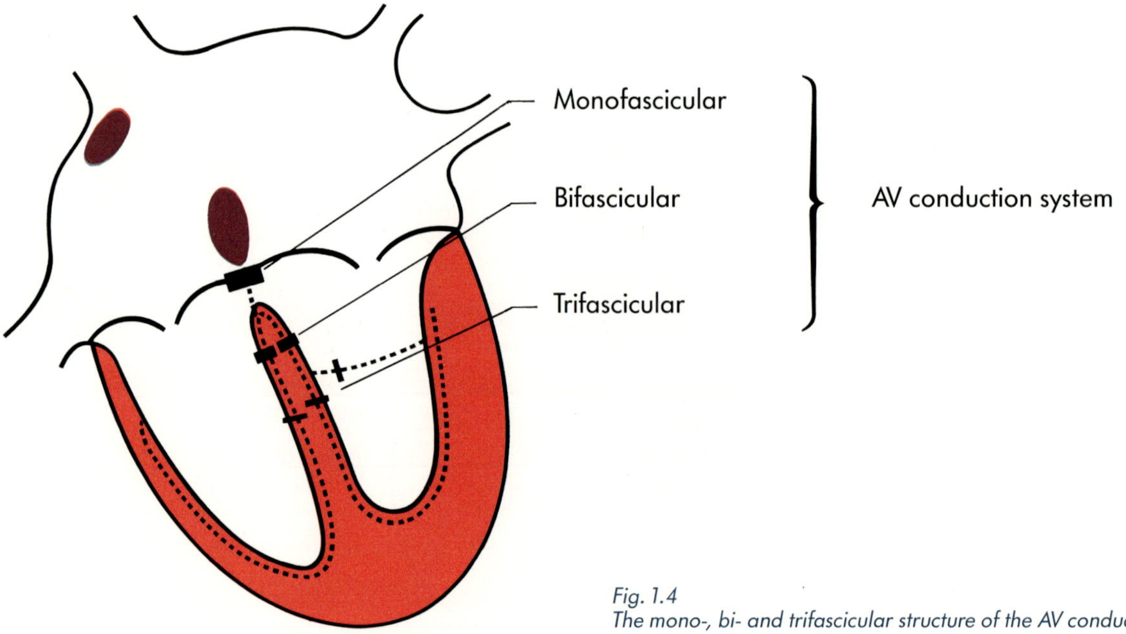

Fig. 1.4
The mono-, bi- and trifascicular structure of the AV conduction

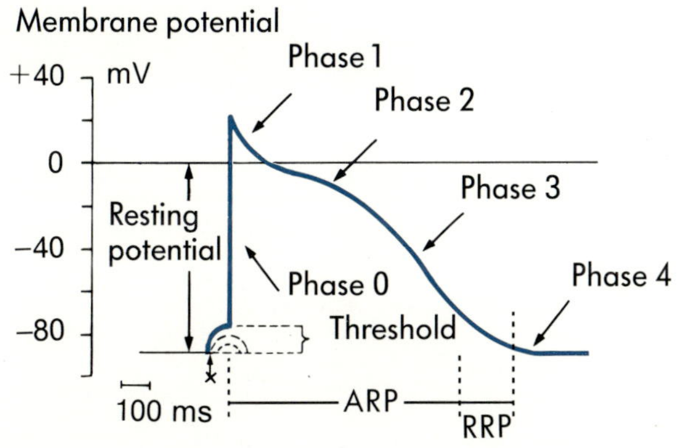

Fig. 1.5
Action potential of the myocardial cell
ARP: Absolute refractory period, RRP: Relative refractory period

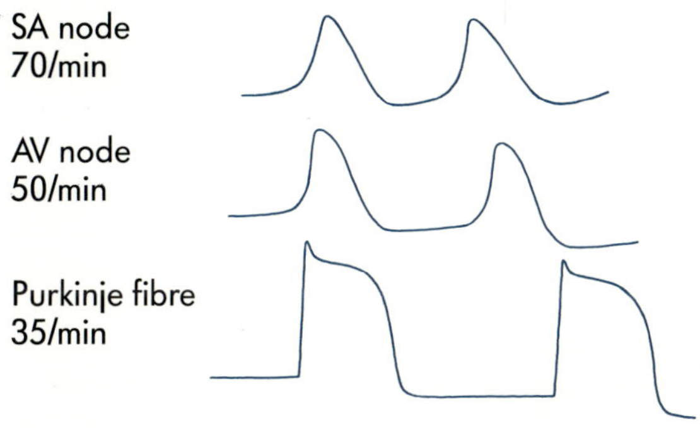

Fig. 1.6
Action potentials recorded from isolated pacemaker cells immersed in a saline bath and firing at their own inherent discharge rates

The action potential [1, 9, 10]

The membrane of the resting cell is polarized with positive charges on the outside and negative charges within, the resting membrane potential being 60–90 mV (Fig.1.5). The cell will contract if activated by a negative electrical current applied to its surface. The application of a very weak electrical current results merely in a transient, moderate reduction of the membrane potential (stipled lines in Fig. 1.5). However, once the membrane potential is reduced beyond a critical level, the *threshold potential,* the cell is activated and contracts. The formerly negative membrane potential rises abruptly to about +30 mV.

This rapid depolarization of the cell membrane (phase 0) is succeeded by a brief period of rapid repolarization towards the zero potential (phase 1), a plateau phase (phase 2) with the membrane potential maintained at or near zero potential. Finally, the activation is terminated by rapid repolarization (phase 3) with restoration of the resting membrane potential. The subsequent diastolic period with a stable membrane potential is known as phase 4.

The entire sequence of potential changes from the beginning of depolarization to the end of repolarization is the *action potential* of the cell (Fig. 1.5). From the start of depolarization until repolarization restores the membrane potential to a critical level, usually about −50 mV, the cell cannot be reactivated by a stimulus of any strength, *the absolute refractory period (ARP).* From then until just before complete repolarization, only strong stimuli can evoke a response, *the relative refractory period (RRP).* The action potential evoked during the RRP is usually of reduced amplitude which may fail to stimulate neighbouring cells with no resultant impulse propagation.

The majority of myocardial cells are ordinary working cells which contract only upon stimulation from an external source. However, cells with a capacity for impulse formation, *pacemaker cells,* are found in the conduction system. In pacemaker cells, full repolarization (end phase 3) is followed by a slow but steady decrease in the resting membrane potential. This period of *diastolic depolarization* (phase 4 of the action potential of the pacemaker cell) eventually reaches the threshold for activation of the cell; a new action potential is evoked, and so the process continues (Fig. 1.6). The steeper the slope of phase 4, the higher the discharge rate of the pacemaker. The steepness (rate of rise) of phase 4 decreases (and ergo the discharge rate) the more peripherally the pacemaker cells are located in the conduction system.

A pacemaker is a group of cells capable of activating the heart. The *pacemaker of the heart* is the cell group which actually activates and so *paces* the heart. Pacemaker cells in the SA node discharge 60–100 times/min, those of the AV node 40–60 times/min and those of the Purkinje fibres 30–40 times/min. Normally the SA node is the pacemaker of the heart as due to its high inherent discharge rate it activates and resets the other pacemakers before their own spontaneous depolarization. The physiological role of the other pacemakers, the *ectopic or subsidiary pacemakers,* is as a standby, ready to take over pacing of the heart if normal impulse generation or propagation should fail.

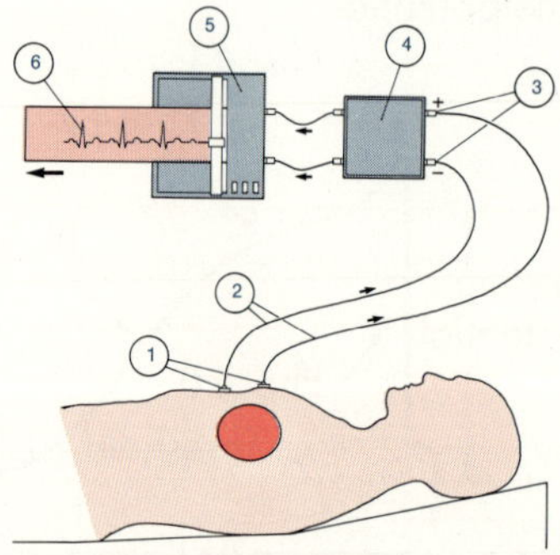

Fig. 1.7
The principal elements of an ECG recording system
1) The electrodes 2) The leads 3) The input terminals of the amplifier 4) The amplifier 5) The recorder and 6) the ECG
Usually, the amplifier and the recorder will be built together in one unit

Principles of electrocardiography [11, 12]

During activation and subsequent repolarization the many cells of the heart behave like electrical generators from which electrical current flows out into the body and back again to the heart producing varying electrical potentials on the body surface. Electrocardiography (ECG) is the technique used for the recording of these electrical manifestations of cardiac activity. The principal elements of an ECG recording system are shown in Fig. 1.7. The voltage difference is measured between two electrodes in immediate contact with the skin (1). Together a pair of electrodes form an ECG lead (2) which is connected to the two input terminals (3) of an ECG amplifier (4). The amplified signal is fed to a recorder (5) or to a TV monitor or an oscilloscope. The resulting curve is the electrocardiogram, the ECG (6).

The ECG represents voltage difference as a function of time. The voltage is indicated along the Y (vertical) axis of the diagram and time along the X (horizontal) axis (Fig. 1.8). When there is no voltage difference between the electrodes of the ECG lead, the ECG records a straight line, an *isoelectric line.* An upward deflection from this line is a *positive deflection* or *wave.* Similarly, a downward deflection from the isoelectric line is a negative *deflection* or *wave.*

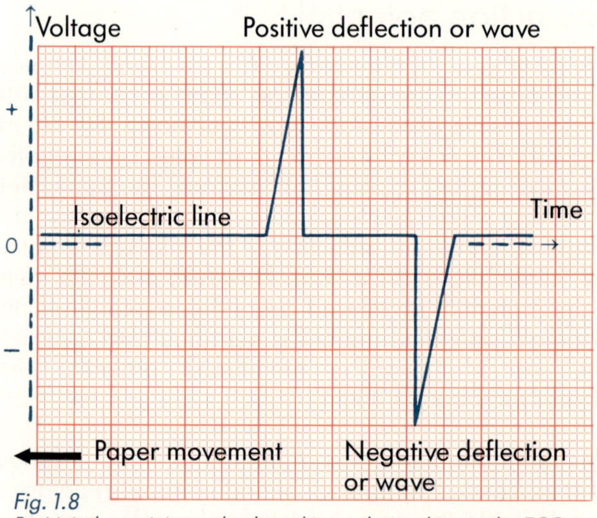

Fig. 1.8
Positivity/negativity and voltage/time relationships in the ECG

Calibration of the ECG [13, 14]

The paper used for ECG recording is divided by thick and thin lines into large (5 x 5 mm) and small (1 x 1 mm) squares (Fig. 1.9). At a paper speed of 25 mm/s which is the most commonly used paper speed and the one preferred in this book, the width of one of the large square corresponds to 0.20 s and that of a small square 0.04 s (Fig. 1.9).

The amplifier is normally calibrated so that the test square wave of 1 mV corresponds to a deflection of 10 mm above the isoelectric line, the height of two large squares (Fig. 1.9). Half amplification, or "half sensitivity" where 1 mV = 5 mm (the height of one large square) is used in the patient whose ECG deflections are too large to be recorded within the normal range of the ECG recorder at normal amplification.

The height of the deflections or waves are by tradition indicated in mm implying that standard amplification has been used (10 mm = 1 mV). If amplification is only "half sensitivity" (1 mV = 5 mm), the measured distances in millimeters have to be converted to "standard millimeters of ECG" by multiplying by two.

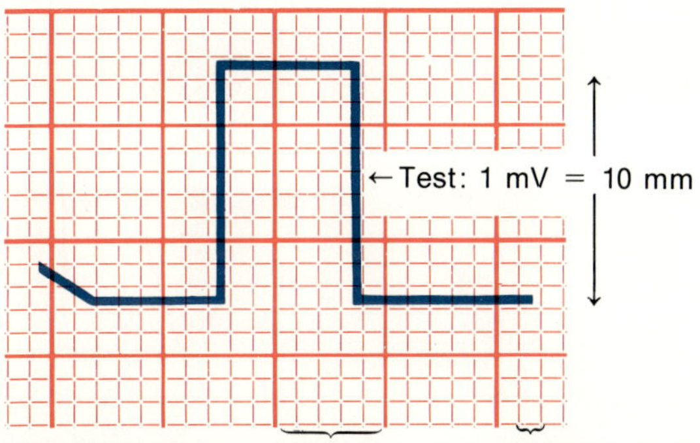

Paper speed 50 mm/s:	0.1 s	0.02 s
Paper speed 25 mm/s:	0.2 s	0.04 s
Paper speed 10 mm/s:	0.5 s	0.10 s

Fig. 1.9
Paper speed and voltage calibration in ECG recording

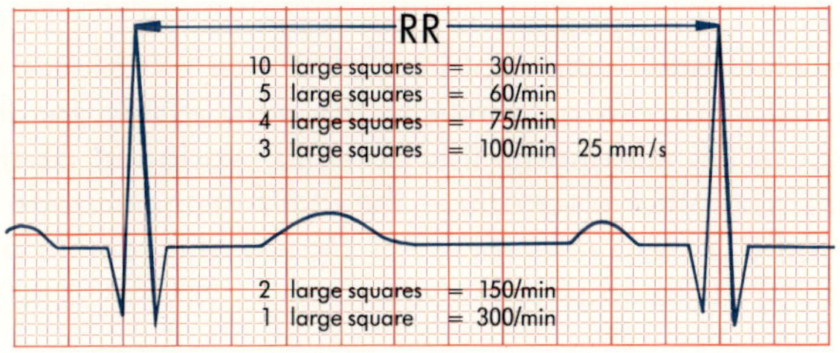

Fig. 1.10
Rapid assessment of heart rate by the "rule of 300"

Measurement of heart rate

A quick estimate of cardiac rate is provided by the "rule of 300" (Fig. 1.10):

$$\text{Heart rate/min} = \frac{300}{\text{RR (PP) measured in large squares}}$$

Search for an R wave (or P wave) falling on a heavy vertical line and measure the distance to the next R wave (or P wave) in numbers of heavy vertical lines. An interval of one line correlates to a rate of 300/1 = 300/min, of two 300/2 = 150/min, of three 300/3 = 100/min and of four 300/4 = 75/min etc.

The isolated muscle strip experiment [11, 12]

An understanding of some of the electrophysiological processes involved in the formation of the ECG is gained by considering the electrical events surrounding the activation and repolarization of an isolated muscle strip cut from the thick free wall of the left ventricle (Fig. 1.11, page 8). The muscle strip, which for an analogy with the clinical situation might represent the heart, is suspended in a vessel filled with an electrolyte solution representing the body. Electrical potential variations occurring in the electrolyte solution are assessed by voltage measurement through a pair of electrodes representing an ECG lead. The two electrodes are connected to a voltmeter/ink recorder unit representing an ECG

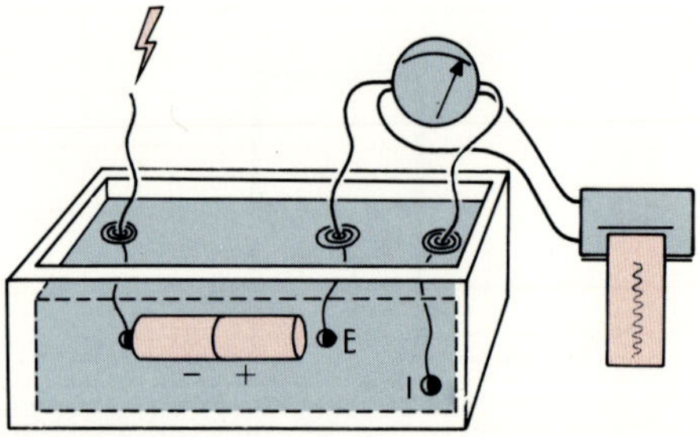

Fig. 1.11
An experimental setting with a muscle strip immersed in a large vessel filled with an electrolyte solution. The voltmeter output is recorded on paper by an ink recorder
E = Exploring electrode
I = Indifferent electrode

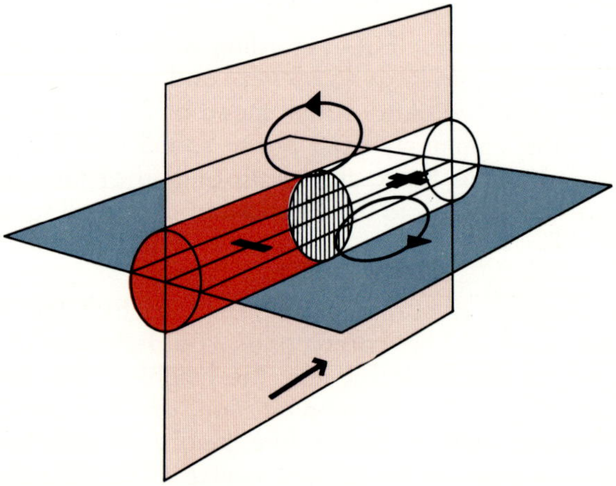

Fig. 1.12
Dipole of the propagating activation wave front with electrical current flowing in curved pathways from the front source to the rear sink. Experimental setting as in Fig. 1.11.

channel with a paper write-out representing the ECG. One electrode – the *exploring electrode* – is placed at point (E) in close proximity to the muscle strip for the purpose of measuring the potential variation at this point. The other electrode – the *indifferent electrode* – is used as a zero reference; it is placed at a remote position (I) at the edge of the vessel.

Activation of the muscle strip is initiated by application of a brief electrical shock to one end of the strip. Once initiated, the activation wave proceeds along the strip until the entire strip has become activated.

The propagating front of the activation wave forms an electrical dipole with a positive front side (the positively charged surface of the still resting muscle) and a negative rear (the negatively charged just activated muscle) (Fig. 1.12). From the source on the front side of this dipole electrical current flows in curved pathways out in the surrounding electrolyte solution and back again to the "sink" on its rear side. The associated potential variations in the electrolyte solution (Fig. 1.13) are sensed by the voltmeter and recorded on the paper write out (the "ECG") from the ink recorder.

Several simple rules for inscribing the deflections (waves) in an ECG recording can be illustrated by this experimental model:

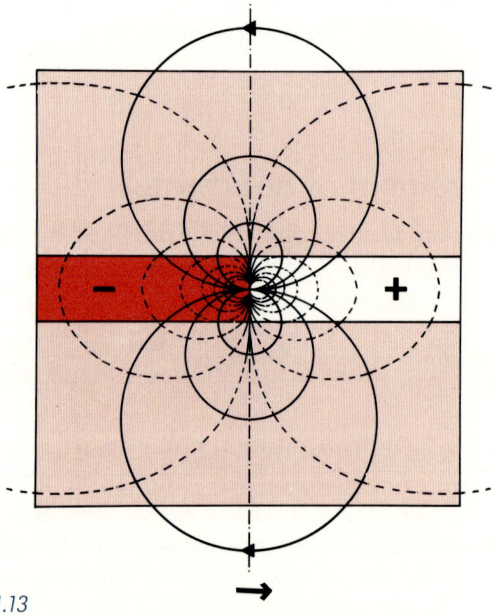

Fig. 1.13
A planar mapping of the current flow field from Fig. 1.12. Solid lines indicate flow of electrical current, stippled lines evoked potential difference (each stippled line is an isopotential which connects points of an equal electrical potential with a change in electrical potential of e. g. 0.1 mV from one line to the next).

An activation wave moving toward the exploring electrode will record a positive deflection (an R wave) on the ECG; the larger the muscle mass the greater the deflection. At the moment of complete activation of the muscle strip (heart), the dipole ceases to exist and the ECG tracing returns abruptly to the isoelectric line (Fig. 1.14).
An activation wave travelling away from the exploring electrode will inscribe a negative deflection (a Q or QS wave) on an ECG; the larger the muscle mass the deeper the deflection. Again when activation of the whole muscle strip (heart) is complete, the ECG tracing returns abruptly to the isoelectric line (Fig. 1.15).

Finally, the pattern of ECG deflections varies with the site of the electrode in relation to the direction of the spread of the activation wave along the long axis of the muscle strip. The determinant is the angle, sometimes called the axis, between the sighting line from the center of the muscle strip to the exploring electrode and the direction of the spread of the activation wave (Fig. 1.16). The maximum deflection on the ECG is recorded with the line of sight (axis) parallel to the spread of the activation wave; a major posi-

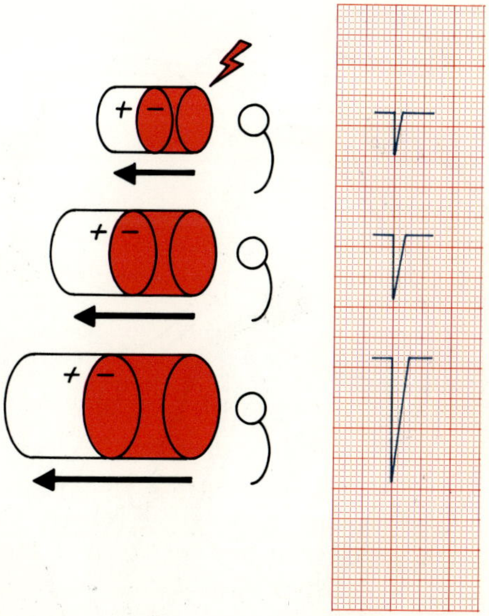

Fig. 1.15
Activation away from the electrode results in a negative deflection. The larger the muscle mass, the deeper the deflection. Same experimental setting as in Fig. 1.11.

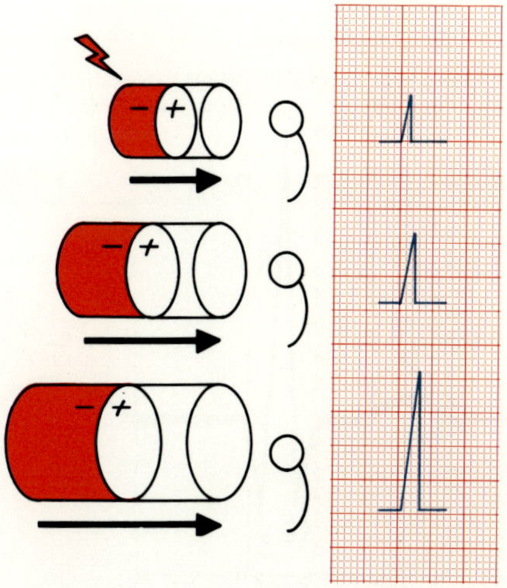

Fig. 1.14
Activation towards the electrode results in a positive deflection; the larger the muscle mass, the higher the deflection. Same experimental setting as in Fig. 1.11

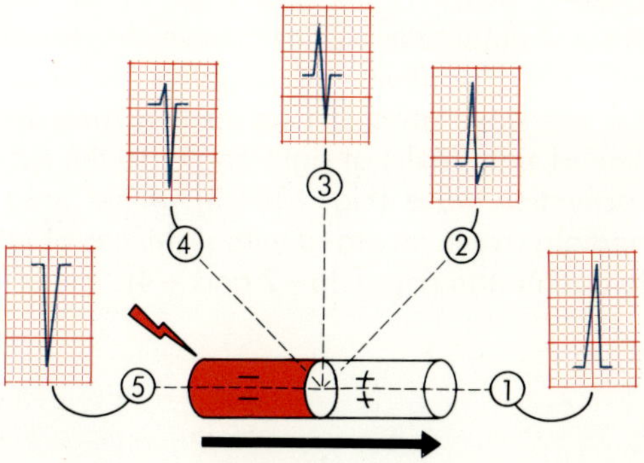

Fig. 1.16
Recording with the exploring electrode placed at a varying angle (axis) to the direction of the spread of the activation wave along the muscle strip. For explanation see text. Same experimental setting as in Fig. 1.11.

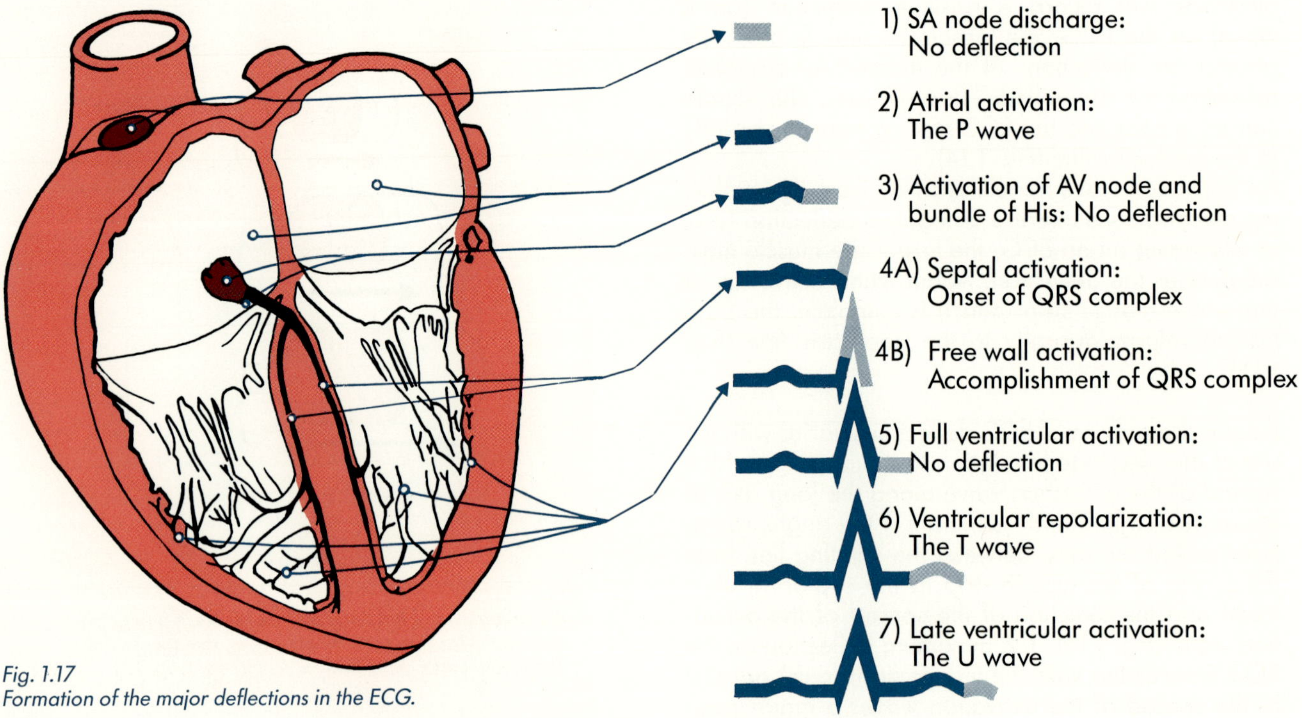

Fig. 1.17
Formation of the major deflections in the ECG.

tive wave is recorded if the spread of activation is towards the electrode and a major negative wave if it is travelling away from it (Fig. 1.16–1 and –5, page 9). A small amplitude biphasic wave composed of an equally sized positive and negative deflection and with a net wave area of near zero is recorded with the line of sight (axis) at right angles to the spread of the activation wave (Fig. 1.16–3). A net area of intermediate size is recorded with sightlines of intermediate orientation (Fig. 1.16–2 and –4).

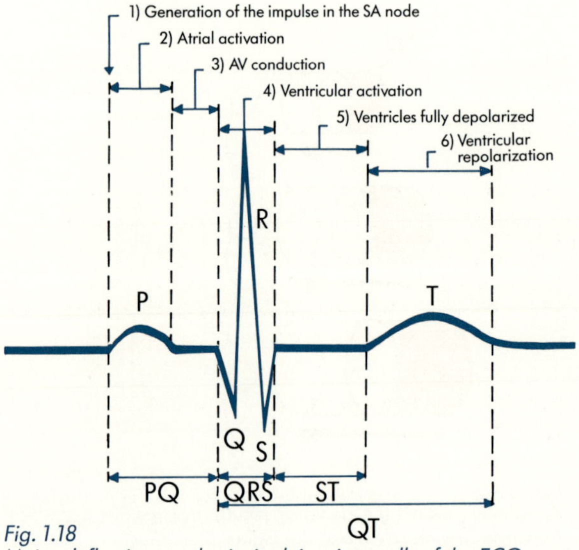

Fig. 1.18
Major deflections and principal time intervalls of the ECG

Major deflections and principal time intervals of the ECG [3, 13, 18]

The formation of the major deflections in the ECG are intimately related to the activation and subsequent repolarization of the atrial and ventricular myocardium (Fig. 1.17):

1 *During impulse formation in the SA node* the ECG records an *isoelectric line*. The electrical current generated by the very small muscle mass of the SA node is too weak to be recorded at the body surface by the exploring electrode.

2 *During activation of the atrial myocardium,* the ECG records a small blunt wave, *the P wave.*

3 *During activation of the AV node and the bundle of His,* the ECG returns to the *isoelectric line,* as activation of these very small structures is usually undetectable on the body surface by the exploring electrode.

4 *During ventricular activation,* with activation of first the septum (A) and then of the free wall of the ventricle (B), the ECG records one or usually two or three major deflections of varying polarity, collectively termed the *QRS complex.*

5 When all parts of the ventricular myocardium are fully activated, the ECG records an isoelectric line, the *ST segment.*

6 *During repolarization of the ventricular myocardium* (correlating with phase 3 of the action potential), the ECG records the *T wave.* As a rule the T wave will be of the same polarity as the major deflection in the QRS complex. Thus, a QRS complex dominated by a major positive deflection, an R wave, is usually followed by a positive T wave and a QRS complex dominated by a negative deflection, a Q or QS wave, by a negative T wave.

7 *During late repolarization of some regions of the ventricular myocardium* (the papillary muscles or Purkinje fibres), the ECG may record a wave after the T wave, a *U wave.*

Such essential variables as heart rate, AV conduction time, total ventricular depolarization time and the duration of ventricular electrical systole can be readily assessed by measuring a few principal time intervals in the ECG (Fig. 1.18):

- The *RR interval* (or PP interval) is the interval between the peaks of two consecutive R waves (or P waves). It varies inversely with the heart rate. If the ventricular rhythm is regular, the RR interval in seconds (or fraction of a second) divided into 60 seconds gives the heart rate per minute.

- The *PR interval* is the time from the onset of the P wave to the onset of the first deflection in the QRS complex. This represents the AV conduction time with the reservation that it also includes the time required for impulse conduction through the atria.

- The *QRS interval* is the interval from the onset of the QRS complex to the termination of the S wave (or the R wave if no S wave is present). This represents ventricular activation time, from the onset of septal activation until all the ventricular myocardium has been activated.

- The *QT interval* starts with the onset of the QRS complex and ends with the termination of the T wave. It represents the total duration of the electrical systole of the ventricles including: ventricular activation (QRS complex), the time during which the ventricular myocardium is fully activated (ST segment) and ventricular repolarization (T wave).

The various ECG leads and their axes [3, 13, 19]

Clinical electrocardiography is based on ECG recordings from several leads, usually twelve. ECG tracings from the various leads can be compared to photographs of the heart taken from different angles (Fig. 1.19). Each lead has its own *lead axis* representing "the line of sight" under which it sees the heart. Like the "ECG tracings" recorded with the exploring electrode placed at a varying angle (axis) to the long axis of the muscle strip in the isolated muscle strip experiment (Fig. 1.16, page 9), each individual lead of the 12 lead ECG preferentially picks up activation and repolarization that occurs parallel to its own axis. Since activation of the ventricular wall occurs from the interiorily located Purkinje network outwards, a lead with an axis pointing directly towards or away from a region will be dominated by the electrical activity of just this region. It is said either *to face* or *to look away* from this same region.

Unipolar and *bipolar* leads should be distinguished. A unipolar lead resembles the lead from the isolated muscle strip experiment (Fig. 1.11, page 8) and is likewise composed of an exploring and an indifferent electrode. The exploring electrode can be placed on a limb (Fig. 1.21, page 14, unipolar limb leads) or, on the chest (Fig. 1.22, page 15, unipolar precordial leads). The stable mean voltage of the indifferent electrode is obtained by shortcircuiting via high electrical resistances the electrodes placed on two or three of the limbs (Figs. 1.22 and 1.23, page 17). The bipolar leads record voltage differences between two electrodes on different limbs (Fig. 1.20, standard leads) or on various parts of the chest (Fig. 3.19, page 54, monitoring leads).

For a unipolar lead *the lead axis* is simply the direction of the line drawn from the exploring electrode to the (electrical) centre of the heart with positive orientation towards the exploring electrode. Electrodes placed on a limb function as if they had been sited at the root of the limb, e.g. in the groin or at the shoulder. For the bipolar standard leads the axes can be constructed by a simple geometrical approach (Einthoven's triangle).

The standard diagnostic ECG usually comprises 12 leads:

3 bipolar standard leads: I, II, III
3 unipolar limb leads: aVR, aVL, aVF
6 unipolar precordial leads: V_1, V_2, V_3, V_4, V_5, V_6.

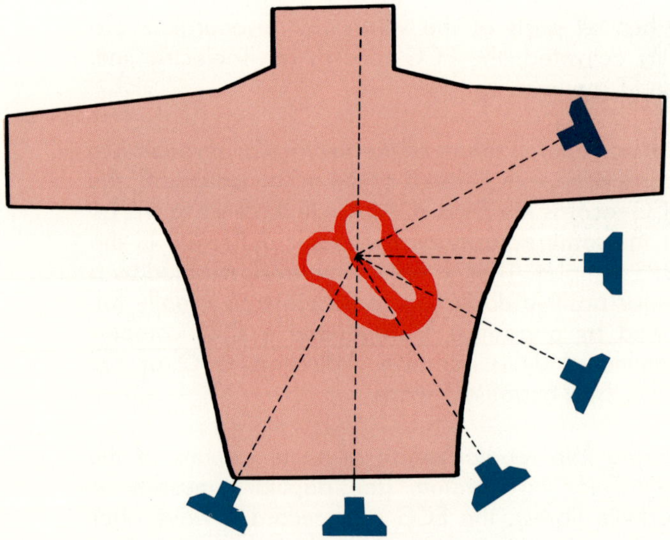

Fig. 1.19
ECG recording in several leads is like photographs of the heart taken from different angles of view with the axis of the individual lead representing the angle of view of the ECG tracing.

Standard leads: I, II and III [3, 13, 19]

The *standard leads* (Fig. 1.20 A) are *bipolar limb leads*, which record voltage differences between the arms or between one arm and the left leg:

I – between the left and right arm
II – between left leg and right arm
III – between left leg and left arm.

All points on the same limb have the same potential, which is that of the adjoining area of the body. The site of the electrode on the limb is therefore of minor importance and the electrodes can for practical clinical purposes be placed at the root of the limb, on the right or left shoulder, and in the left groin or above the symphysis pubis. By convention the left leg is used for electrode placement for ECG recording, the right leg for grounding.

The axes of the standard leads lie along a frontal plane (Fig. 1.20 B); lead I faces the lateral wall of the left ventricle, while leads II and III face the diaphragmatic (the inferior) wall (Fig. 1.23, page 17).

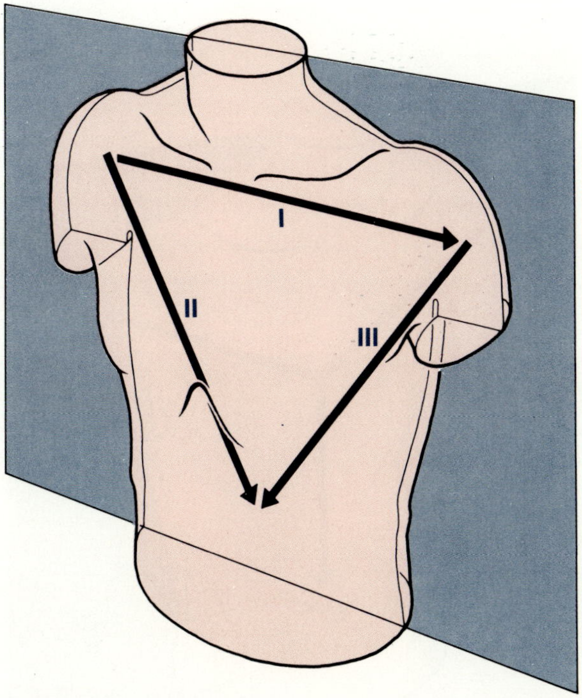

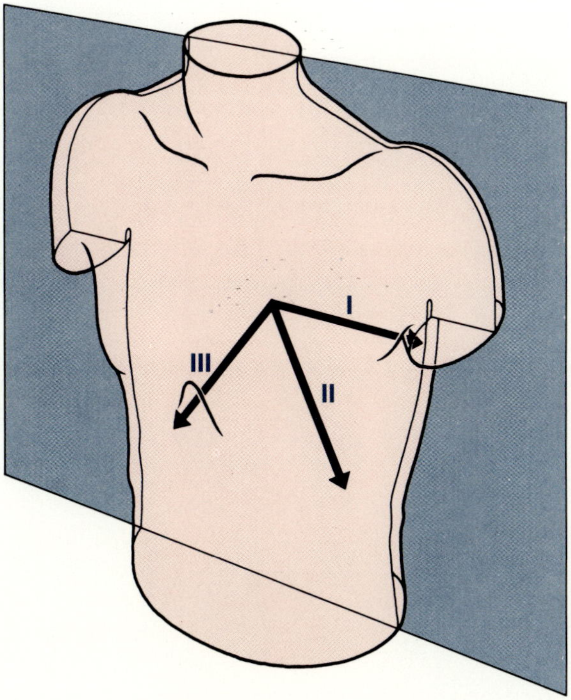

Fig. 1.20
The standard leads and their axes
A. Electrode placement

B. Lead axes

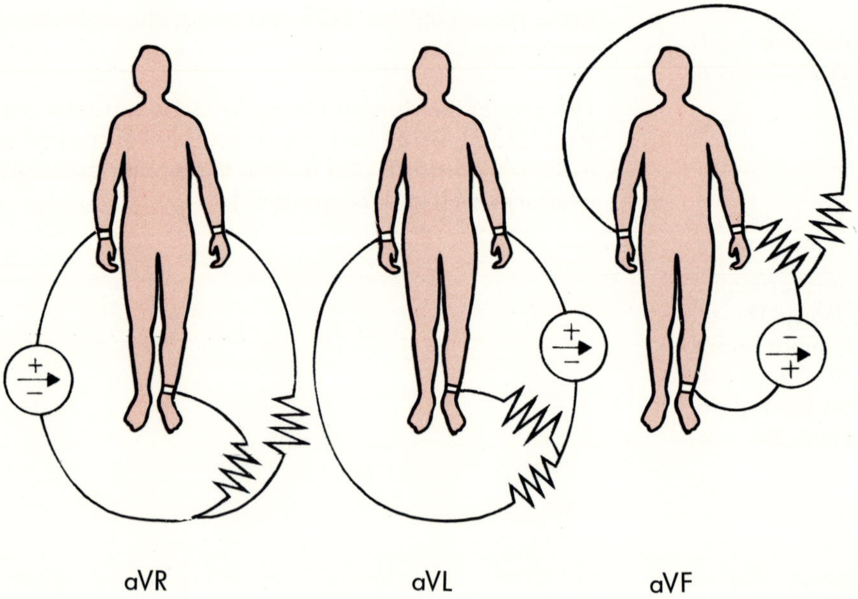

A. Electrode placement

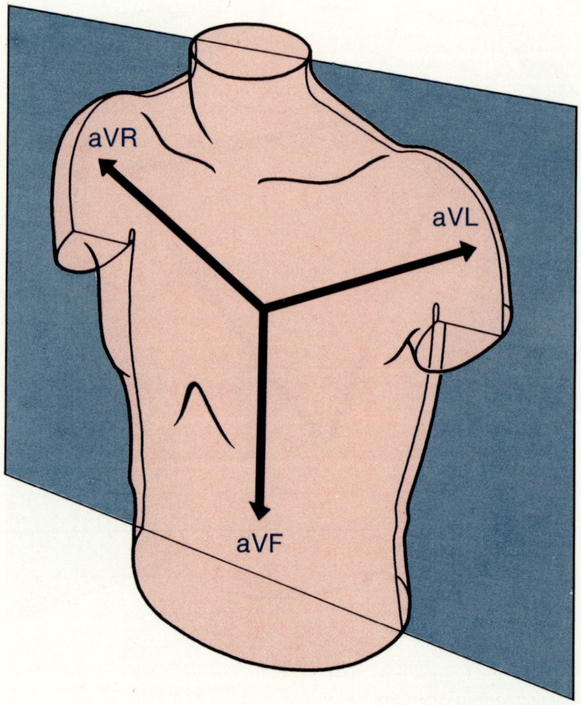

B. Lead axes

Fig. 1.21
The unipolar limb leads and their axes

Unipolar limb leads: aVR, aVL and aVF [3,13,19]

The exploring electrodes of the *unipolar limb leads*, aVR, aVL and aVF (Fig. 1.21 A) are placed on the right arm (aVR), left arm (aVL) and left leg (aVF), or they can be placed on the right or left shoulder and in the left groin or just above the symphysis pubis. The indifferent electrode is formed within the electrocardiograph by connecting together the electrodes placed on the two other limbs. In practice, recordings are made by placing electrodes on the three limbs and setting the dial of the electrocardiograph to "aV", which will then automatically connect the limb electrodes to form the correct indifferent electrode terminals for the unipolar leads. Together with the axes of the standard leads, the axes of the unipolar limb leads lie along a frontal plane parallel with the ventral and dorsal plane of the body (Fig. 1.21 B); lead aVF faces the diaphragmatic (inferior) wall of the left ventricle, whereas aVR and aVL look into the right and left cavities of the heart (Fig. 1.23, page 17).

Unipolar precordial leads: V_1–V_6 [3,13,19]

The exploring electrodes of the *unipolar precordial leads*, V_1 to V_6 (Fig. 1.22 A) are placed on the chest according to the following system:

V_1 – over the 4th intercostal space, just to the right of the sternum
V_2 – over the 4th intercostal space, just to the left of the sternum
V_3 – midway between V_2 and V_4
V_4 – over the 5th intercostal space along the left midclavicular line

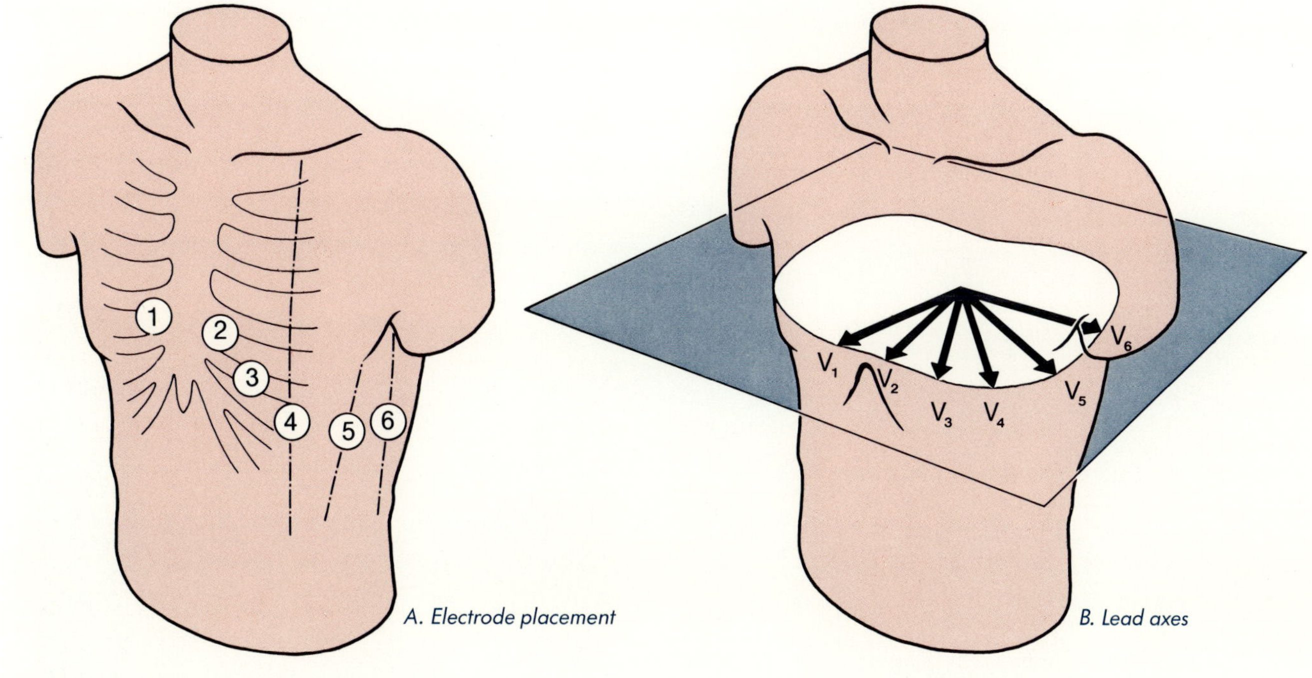

Fig. 1.22
The unipolar precordial leads and their axes

V_5 – the same height as V_4, on the left anterior axillary line
V_6 – the same height as V_4, on the left mid-axillary line.

The indifferent electrode is the same for all six precordial leads. It is created within the electrocardiograph by connecting the electrodes placed on the three limbs. This happens automatically by setting the dial of the electrocardiograph to "V".

The axes of the precordial leads are a horizontal plane (Fig. 1.22 B, page 15); V_1 faces the right ventricle, V_{2-4} the interventricular septum and V_{5-6} the lateral wall of the left ventricle (Fig. 1.23).

Three dimensional orientation of lead axes of the 12-lead ECG [3, 19]

The axes of the standard and unipolar leads lie along a frontal plane parallel with the ventral and dorsal surfaces of the body, whereas the precordial leads are located in a horizontal plane (Fig. 1.23). The intersection between the two planes coincides with the axis of standard lead I, which is thus included in both planes. It follows from the biplanar orientation of the lead axes that the extremity leads form a frame of reference for the propagation of the activation process in the frontal plane; the precordial leads form a corresponding frame of reference in the horizontal plane.

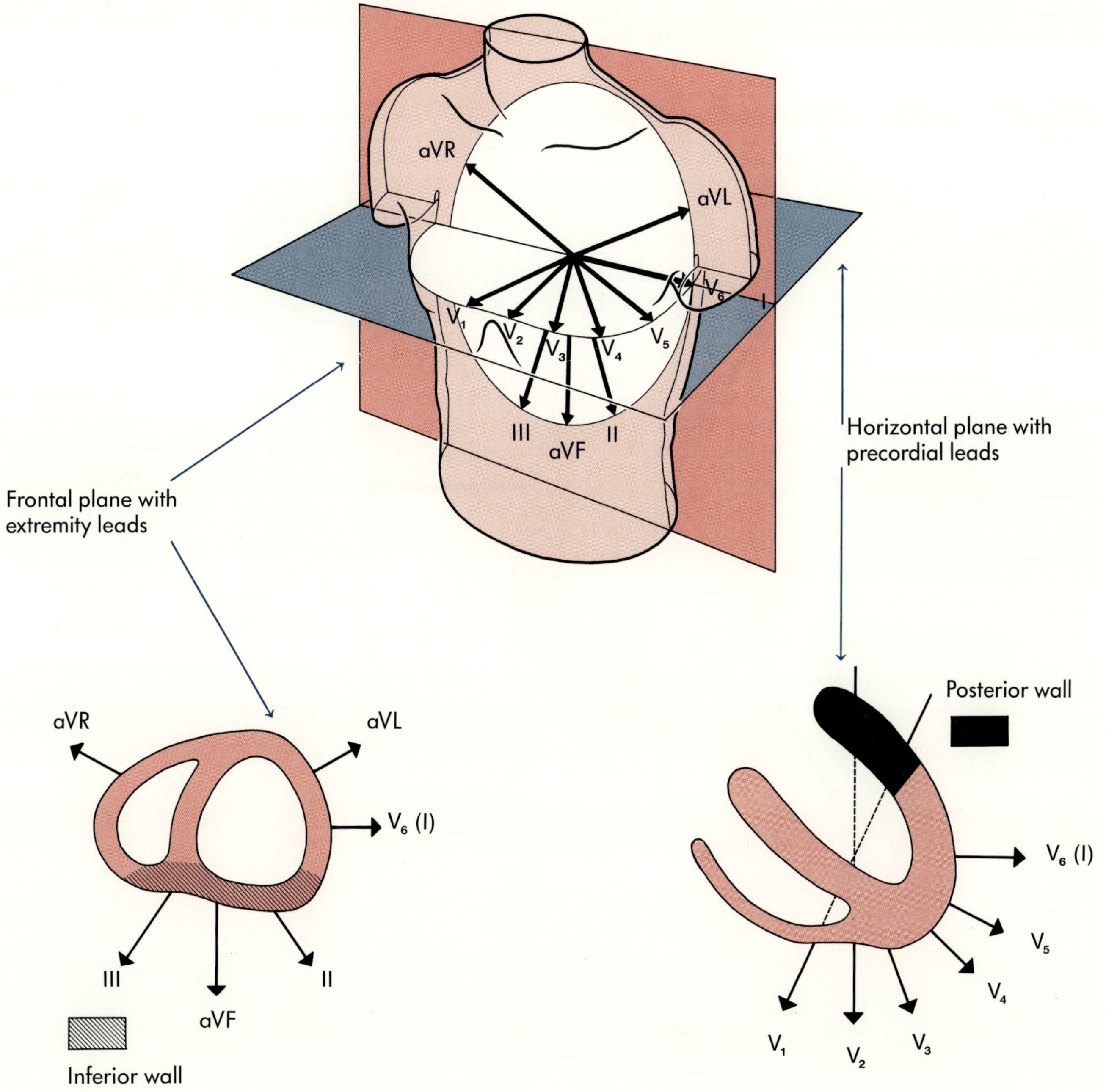

Fig. 1.23
The orientation of the 12 leads to the various parts of the ventricles

The P wave [3, 14–16]

Activation of the atrial myocardium begins high in the right atrium and spreads in every direction. The predominant direction of the spread of atrial activation is to the left and somewhat downwards (Fig. 1.24). Thus, the normal P is positive in I, II and V_{5-6} and usually positive in III and aVF

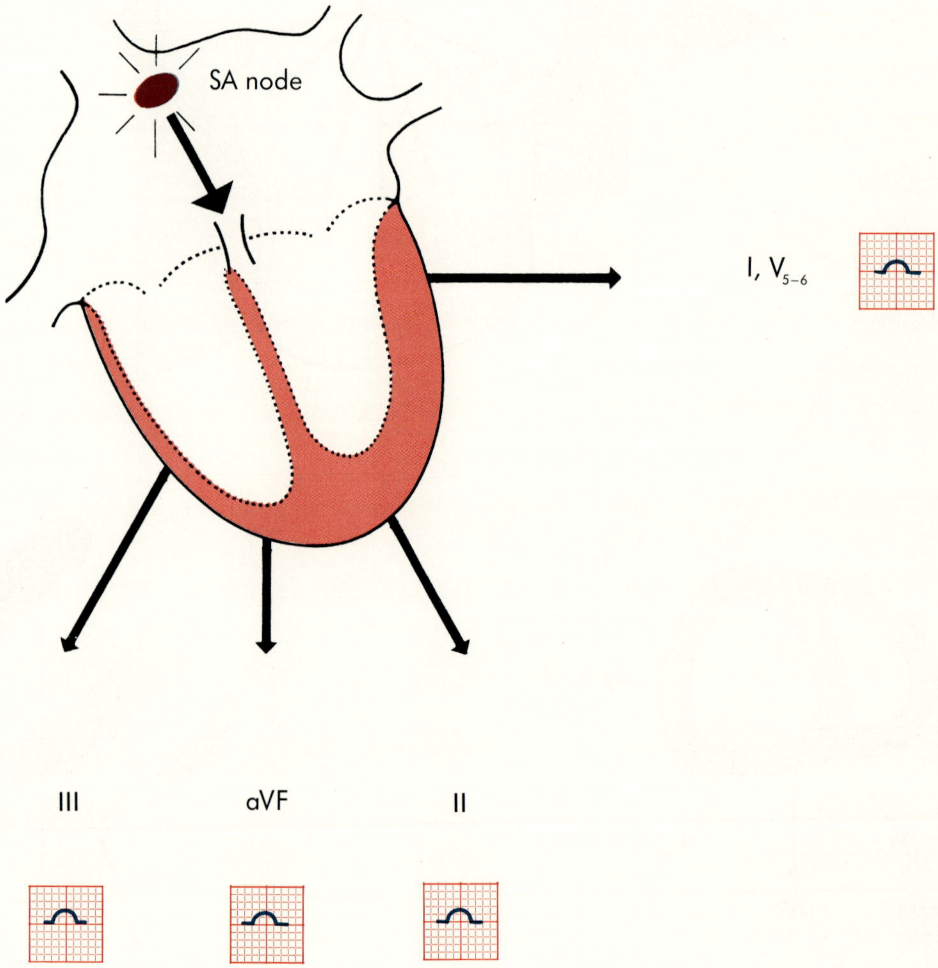

Fig. 1.24
The polarity of the normal P wave

The mean QRS axis [3, 14, 20, 21]

The mean QRS axis should represent the average direction of the spread of the activation wave through the ventricular wall. It is a three dimensional vector but for clinical purposes usually only the mean QRS axis in the limb leads (frontal plane vector) is of interest (Fig. 1.25).

The mean QRS axis can be related to a hexaxial reference system in which the axes of the six frontal leads (I, II, III and aVR, aVL, aVF) are represented on a graded circle surrounding the heart (Fig. 1.26, page 20). The positive pole of lead I is defined as zero degree with a positive clockwise grading of the circle from 0° through 90° to +180° and a negative counterclockwise gradua-

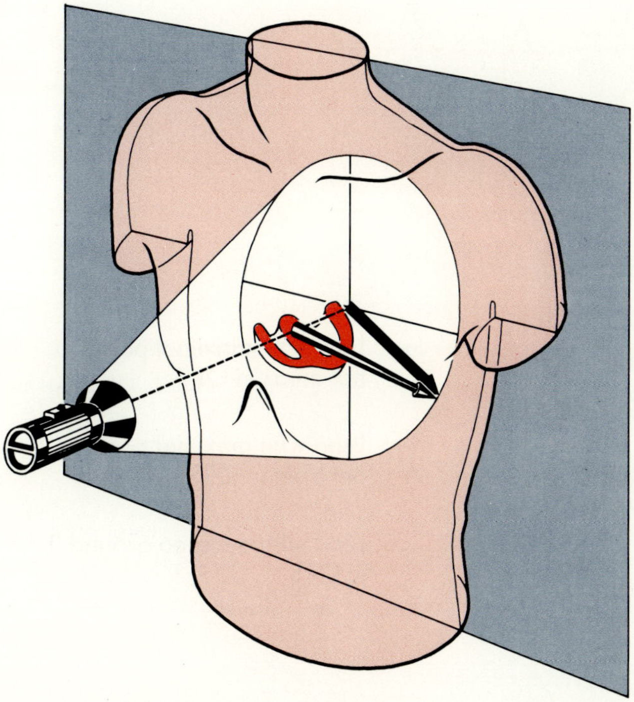

Fig. 1.25
The mean vector of ventricular activation and its projection on the frontal plane which corresponds in axis to the mean QRS axis in the limb leads

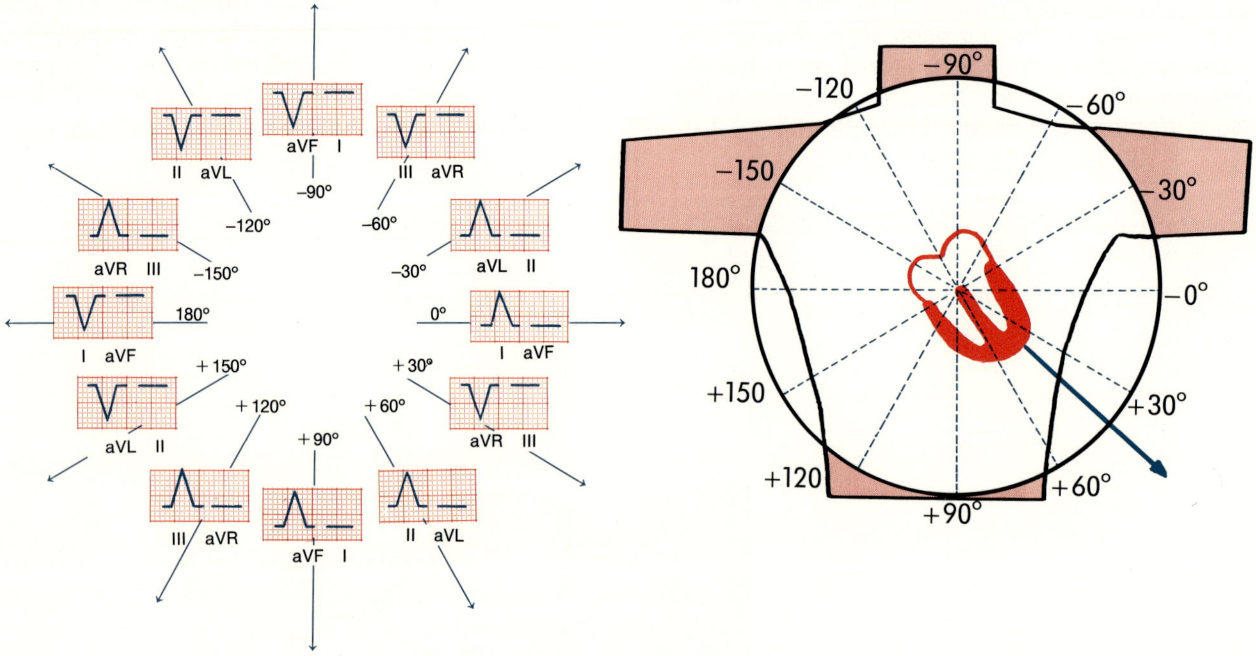

Lead with maximal positive net areas in QRS

Lead with maximal negative net area in QRS

Lead with net area around 0 in QRS

Fig. 1.26
The hexial reference system
Estimation of the mean QRS axis in the limb leads to the nearest 30°

tion from 0° through −90° to −180°. The mean QRS axis is assessed from an estimate of the relative size of the net area of the QRS complex (Fig. 1.27) in the six limb leads. The tallest positive net area is found in the lead with an axis of the same orientation, the major negative net area in a lead with an axis of opposite orientation, and a small biphasic complex with a net area near zero in a lead with an axis at right angle to the QRS axis. In Fig. 1.26 the QRS axis can be estimated to the nearest 30°. The QRS axis usually approximates to +60° with a normal range from −30° to +90°. It appears from Fig. 1.28 (page 22) that a QRS axis within this range is characterized by a positive QRS net area in both leads I and II. The QRS axis will vary somewhat (within the range of normality) depending on the position of the heart in the chest. Asthenic individuals with vertically orientated hearts often have a QRS axis of +90°.

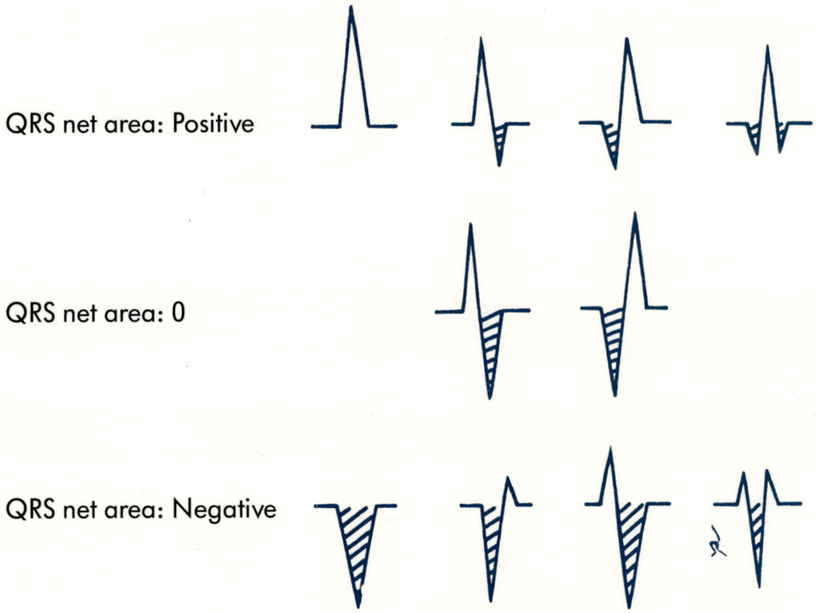

Fig. 1.27
Calculation of the QRS net area. The area below the isoelectric line (hatched) is subtracted from the area above the line.

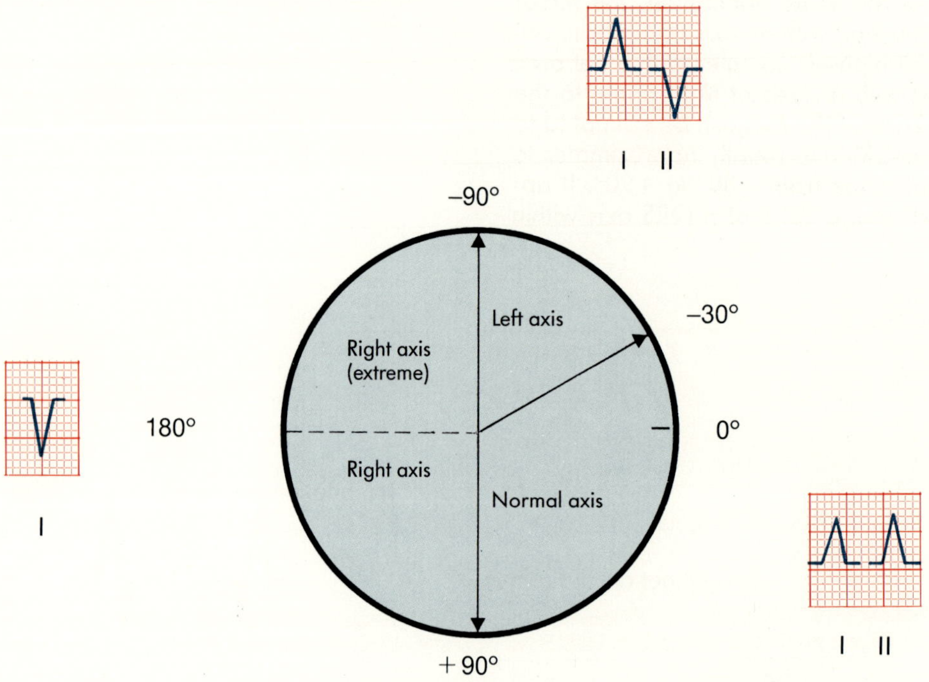

Fig. 1.28
Classification of the mean QRS axis as normal, right-sided or left-sided according to the net area of QRS in leads I and II

The deflections of the QRS complex [13, 14]

The various components of the QRS complex are designated as follows (Fig. 1.29):

Q wave: the initial downward deflection followed by an R wave

R wave: the first upward deflection whether preceded by a Q wave or not

S wave: the downward deflection following the R wave

R′ wave: the second upward deflection

QS: a single negative deflection representing the entire QRS complex.

Capital letters (Q,R,S) refer to relatively large waves (over 5 mm); small letters (q, r, s) refer to relatively small waves (under 5 mm).

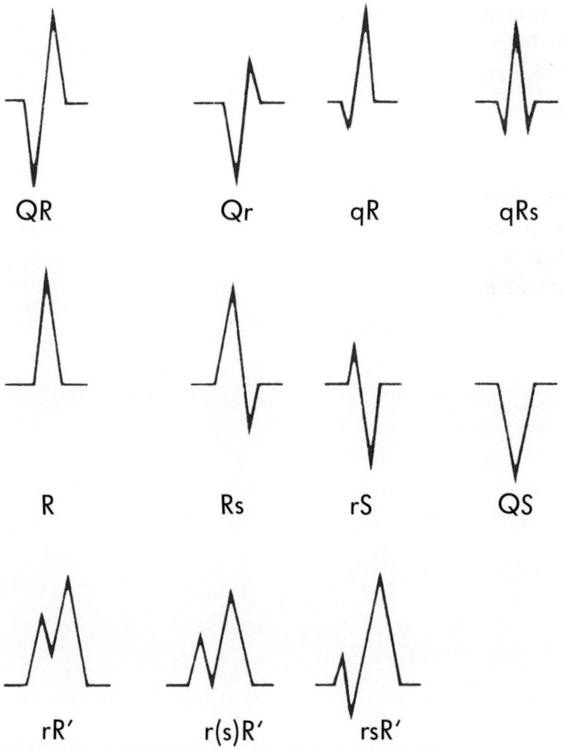

Fig. 1.29
Letter designations of different QRS patterns.
The QRS complexes in the bottom row show bundle branch block patterns with an abnormally wide QRS (≥ 0.12 s wide).

The QRST complex in the precordial leads [3, 13, 14]

The formation of the QRST complex in the precordial leads is illustrated in Fig. 1.30:

A Septal activation: Activation of minor muscle masses towards V_1 and away from V_{5-6}, leading to the recording of a small r wave in V_1 and a small q in V_{5-6}.

B Free wall activation with simultaneous activation of: (1)The smaller muscle mass of the right ventricular wall towards V_1, away from V_{5-6}. (2) The larger muscle mass of the left ventricular wall away from V_1. The opposing activation processes counteract each other but due to the greater muscle mass in the left ventric- ular wall, a deep negative S wave is recorded in V_1 and a tall positive R wave in V_{5-6}. Final activation of more remote parts of the ventricular myocardium may produce a terminal r′ in V_1 and an s in V_{5-6}. The end result is an *rS pattern* in lead V_1 and *qR(s)* in leads V_{5-6}. There is usually a smooth transition from the rS pattern in lead V_1 to an RS in leads V_{3-4} and a qR(s) pattern in leads V_{5-6} (Fig. 1.31, page 26).

C Ventricular repolarization: Following complete ventricular activation an isoelectric ST segment is recorded. Following this, ventricular repolarization occurs and is represented by the T wave, of variable polarity in V_1, but consistently positive in V_{5-6}.

Fig. 1.30
The formation of the QRST complex in the precordial leads

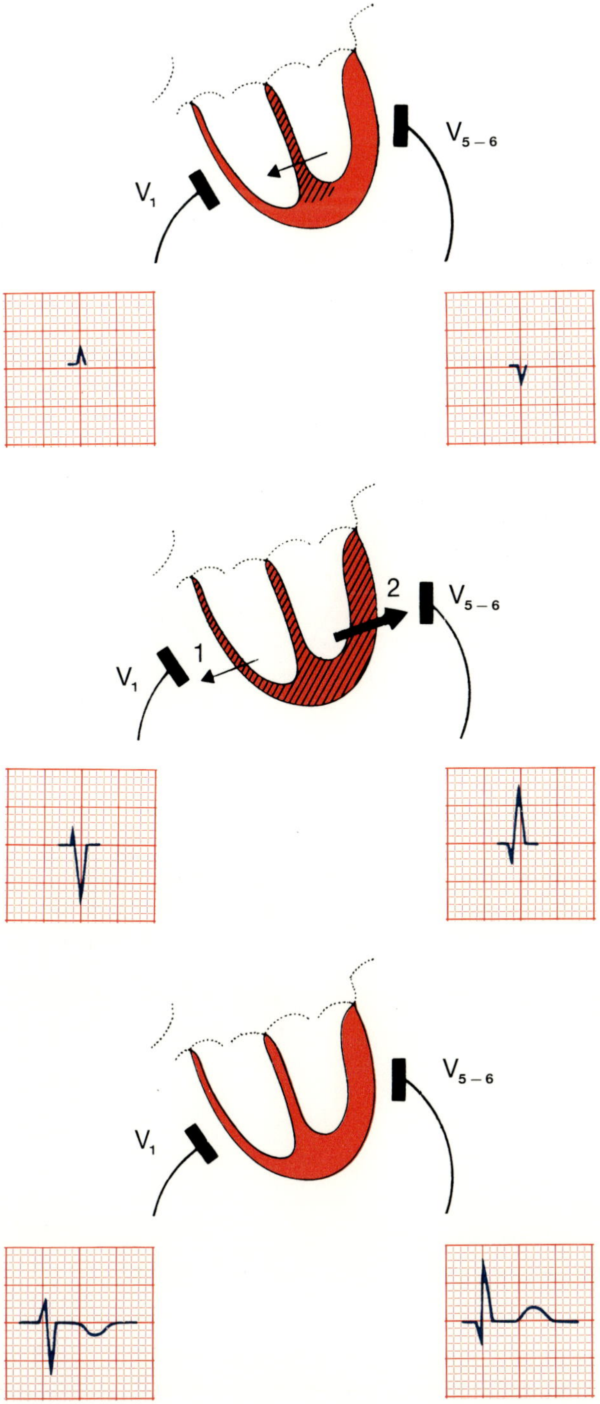

A. Septal activation

B. Free wall activation

C. Ventricular repolarization

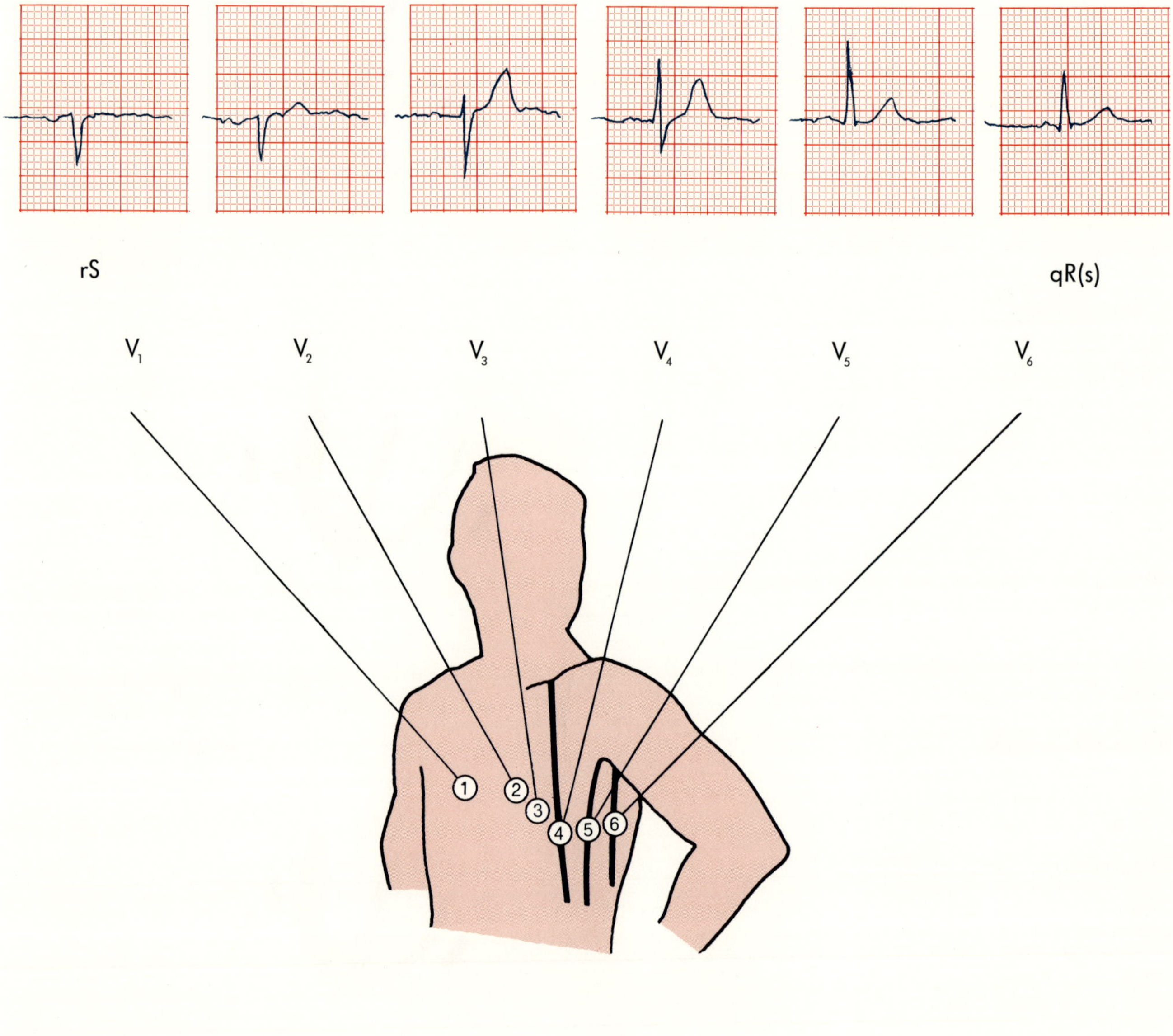

Fig. 1.31
Transition from the rS pattern in V_1 to RS and/or Rs pattern in V_{3-4} to qR(s) pattern in V_{5-6}.

1. Opie LH. The heart. Physiology, metabolism, pharmacology and therapy. London, New York: Grune & Stratton, 1984.
2. Davies MJ., Anderson RH, Becker AE. The conduction system of the heart. London, Boston: Butterworths, 1983.
3. Schamroth L. An introduction to electrocardiography. Oxford, London: Blackwell Scientific Publications, 1976.
4. Rosenbaum MD, Elizari MV, Lazzari JO. The hemiblocks. Oldsmar, Florida: Tampa Tracings, 1970.
5. Kulbertus HE, Demoulin JC. Pathological basis of concept of left hemiblock. In: Wellens HJ, Lie KI, Janse MJ, eds. The conduction system of the heart. Structure, function and clinical implications. Philadelphia; Lea and Febiger, 1976.
6. Kulbertus HE. The hemiblocks. Ten years experience. Ingelheim am Rhein: Boehringer Ingelheim Postgraduate Medical Services, 1978.
7. Demoulin J-C. The conduction system of the heart. Ingelheim am Rhein: Boehringer Ingelheim, 1988.
8. Meijler FL, Janse MJ. Morphology and electrophysiology of the mammalian atrioventricular node. Physiol Rev 1988; 68: 608–47.
9. Bigger JT, Jr. Electrophysiology for the clinician. Europ Heart J 1984; 5 (Suppl. B): 1–9.
10. Gadsby DC, Wit AL. Normal and abnormal electrical activity in cardiac cells. In: Mandel WJ, ed. Cardiac arrhythmias. Their mechanisms, diagnosis and management. Philadelphia: J.B. Lippincott Co., 1987; 53–80.
11. Liebman J, Plonsey R. Basic principles for understanding electrocardiography. Paediatrician 1973; 2: 251–68.
12. Plonsey R. The biophysical basis for electrocardiography. In: Liebman J, Plonsey R, Gillette PC, eds. Pediatric electrocardiography. Baltimore, London: Williams & Wilkins, 1982; 1–14.
13. American Heart Association Report. Recommendations for standardization of leads and of specifications for instruments in electrocardiography and vectorcardiography: Circulation 1975 (August) 52: pages 11–31.
14. Prineas RJ, Crow RS, Blackburn H. The Minnesota code manual of electrocardiography findings: Standards and procedures for measurement and classification. Boston, Bristol, London: John Wright-PSG Inc, 1982.
15. Barr RC. Genesis of the electrocardiogram. In: Macfarlane PW, Veitch Lawrie TD, eds. Comprehensive electrocardiology. Theory and practice in health and disease. New York, Oxford: Pergamon Press, 1989; 129–52.
16. van Dam RTh, Janse MJ. Activation of the heart. In: Mac farlane PW, Veitch Lawrie TD, eds. Comprehensive electrocardiology. Theory and practice in health and disease. New York, Oxford: Pergamon Press, 1989; 101–28.
17. Noble D, Cohen I. The interpretation of the T wave of the electrocardiogram. Cardiovasc Res 1978; 12: 13–27.
18. Lepeschkin E. The U wave of the electrocardiogram. Mod Concepts Cardiovasc Dis 1969; 38: 39–45.
19. Macfarlane PW. Lead systems. In: Macfarlane PW, Veitch Lawrie TD, eds. Comprehensive electrocardiology. Theory and practice in health and disease. New York, Oxford: Pergamon Press, 1989; 316–52.
20. Schamroth L. The electrical axis, its determination and significance. Ingelheim am Rhein: Boehringer Ingelheim Post graduate Medical Servise, 1976.
21. Dubin S, Staib J. Numerical calculation of the mean electrical axis of electrocardiographic deflections. J Electrocardiol 1977; 10: 77–78.

Chapter 2
The normal ECG

Sinus rhythm (Fig. 2.1) [1–3]

One P wave, and only one, preceding each QRS complex. Positive P waves in leads I, II and V_6.

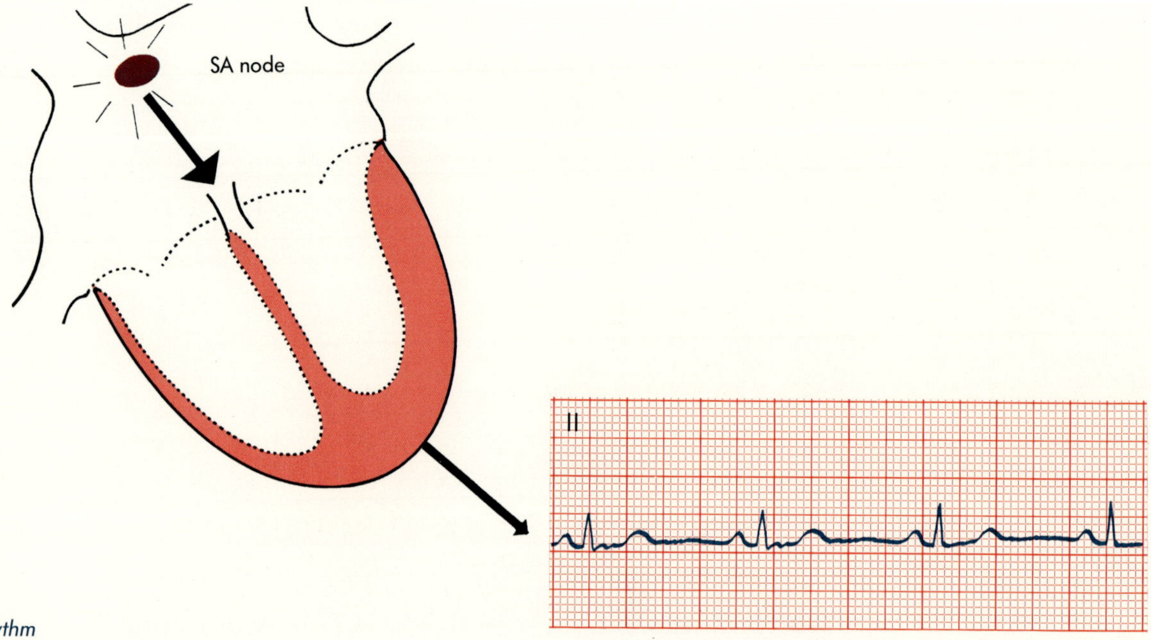

Fig. 2.1
Sinus rhythm

Regular rhythm and heart rate within normal range (Fig. 2.2) [1–3]

Consistent RR and PP interval.

RR (and PP) interval 5–3 large squares = heart rate of 60–100/min.

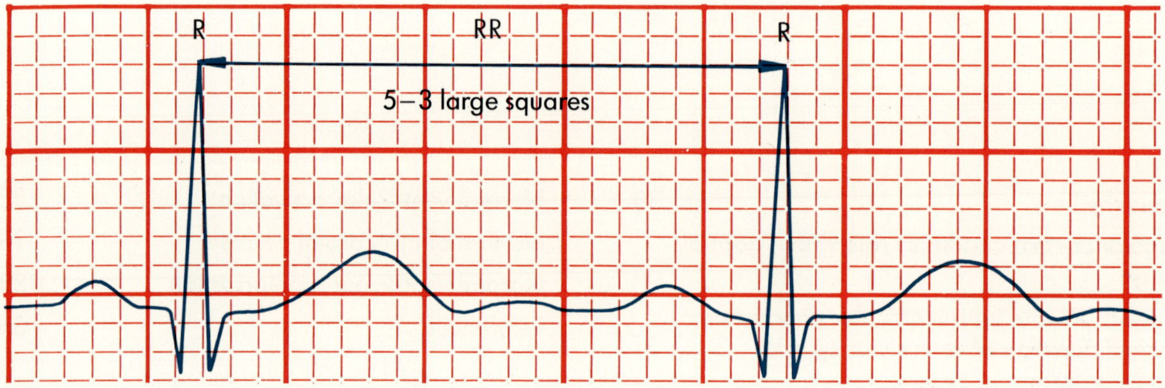

Fig. 2.2
Normal rate and regular rhythm

Normal AV and intraventricular conduction, normal duration of ventricular systole (Fig. 2.3)[1–5]

PR > 0.12 s and < 0.22 s (normal AV conduction).
QRS < 0.12 s (normal intraventricular conduction).
QT within normal limits according to table 2.1 (normal duration of ventricular systole).

Heart rate	QT	Heart rate	QT
40/min	< 0.50 s	80/min	< 0.38 s
50/min	< 0.46 s	90/min	< 0.36 s
60/min	< 0.43 s	100/min	< 0.35 s
70/min	< 0.42 s	110/min	< 0.33 s

Table 2.1
Upper limits of the normal QT interval

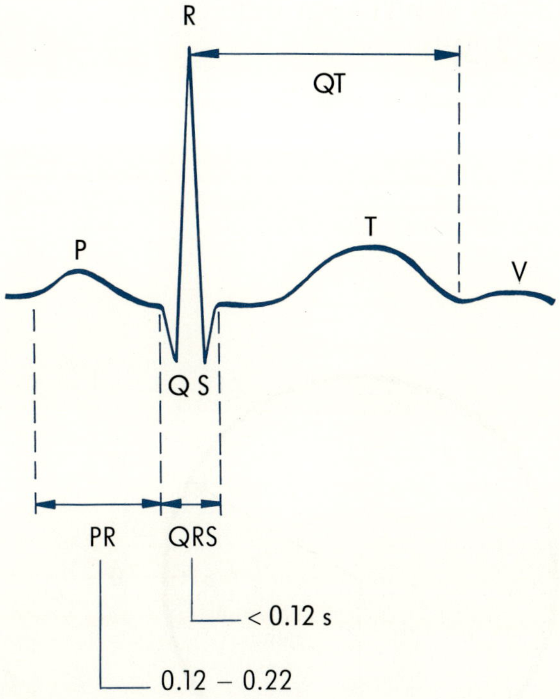

Fig. 2.3
Normal AV conduction (PR 0.12 – 0.22 s) normal intraventricular conduction (QRS < 0.12 s) and normal duration of ventricular systole (QT normal, see Table 2.1)

Normal atrial activation (Fig. 2.4)[1–3]

In lead II a P wave which is less than 2 mm in height and less than 0.12 s in width;
In lead V_1, a P wave which most often is diphasic with an initial positive and a subsequent negative component; the negative component does not exceed that of the preceding positive component, or the P wave is reduced to a small positive deflection.

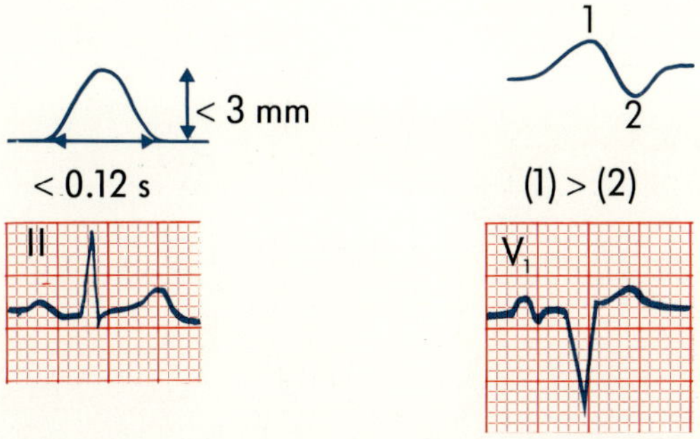

Fig. 2.4
Normal P in II and V_1

Normal ventricular activation (Fig. 2.5) [1–3]

In the limb leads a mean QRS axis between −30° and +90°.

In the precordial leads an rS pattern in lead V_1 and a qR(s) pattern in leads V_{5-6} with $R_{V\,5-6}$ less than 27 mm and $R_{V\,5-6} + S_{V1}$ less than 35 mm.

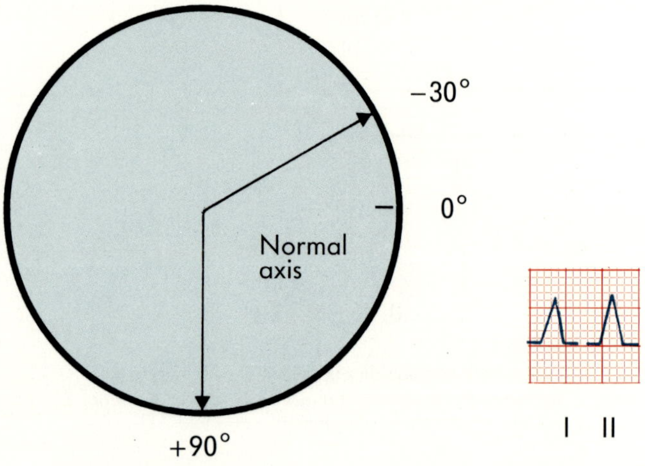

A. Normal QRS axis

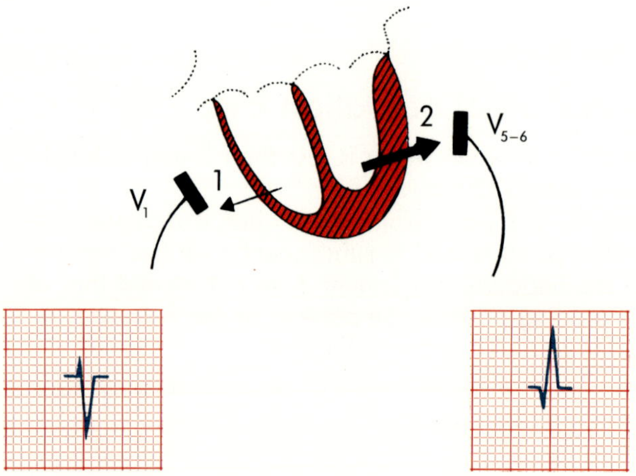

B. rS pattern in V_1 and (q)R(s) pattern in V_6

Fig. 2.5
Normal ventricular activation

No sign of myocardial necrosis (Fig. 2.6)

Q wave less than 0.04 s in width *and* less than 25 % of following R wave in depth provided the R wave itself is larger than 5 mm.

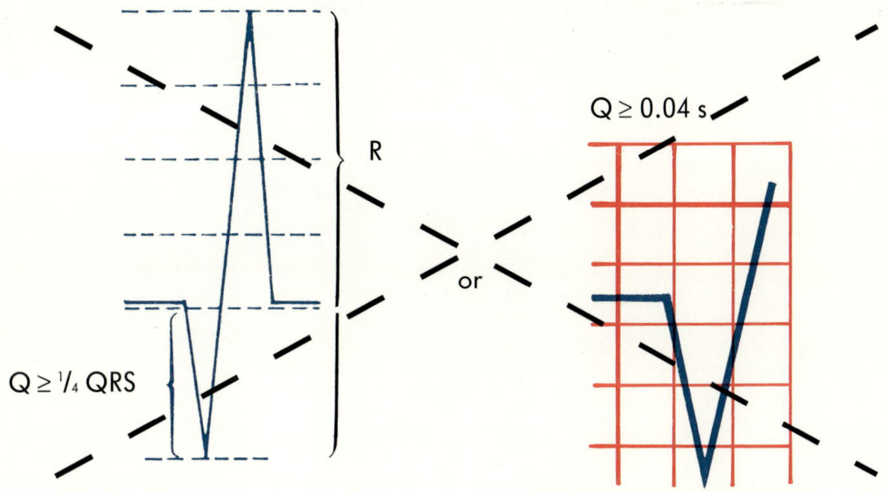

Fig. 2.6
Check for abnormal Q waves indicating myocardial necrosis

Normal ventricular repolarization[1–3]

ST segment: ST elevation < 2 mm (< 4 mm in V_2–V_4).
ST depression < 1 mm.

T wave: Positive T wave in lead I and V_{5-6}.
U wave: If present positive in leads with positive T and U < 25 % of T wave in height or, in V_2–V_4 < 2 mm.

References Chapter 2

1. Macfarlane PW, Veitch Lawrie TD. The normal electrocardiogram and vectorcardiogram. In: Macfarlane PW, Veitch Lawrie TD, eds. Comprehensive electrocardiology. Theory and practice in health and disease. New York, Oxford: Pergamon Press, 1989; 407–58 and 1442–1524.
2. The Criteria Committee of the New York Heart Association. Nomenclature and criteria for diagnosis of diseases of the heart and great vessels. 8th edition. Boston: Little, Brown and Co. 1979.
3. Davignon A, Rautaharju P, Boisselle E, et al. Normal ECG standards for infants and children. Ped Cardiol 1979/80; 1: 123–31.
4. Simonsen E, Cady LD, Woodbury M. The normal Q-T interval. Am Heart J 1962; 63: 747–53.
5. Campbell RWF, Gardiner P, Amos PA, et al. Measurement of the QT interval. Europ Heart J 1985; 6 (Suppl. D): 81–83.

Chapter 3
Cardiac arrhythmias

Cardiac arrhythmias [1, 2]

An arrhythmia is a collective term for any cardiac rhythm which deviates from normal sinus rhythm. The arrhythmia may be due to a disturbance in impulse formation or conduction, or both. Thus, an arrhythmia is a general term for abnormal impulse formation and conduction, not a synonym for irregular heart activity. Impulse formation may be sinus or ectopic, the rhythm regular or irregular and the rate fast, normal or slow.

A review of arrhythmias involving abnormal impulse formation is presented in Fig. 3.1 and involving abnormal conduction (heart block) in Fig. 3.2 (page 39). Included are examples with both abnormal impulse formation and conduction e.g. escapes related to SA and AV block in Fig. 3.1 and escape rhythms related to third degree AV block in Fig. 3.2.

Arrhythmias involving abnormal impulse formation [1–3]

From the site of impulse formation, above or below the bifurcation of His bundle, a differentiation is made between:

- *Supraventricular arrhythmias* (Figs. 3.1-I and 3.10, page 45) with impulse formation in the upper part of the heart above the bifurcation of the bundle of His – somewhere in the atria or AV node.

- *Ventricular arrhythmias* (Figs. 3.1-II and 3.16, page 50) with impulse formation distally to the bifurcation of the bundle of His in the bundle branches or the Purkinje fibres, or rarely in the ordinary working myocardium of the ventricles.

From the rate and irregularity of impulse formation the arrhythmia can be classified as:

Extrasystole: A premature complex (or occasionally two consecutive ones) which besides prematurity is further characterized by a fixed relationship to the preceding complex of the basic cardiac rhythm (Fig. 3.1 A).

Tachycardia: Three or more consecutive impulses from the same pacemaker at a rate exceeding 100/min (Fig. 3.1 B).

Flutter: Rapid (200–400/min) and *regular* electrical activity of the atria or ventricles, characterized in at least one lead by the absence of an isoelectric line between the deflections of the fluttering chamber (Fig. 3.1 C).

Fibrillation: Rapid (300–600/min) and *irregular,* disorganized electrical activity of the atria or ventricles. The ECG deflections of the fibrillating chamber change continuously in shape, duration and amplitude. In atrial fibrillation, the rhythm of the QRS complexes is totally irregular. In ventricular fibrillation QRST complexes are not identifiable (Fig. 3.1 D).

Escape: One or two consecutive impulses arising from the same or occasionally several pacemakers as a result of undue delay in the formation or arrival of the expected impulse of the prevailing rhythm. (Fig. 3.1 E).

Escape rhythm: Three or more consecutive escapes (Fig. 3.2 B, two lower strips).

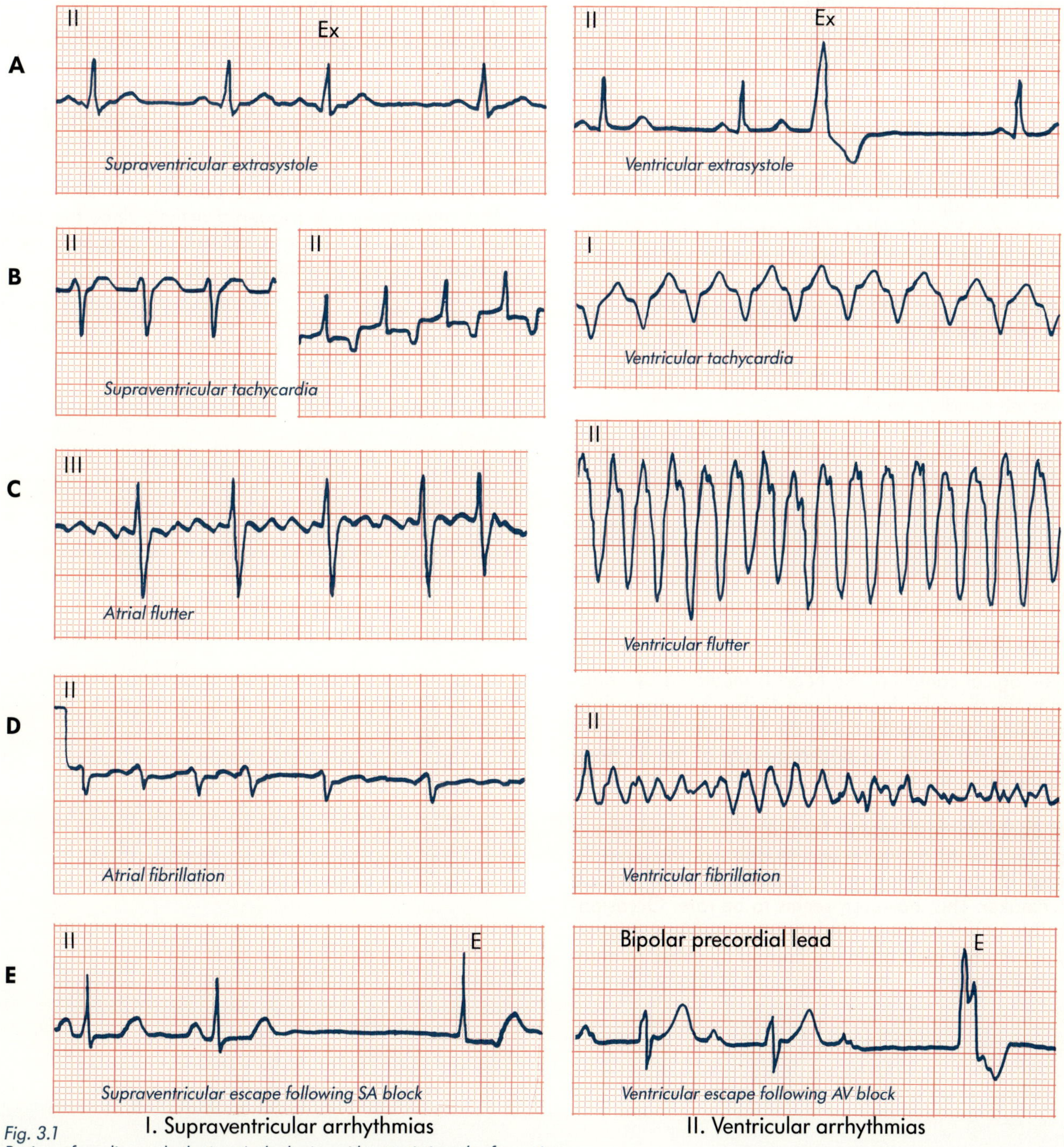

Fig. 3.1
Review of cardiac arrhythmias: Arrhythmias with ectopic impulse formation

Arrhythmias involving abnormal conduction (block) [1–3]

Delay or failure of impulse propagation is named *block*. Blocks are classified according to their anatomical site into (Figs. 3.2 and 3.3, page 40):

A *Sinoatrial (SA) block* with block between the SA node and the adjacent atrial myocardium. *Sinus arrest* which can be difficult to differentiate from SA block is a failure of impulse formation in the SA node.

B *Atrioventricular (AV) block* with block in the AV conduction system.

C *Bundle branch block* with block in either the right or the left bundle branch.

D *Fascicular block* with block in either the anterior or the posterior fascicle of the left bundle branch.

Mechanism of abnormal impulse formation [1–5]

Physiological control of the heart is mediated by variation in the diastolic slope (phase 4) (Fig. 1.5, page 5) of the cellular action potential of the SA node. The steeper the slope, the faster the discharge rate of the SA node and the faster the heart rate.

The abnormal fast impulse formation of an arrhythmia may be due to a similar accentuation of the diastolic phase of the cellular action potential of an ectopic pacemaker. This, however, seems to be rare. Occasionally, abnormal fast impulse formation is due to *triggered activity* but most often it is caused by either *re-entry* or *fibrillation.*

Triggered activity [4–7]

Various pathological conditions, including myocardial ischaemia can cause instability of the membrane potential at the end of an otherwise normal action potential, to produce *afterpotentials.* Such afterpotentials may reach the threshold of the cell and elicit an extrasystole or, if over a period of time they consistently reach threshold they may cause a paroxysm of tachycardia. This phenomenon is *triggered activity* since the abnormal impulse formation is induced or triggered by the preceding action potential.

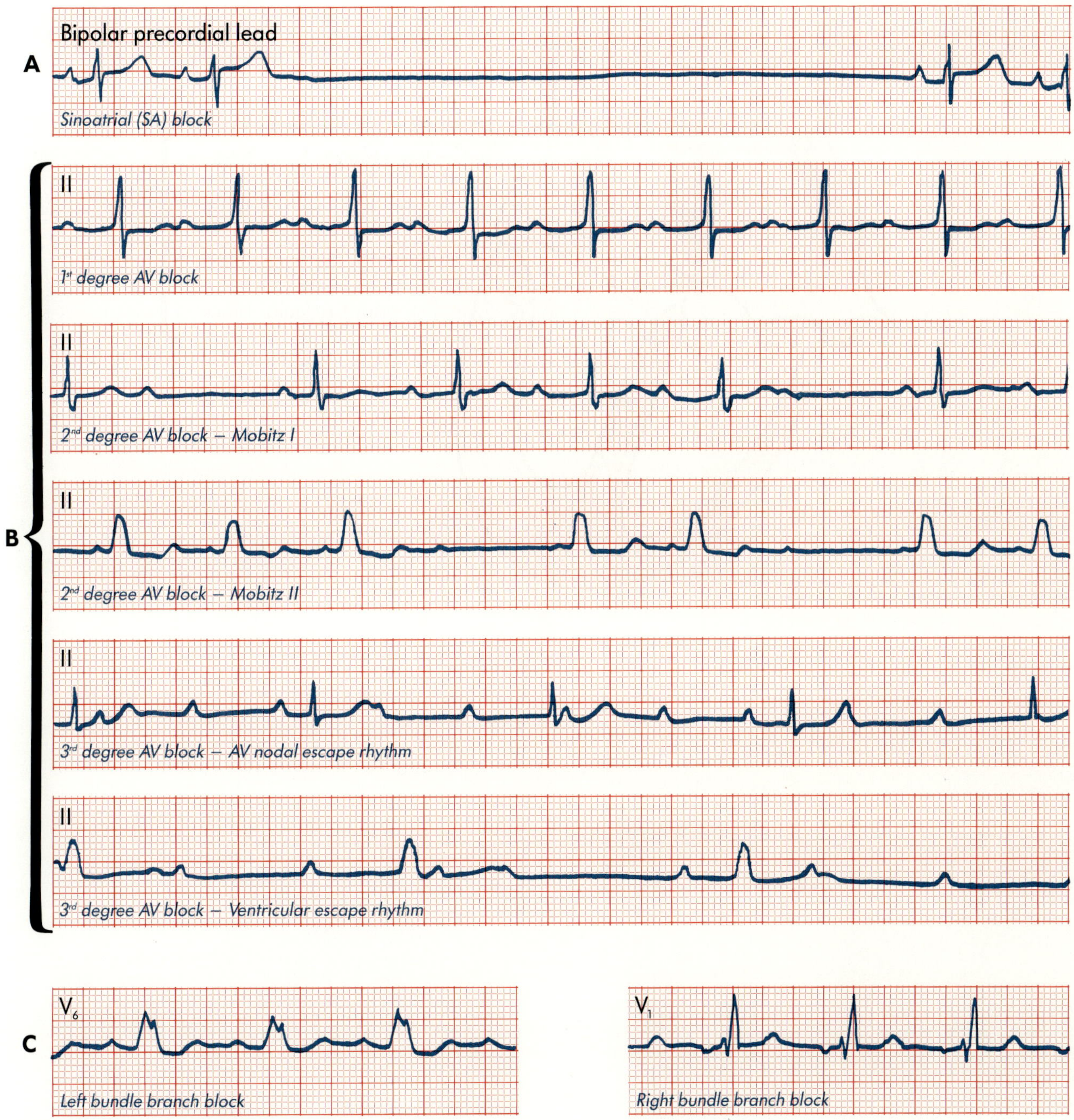

Fig. 3.2
Review of cardiac arrhythmias: Arrhythmias with disturbance in impulse conduction

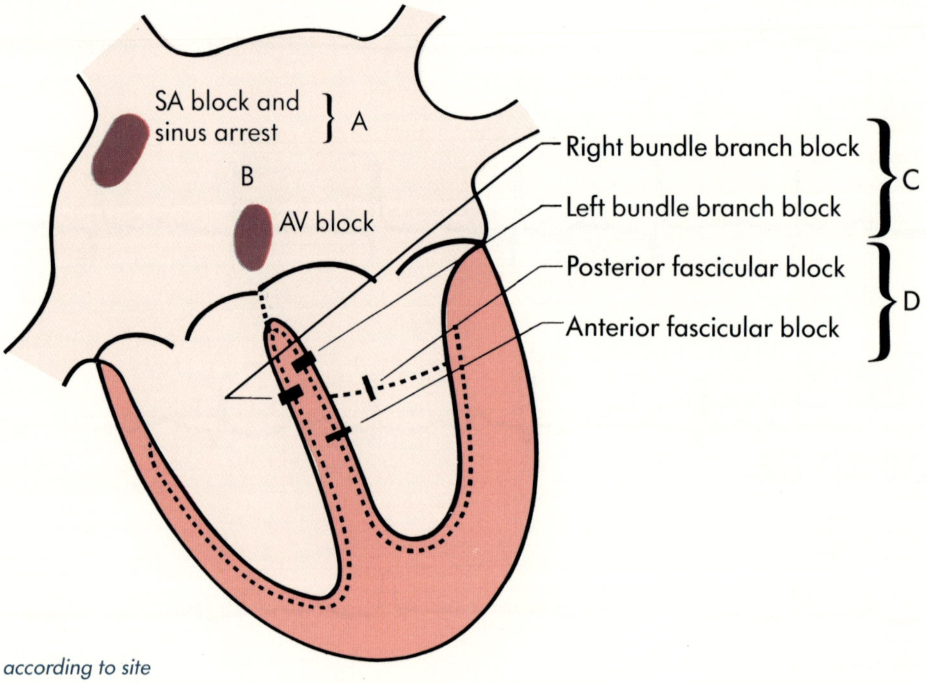

Fig. 3.3
Heart block classification according to site

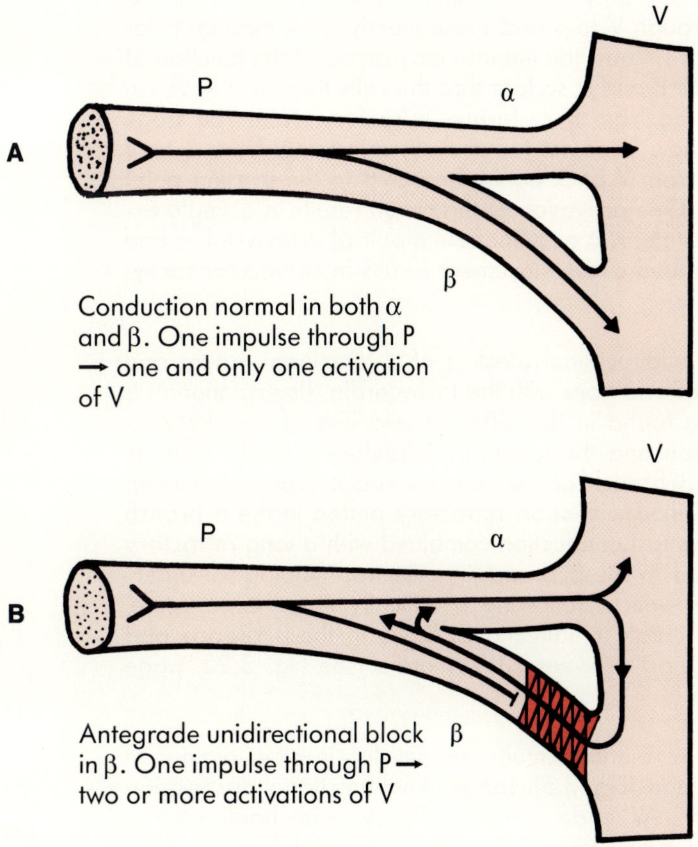

Fig. 3.4
Re-entry in a Purkinje fibre
For explanation see text

Re-entry [4–6]

Re-entry occurs when a single impulse activates the same group of cells two or more times (and from there, the entire heart). A non-homogenous state of conduction in a cross section of the conduction pathway with a localized *unidirectional block* are considered necessary for the phenomenon. Unidirectional block prevents conduction in one direction whereas conduction in the opposite direction is still possible. Anterograde block stops conduction in an anterograde (forward) direction; retrograde block prevents conduction in a retrograde (backward) direction.

Fig. 3.4 A illustrates *normal* impulse conduction from a major Purkinje fibre (P) through its two branches (α and β) to the ventricular wall (V). The conduction in α and β is at the same speed. Activation of V is by the convergence of the two excitation waves originating from myocardial areas adjacent to the α and β branches. At that time further impulse propagation stops due to the common refractory state of all cells in V and the adjacent parts of α and β branches. Fig. 3.4 B shows how the situation changes with the development of unidirectional anterograde block in one Purkinje fibre branch (β) and not in the other (α). Impulse propagation from P to V can now occur through the α branch only. The impulse is propagated from the junction between α and V through V to β and subsequently back through β towards P. Thus, the impulse may arrive at the junction of β with P and α so late that the cells there will have recovered from their former refractory state. The stage has now been set for a *circus movement* from α to V and from V back again through β to the starting point in α. One activation of this circuit results in a single extrasystole; two activations in a pair of extrasystoles; and continued circus movement results in ventricular tachycardia.

The unidirectional block is of a functional nature and comes and goes with the tachycardia. Its explanation is to be found in the different velocities of impulse conduction and the length of refractory periods in the α and β branch of the re-entry circuit (slow conduction combined with short refractory period in the α branch versus fast conduction combined with a long refractory period in the β branch) – electrophysiological differences which, following a critically timed extrasystole, may create unidirectional block in the β branch and thus start a re-entry tachycardia (see Fig. 3.22, page 57).

Similar re-entry circuits can develop in other regions of the heart (Fig. 3.5). Longitudinal functional dissociation of the AV node in two pathways with unidirectional block in one can be the cause of AV nodal extrasystoles and tachycardia (Fig. 3.5 A). The existence of an extra AV conduction pathway, an accessory AV connection, is the basis of attacks of paroxysmal supraventricular tachycardia in the WPW syndrome (Fig. 3.5 B), while atrial flutter is most often caused by a circus movement in the right atrium – a large circuit with a circumference of several centimeters (Fig. 3.5 C).

Fibrillation [8–14]

The cells of the normal myocardium are synchronized or near synchronized in their responsiveness to activation and conduction (Fig. 3.6). An excitation wave therefore spreads uniformly away from its site of origin with a steady speed and a stable front, sharply dividing activated and non-activated muscle. The wave can move only forward because any tendency to backward

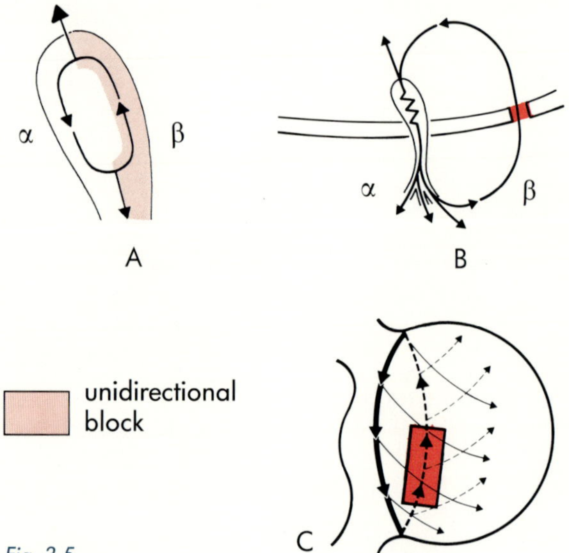

Fig. 3.5
Re-entry tachycardias in various parts of the heart
A AV nodal re-entry
B WPW tachycardia
C Atrial flutter

conduction is stopped by the non-responsiveness of the already activated cells (Fig. 3.6 A2). The activation wave continues until all parts of the myocardium are activated and finally stops because all cells have become refractory (Fig. 3.6 A3). When, however, this normal in-phase functional state of the myocardium becomes out-of-phase and the refractory state between groups of cells is randomly disorganized (Fig. 3.6 B1), then the stage is set for disintegration of the activation wave.

When an excitation wave in an asynchronized myocardium reaches an islet of refractory cells, it splits and surrounds the islet. In this way a single excitation wave becomes two or several smaller wavelets (Fig. 3.6 B2). A vicious circle is started; the cells of the formerly refractory islets pass from their refractory state to a responsive state and are re-excited by the wavelets, and later re-excite the formerly refractory, but now non-refractory cells along the path of the primary wavelets (Fig. 3.6 B3), and so it continues. Fibrillation has been

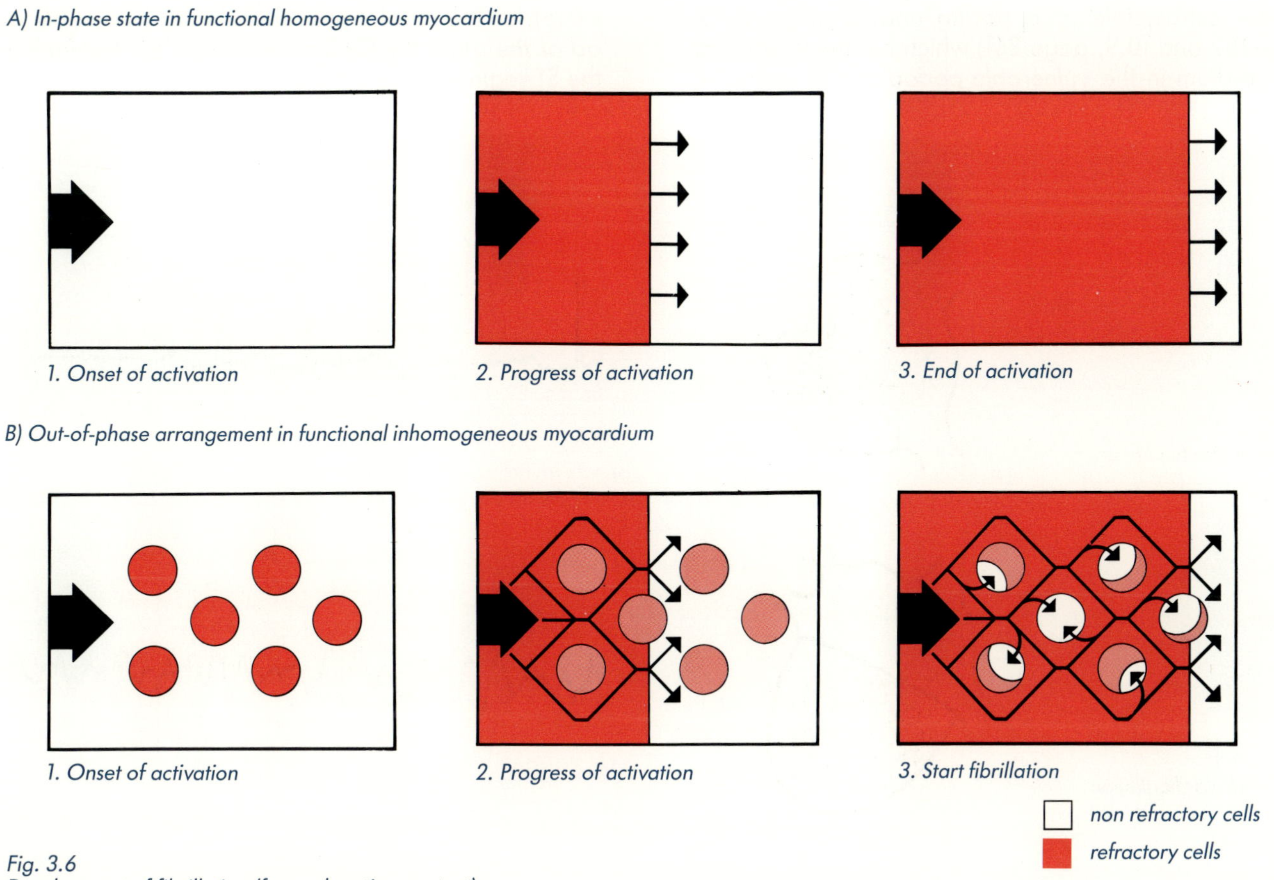

Fig. 3.6
Development of fibrillation (for explanation see text)

started with a very fast and completely irregular disorganized activation of the myocardium. The contractile response to the turbulent activation of the chamber is a continuous worm-like twitching in its wall with loss of pumping activity.

Fibrillation is seen in the ECG as very rapid, irregular deflections. In atrial fibrillation (Fig. 3.7, page 44), the fibrillatory pattern is a background to the QRS complexes which are completely irregular (perpetual arrhythmia); the chaotic, continuous bombardment of the AV node with atrial impulses are normally "processed" by the AV node. Cardiac pumping activity is maintained yet is irregular and often rapid. In ventricular fibrillation the ECG shows no coordinated coherent electrical activity; there are no QRS complexes (Fig. 3.8, page 44). The pumping activity of the heart stops – a cardiac arrest ensues with no pulse, loss of consciousness and if uncorrected, sudden death.

Fibrillation can be induced by rapid repeated stimulation of the atria or ventricles at a rate of e.g. 250–300/min. At these stimulation rates parts of the myocardium are unable to "follow". Functional homogeneity disintegrates and with continued rapid stimulation fibrillation will ensue.

Fibrillation can also start with a single stimulus, a ventricular extrasystole or a pacing impulse (Figs. 6.43, page 182 and 10.9, page 261) which hits the ventricular myocardium in the *vulnerable period of the ventricles,* the ascent and peak of the T wave (first 80 % of the T wave), or the atrial myocardium in the *vulnerable period of the atria,* the QRS complex and the beginning of the ST segment (Fig. 3.9).

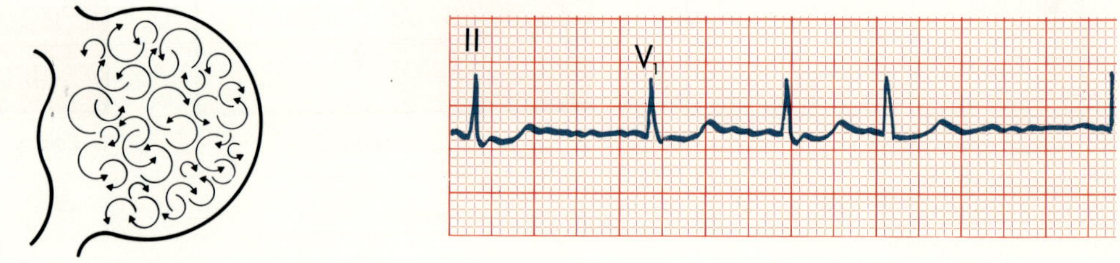

Fig. 3.7
Atrial fibrillation

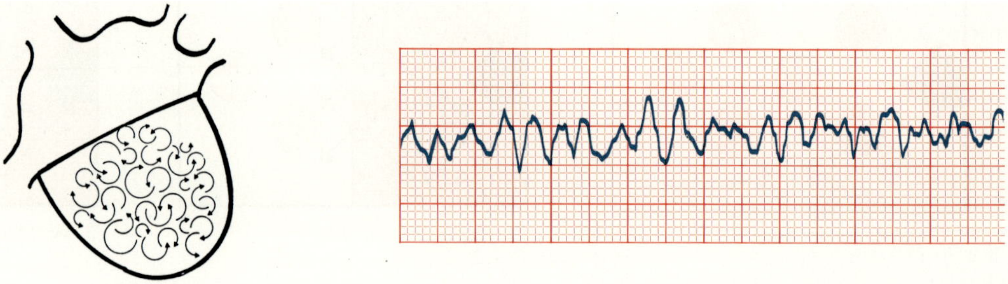

Fig. 3.8
Ventricular fibrillation

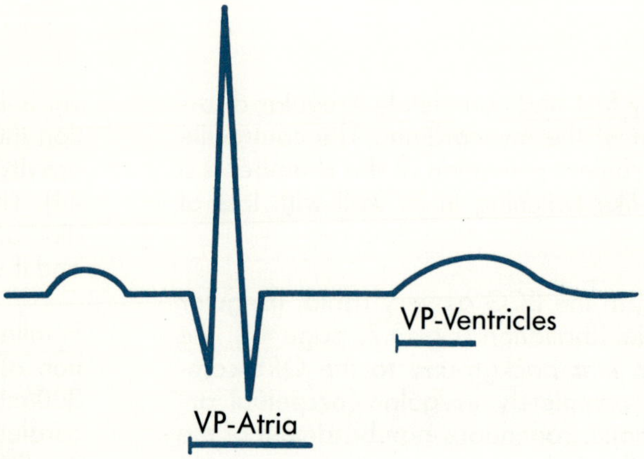

Fig. 3.9
Vulnerable period (VP) of the ventricular and atrial myocardium related to the ECG
VP-Ventricles: Vulnerable period of the ventricular myocardium
VP-Atria: Vulnerable period of the atrial myocardium

Supraventricular arrhythmias: The QRS complex [15–18, 28, 29]

In general, during supraventricular arrhythmias the ventricular myocardium is activated via the normal intraventricular conduction pathway: the bundle of His, the bundle branches and the Purkinje fibres. Occasionally, however, the timing of the activation and repolarization process may be slightly modified. Correspondingly, the common ECG finding in supraventricular arrhythmias is:

– A QRST complex identical to the one recorded in sinus rhythm, usually a narrow complex < 0.12 s wide, followed by an isoelectric ST segment and a blunt T wave which is positive in most leads (Fig. 3.10), or

– A QRST complex similar to the one recorded in sinus rhythm though with minor differences i.e. in the QRS configuration, the QRS axis, the amplitude and/or width (but still a QRS duration of < 0.12 s) and/or a depressed or elevated ST segment and an inverted T wave.

The recording of a wide QRS complex of 0.12 s or more is exceptional but will occur in the patient who in sinus rhythm has QRS widening due to bundle branch block (Figs. 5.10, page 113 and 6.2, page 127). Moreover, the QRS complex may become wider due to "aberrant ventricular conduction".

Aberrant ventricular conduction

The term aberrant ventricular conduction refers to intraventricular conduction disturbances related to change in heart rate. It is a reversible phenomenon which comes and goes with the change in heart rate. In supraventricular extrasystole and tachycardia, aberrant ventricular conduction will occur when supraventricular impulse formation is timed such that the AV conducted impulse reaches the bifurcation of the bundle of His at the point where one bundle branch has just recovered and the other is still refractory to activation. In this situation the impulse spreads through the bundle branch

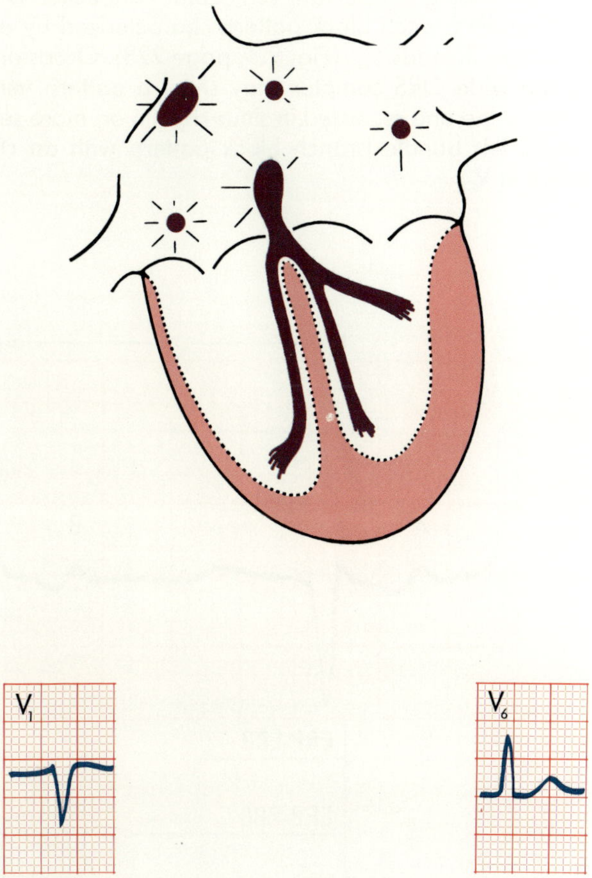

Fig. 3.10
The QRST complex in supraventricular arrhythmia

first to the ventricle which has recovered and then, after some delay, to the other ventricle, producing a wide QRS complex (≥ 0.12 s) with an altered configuration in the form of a so-called bundle branch block (Figs. 3.11, 5.11 C, page 114 and 6.3, page 128/129). Since the refractory period of the right bundle branch is slightly longer than that of the left in most individuals, the most common finding in aberrant ventricular conduction is a right bundle branch block pattern characterized by an rR′ pattern in leads V_{1-2} (Fig. 9.4, page 228). Occasionally the wide QRS complex may show a pattern very similar to the one recorded in sinus rhythm or, more seldom, a left bundle branch block pattern with an rR′ pattern in V_{5-6}.

The duration of the refractory period varies with the length of the preceding RR interval. The longer the preceding cycle, the longer the refractory period and most likely also the greater the difference between the refractory period of the bundle branches. Thus, the long-short sequence of RR intervals in the form of a long RR interval (X) in the basic heart rate and a subsequent short interval (Y) for the following extrasystole or first complex of a tachycardia will favour aberrant ventricular conduction, the Ashman phenomenon (Figs. 3.11, 6.3 B and 6.19, page 146).

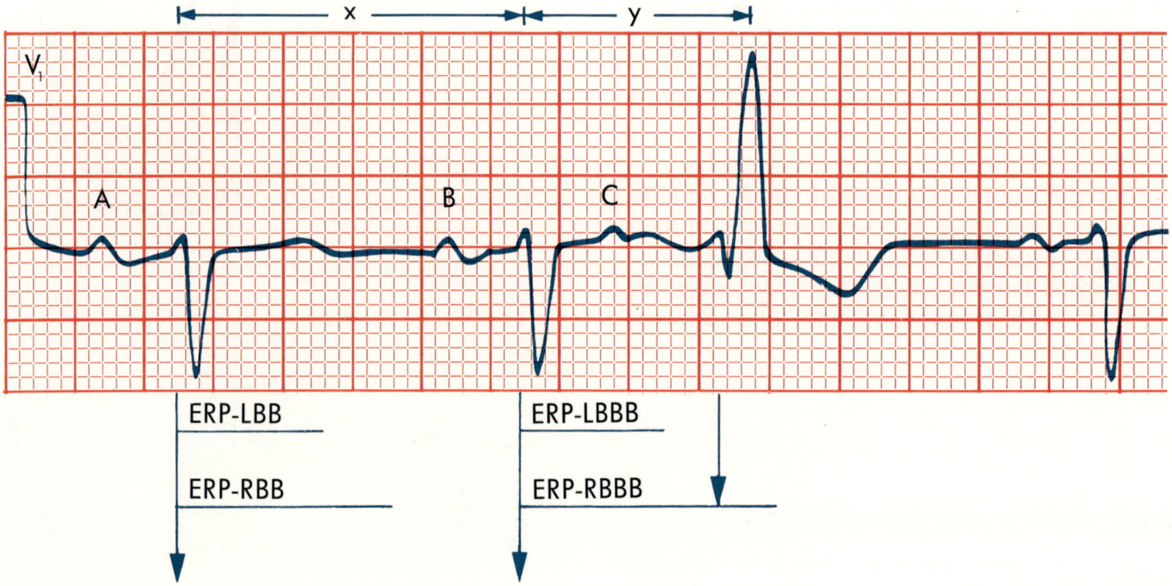

ERP-LBB: Effective refractory period of left bundle branch

ERP-RBB: Effective refractory period of right bundle branch

Fig. 3.11
Aberrant ventricular conduction in supraventricular extrasystole A and B: Normally timed supraventricular impulses. Both bundle branches are fully recovered when the impulse arrives at the bifurcation of the bundle of His: Normal ventricular conduction. Normal QRST complex. C: Premature arrival of the supraventricular impulse before full recovery of the right bundle branch. Activation of the left ventricle through the conducting left bundle branch, delayed activation of the right ventricle from the left ventricle: Right bundle branch block pattern in the ECG. The PR interval will often be prolonged because the AV conduction occurs during the relative refractory period of the AV conduction system.

Supraventricular arrhythmias: The P wave [19–21]

A supraventricular arrhythmia (Fig. 3.12) with the pacemaker site in the SA node or upper part of the right atrium is reflected in the ECG by an upright P wave in lead II, and usually also in leads III and aVF. A pacemaker site in the AV node or lower part of the atrium is characterized by a retrograde activation of the atria with a P wave having a polarity opposite to that of the sinus P, i.e. a negative P in leads II, III and aVF.

In an AV nodal arrhythmia the relative speed of the impulse conduction from the pacemaker site towards the atria and towards the ventricle varies between individuals with corresponding variations in the time relationship between the P wave and the QRS complex (Fig. 3.13, page 48):

A The common finding is the simultaneous recording of the P wave and the QRS complex with the P wave buried in the QRS complex (where it can be identified only by the recording of an oesophageal or intra-atrial ECG lead).

B The P wave may be visible in the ST segment usually immediately after the QRS complex, occasionally further delayed.

C The retrograde P wave may appear at a varying distance before the QRS complex, most often immediately ahead of it, occasionally at an interval approaching or exceeding that of the normal PR interval in sinus rhythm.

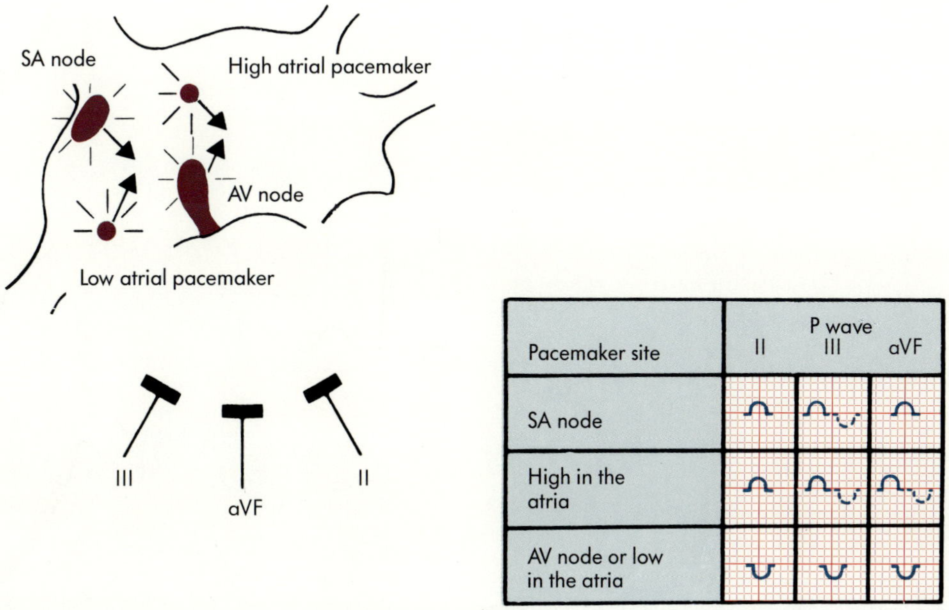

Fig. 3.12
P wave polarity and pacemaker site in atrial and AV nodal arrhythmias (schematic drawing)

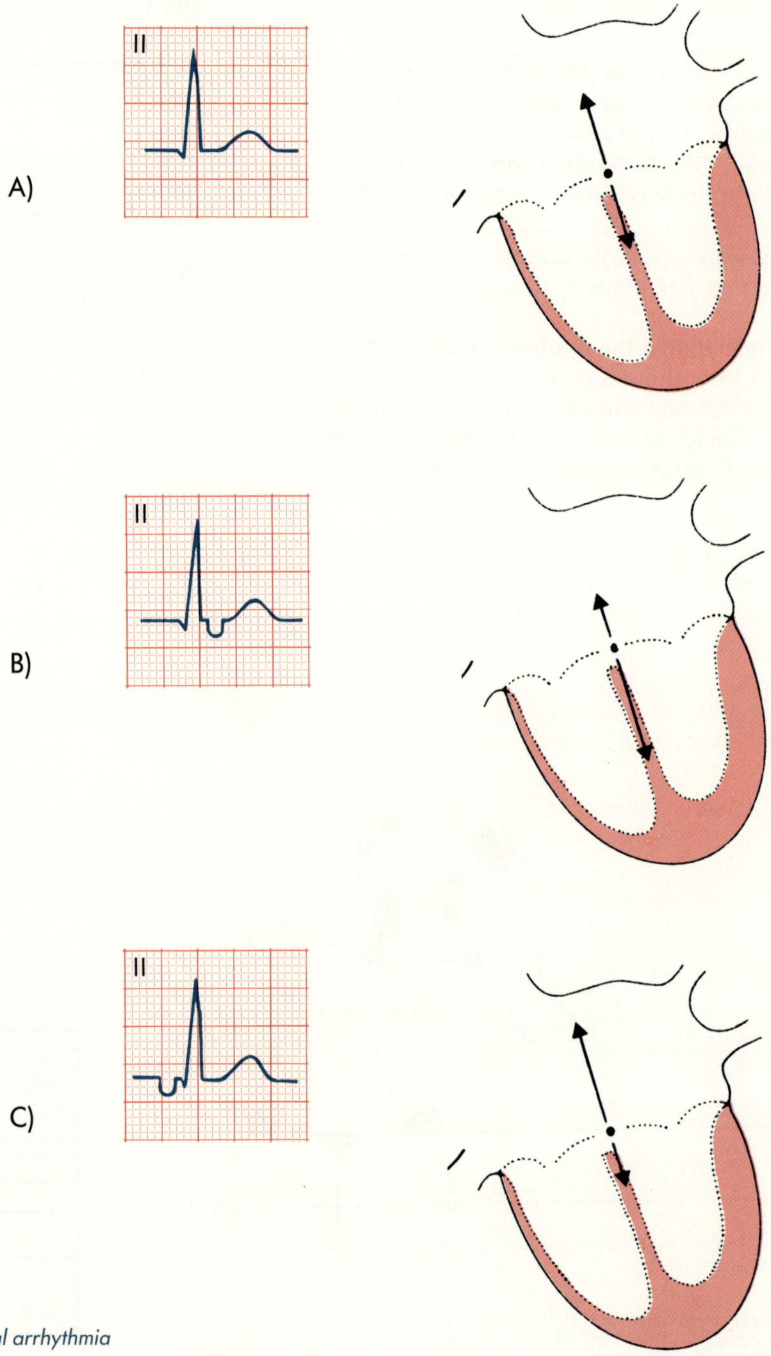

Fig. 3.13
P wave/QRS time relationship in AV nodal arrhythmia
For explanation see text on page 47

Supraventricular arrhythmias: AV conduction [22–24]

The cells of atrial myocardium have a short refractory period and can be excited and can conduct impulses at a significantly higher rate than the AV node which by comparison has a very long refractory period. Thus, the AV conduction of an atrial extrasystole will vary with its timing relative to the preceding complex (Fig. 3.14):

A It will not be conducted through the AV node if its coupling interval is short so that it arrives at the AV node during the effective refractory period, which corresponds to the ST segment and the first part of the T wave; in this situation the atrial extrasystole will be recorded in the ECG as a P wave not followed by a QRS complex (Fig. 5.11 A, page 114).

B It will be conducted by the AV node but with a prolonged PR interval if it arrives at the AV node in the relative refractory period which corresponds to the last half to one third of the T wave (Fig. 5.11 B).

C Later extrasystoles will be normally conducted by the AV node with a normal PR interval.

The long refractory period of the AV node acts as a safeguard, to protect the ventricular myocardium from AV transmission of the very fast atrial activity of atrial fibrillation and flutter (Fig. 3.15). In general, the upper rate limit for AV transmission is low in the elderly and high in children. It varies with the balance between parasympathetic and sympathetic tone and with medication. Individual variations are substantial, however.

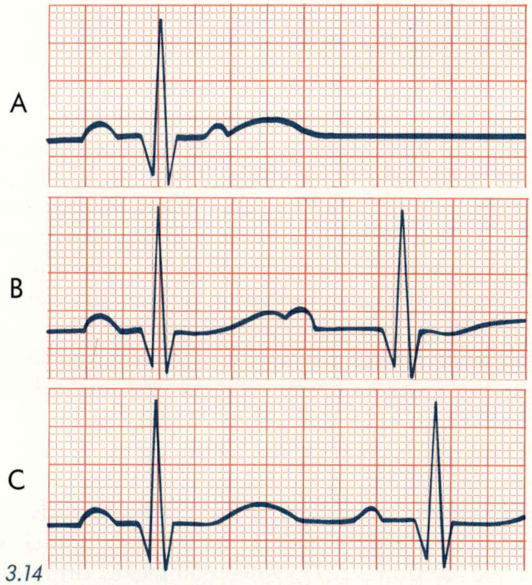

Fig. 3.14
The refractory periods of the AV node
A Premature activation of the atria during the absolute refractory period of the AV node; the P wave of the atrial extrasystole is not AV conducted and, thus, not followed by any QRS complex.
B Premature activation of the atria during the relative refractory period of the AV node. The P wave of the atrial extrasystole is AV conducted but the PR interval is prolonged due to slow AV conduction.
C Premature activation of the atria following full recovery of the AV node; the P wave of the atrial extrasystole is followed by a QRS complex after a normal PR interval.

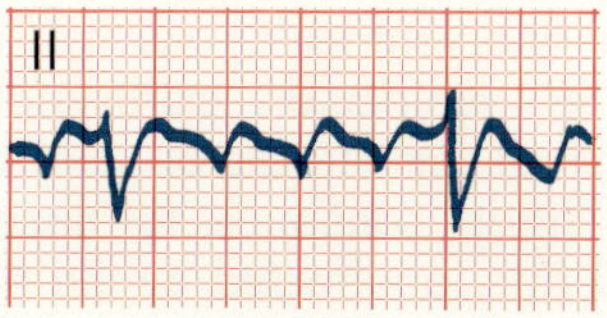

Fig. 3.15
Atrial flutter with 4:1 conduction ratio; one out of four flutter waves conducted to the ventricles

Ventricular arrhythmias: The QRST complex [25–29]

In ventricular arrhythmias the duration and sequence of ventricular activation and repolarization is altered completely producing changes in the QRS complex, the ST segment and the T wave (Fig. 3.16). The QRS complex is wide, always ≥ 0.12 s, and often in the range of 0.15–0.20 s. Variations in morphology are great. Often it is a high amplitude monophasic or biphasic QRS complex. The ST segment usually is shifted away from the isoelectric line (depressed or elevated) in a direction opposite to that of the main deflection in the QRS complex. The T wave usually is broad and peaked with the same polarity as the ST segment shift (and opposite to the main deflection of the QRS complex). QRS complexes originating in the free wall of the right ventricle usually present a positive QRS net area in leads V_{5-6} and I (a QRS polarity similar to left bundle branch block, Fig. 9.3 C, page 227), while complexes originating in the free wall of the left ventricle have a positive QRS net area in leads V_{1-2} (a QRS polarity similar to right bundle branch block, Fig. 9.3 B). Complexes originating in the lower part of the septum can show either pattern irrespective of the side of the septum on which the pacemaker is located.

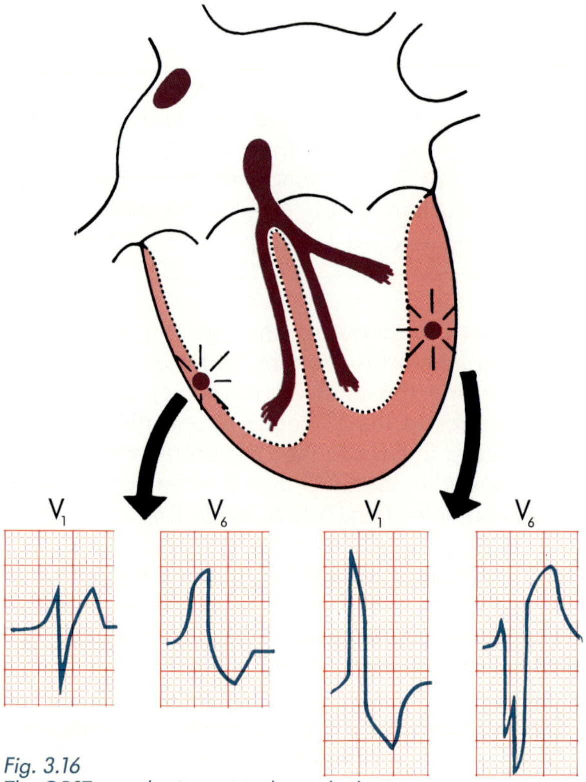

Fig. 3.16
The QRST complex in ventricular arrhythmia

Ventricular arrhythmias: Atrial activity [8, 27–29]

Ventricular extrasystole and tachycardia can be associated with (Fig. 3.17):

A *AV dissociation* with independent or fairly independent atrial and ventricular activity. This is the common finding in ventricular extrasystole and seen in 60–70 % of the attacks of ventricular tachycardia. The SA node continues to discharge at an unchanged rate, unaffected by the simultaneous firing of the ectopic ventricular pacemaker. The SA node impulses are propagated anterogradely in the AV junction towards the ventricles, while ventricular impulses are conducted retrogradely towards the atria. The two activation waves penetrate the upper and

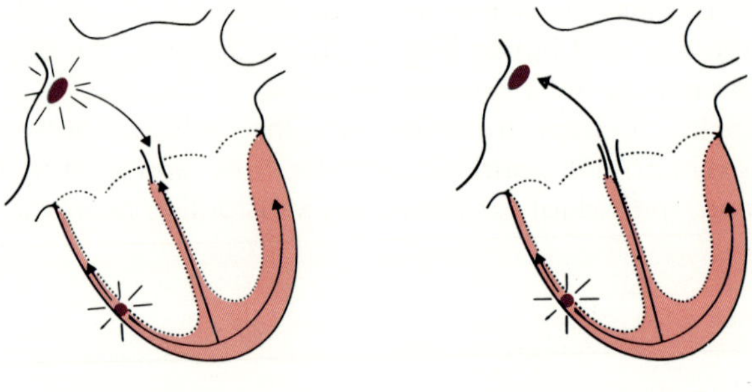

A AV dissociation with antegrade (sinus) atrial activation

B VA conduction with retrograde atrial activation

Fig. 3.17
Atrial activity in ventricular extrasystole and tachycardia. AV dissociation is by far more common (see also Figs. 5.3, p. 111 and 6.27– 6.29, p. 157–159).

lower parts of the AV junction. Somewhere in the AV node/His bundle, however, propagation of one wave is halted by the refractory state created by the other (Fig. 3.17 A). This continuous "concealed" AV/VA impulse collision in ventricular tachycardia may occasionally be interrupted by a supraventricular impulse which succeeds in traversing the AV node and His bundle to the ventricular myocardium where it "captures" the ventricular myocardium to effect a "ventricular capture" (Fig. 6.28, page 158). Alternatively, VA transmission of a ventricular impulse may in the same way capture the atria to achieve "atrial capture".

B *Retrograde atrial activation* with VA conduction of the ventricular impulses. This finding is the exception in ventricular extrasystole (Fig. 5.6, page 112) but occurs in 20 to 30 % of patients with ventricular tachycardia (Fig. 6.29, page 159). The retrograde atrial activation often is associated with intermittent VA block which changes from 1:1 to 2:1 or 3:1 VA conduction (VA conduction of all QRS complexes; one out of two complexes or, one out of three complexes).

Which ECG leads should be recorded in tachycardia?

Whenever possible, all 12 standard ECG leads should be recorded during the arrhythmia, particularly in paroxysmal tachycardia, since:

- The ease of distinguishing atrial activity (P waves) which is essential in the differential diagnosis of tachycardias, varies from lead to lead. Atrial activity can be reflected clearly in one lead and not visible in another.
- The varying contour of the QRS complex in the 12 leads can assist in the differential diagnosis between supraventricular and ventricular tachycardia (Figs. 6.25, page 155 and 6.26, page 155).
- In paroxysmal ventricular tachycardia a 12 lead recording of the spontaneous attack will serve as a reliable "identity card" to distinguish between clinically relevant and "non-clinical" tachycardias induced by programmed electrical stimulation at an electrophysiologic study.

To better clarify atrial activity and its relationship to ventricular activity, an oesophageal recording should be considered when the 12 lead ECG does not provide adequate information.

The oesophageal ECG [30–32]

For several centimeters the lower one-third of the oesophagus lies in immediate contact with the atria, primarily the left atrium. Thus, an electrode placed in the oesophagus at this site will record a high amplitude atrial deflection. At a somewhat lower position the electrode will come in close contact with the "true" posterior wall of the left ventricle and can be used to pick up localized signs of ischaemia or infarction in this part of the heart.

Widely used for oesophageal ECG recording is the "pill electrode" (Fig. 3.18, page 52). The electrode is enclosed in an ordinary 15 mm cylindrical pharmaceutical gelatine capsule and is connected by a twisted pair of very thin teflon insulated steel wires. After lignocaine (lidocaine) spray anaesthesia of the pharynx, the patient swallows the capsule with water while the nurse or technician gradually releases the wire and allows the capsule to descend. Within a few moments the capsule dissolves and peristalsis has lowered the electrode to a level below the left atrium (approximately 40 cm from the teeth).

The wire pair is connected to an electrocardiograph via a differential amplifier. By a gentle pull on the wire the electrode can be manipulated cautiously in the oesophagus until the ECG recording shows a distinct atrial deflection with a three to one ratio between the amplitude of P and QRS deflections (Fig. 3.18). The recording of an oesophageal lead should always be combined with a simultaneous recording of a conventional lead (V_1 or standard lead II). The conventional lead serves as a point of reference for identifying the QRS complex, as it can be difficult to differentiate between atrial and ventricular activity in the oesophageal tracing.

The oesophageal ECGs reproduced in this book have been recorded using a somewhat more complicated technique which permits simultaneous recordings from two or three electrodes placed in a row below each other at intervals of 2–3 cm. They are indicated in the illustrations by Ex where E stands for oesophagus and x indicates the distance of the electrode from cardia (and not from the teeth).

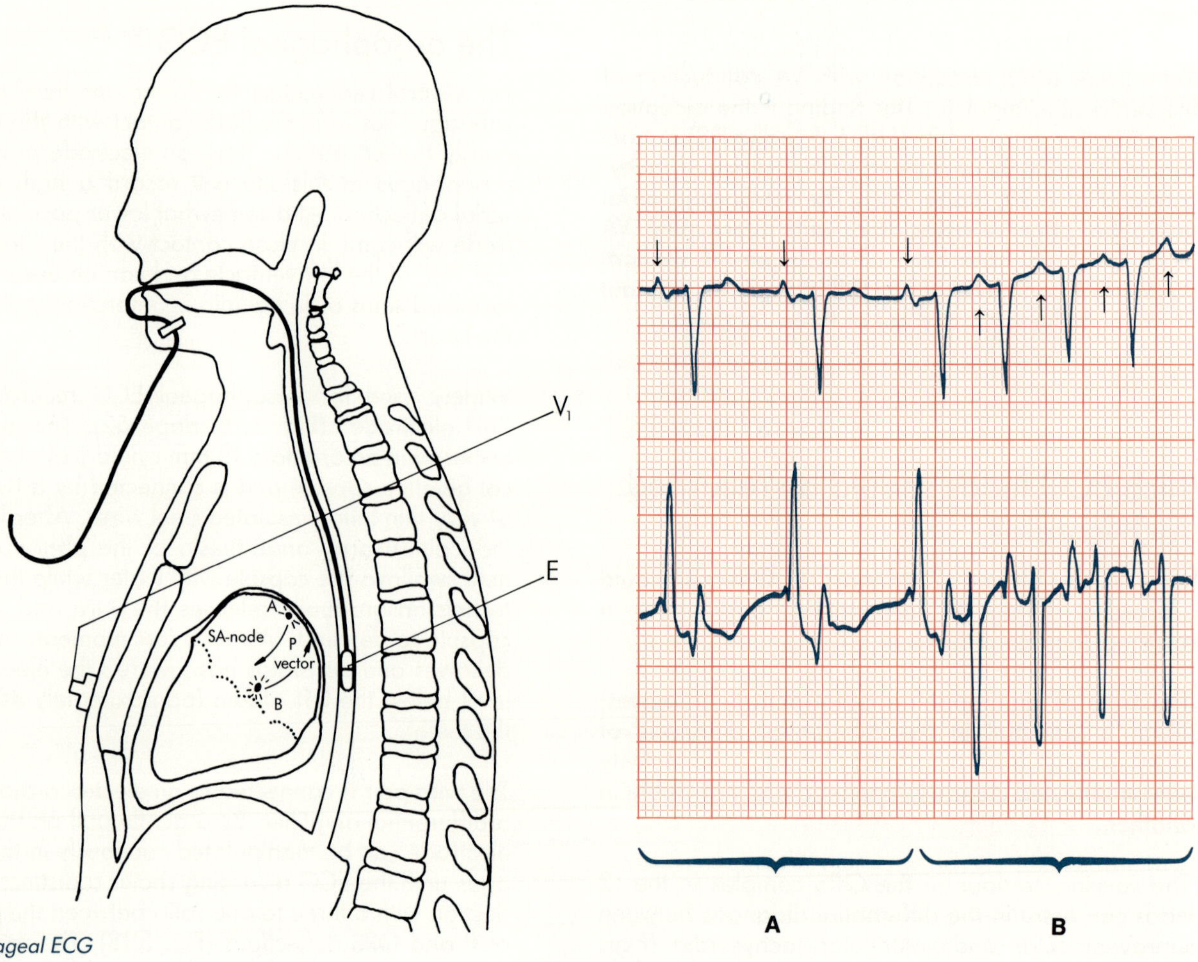

Fig. 3.18
Oesophageal ECG

To the left semidiagramatic drawing of the pill electrode in position in the oesophageal tube. To the right ECG recording with a change from sinus rhythm (A) to a paroxysm of supraventricular tachycardia (B) with retrograde atrial activation manifested by a change in P wave polarity in the oesophageal ECG (E)

Capturing the ECG of an arrhythmia in the patient with few and unpredictable attacks [32–39]

Cardiac arrhythmias vary greatly in their recurrence interval. Some variations are related to stress, exercise or time of the day while others, the majority, seem totally unpredictable. Periods of repeated and long-lasting attacks often alternate with long intervals of normal cardiac rhythm.

To obtain an ECG recording of the arrhythmia in such a patient with rare attacks can be extremely difficult. A simple and inexpensive solution is to advise the patient to seek medical assistance (and an ECG recording) without delay at the very onset of the next attack. This approach is inappropriate when attacks are shortlasting or very disabling. In such circumstances an ECG recording of the arrhythmic event can be obtained by:

- A *mini ECG-event-recorder.* This is about the size of a cigarette packet and contains a solid state memory to store up to 15 min ECG recording. When an attack occurs, the patient activates the device and makes connection with the ECG recorder by pressing his moistened fingers on each hand against two electrodes on the top of the recorder. The recorded ECG can be replayed later, from the solid state memory of the device.

- *24 hour ambulatory ECG monitoring* by small portable tape recorders, named *Holter monitoring* after its inventor, Norman Holter. The recorded tape can be analyzed automatically by computer or, semiautomatically involving a combination of computer analysis and visual scanning.

- *Admission to a Coronary Care Unit (CCU).* This is indicated for the patient with attacks of life threatening arrhythmias or those suspected to suffer from such arrhythmias. In a CCU ECG monitoring is usually performed by *cable connection of the patient to a bedside ECG* amplifier. Ambulant patients can be monitored by *radiotelemetry.* The ECG signal is transmitted from a light-weight amplifier/radiotransmitter worn an a belt. The transmitted signal is received by antennae placed in strategic positions in the ward or in a larger area of the hospital in which the patient is allowed to move freely. In both situations the ECG is continuously displayed on a central display where it is watched by the nurse on duty and, in addition, may be continuously analyzed by a computer. The safety of the patient is ensured by the availability of skilled personnel to intervene immediately in the case of a life threatening arrhythmia.

- *An exercise ECG.* This is indicated in the patient with a history of effort induced arrhythmic events (Figs. 6.41, page 178/179 and 14.22, page 336/337).

The time relationship between the symptoms experienced by the patient and the ECG events recorded is important. Corroborating symptoms with the ECG recording of an arrhythmia confirms the arrhythmogenic background of the symptoms, whereas a normal ECG recording at the time when the patient experiences symptoms excludes this possibility.

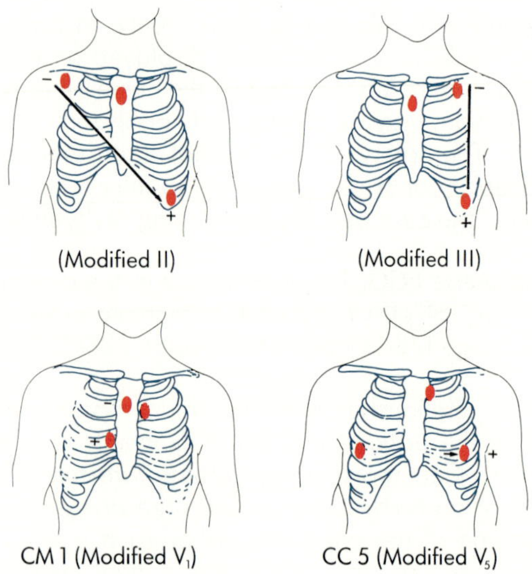

Fig. 3.19
Bipolar chest leads for long-term ECG monitoring

ECG leads for ECG monitoring [33–35]

ECG leads suitable for long-term ECG monitoring are shown in Fig. 3.19. Electrode locations have been chosen to minimize the risk of muscle "noise", interference and movement artifacts. The ECG tracings obtained from these leads will resemble but will not be identical to those of leads II, III, V_1 and V_5. For practical reasons ECG monitoring most often involves only one lead. For 24-hour ambulatory ECG recording, however, a two-lead system is advantageous. The two-lead recording makes artifact arrhythmias more readily recognizable. Moreover, it adds a margin of safety against monitoring failure due to a faulty single electrode, or when a QRS axis shift produces a small amplitude QRS complex recording in one lead.

In ECG monitoring for ischaemia signalled by ST segment deviation the use of a two lead system is mandatory. The lead axes of the two monitoring leads preferably should be perpendicular to each other.

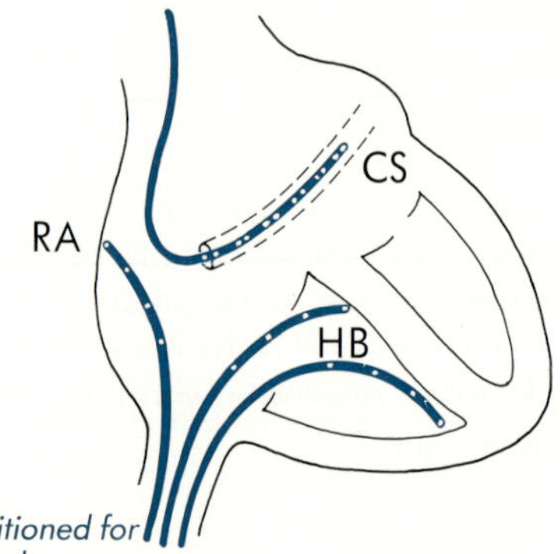

Fig. 3.20
Catheter electrodes positioned for an electrophysiologic study
RA: Right atrium
CS: Coronary sinus
HB: His Bundle

The electrophysiologic study [4–39, 46]

The electrophysiologic study should be performed in the catherization laboratory of a department specialized in cardiology. It is done under sterile conditions in the minimally sedated patient under local anaesthesia. With fluoroscopic guidance, intravenous catheter electrodes are introduced into specific regions of the heart (Fig. 3.20). The catheter electrodes are usually multipolar to permit both recording of local electrograms (electrogram = intracardiac ECG) and electrical stimulation (pacing). Depending the type of arrhythmia the study may focus on the recording of a His bundle electrogram (HBE), sinus node recovery time (SNRT), programmed electrical stimulation (PES) or arrhythmia mapping, or it may involve two or more of these procedures.

His bundle electrogram (HBE) [4, 40–43]

A catheter electrode introduced via the femoral vein can be manipulated to lie across the septal leaflet of the tricuspid valve. The uninsulated tip of the catheter electrode is manœuvered to the His bundle. The correct position is seen on the electrogram by the recording of a sharp deflection, a His spike, between the atrial and ventricular activity. The capital letters A, H and V are

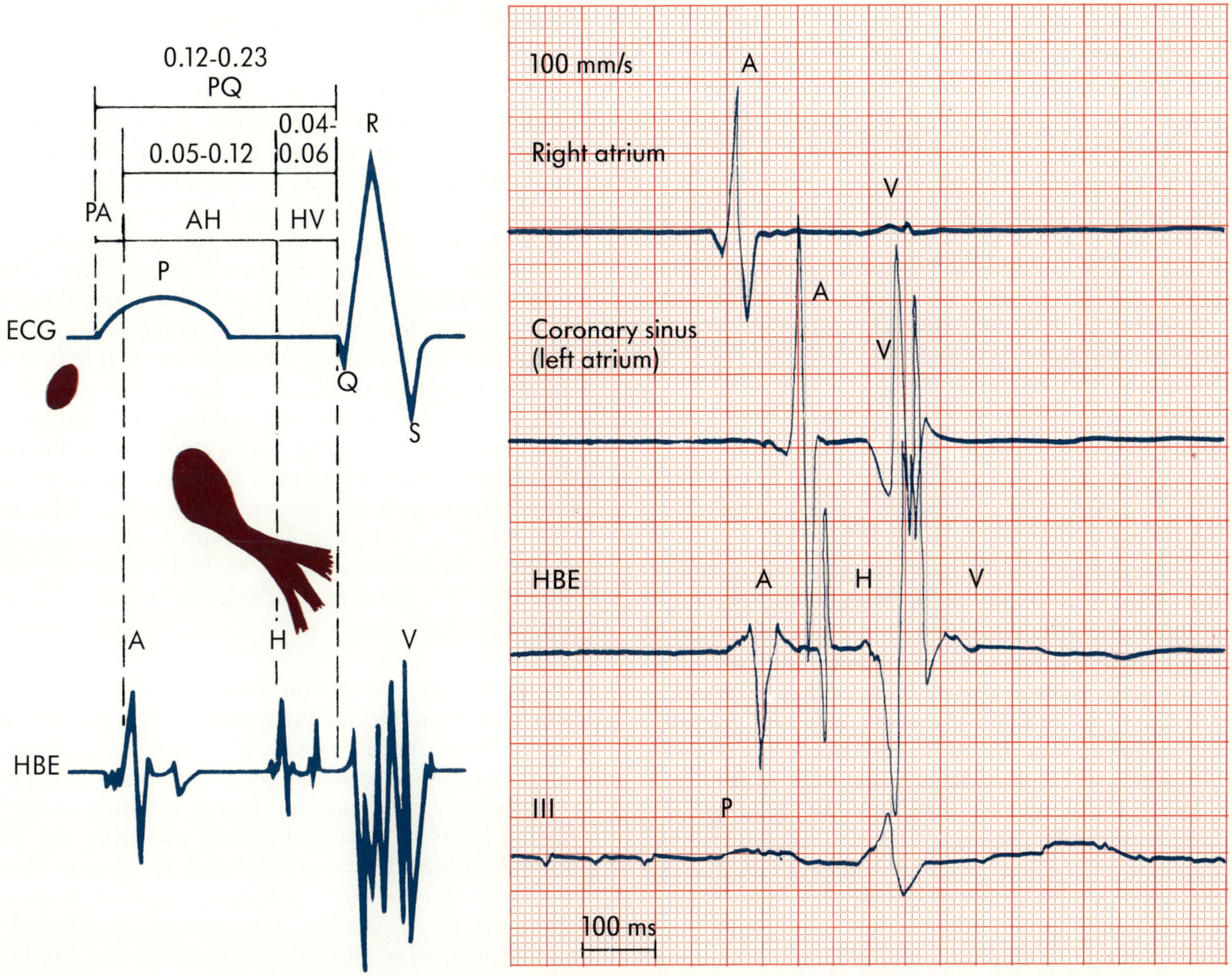

Fig. 3.21
His bundle electrogram (HBE). To the left schematic drawing, to the right an HBE tracing with simultaneous recordings of electrograms from the right atrium and coronary sinus and a surface ECG from lead III.

used as designations for the major deflections of the HBE (Fig. 3.21): A for onset of atrial activity, H for the His spike and V for the onset of ventricular activation. Whereas the PR interval of the surface ECG expresses total AV conduction time, the His bundle electrogram enables the investigator to subdivide this period into:

- The AH interval which reflects conduction time through the AV node to the bundle of His (suprahisian AV conduction time), and

- The HV interval which reflects conduction from the His bundle through the first part of the bundle branches until the onset of septal activation (infrahisian AV conduction time).

His bundle electrograms have been used primarily in patients with AV conduction disturbances in order to determine whether the site of the AV block is above or below the bundle of His and thus classify AV blocks as either proximal (suprahisian) blocks with prolonged AH interval or distal (infrahisian) blocks with prolonged HV interval (Fig. 10.1, page 247). His bundle electrography can be used also in the differential diagnosis of supraventricular and ventricular arrhythmias. The QRS complex in supraventricular arrhythmias is preceded by an H deflection, while the inability to record His bundle activity suggests a ventricular origin.

Sinus node recovery time (SNRT) [4, 40–47]

Rapid atrial pacing is performed for a period of 30–60 s to establish a steady state of sinus suppression. When atrial pacing is discontinued, a pause occurs before sinus rhythm is resumed; this postpacing pause is called the sinus node recovery time (SNRT). A significantly prolonged SNRT in a patient who has fainted strongly suggests that the faint was caused by paroxysms of sinoatrial block or sinus arrest (Figs. 11.3–11.7, page 281–287). A normal SNRT, however, does not by any means preclude sinus node disease since a negative outcome of the test has been observed in about half the patients with recurrent fainting due to SA block or sinus arrest.

To reduce the spontaneous variability in sinus node recovery time most investigators "correct" the measured sinus node recovery time by subtracting the prepacing sinus cycle length to achieve the so-called *corrected sinus node recovery time.* The normal corrected sinus node recovery time is about half a second (500 ms) or less.

Programmed electrical stimulation (PES) [39–42]

In most patients with paroxysmal tachycardia of re-entry type (both supraventricular and ventricular tachycardia) an attack of tachycardia can be provoked by programmed electrical stimulation (PES) (Fig. 3.22). PES starts with the introduction of a pacing impulse late in diastole. It is then gradually moved earlier towards the T wave of the preceding complex until tachycardia is initiated or until refractoriness is encountered. Pacing with double extra stimuli (two pacing impulses, one shortly after the other) and eventually triple extra stimuli may be necessary if a single stimulus fails to initiate the tachycardia. PES is performed at several sites and usually both in sinus rhythm and in paced rhythms at various rates of pacing. Once initiated, the tachycardia usually can be terminated by repeating the PES with the electrode in the same position (see Fig. 4.12, page 88). Atrial or ventricular fibrillation which occasionally develops as a complication to PES cannot be terminated by PES, but requires defibrillation by a DC countershock.

A major problem in the study of the patient with paroxysmal ventricular tachycardia is the risk of induction of "non-clinical" attacks of ventricular tachycardia, a risk which increases with more aggressive stimulation programmes including four, five or a whole "burst" of pacing impulses delivered rapidly one after the other. For this reason it is most essential to have a 12 lead ECG recording of the spontaneous attack available for comparison to decide the relevance (clinical or non-clinical) of a PES-induced tachycardia. The induction of multiform ventricular tachycardia and ventricular fibrillation usually are considered as non-specific end points.

The PES induction of a re-entry tachycardia is valuable for:

1 *Assessment of the mechanism of the arrhythmia.* A tachycardia which can be induced and subsequently terminated by critically timed pacing impulses is most likely of re-entry type, though tachycardias related to triggered automaticity may occasionally be induced and terminated in a similar way.

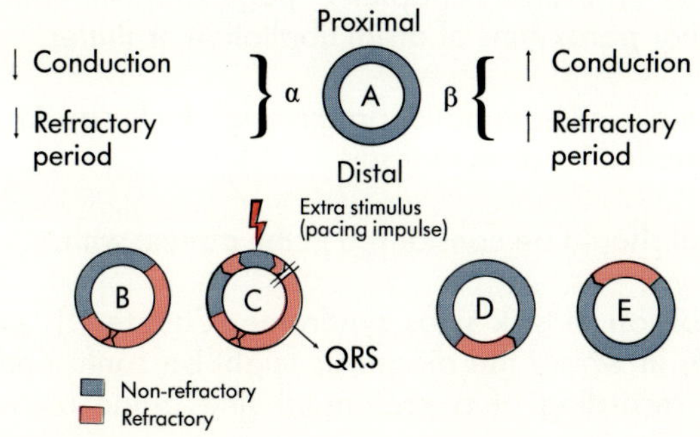

Fig. 3.22
A simplified model of the principle inprogrammed electrical stimulation (PES). The figure represents in diagram form the electrophysiological events which may underlie the induction of re-entry tachycardia in one of the re-entry substrates depicted in Figs. 3.4 and 3.5 (p. 41, 42) as it can occur during PES in the Cardiac Laboratorium or following extrasystole in the daily life of the patient. The figures presents only one out of a multitude of possibilities of how a premature activation may interact with the electrophysiological inhomogeniety of the re-entry substrate and thus start an attack of re-entry tachycardia.

A *The re-entry substrate in diastole with indications of the differences in the electrophysiological properties of the α and β branch of the re-entry substrate.*

B *The re-entry substrate shortly after a normal activation; the proximal part of the α pathway has recovered, whereas the proximal part of the β pathway is still in the refractory state.*

C *During the pace scan of the diastole, a pacing impulse just happens to be "critically" timed to arrive at the proximal end of the re-entry substrate during the brief moment of simultaneous α non-refractoriness and β refractoriness depicted in (B); thus, whereas the pacing induced activation wave moves freely but slowly down the α branch, it is blocked and halted by the refractoriness of the β branch.*

D *When the pacing impulse eventually arrives at the distally located junction between the α and β branches, the β branch may have had time to recover, so that the impulse can be conducted centrally via the β branch to the proximal junction of the α and β branches.*

E *From the proximal junction between α and β branches the impulse will move distally via the α and then back again via the β branch, and so on.*

2 *Selection of an optimal antiarrhythmic drug regime.* PES is performed with the intention of deliberately provoking the arrhythmia before and after drug administration to test the antiarrhythmic efficiency of chosen drug treatment. Therapy guided by PES is probably the most effective method for identifying the appropriate antiarrhythmic medication in the patient. In this controlled situation, antiarrhythmic drugs can be studied serially. Any drug which prevents initiation of the tachycardia will likely prove effective; long-term and successful prevention of the arrhythmia can be expected.

PES for induction of supraventricular, but not for ventricular tachycardia, can be performed non-invasively by pacing via an oesophageal lead (the pill electrode). Thus, PES (and burst pacing) via an oesophageal lead has been used in the electrophysiological assessment of the patient with the WPW syndrome (Chapter 7, page 188).

Electrophysiologic mapping [39–41]

The basic mapping procedure involves the simultaneous recording of electrograms from strategically selected sites in the atria or ventricles or, if simultaneous recording is not possible, sampling of local electrograms timed against a reference electrogram recorded from one and the same site in the heart every time. Mapping preferably is performed during a sustained paroxysm of reentry tachycardia induced by PES. The aim of mapping is to find the *point of earliest myocardial activation* for instance to locate:

- The site of the accessory AV pathway in the WPW syndrome which in tachycardia with VA conduction over the accessory pathway (the common form of WPW tachycardia) would correspond to the earliest point of left or right atrial activation during the tachycardia.

- The site of origin of a ventricular tachycardia which would correspond to the point of earliest endocardial activation in the left (or rarely the right) ventricle.

Electrophysiological mapping performed in the catherization laboratory usually is too inaccurate to form the basis for a surgical intervention. Thus, in the patient referred for operation, mapping will be repeated in the theatre with the tachycardia initiated by programmed pacing and with electrogram recordings from electrodes placed on the exposed heart (epicardial and/or endocardial).

Who should be referred for electrophysiologic studies? [39–41]

Referral for electrophysiological studies is indicated for the patient with:

- Paroxysmal sustained (> 30 s or causing collapse) ventricular tachycardia not associated with acute myocardial infarction

- Sudden cardiac arrest (ventricular fibrillation) not associated with acute myocardial infarction

- WPW syndrome (Chapter 7, page 188) with fainting and/or paroxysms of atrial fibrillation or flutter

- Severely symptomatic paroxysmal tachycardia not controlled by drug therapy.

Referral should be considered in the patient with:

- Suspicion of sick sinus syndrome (Chapter 11, page 286) in whom the diagnosis might be confirmed by the recording of a prolonged sinus node recovery time

- Syncope of unknown aetiology after all causes, including vascular, neurologic and metabolic, have been excluded and a comprehensive cardiac evaluation has been unrevealing

- AV block of first or second degree to localize the site of block for prognostic reasons (Chapter 10, page 248).

Ventricular late potentials [47–49]

Ventricular late potentials (Fig. 3.23) are low amplitude signals at the microvolt level, 1–25 microvolt, containing a relatively high frequency of waveforms, > 25 Hz. They are a continuation of the QRS complex and persist for tens of milliseconds into the ST segment. They are thought to arise from regions of delayed conduction in the border zone of an old myocardial infarction. Thus, it is probable that they may be used to identify tissue with tachycardia generating properties.

The major problem in the recording of these small bioelectric cardiac signals is interference from extraneous noise. Environmental sources of noise include skeletal muscle activity, electrodes, amplifiers and 50 Hz power interference. The problem of noise contamination may be overcome by feeding the highly amplified signal to a signal averaging device. The averaging process allows elimination of random noise not synchronized with the consistent waveform of the QRS complex (extrasystoles of varying configuration are rejected). Eventually, the signal averaged ECG is high-pass filtered to emphasize the high frequency waveforms of cellular activation and

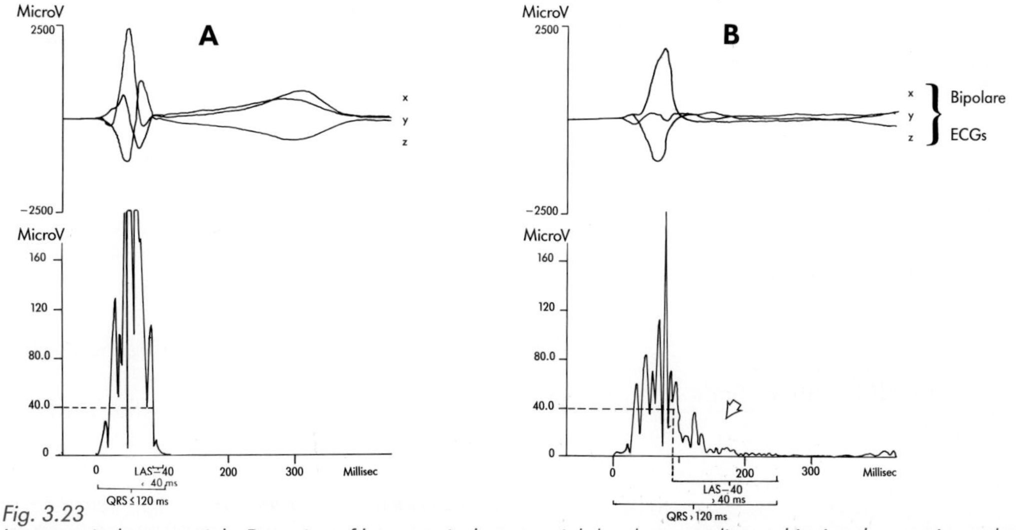

A Signal averaged ECG from a normal individual without late potentials

B Signal averaged ECG from a postinfarction patient with paroxysms of ventricular tachycardia. The arrow points at the very distinct late potentials.

Fig. 3.23
Late ventricular potentials. Detection of late ventricular potentials by electrocardiographic signal averaging technique. ECG recordings are from three bipolar surface leads, usually modifications of the so called orthogonal leads, x, y and z (upper part of figure). The highly amplified and signal averaged ECG from the three orthogonal leads are combined by computing them into one single averaged "vector" = $\sqrt{x^2 + y^2 + z^2}$ *(lower part of figure). Late potentials are considered present if: – The duration of the QRS complex of the signal averaged vector exceeds 120 milliseconds (in the absence of bundle branch block) and/or – The low amplitude terminal component of the complex with an amplitude of less than 40 mV (LAS–40) exceeds 40 milliseconds and/or – The mean amplitude of the terminal 40 milliseconds of the QRS complex (RMS–40) is under 25 microvolt.*

to minimize the low frequencies corresponding to repolarization.

The high-pass filtering should aid the detection of microvolt level waveforms arising from activation of small areas of myocardium. However, techniques of recording and analysis of ventricular late potentials are complicated and varying. Rules of standardization have to be established, but seem to be on the way to being resolved.

The clinical and prognostic significance of ventricular late potentials has not been clarified. A high incidence (71–92 %) of late potentials have been recorded in the survivors of myocardial infarction who suffer attacks of ventricular tachycardia. A significantly lower incidence of late potentials (7–34 %) has been recorded in the infarction survivor without attacks of ventricular tachycardia and a very low incidence (0–6 %) in the individual without former infarction or attacks of ventricular tachycardia. For the myocardial infarction patients studied during the first 4 to 8 weeks after the acute infarction, ventricular late potentials portend an increased risk for the subsequent occurrence of symptomatic attacks of ventricular tachycardia and sudden death. However, in the patient studied with ECG signal averaging techniques later than two months after the acute myocardial infarction, the recording of late potentials has been associated with a much lower incidence of arrhythmic events.

The question arises whether treatment with antiarrhythmic drugs or antitachycardia surgery can modify these low amplitude potentials to an extent that the antiarrhythmic efficacy of the intervention can be assessed. In clinical studies there has been no uniform response of the signal averaged ECG to therapy with antiarrhythmic drugs. Elimination of late potentials following antitachycardia surgery, however, has been shown to correlate with a successful outcome of the procedure.

Aetiology of arrhythmias [49–79]

A variety of cardiac arrhythmias occur in the normal healthy individual. Thus, in 24 hour ambulatory ECG monitoring the following findings should be considered within normal limits:

- Supraventricular extrasystoles up to 100/24 hours and episodes of supraventricular tachycardia up to 10 consecutive complexes (individuals above the age of 40 years)
- Ventricular extrasystoles up to 200/24 hours and ventricular extrasystolic pairs up to 50/24 hours (individuals above the age of 50 years)
- Pauses in the heart rate of up to 2 s
- Bradycardia of 40–60/min (mean heart rate over one min)
- SA block of second degree and AV block of first degree or second degree Mobitz type II recorded during sleep.

Cardiac arrhythmias of clinical significance can from an aetiological point of view be grouped as follows:

A *Arrhythmogenic syndromes* associated with paroxysmal or chronic arrhythmias in the otherwise apparently healthy individual without concomitant heart disease:

- Paroxysmal tachycardia in the WPW syndrome (Fig. 7.9, page 196) paroxysmal re-entry nodal tachycardia (Fig. 6.10, page 135), lone atrial fibrillation, the congenital long QT syndromes (Fig. 6.35, page 168/169) and paroxysmal ventricular tachycardia in the young (Figs. 6.39–6.41, page 176 – page 178/179)
- Paroxysmal or chronic heart block in the sick sinus syndrome (Fig. 11.7, page 287) and Stokes-Adams syndrome (Figs. 10.10, page 263 and 10.11, page 265).

B *Cardiac disease:* Any cardiac disease can cause cardiac arrhythmias for instance acute myocardial infarction, chronic ischaemic heart disease, hypertensive heart disease, valvular disease, cardiomyopathy and in the child congenital heart disease. In congestive heart failure neurohumoral activation (increased plasma norepinephrine level) and ventricular stretch may act as potential arrhythmogenic factors.

C *Non-cardiac arrhythmia precipitating factors.* These are particularly prone to cause arrhythmias in patients with heart disease. They include:

- *Acute infections* particularly those affecting the lungs
- *Hypotension, shock and anaemia* in the postoperative patient
- *Drug overdosage and intoxication* for instance with digitalis (Chapter 12, page 292), antiarrhythmic drugs of any type but particular drugs of Class IA and IC (Chapter 4, page 71), tricyclic antidepressants, thioridazine (Fig. 6.34, page 167) and sympathomimetic, parasympathomimetic and parasympatholytic drugs
- *Electrolyte derangements,* both hypo- and hyperkalaemia may precipitate arrhythmias whereas hypomagnaesemia and hypercalcaemia act primarily by amplifying the arrhythmogenic effect of hypokalaemia (Chapter 13, page 298).

D *Endocrine disorders* primarily thyrotoxicosis, rarely phaeochromocytoma and hyperparathyroidism.

E *Catheters and catheter electrodes introduced into the cavities of the heart* can induce extrasystoles, tachycardia or fibrillation either by the scraping of the tip against the atrial or ventricular wall or by the transmission of electrical current to the myocardium. All electrical apparatus and equipment used in connection with intracardiac catheters and electrodes should therefore be safeguarded against "leakage" of even very weak electrical current to the heart.

F *Changes in the autonomic nervous tone to the heart.* In general, vagal tone aggravates while sympathetic tone ameliorates any tendency for supraventricular bradycardia, sinoatrial block or AV block of the proximal type (Chapter 10). An increase in vagal tone can elicit atrial fibrillation in the predisposed individual, most likely due to an uneven distribution of the vagal fibres to the various parts of the atria. A high sympathetic tone may predispose to ventricular extrasystole, tachycardia and fibrillation.

Cardiac arrhythmias often are of multifactorial origin. Thus arrhythmia management should be based on a careful search not only for underlying heart disease but also for potential arrhythmogenic factors in the environment such as electrolyte derangements, antiarrhythmic drug treatment, infection etc.

Signs and symptoms [80–86]

The clinical manifestations of cardiac arrhythmias encompass the triad: Arrhythmic complaints, haemodynamic complications and neurological symptoms.

Arrhythmic complaints. The perception of the arrhythmic heart beat, varies greatly from one individual to another. A brief "slight" arrhythmia may cause severe distress and anxiety in one patient while a sustained, serious arrhythmia in another patient may occur unnoticed. In nervous patients especially extrasystoles result in an "extrasystolic sensation", described as the heart turning cartwheels, standing still for a moment, or occasionally beating very hard. Some patients feel even a single extrasystole, while others may have many with no sense of discomfort. In tachycardia, there is often a feeling of rapid heart beat or fluttering in the chest and/or a variety of symptoms such as anxiety, breathlessness, fatigue or dizziness. Some patients do not recognize the rapid heart rate at all, complaining only of vague symptoms. The paroxysms may be followed by or sometimes accompanied by frequent micturation (urina spastica). A slow heart rate is rarely, if ever, sensed as such by the patient.

Haemodynamic complications. The haemodynamic consequences of an arrhythmia are related not only to the severity of the arrhythmia, but also to the functional states of the myocardium and circulatory system. In an individual with a healthy myocardium and normal coronary arteries, an increase in heart rate up to 200/min or more often will produce only minor symptoms of palpitation, fatigue and a feeling of physical distress, while in a patient with a severely diseased myocardium or severe coronary artery disease, even a moderate increase in heart rate to about 140–150/min may induce congestive failure, pulmonary oedema or anginal pain. Bradycardia down to 25–30/min is well tolerated in the individual with a well preserved myocardium but may cause shock or congestive failure in acute myocardial infarction, severe chronic ischaemic heart disease or valvular heart disease.

Neurological symptoms. During attacks of tachycardia, or sometimes bradycardia, episodes of confusion, dizziness or mental tiredness may occur particularly in elderly patients. The most serious neurological conditions caused by arrhythmias are Stokes-Adams attacks and sudden death related to cardiac arrest.

Cardiac arrest, sudden death and Stokes-Adams attacks [87–89]

Cardiac arrest is the sudden cessation of the pumping activity of the heart. It is most often caused by the acute onset of an arrhythmia, but more rarely can be due to sudden failure of the pumping ability of the cardiac muscle (primary pump failure). The arrhythmias which can cause cardiac arrest range from tachycardia and fibrillation with fast but ineffective ventricular activity to AV block or SA block complicated by ventricular arrest. The cardinal clinical signs in cardiac arrest are the sudden loss of consciousness associated with the disappearance of the arterial pulse. Since the cells of the cerebral cortex are very sensitive to lack of oxygen they cease to function 8–20 s after the interruption of the blood flow (sooner in the old, later in the young). The initially reversible suppression of nerve cell function becomes irreversible with sustained cerebral ischaemia. The end result of cardiac arrest beyond a few minutes, usually 4–6 min, is *death*. The complete acute process is called "sudden death". In acute myocardial infarction, cardiac arrest may be preceded by intense pain behind the sternum, but usually a cardiac arrest including arrest due to acute myocardial infarction occurs without preceding symptoms in the chest. The patient merely perceives that he is becoming distant, or occasionally he feels as if something is "running down" in him, then all is black and he loses consciousness without being able to call for help. A bystander would see the patient suddenly collapse. The face of the unconscious patient would be pale or cyanotic. The pupils often but not invariably are dilated. Respiration stops immediately or within a short time. The arterial pulses cannot be felt.

Stokes-Adams attacks are attacks with sudden loss of consciousness related to brief episodes of cardiac arrest with spontaneous recovery. Depending on how rapidly the heart starts again, the state of unconsciousness ranges from momentarily impaired consciousness to black out and fainting. Clonic or tonic seizures may occur. Trauma is frequent. Brief attacks of cardiac arrest with spontaneous recovery often presage later longer-lasting or fatal cardiac arrest. Thus, a Stokes-Adams attack is a clinical event which should always be taken seriously, since it can portend sudden death. Differential diagnosis in Stokes-Adams attacks includes transitory cerebral ischaemia and in the case of seizures, epilepsy.

1. WHO/ISFC Task Force. Definition of terms related to cardiac rhythm. Am Heart J 1978; 95: 796–806.
2. WHO/ISFC Task Force. Classification of cardiac arrhythmias and conduction disturbances. Am Heart J 1979; 98: 263–67.
3. Surawicz B, Uhley H, Borun R, et al. Optimal electrocardiography. Task force I: Standardization of terminology and interpretation, Bethesda Conference Report. Am J Cardiol 1978; 41: 130–45.
4. Singh BN, Opie LH, Harrison DC, et al. Antiarrhythmic agents. In: Opie LH, ed. Drugs for the heart. Orlando, New York, London: Grune & Stratton, Inc., 1987; 54–90.
5. Bigger JT, Jr. Electrophysiology for the clinician. Europ Heart J 1984; 5 (Suppl. B): 1–9.
6. Gadsby DC, Wit AL. Normal and abnormal electrical activity in cardiac cells. In: Mandel WJ, ed. Cardiac arrhythmias. Their mechanisms, diagnosis, and management. 2nd edition. Philadelphia: J. B. Lippincott Co., 1987; 53–80.
7. Gorgels APM, Vas MA, Brugada P, Wellens HJJ. The clinical relevance of abnormal automaticity and triggered activity. In: Brugada P, Wellens HJJ, eds. Cardiac arrhythmias: Where to go from here? Mount Kisco, New York: Futura Publishing Co., 1987; 147–69.
8. Scherf D, Schott A. Extrasystoles and allied arrhythmias. London: William Heinemann, 1973; 397–402.
9. Moe GK, Rheinholdt WC, Abildskov JA. A computer model of atrial fibrillation. Am Heart J 1964; 67: 200–20.
10. Allessie MA, Lammers WJEP, Rensma PL, Bonke FIM. Flutter and fibrillation in experimental models: What has been learned that can be applied to humans? In: Brugada P, Wellens HJJ, eds. Cardiac arrhythmias: Where to go from here? Mount Kisco, New York: Futura Publishing Co., 1987; 67–82.
11. Olsson SB, Dohnal M. Is atrial fibrillation propencity linked to intrinsic AV-nodal Function? New Trends Arrhythmias 1988; 4: 569–74.
12. Surawicz B. Ventricular fibrillation. Am J Cardiol 1971; 28: 268–85.
13. Josephson ME, Spielman SR, Greenspan AM, Horowitz LN. Mechanism of ventricular fibrillation in man. Observations based on electrode catheter recordings. Am J Cardiol 1979; 44: 623–331.
14. Wiggers CJ, Wegreia R. Ventricular fibrillation due to single localized induction and condenser shocks applied during the vulnerable phase of ventricular systole. Am J Physiol 1940; 128: 500–05.
15. Marriott HJL, Conover MH. Advanced concepts in arrhythmias. Aberrant ventricular conduction: 244–67; Phase 3 and phase 4 block: 155–66. St. Louis: The C.V. Mosby Co., 1983.
16. Blondeau M. Aberrant ventricular conduction. (Functional, pardoxical and intermittent bundle branch block.) In: Puech P, Siama R, eds. The cardiac arrhythmias by the arrhythmia working group of the French Cardiac Society. Paris: Corbière and Roussel, 1979; 127–38.
17. Pick A, Langendorf R. Interpretation of complex arrhythmias. Philadelphia: Lea & Febiger, 1979; 367–90.
18. Schamroth L. Aberrant ventricular conduction. Ingelheim am Rhein: Boehringer Ingelheim Postgraduate Medical Services, 1983.
19. Puech P. The P wave: Correlation of surface and intraatrial electrograms. Cardiovasc Clin 1974; 6; 43–68.
20. Josephson ME. Paroxsysmal supraventricular tachycardia: An electrophysiologic approach. Am J Cardiol 1978; 41: 1122–26.
21. Kuchar DL, Thorburn CW, Sammel NL, et al. Surface electrocardiographic manifestations of tachyarrhythmias: Clues to diagnosis and mechanism. Pace 1988; 11: 61–82.
22. Wit AL, Weiss MB, Berkowitz WD, et al. Patterns of atrioventricular conduction in the human heart. Circulat Res 1970; 32: 345–57.
23. Meijler FL, Fisch C. Does the atrioventricular node conduct ? Br Heart J 1989; 61: 30915.
24. Pick A, Langendorf R. Interpretation of complex arrhythmias. Philadelphia: Lea & Febiger, 1979; 471–541.
25. Josephson ME, Waxman HL, Marchinski FE, et al. Relation between site of origin and QRS configuration in ventricular rhythms. In: Wellens HJJ; Kulbertus HE, eds. What's new in electrocardiography. The Hague, Boston, London: Martinus Nijhoff Publishers, 1981; 200–28.
26. Josephson ME. The origin of premature ventricular complexes – role and limitation of the 12-lead electrocardiogram. Int J Cardiol 1982; 2: 87–90.
27. Kuchar DL, Ruskin JN, Garan H. Electrocardiographic localization of the site of origin of ventricular tachycardia in patients with prior myocardial infarction. Pace 1989; 13: 893–900.
28. Wellens HJJ, Brugada P. Diagnosis of venticular tachycardia from the 12-lead electrocardiogram. Cardiol Clin 1987; 5: 511–25.
29. Akhtar M, Shenasa M, Jazayeri M, et al. Wide QRS complex tachycardia. Reappraisal of a common clinical problem. Ann Int Med 1988; 109: 905–12.
29.A Gouaux JL, Ashman R. Auricular fibrillation with aberration simulating ventricular paroxysmal tachycardia. Am Heart J 1947; 34: 366.
30. Schnittger I, Rodriguez IM, Winkle RA. Esophageal electrocardiography: A new technology revives an old technique. Am J Cardiol 1986; 57: 604–07.
31. Guarnieri T. Eophageal recording and pacing. In: Zipes DP, Rowlands DJ, eds. Progress in cardiology. Philadelphia: Lea & Febiger, 1988; 305–15.
32. Brown AP, Dawkins KD, Davies JG. Detection of arrhythmias: Use of a patient-activated ambulatory electrocardiogram device with a solid-state memory loop. Br Heart J 1987; 58: 251–53.
33. Campbell RWF, Murray A. Dynamic electrocardiography. Edin burgh, London, New York: Churchill Livingstone, 1985.
34. Leclercq JR, Coumel Ph. Ambulatory electrocardiogram monitoring. In: Macfarlane PW, Veitch Lawrie TD, eds. Comprehensive electrocardiology. Theory and practice in health and disease. New York, Oxford: Pergamon Press, 1989; 1063–66.
35. Knoebel SB, Crawford MH, Dunn MI, et al. Guidelines for ambulatory electrocardiography. A report of the American College of Cardiology/American Heart Association Task Force on assessment of diagnostic and therapeutic cardiovascular procedures (Subcommittee on ambulatory electrocardiography). ACC/AHA Task Force, Br Heart J 1982; 47: 213–20.
36. Arndal P, Damgaard Andersen J. Ten years experience with routine use of radiottelemetry in a coronary care unit. In: Cathignol P, Faust U, Kimmich H, eds. Medical wireless telemetry. Luxembourg: Comm Europ Comm 1983; 3–6.

37. Coumel P, Cokkinos DV, eds. Symposium on exercise in the diagnosis and evaluation of treatment of arrhythmias. Europ Heart J 1987; 8 (Suppl. D).
38. Podrid PJ, Venditti FJ, Levine PA, Klein MD. The role of exercise testing in evaluation of arrhythmias. Am J Cardiol 1988; 62: 24–33.
39. Josephson ME, Seides ST. Clinical cardiac electrophysiology. Techniques and interpretations. Philadelphia: Lea & Febiger, 1979.
40. Ward DE, Camm AJ. Clinical electrophysiology of the heart. London: Edward Arnold, 1987.
41. Rahimtoola SH, Zipes DP, Akhtar M, et al. Consensus statement of the conference on the state of the art of electrophysiologic testing in the diagnosis and treatment of patients with cardiac arrhythmias. Circulation 1987; 75 (Suppl. III): 3–11.
42. Horowitz LN, Kay HkR, Kutalek SP, et al. Risks and complications of clinical cardiac electrophysiologic studies: A prospective analysis of 1,000 consecutive patients. JACC 1987; 9: 1261–68.
43. Bloch Thomsen PE. Intracardiac electrography in patients with bifascicular bundle branch block. Acta med scand 1981; Suppl. 653.
44. Reiffel JA. Electrophysiologic evaluation of sinus node function. Cardiol Clin 1986; 4: 401–16.
45. Simonsen E. Sinus node dysfunction. A prospective clincal study with special reference to the diagnostic value of ambulatory electrocardiography, electrophysiologic study and exercise testing. Odense: CAVI, 1987.
46. Fujimura O, Yee R, Klein GF, et al. The diagnostic sensitivity of electrophysiologic testing in patients with syncope caused by transiet bradycardia. New Engl J Med 1989; 321: 1703–07.
47. Simson MB. Signal averaging. Circulation 1987; 75 (Suppl. III): 69–73.
48. Breithardt G, Borggrefe M. Recent advances in the identification of patients at risk of ventricular tachyarrhythmias: Role of ventricular late potentials. Circulation 1987; 75: 1091–96.
49. Cripps TR, Camm AJ, Bennett ED, Ward DE. Prediction of serious post-infarction cardiac arrhythmias. Lancet 1989; ii: 845–47.
50. Chamberlain DA, Kulbertus H, Mogensen L, et al, eds. Cardiac arrhythmias in the active population. Prevalence, significance and management. Mölndal: Hässle, 1980.
51. Bjerregaard P. Premature beats in healthy subjects 40–79 years of age. Europ Heart J 1982; 3: 493–503.
52. Bjerregaard P. Mean 24-hour heart rate, minimal heart rate and pauses in healthy subjects 40–79 years of age. Europ Heart J 1983; 4: 44–51.
53. Ingerslev J, Bjerregaard P. Prevalence and prognostic significance of cardiac arrhythmias detected by ambulatory electrocardiography in subjects 85 years of age. Europ Heart J 1986; 7: 570–75.
54. Viitasalo MT, Kala R, Eisalo A. Ambulatory electrocardiographic findings in young athletes between 14 and 16 years of age. Europ Heart J 1984; 5: 2–6.
55. Viitasalo MT, Kala R, Eisalo A. Ambulatory electrocardiographic recording in endurance athletes. Circulat Res 1989; 79: 206–15
56. Bigger JD Jr, Dresdale RJ, Heissenbuttel RH, et al. Ventricular arrhythmias in ischemic heart disease: Mechanism, prevalence, significance, and management. Cardiovasc Dis 1977; 19: 255–300.
57. Pantridge JF, Webb SW, Adgey AAJ. Arrhythmias in the first hours of acute myocardial infarction. Cardiovasc Dis 1981; 23: 265–78.
58. Rehnqvist N, Ericsson C-G, Erhardt L, Olsson G. Arrhythmias in acute myocardial infarction: Special considerations in treatment and monitoring. Europ Heart J 1988; 9 (Suppl. B): 547–61.
59. Møller M, Nielsen BL, Fabricious J. Paroxysmal ventricular tachycardia during 24-hour ambulatory ECG tape recording in postmyocardial infarction patients. Br Heart J 1980; 43: 447–53.
60. Borggrefe M, Kuhn H, Königer HH, et al. Arrhythmias in hypertrophic obstructive and non-obstructive cardiomyopathy. Europ Heart J 1983; 4 (Suppl. F): 245–51.
61. McKenna WJ. Sudden death in hypertrophic cardiomyopathy: Identification of the „high risk" patient. In: Brugada P, Wellens HJJ, eds. Cardiac arrhythmias: Where to go from here? Mount Kisco, New York: Futura Publishing Co., 1987; 353–65.
62. Olshausen KV, Stienen U, Math D, et al. Long-term prognostic significance of ventricular arrhythmias in idiopathic dilated cardiomyopathy. Am J Cardiol 1988; 61: 146–51.
63. Shih HT, et al. Frequency and significance of cardiac arrhythmias in chronic obstructive lung disease. Chest 1988; 94: 44–8.
64. Campbell RWF, Godman MG, Fiddler GI, et al. Ventricular arrhythmias in syndrome of ballon deformity of mitral valve. Definition of possible high risk group. Br Heart J 1976; 38: 1053–57.
65. Savage DD, Levy D, Garrison RJ, et al. Mitral valve prolapse in the general population. 3. Dysrhythmias: The Framingham study. Am Heart J 1983; 106: 582–86.
66. Parmley WW. Factors causing arrhythmias in chronic congestive heart failure. Am Heart J 1987; 114: 1267–72.
66.A Captopril-Digoxin Multicenter Research Group: Comparative effects of therapy with captopril and digoxin in patients with mild to moderate heart failure. JAMA 1988; 259: 539–544
67. Angelini P, Felman MI, Lufschanowski R, et al. Cardiac arrhythmias during and after heart surgery: Diagnosis and management. Prog Cardiovasc Dis 1974; 26: 469–95.
68. Goldman L. Supraventricular tachyarrhythmias in hospitalized adults after surgery: Clinical correlates in patients over 40 years of age after major noncardiac surgery. Chest 1978; 73: 450–54.
69. Hultén B-Å, Health A. Clinical aspects of tricyclic antidepressant poisoning. Acta med scand 1983; 213: 275–78.
70. Brorson L, Wennerblom B. Electrophysiological methods in assessing cardiac effects of the tricyclic antidepressant imipramin. Acta med scand 1978; 203: 429–32.
71. Montalescot G, Levy Y, Hatt PY. Serious sinus node dysfunction caused by therapeutic doses of lithium. Int J Cardiol 1984; 5: 94–6.
72. Surawicz B, Mangiardi ML. Electrocardiogram in endocrine and metabolic disorder. In: Rios JD, ed. Clinical-electrocardiographic correlations. Cardiovasc Clin 1977; 8/3: 243–66.
73. Voukydis PC, Cohen SI. Catheter-induced arrhythmias. Am Heart J 1974; 88: 588–92.
74. Whalen RE, Starmer CF. Electric shock hazards in clinical cardiology. Mod Concepts Cardiovasc Dis 1967; 36: 7–12.

75. Raftery EB, Green HL, Yacoub MH. Disturbances of heart rhythm produced by 50 Hz leakage currents in human subjects. Cardiovasc Res 1975; 9: 263–65.
76. Geselowitz DB, Arzbaecher RC, Barr RC, et al. Electrical safety standards for electrocardiographic apparatus. Circulation 1980; 61: 669–70.
77. Verrier RL. Autonomic stubstrates for arrhythmias. In: Zipes DP, Rowlands DJ, eds. Progress in cardiology. Phila delphia: Lea & Febiger, 1988; 65–81.
78. Schlepper M. The automatic nervous system and supraventricular rhythm disturbances. (Einflüsse des autonomen Nervensystems bei supraventrikulären Rhythmusstörungen). Z Kardiol 1986; 75 (Suppl. 5): 35–40.
79. Malliani A, Schwartz PJ, Zanchettei A. Neural mechanisms in life-threatening arrhythmias. Am Heart J 1980; 100: 705–15.
80. Samet P. Hemodynamic sequelae of cardiac arrhythmias. Circulation 1973; 47: 399–407.
81. Godberg AD, Raftery EB, Cashman PMM. Ambulatory electrocardiographic records in patients with transient cerebral attack or palpitation. Br Med J 1975; 4: 569–71.
82. Abdon N-J, Malmcrona R. High pacemaker implantation rate following "cardiogenic neurology". Results in 120 consecutively paced patients. Acta med scand 1975; 198: 455–61.
83. Johansson BVW. Long-term ECG in ambulatory clinical practice: Analysis and 2-year follow-up of 100 patients studied with a portable ECG tape recorder. Europ J Cardiol 1977; 5: 39–48.
84. Beder SD, Cohen MH, Reimenschneider TA. Occult arrhythmias as the etiology of unexplained syncope in children with structurally normal hearts. Am Heart J 1985; 109: 309.
85. Camm AJ, Lau CP. Syncope of undetermined origin: Diagnosis and management. In: Zipes DP, Rowlands DJ, eds. Progress in Cardiology. Philadelphia: Lea & Febiger, 1988; 139–56.
86. Ringqvist I, Jonason T, Nilsson G, et al. Diagnostic value of longterm ambulatory ECG in patients with syncope, dizziness or palpitations. Clin Physiol 1989; 9: 47–55.
87. Jensen G, Sigurd B, Meibom J, Sandøe E. Adams-Stokes syndrome caused by paroxysmal third-degree atrio-ventricular block. Br Heart J 1973; 35: 516–20.
88. Editorial. Both ends of the stethoscope: Cardiac arrest. Lancet 1969; ii: 262–64.
89. Wellens HJJ, Brugada P. Sudden cardiac death: A multifactorial problem. In: Brugada P, Wellens HJJ, eds. Cardiac arrhythmias: Where to go from here? Mount Kisco, New York: Futura Publishing Co., 1987; 391–99.

Chapter 4
Management of cardiac arrhythmias

When to treat and when not? [1, 2]

Malignant cardiac arrhythmias which cause pulmonary oedema, shock or cardiac arrest need immediate intervention to save life. There are other arrhythmias with troublesome symptoms or serious prognostic implications for which long-term antiarrhythmic medication with risk of serious side effects can be justified. Finally, there are benign arrhythmias with few or no symptoms and without prognostic implications for which antiarrhythmic medication would act only as an ECG cosmetic and would do little or no good to the patient. Indeed side effects might affect life quality and even endanger life.

Thus, the decision to treat or not to treat should be based on firm evidence about the clinical significance of the arrhythmia considering:

- *ECG diagnosis* and *differential diagnosis.* Does ECG evidence support the arrhythmia diagnosis? Which other arrhythmias might present with the same or similar ECG findings?

- *Symptoms.* Does the arrhythmia affect life quality? What are the haemodynamic consequences of the arrhythmia? Will it provoke congestive failure or shock or maybe cause neurological symptoms: dizziness, blackout or fainting?

- *Aetiology.* What is the cause of the arrhythmia: "arrhythmogenic cardiac disorder", underlying heart disease or is it due to non-cardiac arrhythmia precipitating factors?

- *Prognosis.* What is the risk of sudden death, Stokes-Adams attacks, congestive failure, shock and embolism?

Examination of an arrhythmia patient will routinely include a clinical history, physical examination, a 12-lead between-attack ECG, x-ray of the chest, often an echocardiogram and a variety of simple laboratory tests (haemoglobin, serum potassium and serum creatinine); Depending upon the individual arrhythmia *additional investigations* may be needed to clarify the aetiology and clinical significance of the arrhythmia e.g. thyroid parameters, exercise ECG, 24 hour ambulatory ECG monitoring, referral for an electrophysiological study.

Search for tachycardia precipitating factors

A careful search for tachycardia precipitating factors is a fundamental element in the management of tachycardia. Among the many tachycardia precipitating factors amenable to correction or suppressive therapy are:

A *Congestive heart failure (CHF).* In the failing heart neurohumeral activation (e.g. increased plasma norepinephine level) and ventricular stretch may act as potential arrhythmogenic stimuli. Thus, in the CHF patient treatment of arrhythmias should always as a primary element include an optimation of the CHF therapy with diuretics, vasodilating agents (angiotensin converting enzyme inhibitors) and/or digitalis.

B *Ventilatory problems, infection, anaemia, hypotension and schock.* Attacks of supraventricular tachycardia in the postoperative state are better managed by correction of the postoperative complication which precipitated the arrhythmia than by specific antiarrhythmic drug treatment.

C *Drug overdosage/intoxication* e.g. antiarrhythmic drugs, Class IC drugs (flecainide, propafenone) and IA drugs (quinidine, disopyramide, procainamide); digitalis; and tricylic antidepressants; thioridazine and, possibly, theophylline preparatous.

D *Serum electrolyte derangements* in particular hypo- and hyperkalaemia, rarely hypomagnaesemia and hypercalcaemia.

E *Arrhythmogenic cardiac disorders* manifest on the ECG as a WPW pattern (Fig. 7.3, page 191) or a long QT (Fig. 6.34, page 167)

F *Effort induced ventricular tachycardia* (Fig. 6.41, page 178/179 and 14.20, page 334) where the clue to the diagnosis and specific treatment (with beta blockade or in ischaemic heart disease myocardial revascularization) is given by the close correlation between physical strain and the attack of tachycardia.

G *Thyrotoxicosis* which can precipitate atrial fibrillation or, sometimes atrial flutter, often with the arrhythmia as the prevailing clinical symptom of the disease.

Treatment of tachycardia and fibrillation

Treatment of tachycardia and fibrillation has two aspects, termination of the acute attack and prophylaxis of recurrence.

The therapeutic spectrum of modalities to terminate the acute attack encompasses: Vagal manoeuvers, DC countershock, antiarrhythmic drugs, digitalis and defibrillation or cardioversion.

For long-term prophylaxis of recurrent paroxysmal tachycardia or fibrillation pharmacological antiarrhythmic medication has been and still is the prevailing therapy. Alternative non-pharmacological approaches of treatment introduced during recent years are becoming increasingly important. They include: Antitachycardia surgery, catheter ablation of the His bundle, the implantable automatic cardioverter/defibrillator (AICD implant) and antitachycardia pacemakers.

Vagal manoeuvres [3–5]

Vagal manoeuvres reflexly increase vagal tone. The manoeuvres can be highly efficient in terminating supraventricular tachycardia. Atrial flutter and fibrillation are not stopped by the manoeuvres but usually show transient slowing of the ventricular rate which may assist in the ECG diagnosis of the arrhythmia by disclosing formerly hidden flutter or fibrillatory activity. Ventricular tachycardia does not respond to an increase in vagal tone.

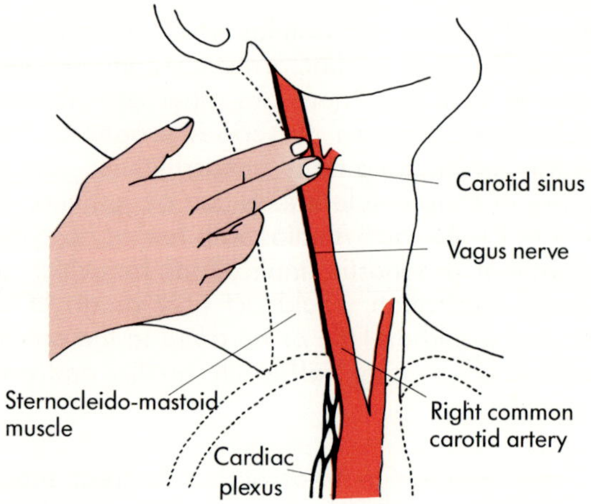

Fig. 4.1
Carotid sinus massage

There is a choice of vagal manoeuvres:

A *Carotid sinus massage* (Fig. 4.1) is performed with the patient in a supine position with the head turned slightly to one side comfortably supported by a pillow. A gentle massaging motion by a pair of fingertips is applied to the area just below the angle of the mandible and just in front of the sternocleido-mastoid muscle where the pulsation of the carotid artery is most clearly felt. The pressure is applied only on one side at a time and for a period of no more than 5–10 s. Usually massage is attempted first on the right side, and if ineffective on the left side. Prior to massage, the carotid arteries should be auscultated. The presence of a murmur contraindicates carotid sinus massage because it implies arteriosclerotic changes in the vessel wall with a risk of dislodging arteriosclerotic matter into the blood stream by the massage.

B The *Valsalva manoeuvre* with forced and sustained expiration against a closed glottis.

C *Finger down the throat* ("gag reflex").

D *Postural changes* that increase venous return, stroke volume and the arterial blood pressure and via the baroceptors induce an increase in vagal tone such as squatting or elevation of the legs against the wall ("upside-down-position"). The combined performance of the Valsalva manoeuvre can often significantly increase the vagotonic effect of these procedures.

E *Submerging the face in ice water* for a few seconds or just taking a drink of cold water induces strong vagal stimulation ("dive reflex"). It has been reported sucessful in terminating supraventricular tachycardia in children but has hitherto not gained extensive use in the adult cardiac clinic.

The use of eyeball pressure to increase vagal tone is discouraged because of the associated risk of initiating retinal detachment.

Individual responses to the different manoeuvres vary greatly and the patient should experiment to find the manoeuvre or combination of manoeuvres which works most efficiently for him/her. The therapeutic potential of vagal manoeuvres is by far greatest in the first minutes of the attack, so the patient should be instructed to use these manoeuvres at the very onset of symptoms.

Antiarrhythmic drugs [6–8]

With only a few exceptions the antiarrhythmic drugs used in the treatment of the acute arrhythmia are the same as those used for the prophylaxis of recurrences. For an acute attack the drug usually is administered as an intravenous bolus which produces a transistory, and, thus, tolerable high peak concentration, which will often terminate the tachycardia. Long-term prophylaxis, however, involves oral medication with a lower serum concentration of the drug. This may explain the relatively low success rate of long-term prophylaxis with antiarrhythmic drugs (usually no more than 30–35 %).

According to their effect on the action potential of the cardiac cell, the antiarrhythmic drugs are grouped in four classes. This classification is based on drug effects on an animal cardiac fiber suspended in an electrolyte bath to which the drug is added. The electrophysiologic characteristics of the four classes are as follows (Fig. 4.2, page 72):

Class I drugs. The common action of these drugs is depression of the rate of rise of phase zero of the action potential. Inhibiting the fast sodium channel they act as membrane stabilizing agents. According to their additional effects on the duration of the action potential the Class I antiarrhythmic drugs are subdivided into:

- *Class IA drugs* [7–10] prolong the duration of the action potential. To this class belong quinidine, disopyramide and procainamide.

- *Class IB drugs* [8, 9, 11–18] shorten the duration of the action potential. Examples are lignocaine (lidocaine), mexiletine and tocainide. Diphenylhydantoin which has a reputation for suppressing digitalis induced tachycardias, also belongs to this group.

- *Class IC drugs* [7, 8, 19–23] do not affect the duration of the action potential. This class includes propafenone and flecainide. Other drugs of this class are under investigation and in some countries have already received regulatory approval. They include encainide, lorcainide and ajmaline.

Class II drugs [7, 8, 24] are the beta blocking agents. They inhibit the influence of sympathomimetic agents on the

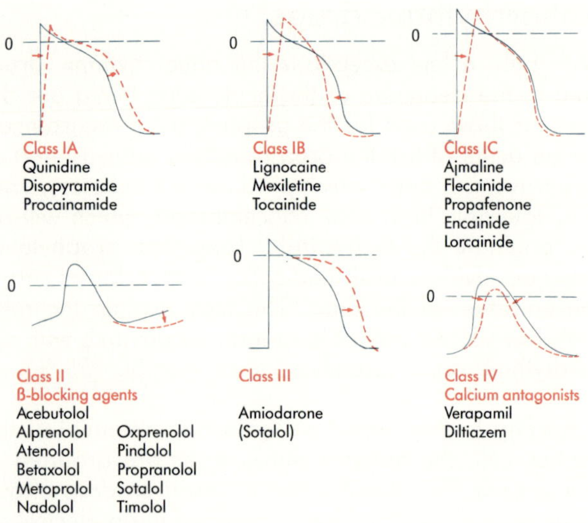

Fig. 4.2
Basic classification of the antiarrhythmic drugs from their dominant effect on the action potential. The figure shows the effect of Class I and III drugs on the action potential of ventricular cells, of Class II drugs on the action potential of SA nodal cells and Class IV drugs on that of AV nodal cells.

action potential. The addition of a sympathomimetic agent to the electrolyte bath in which the cardiac fiber is suspended increases the rate of rise of phase zero and steepens the slope of phase 4 (diastole) of the pacemaker cell. The subsequent addition of a Class II drug will tend to neutralize these sympathomimetic actions e.g. decrease the rate of rise of phase zero and flatten the slope of phase 4 (diastole) of the pacemaker cell.

Class III drugs [7, 8, 25–29] prolong the duration of the action potential without affecting the rate of rise of phase 0. Amiodarone is the only drug currently available for long-term therapy possessing a predominant action of this type. Besides its beta blocking properties, sotalol also prolongs the action potential. Bretylium, a drug primarily used against ventricular fibrillation, possesses a Class III effect but due to side effects in form of orthostatic hypotension is useful only for acute therapy in the supine position.

Class IV drugs [7, 8] are calcium channel blocking agents which affect the calcium flux across the cell membrane. This mechanism particularly influences the activity of the pacemaker cells of the AV node which are dependent more on the slow influx of calcium than that of sodium. Verapamil and diltiazem belong to this class. Other calcium channel blockers e.g. nicardipine and nifedipine are not antiarrhythmic drugs insofar as they exert little effect on the calcium flux across the membrane of the cardiac cell.

The antiarrhythmic drugs are numerous and new compounds are on their way. To accumulate experience with their mode of administration, efficacy and side effects each clinician should decide upon a limited "testing battery" of drugs encompassing one or two drugs from each of the seven antiarrhythmic "classes" (Class IA, IB, IC, II, III and IV) plus a digitalis glycoside – usually digoxin or digitoxin.

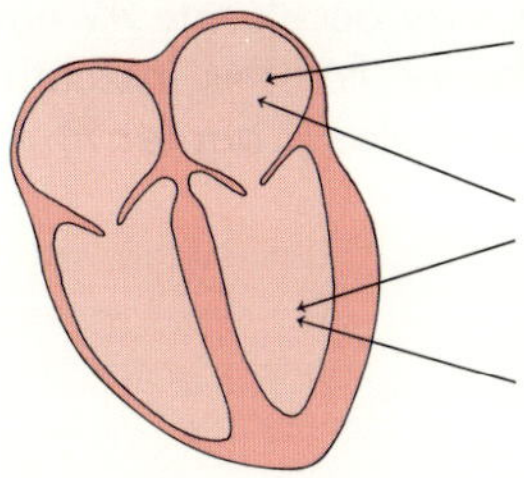

Fig. 4.3
Narrow spectrum and wide spectrum drugs

Specificity of antiarrhythmic drugs [7, 8, 29, 31]

With reference to their therapeutic potential in treating supraventricular and ventricular arrhythmias, the antiarrhythmic drugs can be divided into *narrow* and *wide spectrum drugs* (Fig. 4.3):

I Narrow spectrum drugs with effect on *either* supraventricular *or* ventricular extrasystole and tachycardia:

A Drugs with primary effects on supraventricular extrasystoles and tachycardias and no effect on ventricular arrhythmias: Class IV drugs, the calcium antagonists verapamil and diltiazem. The two and only exceptions to the non-efficacy of these drugs in ventricular tachycardia might be ventricular tachycardia of the fascicular type (Fig. 6.40, page 177) and, possibly, repetitive monomorphic ventricular tachycardia in the young (Fig. 6.39, page 176).

B Drugs with a primary effect on ventricular extrasystoles and tachycardia, and no effect on supraventricular arrhythmias: Class IB drugs, lidocaine, mexiletine and tocainide.

II Wide spectrum drugs with effects on both supraventricular and ventricular extrasystoles and tachycardias i.e. Class IA drugs, quinidine, disopyramide and procainamide, Class IC drugs, ajmaline, propafenone and flecainide, Class II drugs, the beta blocking agents and the Class III drug amiodarone.

Amiodarone probably is the most effective drug of all, but in some aspects is the most toxic. Many physicians (including the authors) tend to consider it the drug of "last resort". Amiodarone's powerful therapeutic effects, however, have made it the drug of first choice for life threatening cardiac arrhythmias:

- In cardiomyopathy, especially hypertrophic cardiomyopathy, with paroxymsal ventricular tachycardia or fibrillation.
- In the WPW syndrome with frequent attacks of atrial fibrillation and flutter until surgery can be arranged.
- In chronic ischaemic heart disease with paroxysmal ventricular fibrillation (aborted cardiac death syndrome) when use of an automatic implantable cardioverter/defibrillator (AICD implant) is not feasible.
- In chronic ischaemic heart disease with paroxysmal ventricular tachycardia if the patient is unsuitable for surgery or for an automatic implantable cardioverter/defibrillator (AICD implant).

For WPW tachycardias, Class IC drugs (ajmaline, propafenone, flecainide) and the more toxic Class III drug amiodarone are considered the most effective antiarrhythmic medication (Chapter 7).

For the long QT syndrome with attacks of torsade de pointes ventricular tachycardia (Fig. 6.35, page 168/169) and for *effort induced ventricular tachycardia* (Fig. 6.41, page 178/179) beta blocking agents (Class II drugs) are the drugs of first choice.

In the *acute treatment of ventricular tachycardia* intravenous lignocaine has become the drug of first choice due to its high efficacy, its low toxicity and its short halflife.

Whereas most antiarrhythmic drugs can be administered both intravenously and orally, the Class IB drug lignocaine and the Class IC drug ajmaline are for intravenous use only.

Slowing of the ventricular rate in atrial fibrillation and flutter [32–37]

Digitalis, verapamil, diltiazem, beta blocking agents and amiodarone inhibit AV impulse transmission and slow the ventricular rate in atrial fibrillation and flutter (Fig. 4.4). Digitalis is usually the drug of choice because it combines a slowing effect on the ventricular rate with a positive inotropic effect. In atrial fibrillation and flutter complicating the WPW syndrome, however, digitalis is contraindicated as it may accelerate AV conduction via the accessory pathway. For this indication amiodarone may be the drug of choice (Chapter 7).

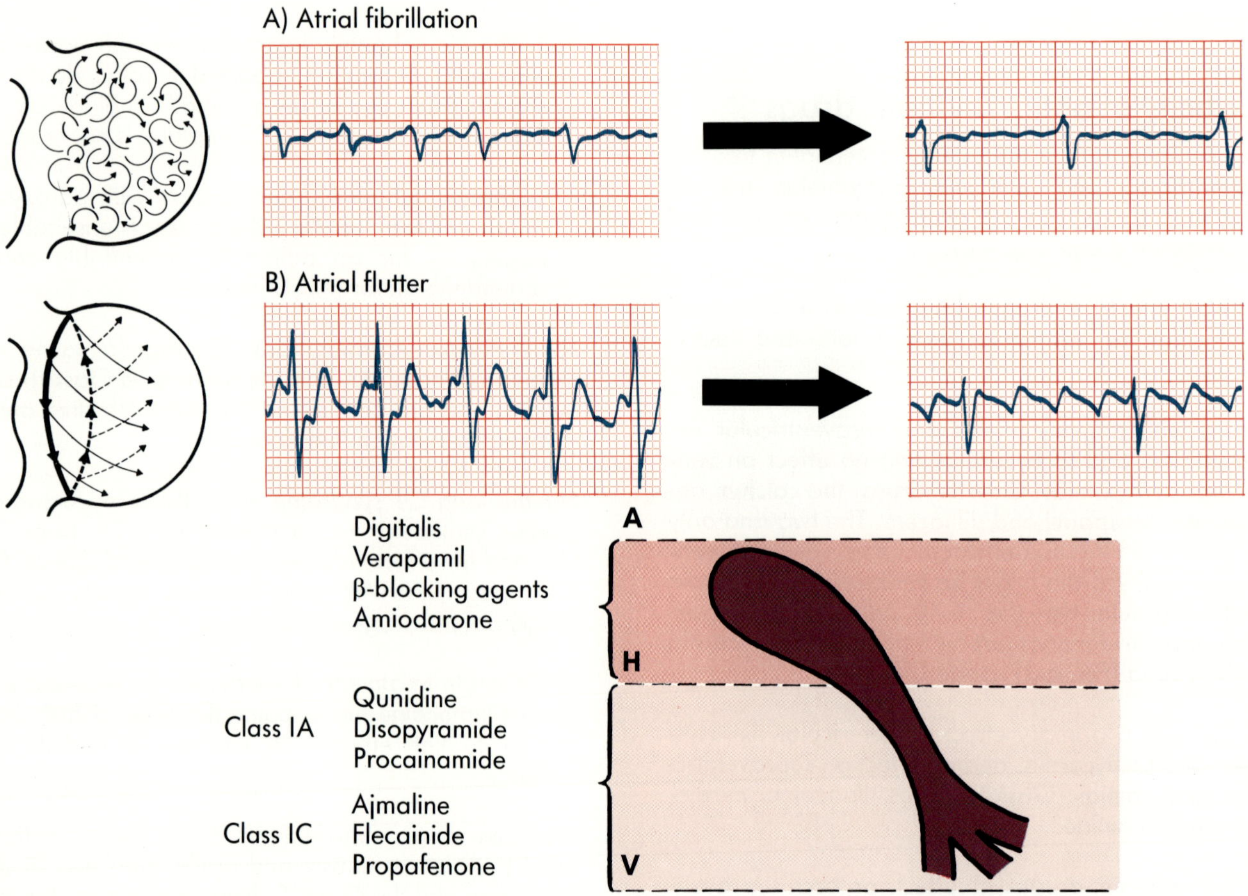

Fig. 4.4
Action of antiarrhythmic drugs on the AV conduction system. Only drugs which prolong the AH interval in the His bundle electrogram (Fig. 3.21, p. 55) have the potential of slowing the ventricular rate in atrial fibrillation and flutter. An increase in ventricular rate in atrial fibrillation and flutter can be seen during treatment with quinidine and disopyramide due to a vagolytic effect.

Effect of antiarrhythmic drugs on the ECG [38]

Antiarrhythmic drug treatment is usually associated with specific changes in the ECG. The changes seen with therapeutic (non-toxic) doses of the antiarrhythmic drugs include (Fig. 4.5):

The heart rate. A reduction in heart rate due to a sinus bradycardia of 40–60/min is a frequent occurrence during treatment with Class II drugs (beta blocking agents), and can be seen during treatment with Class III drugs (amiodarone) and Class IV drugs (verapamil and diltiazem). A slight acceleration in the sinus rate is often seen during treatment with quinidine or disopyramide.

The PR interval. PR prolongation by 0.02–0.04 s is common during treatment with digitalis, Class II drugs (beta blocking agents), Class IV drugs (verapamil and diltiazem), Class III drugs (amiodarone) and can be seen with Class IC drugs (e.g. flecainide and propafenone).

The QRS complex. The width of the QRS complex is often increased by 10–20 % during treatment with Class IA drugs (quinidine, disopyramide and procainamide) or Class IC drugs (flecainide and propafenone). A QRS widening of 25–50 % or a widening to 0.14 s or more forewarns impending arrhythmic complications and calls for withdrawal of the drug or a dose reduction.

The QT interval. A significant prolongation of the QT interval is a consistent finding in amiodarone treatment. Varying degrees of QT prolongation are observed with Class I drugs especially Class IA drugs (quinidine and disopyramide) and sotalol.

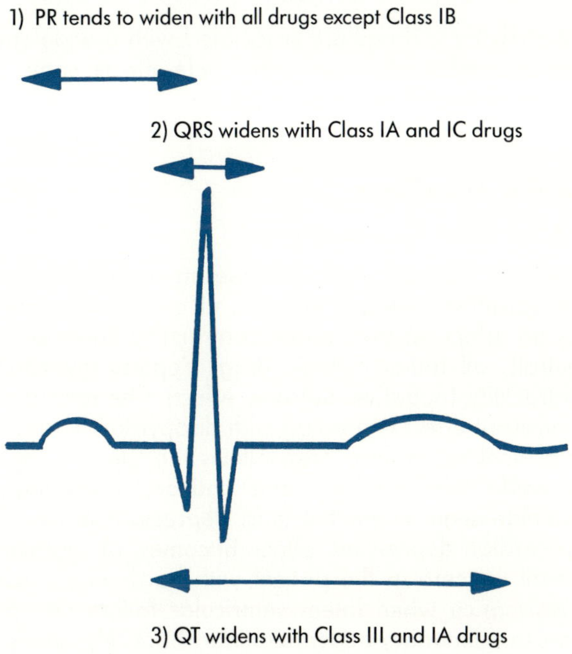

Fig. 4.5
ECG changes during antiarrhythmic treatment

Side effects of antiarrhythmic drugs

Antiarrhythmic drugs are associated with a wide spectrum of cardiac and non-cardiac side effects, some are troublesome and of a serious nature.

Cardiac side effects

A *Myocardial depressant effect* [39–42]

Except for digitalis which increases myocardial contractility (positive inotropic effect) and amiodarone which has no effect on myocardial contractility (inotropically neutral), all antiarrhythmic drugs depress myocardial contractility (negative inotropic effect). The myocardial depressant effect is greatest with disopyramide and the beta blocking agents, next follows the Class IC agent flecainide, whereas lignocaine and oral mexiletine or tocainide seem to be the least depressant drugs. The myocardial depressant effect becomes of particular clinical concern in the patient with borderline cardiac performance when latent ventricular failure can progress to pulmonary oedema and/or shock. Hypotension or shock due to peripheral vasodilatation is seen in relation to an administration of procainamide and quinidine.

B *Block, bradycardia and ventricular arrest* [43–44]

SA block and AV block of proximal type may occur with beta blocking agents, verapamil diltiazem and amiodarone. AV block of distal type occurs primarily with Class IA and IC drugs, while the Class IB drugs (lignocaine, mexiletine and tocainide) are less likely to cause conduction disturbances. The particular at risk situation is the patient with a history of fainting attributable to paroxysms of AV or SA block (Chapters 10 and 11) in whom almost all antiarrhythmic drugs can worsen the tendency for block induced Stokes-Adams attacks. The recording of a bundle branch block in a patient without concomitant signs of AV block or a history of fainting is not a contraindication to the initiation of antiarrhythmic drug therapy, but Class IB drugs (mexiletine and tocainide) might be preferred as drugs of first choice since they have little or no effect on intraventricular conduction.

C *Arrhythmogenesis* [45–65]

Whereas the purpose of antiarrhythmic drugs is to suppress and prevent attacks of tachycardia and extrasystole, occasionally the same agents may act arrhythmogenically and either aggravate the arrhythmia they were meant to treat or create new and often more serious arrhythmias.

Aggravation of existing arrhythmias. Treatment with an arrhythmic drug may worsen the frequency and complexity of extrasystoles. In tachycardia treatment, the unwanted effect of the antiarrhythmic treatment may take the form of an acceleration in rate, of more frequent or more sustained attacks, of progression from paroxysmal to incessant tachycardia, or of degeneration of a monomorphic tachycardia to multiform tachycardia or fibrillation.

Creation of new arrhythmias. Antiarrhythmic drug treatment may cause a wide variety of ventricular arrhythmias varying from asymptomatic benign arrhythmias to malignant potentially lethal arrhythmias. Examples might be ventricular extrasystole of varying complexity and frequency, ventricular tachycardia and fibrillation. Multiform ventricular tachycardia (Fig. 6.36, page 171) with an ECG appearance during tachycardia similar to that of torsade de pointes ventricular tachycardia (page 163) having a high risk of degeneration to fibrillation can occur with all Class I drugs. The Class IC agents flecainide and encainide may carry the highest risk but Class IA drugs, and to a minor degree, Class IB drugs are not devoid of risk. However, torsade de pointes ventricular tachycardia preceded by significant QT prolongation in sinus rhythm before the attack (and thus more completely fulfilling the traditional criteria for torsade de pointes ventricular tachycardia presented in this book, page 163) occurs primarily with the Class IA drugs, quinidine, disopyramide and procainamide (Fig. 4.6) and (though rarely) with the Class III agents, amiodarone and sotalol.

Arrhythmogenesis has been particularly associated with antiarrhythmic drug use in elderly patients, patients with low potassium concentrations and patients already taking a multiplicity of drugs including antiarrhythmic agents. Patients with serious life threatening previously drug refractory ventricular tachycardias are more likely to suffer arrhythmogenesis than patients with supraventricular tachycardia or ventricular extrasystole without underlying heart disease. Survivors of acute myocardial infarction with a high incidence of complex ventricular extrasystole may present a high risk group for arrhythmogenesis as shown in a recent multicenter trial (CAST study: 2-year mortality 5.1 % in patients treated with flecainide or encainide versus 2.3 % in placebo treated group).

ECG changes and risk of arrhythmogenesis. With all Class I drugs (Class IA, B and C) progressive QRS widening may signal an increased risk of arrhythmogenesis. More often than not, however, the arrhythmia complications develop without preceding significant ECG changes.

With the Class IA drugs, and with amiodarone and sotalol the attacks of torsade de pointes ventricular tachycardia (page 163) usually is preceded by prolongation of the QT interval. But then again, prolongation of the QT interval is a consistent and expected feature of the antiarrhythmic action of these drugs with no relationship between the risk of torsade de pointes ventricular tachycardia and a critical QT value or increment in the QT interval. Over and above QT prolongation per se, quinidine syncope has been associated with the development of prominent and abnormal U waves (though again without a clear definition of a high risk threshold).

Plasma drug concentration and risk of arrhythmogenesis. Arrhythmogenic complications are more likely to develop with drug concentrations exceeding the normal therapeutic range but only. A minority of clinical reports of arrhythmogenesis reflect toxicity. In the majority of cases arrhythmogenic effects arise with drug concentrations within the therapeutic range. Consequently, plasma drug concentrations, although important in detecting toxicity, are of limited value for predicting arrhythmogenic side effects.

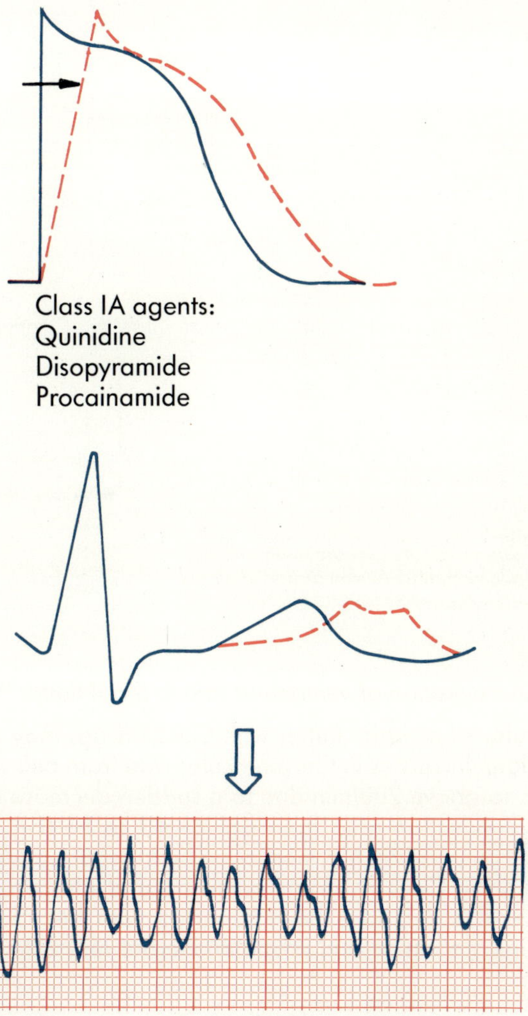

Fig. 4.6
QT prolongation with attack of torsade de pointes ventricular tachycardia induced by Class IA drugs (quinidine, disopyramide, procainamide). Prolongation of the QT interval is a consistent accompaniment to treatment with Class IA drugs. Whereas one series reports uncorrected QT interval prolongation to 0.60 s to signal an imminent attack of torsade de pointes ventricular tachycardia, others have not been capable of defining such a critical value for the QT prolongation. More than with QT prolongation per se quinidine syncope has been associated with the development of abnormal U waves, though again without any clearly defined high risk limit.

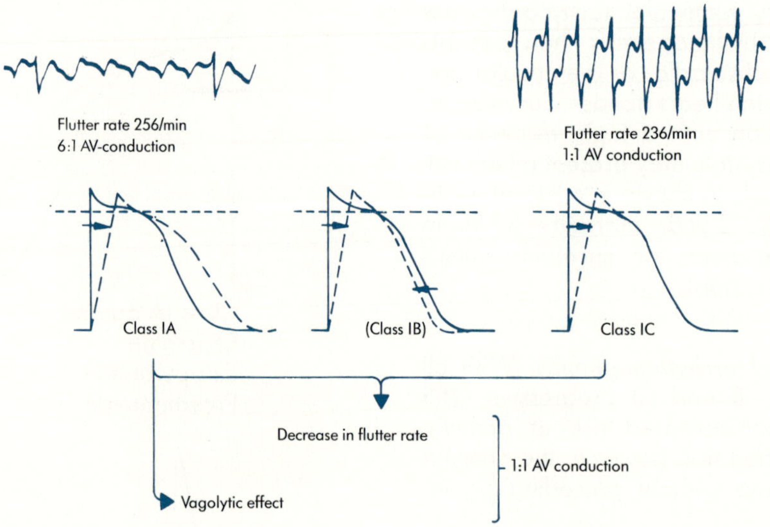

Fig. 4.7
Ventricular rate increase in atrial flutter.
Induction of 1:1 AV conduction in atrial flutter with catastrophic acceleration of the ventricular rate during treatment with Class I drugs.

D *Acceleration of ventricular rate in atrial flutter* [66–69]

Treatment of atrial flutter with Class I drugs may cause sudden increases in the ventricular rate from below 100/min to above 200/min due to a sudden decrease in the AV conduction ratio from e.g. 6–4:1 to 1:1 (Fig. 4.7). The complication has most often been reported with the vagolytic Class IA drugs quinidine and disopyramide. Several cases have been reported with the Class IC drugs, flecainide and propafenone but only a few with the Class IB drug, lignocaine. The explanation of this complication is primarily a reduction in the flutter rate with a corresponding decreased tendency for concealed AV conduction of the atrial impulses. Moreover quinidine and disopyramide have vagolytic actions on the AV node. The risk of 1:1 conduction can be reduced by digitalization prior to treatment with Class IA or C drugs.

Non-cardiac side effects[25, 70–73]

Some of the more common non-cardiac side effects of Class I drugs are listed in Table 4.1. The non-cardiac side effects of Class II (beta blocking agents) and Class IV (verapamil, diltiazem) are few and well known and will not be discussed here.

Disopyramide:	Dryness of the mouth, difficulty in micturition, urinary retention, blurred vision, constipation, nausea, gastric pain, vomiting, skin rashes
Flecainide:	Giddiness, dizziness, light-headedness, double vision, blurring of vision, nausea, vomiting
Lignocaine:	Drowsiness, Paraesthesia, disordered speech, disorientation, focal or grand mal seizures
Mexiletine:	Nausea, nystagmus, drowsiness, paraestesiae, ataxia, tremor
Procainamide:	Arthralgia, systemic lupus erythematosis, skin rashes, fever, flushing, mental depression, giddiness, headache, convulsions
Propafenone:	Gastrointestinal disturbances, disorientation, headache, cholestasis, convulsions
Quinidine:	Diarrhoea, nausea, tinnitus, hearing impairment, vertigo, diplopia, photothobia, skin rashes, fever, petechial bleedings, thrombocytopenia

Table 4.1
Non-cardiac side effects of Class I antiarrhythmic drugs. For side effects of digitalis see page 82.

Non-cardiac side effects of the Class III agent amiodarone are common, are often troublesome and sometimes life threatening. Several organ systems can be affected:

Eyes: During long-term treatment corneal microdeposits are observed in almost all patients, but these rarely interfere with vision, are dose related and disappear after some time when treatment is discontinued. Routine ocular examinations are not neccessary.

Skin: Photosensitivity with rashes or dermal pigmentation is seen in approximately 20 % of patients. Bluish colouration of the face (particularly of the nose) is observed in a few.

Thyroid gland: Goitre or myxoedema develops occasionally. The incidence of thyrotoxicosis has been reported as from 2 to 10 %. Thyroid function monitoring is essential in all patients on long-term therapy with amiodarone. The monitoring should be continued for some time after the termination of chronic treatment since thyrotoxicosis can develop with a time delay of several months (6–8 months).

Central nervous system: Tremor, ataxia, sleep disorders, tiredness.

Peripheral nerves: A peripheral neuropathy with severe sensorimotor symptoms occurs as a late symptom, usually in patients on high maintenance doses.

Liver: Often a rise in liver enzymes, rarely hepatitis.

Lungs: Interstitial pneumonitis progressing to pulmonary fibrosis is a rare but serious hazard of amiodarone treatment. The complication is seen primarily with high dosage (400 to 800 mg daily) and long-term therapy. Early symptoms include exertional dyspnoea, non-productive cough and occasionally low grade fever. Radiographic findings consist of diffuse bilateral interstitial changes and diffuse or patchy alveolar infiltrations. Spontaneous resolution may be seen following discontinuation of the drug. Cortico-steroid therapy is recommended and has been used seemingly with success in several patients. X-ray control every month is advised for patients placed on a high dose amiodarone regime. Aggressive attempts should be made to reduce long-term doses to a minimum once control of the arrhythmia is achieved.

Combined antiarrhythmic drug therapy [7, 74, 75]

Combined antiarrhythmic drug therapy is taken into use on the supposition that added antiarrhythmic potency may be achieved at the same time that side effects remain minimal or not significantly increased. Beneficial antiarrhythmic interaction has been reported with the combination of a Class I drug (quinidine or mexiletine) and a beta blocking agent; with a Class IA drug (quinidine) and a Class IB drug (mexiletine); and with amiodarone and a Class IB drug (mexiletine). With the use of most other drug combinations, and even the just mentioned combinations, the risk of adverse interactions warrants careful attention. A useful guide rule is to refrain from the combination of agents with similar and thus potentially additive side effects such as:

- Agents of the same subclasses
- Proarrhythmic agents (Class IA and Class IC agents)
- Agents which prolong the QT interval (Class IA agents, sotalol and amiodarone)
- Agents with significant negative inotropic action (disopyramide, beta blocking agents and possibly verapamil).

The combination of digoxin therapy with quinidine, amiodarone or verapamil administration reduces the renal excretion of digoxin by approximately 50, 30 and 10–15 % respectively. Thus, daily digoxin dosage has to be reduced correspondingly to avoid the development of digoxin intoxication.

Table 4.2 provides an outline of potential adverse interactions between the various antiarrhythmic drugs and between antiarrhythmic drugs and other therapeutical agents.

Drug	Interaction with	Result
Quinidine	Digoxin	Increased digoxin level
	Other Class IA agents	Added negative inotropic effect and/or depressed AV conduction
	Class IC agents	Arrhythmogenesis, depressed SA and AV conduction, added negative inotropic effect
	b-blockers, verapamil	Hypotension, added negative inotropic effect
	Amiodarone, sotalol	Increased risk of torsade de pointes ventricular tachycardia
	Diuretics	If hypokalaemia, risk of torsade de pointes ventricular tachycardia
	Verapamil	Increased quinidine level
	Warfarin	Enhanced anticoagulation
Disopyramide	Other Class IA agents	Added negative inotropic effect and/or depressed AV conduction
	β-blockers, verapamil	Hypotension, added negative inotropic effect
	Anticholinergics	Exaggerated anticholinergic effect
	Pyridostigmine	Decreased anticholinergic effect
Lignocaine	β-blockers Cimetidine Halothane	Reduced hepatic clearance of lignocaine; lignocaine toxicity
Tocainide	Few adverse interactions	
Mexiletine	Few adverse interactions	
Flecainide	β-blockers, verapamil, diltiazem, digoxin	Added depressed SA and AV conduction depression
	β-blockers, quinidine, disopyramide	Added negative inotropic effect
	Class IA agents	Arrhythmogenesis, depressed SA and AV conduction and/or added negative inotropic effects
	Amiodarone	Increased flecainide levels
Propafenone	As for flecainide but amiodarone interaction not reported	As for flecainide
Sotalol	Diuretics, Class IA agents, amiodarone, tricyclic antidepressants, phenothiazines	Risk of torsade de pointes ventricular tachycardia
Amiodarone	Diuretics, Class IA agents, sotalol, tricyclic antidepressants, phenothiazines	Risk of torsade de pointes ventricular tachycardia
	Digoxin	Digoxin level increased
	Flecainide	Flecainide level increased
Verapamil	β-blockers, excess digoxin	Added depressed SA and AV conduction
	Digoxin	Slight increase of digoxin level

Table 4.2
Adverse interaction of antiarrhythmic drugs

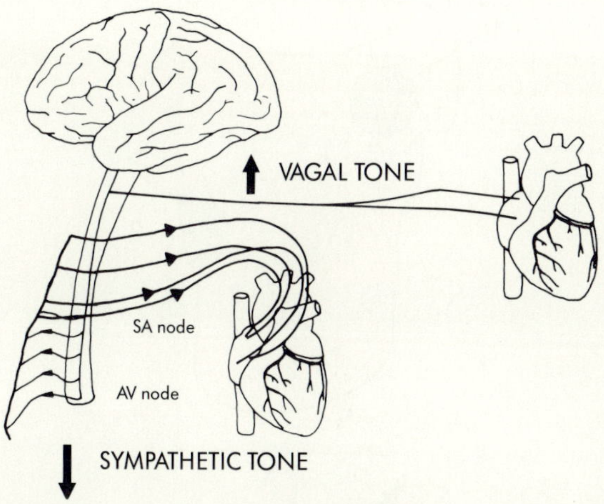

Fig. 4.8
The antiarrhythmic effect of digitalis mediated via the central nervous system.

Digitalis [7, 32, 76, 77]

Mode of action

The antiarrhythmic effects of digoxin and digitoxin and other digitalis compounds are medicated via the central nervous system (Fig. 4.8). These drugs increase vagal tone and decrease sympathetic tone both to the AV node and to the SA node.

Indication

Through its inhibitory effect on AV conduction digitalis slows the ventricular response to atrial fibrillation and flutter. For this reason, and for its positive inotropic action digitalis has become the drug of first choice for the control of the ventricular rate in both acute and chronic atrial fibrillation and flutter. Digitalis is also used in the long-term treatment of paroxysmal atrial fibrillation and flutter. Digitalis medications usually do not prevent recurrences but may ensure a reasonably acceptable ventricular rate during new attacks. For paroxysmal atrial flutter treated by a Class I drug digitalization may be a safeguard against 1:1 AV conduction (Fig. 4.7, page 78). In the WPW syndrome, digitalis may accelerate conduction in the accessory AV pathway, and as a rule should not be given to such patients. An exception is infancy where digitalis appears well tolerated and highly effective.

Pharmacology

Digoxin is the most widely used digitalis compound. It has a short serum halflife of 1.5 days. The drug is primarily excreted unaltered by the kidneys, and only about 20 % via non-renal routes. The alternative drug, digitoxin, has a long half-life of 6–7 days rendering treatment of toxicity more complicated. Digitoxin is chiefly metabolized in the liver or excreted in the gut.

Dosage

Digoxin: On urgent indications a loading dose is required to saturate digitalis receptors in the skeletal muscle throughout the body and for tissue penetration. The loading dose is divided into 3–4 doses given over 24 hours. In the absence of an urgency for immediate effect, the loading dose may be omitted and replaced by the initiation of a daily maintenance dosage. Steady state will usually be reached within one week in a patient with normal renal function. The most important determinamt of the daily maintenance dosage is renal function. An estimate of the maintenance dosage required can be derived from tables based on the relationship between serum creatinine, age, body weight and sex on the one hand and creatinine clearance on the other. There are substantial individual variations, and the dosage must under all circumstances be adjusted individually according to the observed effect and the side effect(s) of the drug.

Digitoxin: Digitalization with digitoxin is usually always started with a loading dose since it would otherwise take over a month to reach a steady state plasma level. The maintenance dosage is usually not much influenced by poor renal function.

Side effects

The cardiac arrhythmias seen as digitalis toxicity are discussed in Chapter 12 (Digoxin and the ECG, page 292). Common non-cardiac side effects include distaste for food, nausea, vomiting, diarrhoea, blurred vision or sometimes green or yellow tinted vision. Gynecomastia (bilateral or unilateral) has been reported but is a very rare complication. Low serum potassium, low serum magnesium and high serum calcium increase digitalis sensitivity and the risk for the development of cardiac arrhythmias.

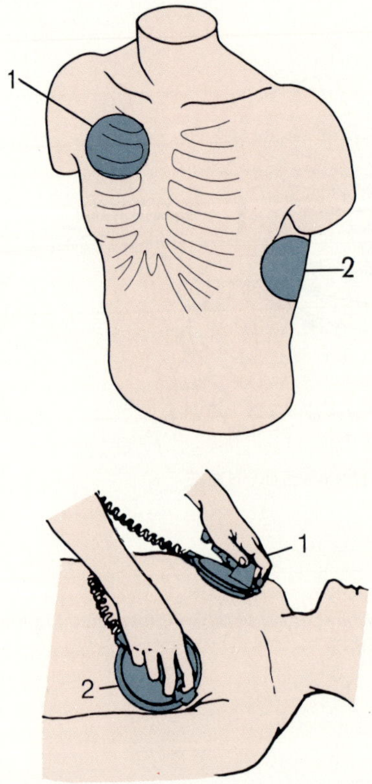

Fig. 4.9
Placement of electrodes in defibrillation and cardioversion. the anterior electrode (1) is placed just to the right of the upper sternum over the second and third intercostal spaces. The lateral electrode (2) is placed on – or just anterior to the left midaxillary line over the fifth intercostal space.

The DC counter shock [77–79]

A DC countershock is a high energy direct current (DC) electrical impulse delivered through the chest (and thus the heart) for a very brief moment. The mechanism of electrical defibrillation is not definitely known. Possibly, the intensive electrical impulse causes momentary activation of all, or almost all non-refractory cells in the heart. With no excitable cells left over, the disorganized turbulent activation of the myocardium must stop and, thus, fibrillation is brought to a halt. Following the shock, the SA node becomes reestablished as the pacemaker of an at least temporarily fully synchronized myocardium.

The DC countershock is delivered by a *defibrillator* or, a *cardioverter*, the latter apparatus being capable of synchronizing the DC countershock with the QRS complex (see next section).

The DC countershock is applied to the chest by a pair of paddles. Each paddle consists of a circular metal plate, the *electrode*, provided with a well insulated handle. An electrode diameter of 8–10 cm is used for adults and larger children. A smaller electrode diameter of 4–5 cm ensures complete contact between the surface of the electrode and that of the arched chest of the small child below 5 kg b.w. (avoiding spark formation resulting in skin burns). The electrodes usually are placed in an *anterior lateral position* with their interconnecting line in parallel with the longitudinal axis of the heart (Fig. 4.9). To ensure good contact between the skin and the electrodes and thus prevent burns, gelatine pads (delivered ready for use in aluminium foil) are placed on the chest at the site of the intended placement of the electrodes for DC defibrillation/cardioversion. Alternatively, burns can be prevented by covering the surface of the electrodes with an abundant layer of electrode paste.

With the paddles pressed firmly against the patient's chest, the DC countershock is discharged. The release of the shock induces a twitching of the chest muscles and a jerking of the arms. The ECG monitoring is usually lost for a few seconds, and when it returns it may already show restoration of sinus rhythm or sinus rhythm may return after a short or sometimes longer episode of bradycardia or ventricular arrest.

Cardioversion [79]

In the treatment of rhythm disorders other than ventricular fibrillation the risk of inducing ventricular fibrillation by the DC countershock is lessened by synchronizing the discharge of the DC countershock with the R wave of the ECG. Usually the DC discharge is timed to occur 0.02–0.04 s after the R wave. Thus, the shock falls outside the vulnerable phase of the ventricles which is restricted to the first four fifths of the T wave (Fig. 3.9, page 44).

The term *defibrillation* applies to the use of non-synchronized DC countershock therapy in ventricular fibrillation and the term *cardioversion* applies to that of synchronized DC countershock therapy in supraventricular tachycardia including atrial fibrillation and flutter and ventricular tachycardia.

Indications for cardioversion [79]

DC cardioversion is used for the acute termination of *an attack of supraventricular or more often of ventricular tachycardia* either because the tachycardia continues despite appropriate antiarrhythmic drug treatment, or because the haemodynamic state of the patient is deteriorating. In *chronic atrial fibrillation* DC cardioversion may be attempted in the rare case in which the long-term prospects for the maintenance of sinus rhythm seem favourable.

In *chronic atrial flutter* an attempt at DC cardioversion is usually a worthwhile undertaking. It may improve the condition of the patient either by restoring sinus rhythm or by converting the chronic atrial flutter to atrial fibrillation, an arrhythmia which is more readily controlled by digitalization than is flutter.

Pretreatment and precautions in cardioversion [79–85]

Anticoagulant therapy. Though controlled trials are lacking, anticoagulant therapy with warfarin or a similar drug is often instituted some time prior to cardioversion of chronic atrial fibrillation to reduce the embolization risk (the prothrombin level should be kept within the therapeutic range for a period of at least some days and preferably 1 to 2 weeks). Other forms of tachycardia do not require anticoagulant therapy prior to the DC cardioversion.

Anaesthesia. Because the procedure is painful it has to be performed under anaesthesia. An adequate anaesthesia is best achieved by the intravenous administration of a short acting barbiturate or of etomidate fentanyl. Diazepam is an often recommended alternative but vivid and traumatic recollections of the electrical discharge are common after this type of anaesthesia.

Digitalis medication. Ventricular fibrillation occurring minutes or even hours after the cardioversion may occur in the over-digitalized patient. Such "late" ventricular fibrillation is more liable to occur in the hypokalaemic state and following DC cardioversion with a shock of a high energy. DC cardioversion should therefore be postponed in the patient suspected to be suffering from digitalis intoxication; hypokalaemia should be corrected prior to cardioversion, and the energy setting should not be higher than required to restore sinus rhythm.

Implanted pacemakers. Rarely, the electronics of implanted pacemakers can be damaged by DC countershock therapy. The risk of pacemaker damage is minimized by using a low energy setting and by delivering the DC countershock with the paddles placed at a distance of at least 10 cm from the implanted pulse generator.

Energy setting in cardioversion and defibrillation [79, 86, 87]

A fairly low energy shock should be used at first, and if this is unsuccessful repeated shocks should be given at an increased energy. The initial energy is varied according to the type of tachycardia. Atrial flutter is most sensitive and usually responds to 25–50 J. Atrial, AV nodal and WPW tachycardia can be terminated by 50–100 J, whereas atrial fibrillation and ventricular tachycardia often require 100–200 J.

In cardiac arrest with ventricular fibrillation the recommended energy settings are: 200 + 200 + 360 J. The dose for children below 30 kg of body weight is 0.25 up to 1 J per kg body weight.

Antitachycardia surgery [88–91]

The combination of tachycardia induction by programmed electrical stimulation (PES) and electrophysiologic mapping from electrodes placed directly on the endocardial surface of the opened heart, has opened the way for intraoperative localization of the anatomical substrates responsible for the various types of re-entry tachycardia (Figs. 3.4, page 41, and 3.5, page 42). Localization of the site of the re-entry needs the close teamwork of the electrophysiologist and the surgeon. Surgical ablation of the re-entry substrate is made possible, and by repeated PES it can be shown that attacks of tachycardia can no longer be induced.

With refinements in surgical techniques, surgical intervention for paroxysmal supraventricular tachycardia is being used for wider indications than just the WPW syndrome (Chapter 7, page 188); recently AV nodal re-entry tachycardia has been tackled (Chapter 6). In chronic ischaemic heart disease with paroxysmal ventricular tachycardia optimal candidates for surgery are patients with a circumscribed ventricular aneurysm and monomorphic ventricular tachycardia. Combined with an endocardial resection of ventricular myocardium guided by electrophysiological mapping, the surgeon may perform an aneurysmectomy and myocardial revascularization by coronary artery bypass grafting. Poor candidates for surgery with high operative mortality and high postoperative tachycardia recurrence rate are those with diffuse left ventricular dysfunction, or multiform ventricular tachycardia and/or early degeneration of the tachycardia to ventricular fibrillation. (This leaves inadequate time for tachycardia mapping and localization of the re-entry).

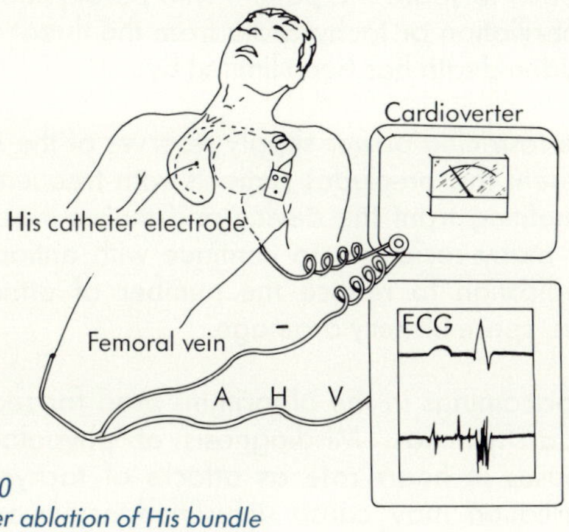

Fig. 4.10
Catheter ablation of His bundle

Catheter ablation of His bundle [88–90, 92]

Drug refractory supraventricular tachycardias, particularly atrial fibrillation and flutter with an uncontrollable ventricular rate can be managed by electrical ablation of the His bundle. The intervention aims to create third degree complete AV block and thereby isolate the supraventricular arrhythmogenic focus or foci from the ventricles. Maintenance of ventricular activation is ensured by the implantation of a pacemaker, preferably a rate responsive pacemaker to allow for a physiological variation in ventricular rate with exercise.

The procedure is performed in the cardiac laboratory (Fig. 4.10). A catheter electrode is inserted via the femoral vein and under fluoroscopy guided into the right atrium and manipulated to record a His bundle electrogram with a distinct His spike (Figs. 3.21, page 55). The electrode is connected to the cathode of a defibrillator while the anode of the defibrillator is connected to an electrode placed on the back of the patient (or a paddle pressed against the left side of the chest). Under general anaesthesia one, or, if required, several shocks of 100–360 J are delivered via the catheter electrode. The success rate is high with 75 % stable AV block after the first intervention and 80–90 % if the procedure is repeated.

It is a fast and safe procedure with immediate and usually lasting effects. It is suited for the elderly patient with drug refractory, frequent attacks of atrial fibrillation or flutter with a rapid ventricular rate. Naturally, it can be used also in the younger patient with chronic atrial fibrillation or flutter and an uncontrollable ventricular rate. His bundle ablation, however, may make the patient pacemaker dependent, so that pacemaker failure (happily a rare event, thanks to modern pacemaker technology) could pose a risk of sudden death.

Catheter ablation may also destroy arrhythmogenic structures in the heart. It has been used in patients with the WPW syndrome to interrupt the accessory AV pathway and in patients with paroxysmal ventricular tachycardia to ablate the arrhythmogenic ventricular focus. Varying rates of success and complications have been reported. Techniques that allow for more controlled destruction using for instance laser or radio frequency energy might in the future yield better results.

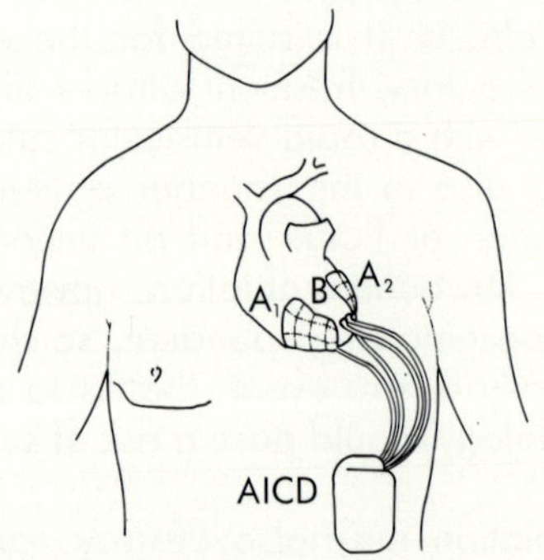

Fig. 4.11
Automatic implantable cardioverter/defibrillator (AICD)
A_1 A_2: Patch electrodes for defibrillation
B_1 B_2: Sensing electrodes for electrogram

The automatic implantable cardioverter/defibrillator (AICD)[88–90, 93, 94]

By miniaturization of the circuits of the defibrillator it has been possible to construct an automatic implantable cardioverter/defibrillator (AICD). It approximates in size to a first generation pacemaker, 10 cm in width and 3 cm in height, and can be implanted in a subcutaneous pocket in the abdominal wall (Fig. 4.11). The AICD unit can continuously monitor cardiac rhythm and will automatically deliver a DC countershock of 25–30 J to the heart whenever fibrillation or tachycardia is detected. It is powered by lithium ioidide cells sufficient for 300+ shocks. The shocks are delivered via two patches (10–20 cm in diameter) placed on the heart through a thoracotomy. The electrogram is sensed by two additional electrodes screwed into the myocardium.

Current candidates for an AICD implant are:

- Cardiac arrest survivors with chronic ischaemic heart disease (aborted cardiac death syndrome) and recurrent ventricular fibrillation.

- Paroxysmal ventricular tachycardia in chronic ischaemic heart disease not amenable to antitachycardia surgery due to diffuse left ventricular dysfunction or with multiform or unstable tachycardia which degenerates to early ventricular fibrillation.

The application of this ingenious non-pharmacological approach to spare the patient with paroxysmal ventricular fibrillation or tachycardia from the threat and fear of sudden death has been limited by:

- The restricted power supply reserves of the AICD. At present this precludes patients with frequent attacks benefiting from the device and makes it neccessary for many recipients to continue with antiarrhythmic medication to reduce the number of attacks and, thus, spare battery drainage.

- Shortcomings in the algorithms used for recognition of arrhythmias. Misdiagnosis of physiological increases in hearт rate as attacks of tachycardia or fibrillation may cause unjustified activation of the device.

- Last, but not least, the device is expensive, currently 9–10.000 pounds sterling.

Antitachycardia pacemakers[88–90, 95–97]

Attacks of re-entry tachycardia can be both started and terminated by pacing applied in the form of programmed electrical stiumulation (PES). Use of PES for the provocation (and termination) of re-entry tachycardia in electrophysiologic studies has been described in Chapter 3, page 56. The principle of PES can be used for the automatic termination of paroxysmal re-entry tachycardias in selected patients with recurrent attacks. Specific types of pacemakers, *antitachycardia pacemakers*, are available for this purpose. The antitachycardia pacemaker monitors a cardiac electrogram via its pacing electrode. When an attack of tachycardia is detected, it automatically starts PES and "scans" diastole for a non-refractory "window" in which the pacing impulse or impulses can penetrate the re-entry circuit and stop the impulse ciculation (Fig. 4.12, page 88). It is prerequisite for successful termination of the tachycardia, however, that the tip of the pacing electrode of the antitachycardia pacemaker be located near the site of the re-entry. Antitachycardia pacemakers have been used with some limited success in AV nodal re-entry tachycardia and the WPW syndrome. They should not be used for paroxysmal ventricular tachycardia as there is a risk of accelerating the arrhythmia with degeneration to ventricular fibrillation.

A future development will be a combined antitachycardia pacemaker and automatic cardioverter/defibrillator. Such a device might solve the critical power supply problem of the AICD implant; most paroxysms of tachycardia would be terminated by the antitachycardia pacemaker which uses very little power while the cardioverter/defibrillator would act only as a safety device to be activated on the rare occasion when the programmed pacing has failed or has caused tachycardia acceleration or induced fibrillation.

When and how to treat block/bradycardia

In patients with AV block or SA block, treatment for or prevention of Stokes-Adams attacks due to sustained episodes of ventricular arrest or torsade de pointes ventricular tachycardia is the primary concern.
Acute intervention strategies encompass:

1 If required, *immediate resuscitation with cardiac massage and artificial ventilation; a sharp blow to the chest* can sometimes restart the heart.

2 *Intravenous medication* with a parasympathicolytic or a sympathomimimetic may prove life saving. Intravenous atropine or ipratropium bromide can be effective in SA block and in AV block of proximal type. Intravenous adrenaline and/or an infusion of isoprenaline might prove effective in both SA block and in AV block of proximal and distal type. Due to the counterbalancing effect of the calcium ion on the action of the potassium on the cardiac cell, calcium salts (chloride or gluconate) as an intravenous bolus may be worthwhile for treating AV block secondary to hyperkalaemia.

3 *Temporary pacing,* transthoracic or when it can be arranged external transvenous pacing (see later).

Before planned major surgery on an individual with second or third degree AV block of proximal or distal type, insertion of a ventricular pacing electrode and the initiation of temporary artificial pacing has become standard practice to prevent block/bradycardia induced operative and postoperative complications.

Long-term prevention of Stokes-Adams attacks is primarily achieved by pacemaker implantation. Oral drug treatment (atropine, ipratropium bromide, isoprenaline or orciprenaline) is an unreliable preventative measure in the patient with Stokes-Adams attacks and normally not a worthwhile undertaking.

In the patient with third degree AV block or 2:1 AV block complicated by *chronic* congestive heart failure pacemaker implantation with acceleration of the heart rate from the level of only 30–40/min up to 70–90/min can

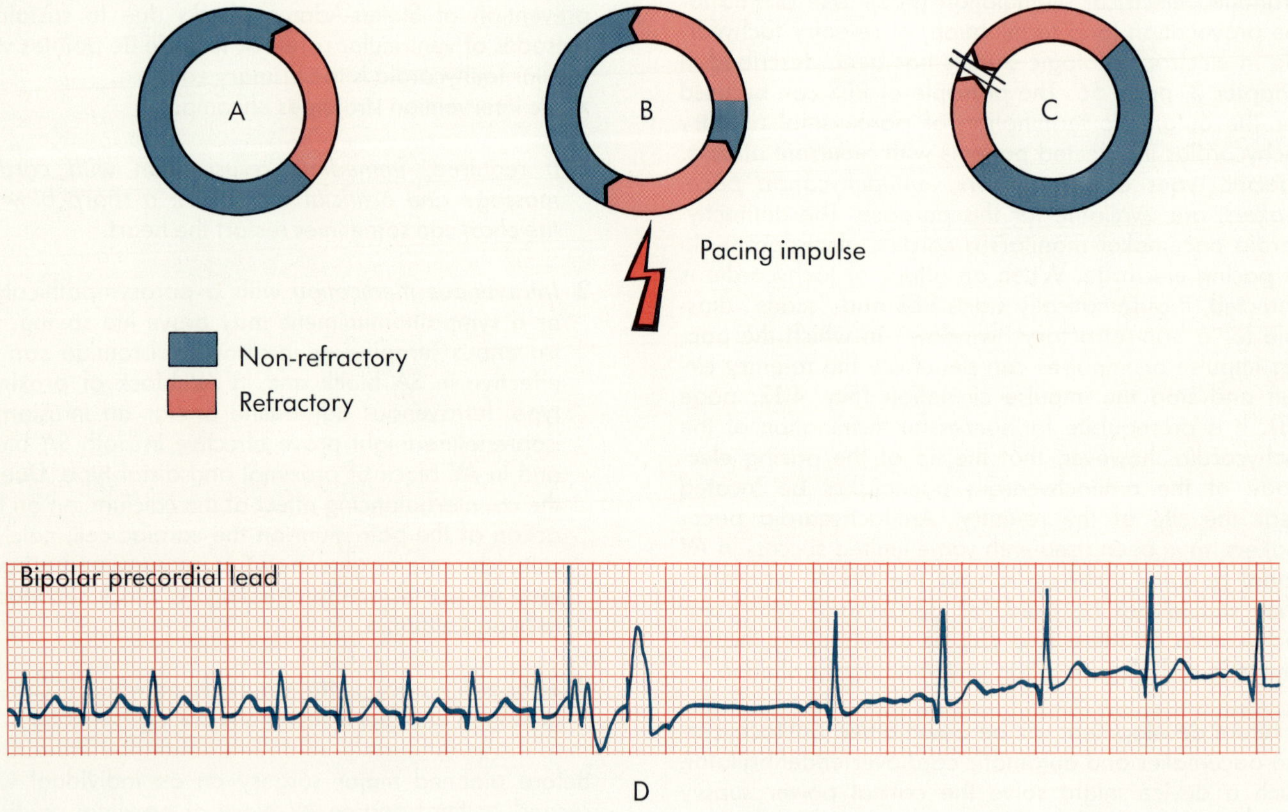

Fig. 4.12
Working principle of the antitachycardia pacemaker

A Re-entry tachycardia; there is a window of non refractory tissue in between the advancing front of the circulating impulse and its tail

B The activation induced by the pacing impulse penetrates into the non-refractory window of the re-entry pathway

C The pacing induced activation closes the non-refractory window and terminates the impulse caroussel

D An ECG recording of a paroxysm of AV nodal tachycardia terminated by a pair of pacing impulses from an antitachycardia pacemaker often increase the cardiac output and ameliorate symptoms. The best results are usually achieved by dual chamber pacing (DDD), or in third degree AV block combined with atrial fibrillation or flutter by rate responsive ventricular pacing (VVI-R).

Contraindications to pacemaker implantation

Pacemaker implantation should be undertaken only:

- If it is considered likely that the patient will survive for a significant period of time afterwards; and
- If the patient is considered to have a prospect of a bearable, tolerably good existence *without* chronic severe pain, congestive failure or intellectual reduction.

Senility, intractable heart disease with severe angina pectoris or severe heart failure unalleviated by temporary pacing, or advanced malignant disease may be contraindications to pacemaker implantation.

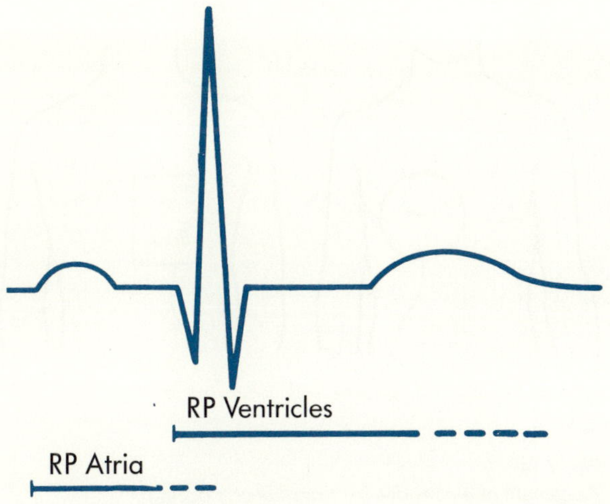

Fig. 4.13
Refractory period of the ventricular and atrial myocardium related to the ECG

RP Ventricles: Refractory period of the ventricular myocardium

RP Atria: Refractory period of the atrial myocardium. Stippled lines indicate individual variation

Pacing [98–100]

Like the individual cardiac cell (Fig. 1.5, page 5), the ventricles or the atria, can be activated (paced) by an electrical impulse, a *pacing impulse* or *pacing pulse*, which exceeds the *myocardial threshold for pacing*. With a pacing impulse of about 1 ms duration and with direct contact between the myocardium and the uninsulated tip of the conductor *(pacing electrode)* the threshold for pacing will usually be in the order of 1/2 – 1 volt or 5–10 milliamp. For pacing through the skin and thorax, *(transthoracic pacing)*, a much longer duration of pacing impulse and much greater electrical energy will be required.

Activation of the ventricle or atrium is followed by a *refractory period* where the chamber cannot be reactivated by renewed pacing. The *refractory period of the ventricles* (Fig. 4.13) starts with the QRS complex and ends at or just after the peak of the T wave. The *refractory period of the atria* (Fig. 4.13) starts with the P wave and ends at the onset or shortly before the QRS complex. Due to the prolonged refractory period of the AV node AV conduction of a pacing induced P wave will be possible only if the P wave occurs in the last part of the T wave or later (Fig. 3.14, page 49).

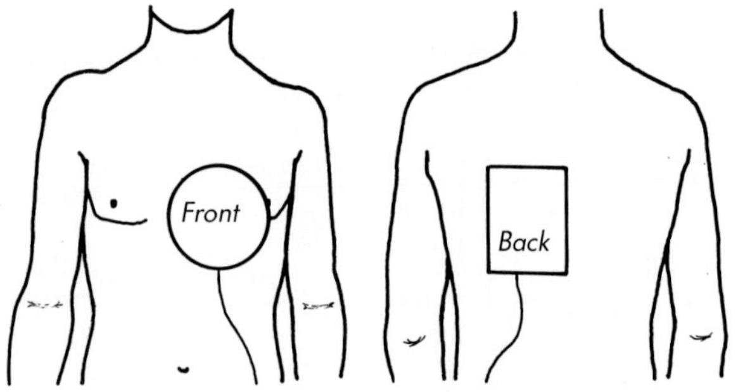

Fig. 4.14
Placement of electrodes for transthoracic pacing

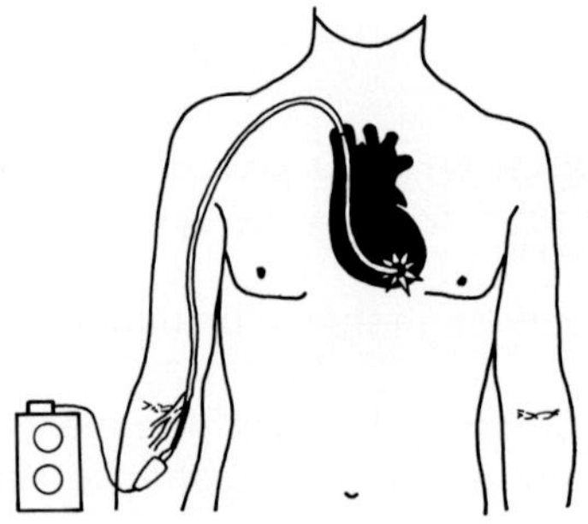

Fig. 4.15
External i. v. pacing

Temporary pacing [99, 100]

In the emergency situation of a cardiac arrest, cardiac pacing by transthoracic pacing can be established within minutes and external transvenous pacing within 10 minutes to half an hour provided that the neccessary equipment and expertise are at hand.

Transthoracic pacing (Fig. 4.14) [101]

The equipment comprises a transthoracic pulse generator ("the noninvasive transcutaneous Zoll pacemaker") and stick-on pacing electrodes (diameter 25–45 cm). One electrode is placed on the front of the chest just to the left of the lower part of sternum, the other electrode on the back, to the left of the spine below the left scapula. Pacing is usually achieved at an output varying from 30 J up to 80 J with a duration of the pacing impulse of 40 ms. Most conscious patients complain of discomfort or pain during the transcutaneous pacing so heavy sedation is often required.

External transvenous pacing (Fig. 4.15) [99, 100]

A pacing electrode is inserted via a peripheral vein or, through a percutaneous needle puncture of the subclavian vein. Under fluoroscopic guidance, the electrode is passed to the right atrium and into the right ventricle where it is embedded in the trabecular network of the apical region. Once in a stable pacing position, the external part of the electrode is tethered to the skin, covered with a sterile bandage and is connected to an external pulse generator. The pulse generator is powered by alkaline batteries which with the electronic components of the generator are contained in a small box. The external pulse generator is placed at the bedside or is worn by the patient attached to a belt or placed in a pocket. External transvenous pacing can provide painless, stable right ventricular pacing for a period of one to several weeks.

The implantable pacemaker [98–100, 102]

The implantable pacemaker consists of a *pulse generator,* the electronic part which generates the pacing impulses, and a *pacing electrode,* which conducts the pacing impulses to the ventricular or atrial myocardium.

The *pulse generator* is a small compact unit with a lightweight lithium battery and encased in metal. It is implanted in a subcutaneous "pocket", usually in the pectoral region. From its point of insertion in the vein, the pacing electrode is tunnelled through the subcutaneous tissue to the pacemaker pocket and connected to the pulse generator. The *pacing electrode* contains one or two conductors insulated in a plastic shielding but with an uninsulated tip that brings the pulse generator in contact with the endocardial side of the myocardium.

The pacing electrode is usually inserted by the *transvenous technique (the endocardial approach).* The procedure is performed under local anaesthesia. The cephalic vein or the external jugular vein is exposed, or the subclavian vein is punctured and a pacing lead inserted into the vein. Under fluoroscopic guidance, the pacing lead is passed to the right atrium and:

- For *ventricular pacing* (Fig. 4.16 A, page 92) into the right ventricle where the pacing electrode is embedded in the trabecular network of the apical region, or

- For *atrial pacing* (Fig. 4.16 B) into the right atrial appendage.

Most modern pulse generators are provided with a programming option which allows a range of technical variables to be altered non-invasively after implantation.

A code consisting of three to five letters (Table 4.3) has been internationally adopted for describing pacemaker type and function. The first letter indicates the chamber(s) paced, the second letter the chamber(s) in which electrical activity is sensed and the third letter, the response to a sensed signal. The additional fourth and fifth letters of the pacing code reflect respectively rate responsiveness, programability and antitachycardia functions. The first three letter codes are used in this book and are occasionally combined with an R in the fourth position to indicate rate responsiveness.

Position	Category	
I	Chamber(s) Paced	O = None A = Atrium V = Ventricle D = Dual (A + V)
II	Chamber(s) Sensed	O = None A = Atrium V = Ventricle D = Dual (A+ V)
III	Response to Sensing	O = None T = Triggered I = Inhibited D = Dual (T + I)
IV	Rate Responsiveness, Programmability	O = None R = Rate Responsiveness M = Multiprogrammable C = Communicationg
V	Antitachyarrhythmia Function(s)	O = None P = Pacing (antitachyarrhythmia) S = Shock D = Dual (P + S)

Table 4.3
International pacemaker code

The pacemaker ECG [103, 104]

The pacing impulse causes a rapid deflection on the ECG in the form of a vertical line referred to as the *pacemaker spike*. In *ventricular pacing*, the most common form of pacing (Fig. 4.16 A) the spike is immediately followed by a wide QRS complex of ventricular type. In *atrial pacing* (Fig. 4.16 B) the spike is followed by a P wave which with the electrode positioned in the right atrial appendage will be positive in lead II and in the patient without AV or intraventricular conduction disturbances after a normal PR interval will be followed by a normal narrow QRS complex.

In ventricular pacing with a *fixed rate* the ECG findings will vary depending on the relationship between the spontaneous heart rate and the pacing rate. If the spontaneous rate is slow and consistently lies below the pacing rate, then the pacemaker will become "the pacemaker of the heart" and suppress the spontaneous cardiac activity. The result will be a stable pacemaker rhythm (Fig. 4.17). If, however, the spontaneous heart rate and the pacing rate lie in the same range, then the two rhythms will interfere and compete all the time. The result is a chaotic heart rhythm (Fig. 4.18, page 94) and, at times pacing will occur in the vulnerable period of the ventricles, – an event which in the patient with acute myocardial infarction can induce ventricular fibrillation (Fig. 10.9, page 261).

Inhibited pacing (Fig. 4.19, page 95), which is the common mode of pacing today, tends to overcome this problem. The pulse generator in addition to its pacing

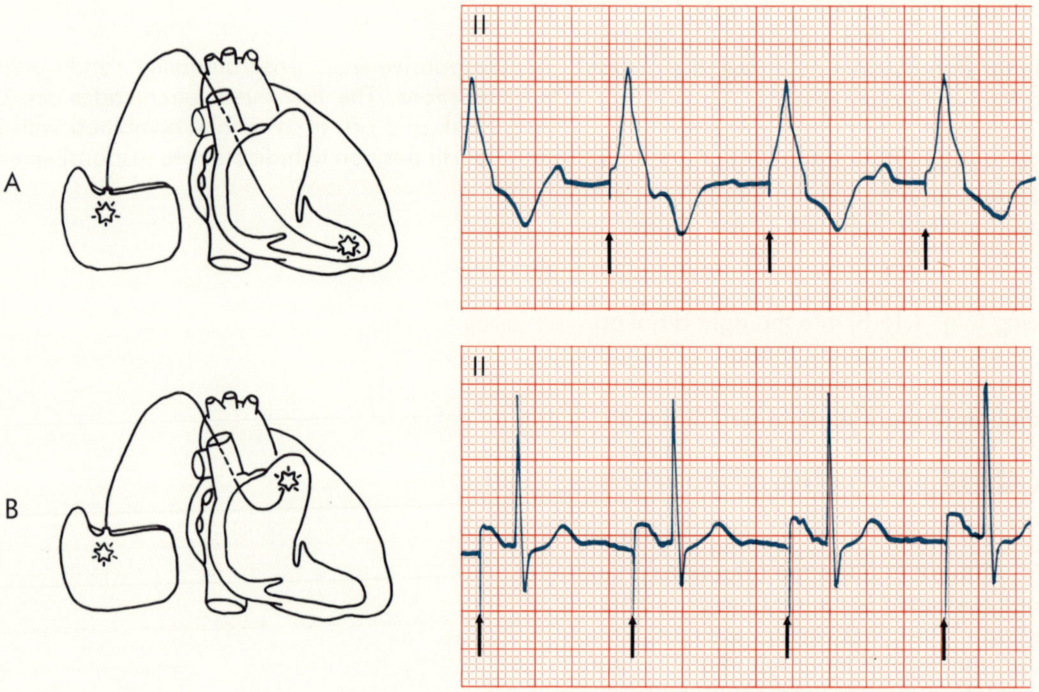

Fig. 4.16
Ventricular pacing (A) and atrial pacing (B)

A

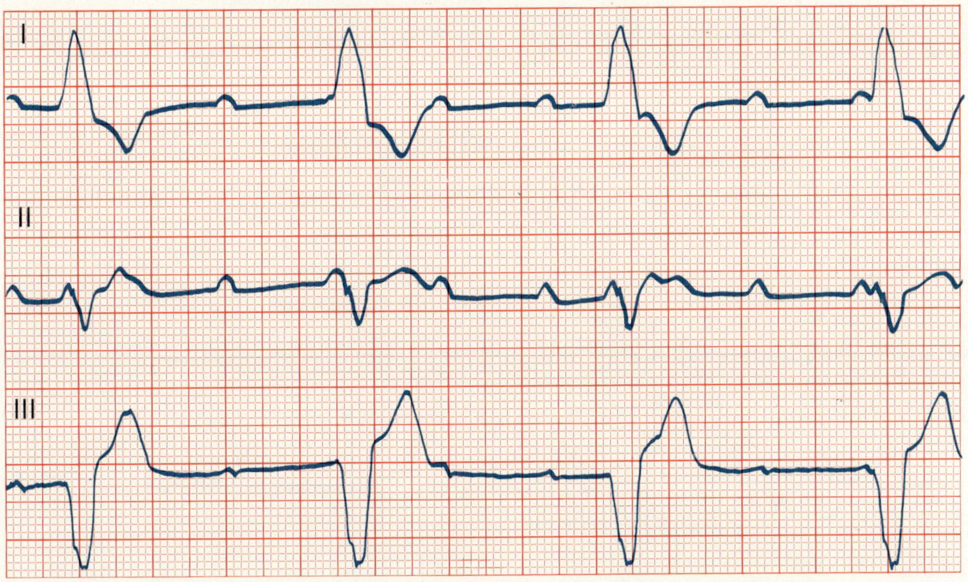

B

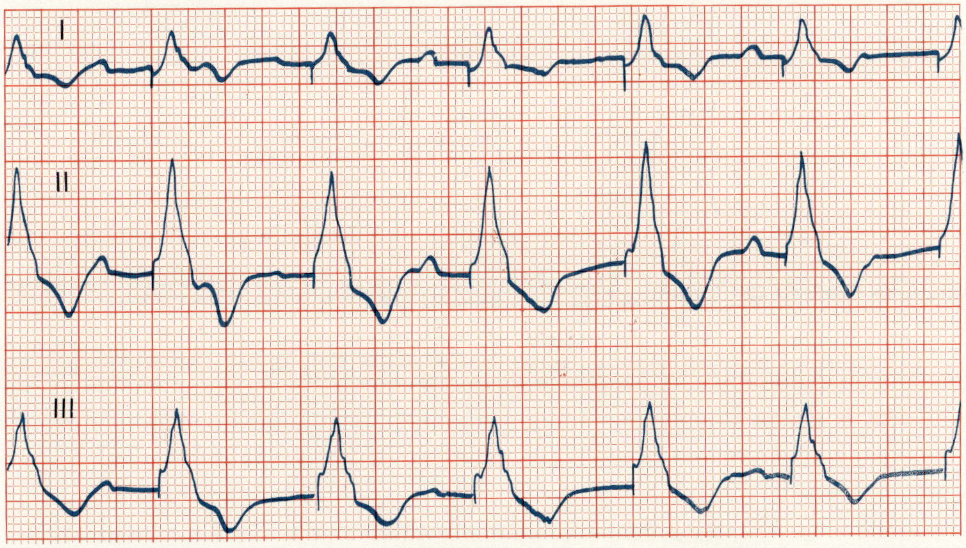

Fig. 4.17
Ventricular pacing. Fixed rate pacing (VOO pacing). The spontaneous heart rate (ventricular escape rhythm) is lower than the pacing rate

A ECG before pacing. Third degree AV block, P waves at a steady rate of 104/min. QRS complexes of ventricular type at a slower independant rate of 41/min (Chapter 10)

B ECG after pacemaker implantation. Paced QRS complexes at a rate of 70/min, P waves at an unchanged rate of 100/min; no spontaneous ventricular activity.

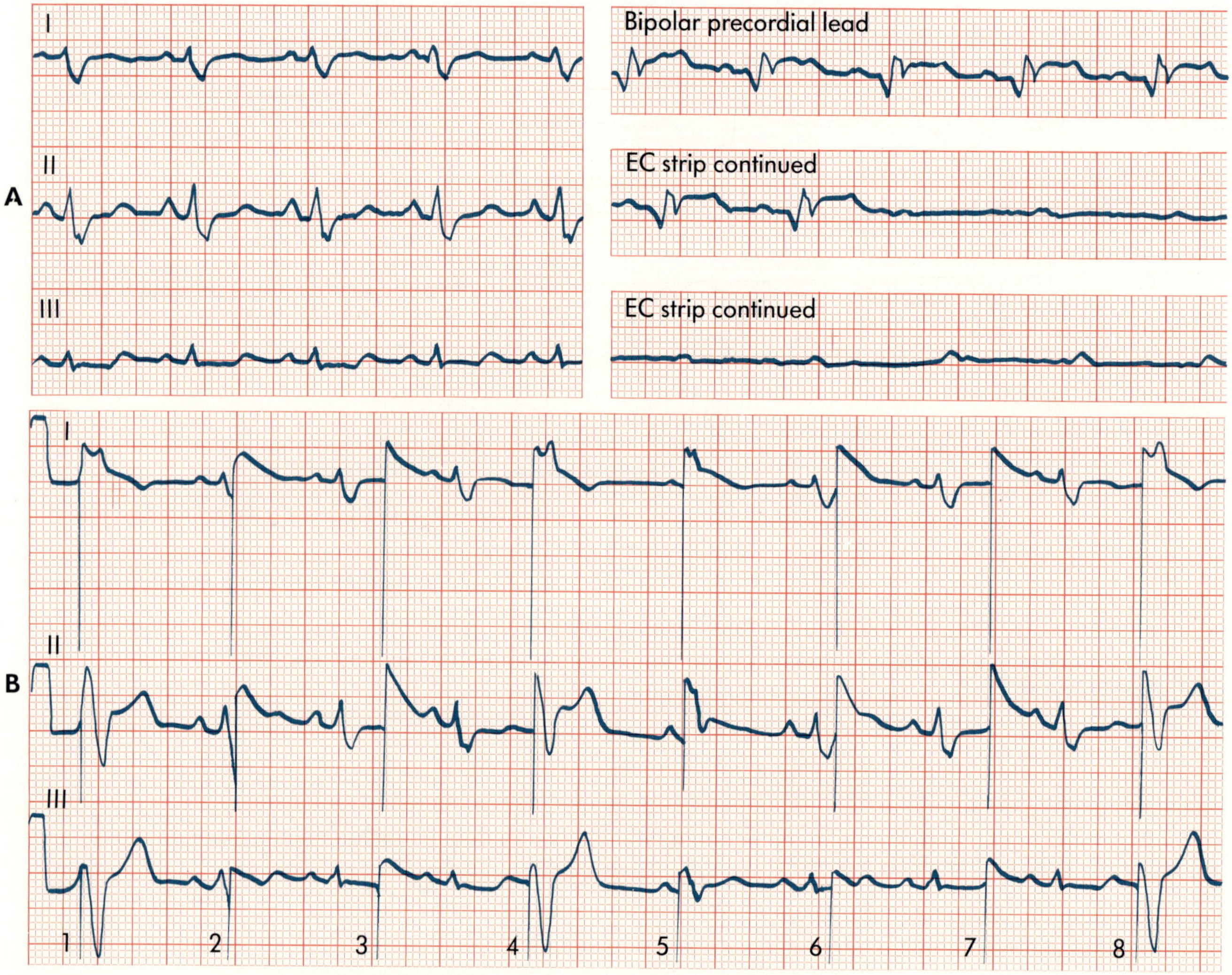

Fig. 4.18
Vetricular pacing. Fixed rate pacing (VOO pacing). The spontaneous heart rate (sinus rhythm) is in the same range as the pacing rate.

A ECG before pacemaker implantation. There is sinus rhythm with right bundle branch block (ECG to the left) between episodes of third degree AV block with ventricular arrest (ECG to the right) necessitating pacemaker implantation.

B ECG after pacemaker implantation. Fixed rate pacing with pacemaker spikes at a consistent rate of 68/min against a background of sinus rhythm. The outcome of pacing varies with the timing of the pacemaker spike:

- *Spikes 1, 4 and 8 are followed by paced QRS complexes as the spikes fall outside the QRST complex (outside the refractory period)*
- *Spike 5 is followed by a fusion complex as the spike falls soon after the sinus P wave*
- *Spikes 2, 3, 6 and 7 are not followed by any QRS complex as they fall on the QRS complex (2), on the ST segment (6) or on the very first part of the T wave (3, 7) (the refractory period of the ventricular myocardium Fig. 4.13); spike 2 represents an example of coincidental QRS/pacemaker spike recording*

circuit is equipped with a sensing circuit which senses the spontaneous QRS complexes (or in atrial pacing the spontaneous P waves). If spontaneous activity is sensed, then the firing of the next pacing impulse is postponed. Thus, the pacing is adapted not to interfere with spontaneous cardiac activity (Figs. 4.20 and 4.21, page 96). The pulse generator remains silent as long as the sensing circuit registers spontaneous QRS complexes (or in atrial pacing spontaneous P waves) at a faster rate than the rate of the pulse generator. Pacing activity resumes if the pause following a sensed QRS complex (or in atrial pacing a sensed P wave) exceeds the basic interval of the preset pacing rate.

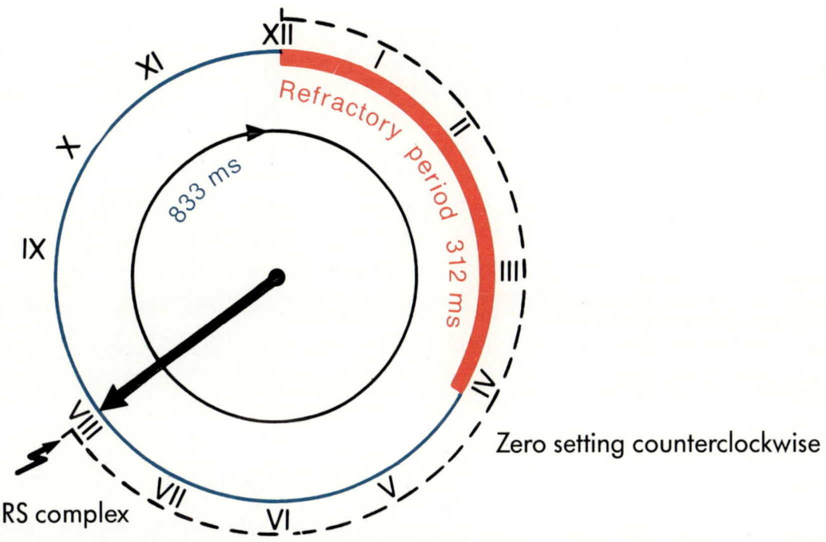

Fig. 4.19
The working principle of inhibited ventricular (VVI pacing). The working principle of the pulse generator can be represented by a clock with one hand. Continuous passage of the hand over the dial will result in a steady paced rhythm at the basic rate of the pulse generator with the emission of a pacing impulse every time the hand passes XII on the dial; thus, one uninterrupted passage of the hand over the dial corresponds to the length of one cycle at the basic rate. If the basic rate of the generator is 72/min, one undisturbed passage is 60/72 s = 833 milliseconds (ms). The very first section of the dial e. g. from "XII" to "IV" represents the refractory period of the pulse generator. It covers a short period of time (200–500 ms) in which the pulse generator is insensitive to cardiac activation. From then on QRS complexes (or in atrial pacing, P waves) generated during the onward passage of the "hand" towards "XII" will be sensed by the pulse generator and will reset the "hand" in a counterclockwise direction to "XII" from where it will start a new cycle without having emitted a pace impulse. In this way, the "hand" controlling the release of pacing impulses continues its cycle:

– Until it is reset in a counterclockwise direction by spontaneous cardiac activity occurring between "IV" and "XII"; or

– Until it passes "XII" and a pacing impulse is emitted

In both situations the hand immediately starts a new passage around the dial. The refractory period of most pulse generators in use today is subdivided into two intervals. During the first interval – the absolute refractory period – the pulse generator is unable to sense impulses. During the following interval – the relative refractory period – the pulse generator is able to sense impulses. However, the sensing of a QRS complex during the relative refractory period immediately initiates a new refractory period including both an absolute and a relative refractory period. In other words, there will be no postponement of the emission of the next pacing impulse. This mode of construction protects the pacemaker from being inhibited by interference from continuous pulsating electrical signals of the type produced by most commonly used electrical devices (50 Hz AC interference). If such a signal should happen to penetrate the filters of the pulse generator, there is a perpetuation of the refractory state of the pacemaker with a shift in the pacing mode from that of inhibited to fixed rate pacing.

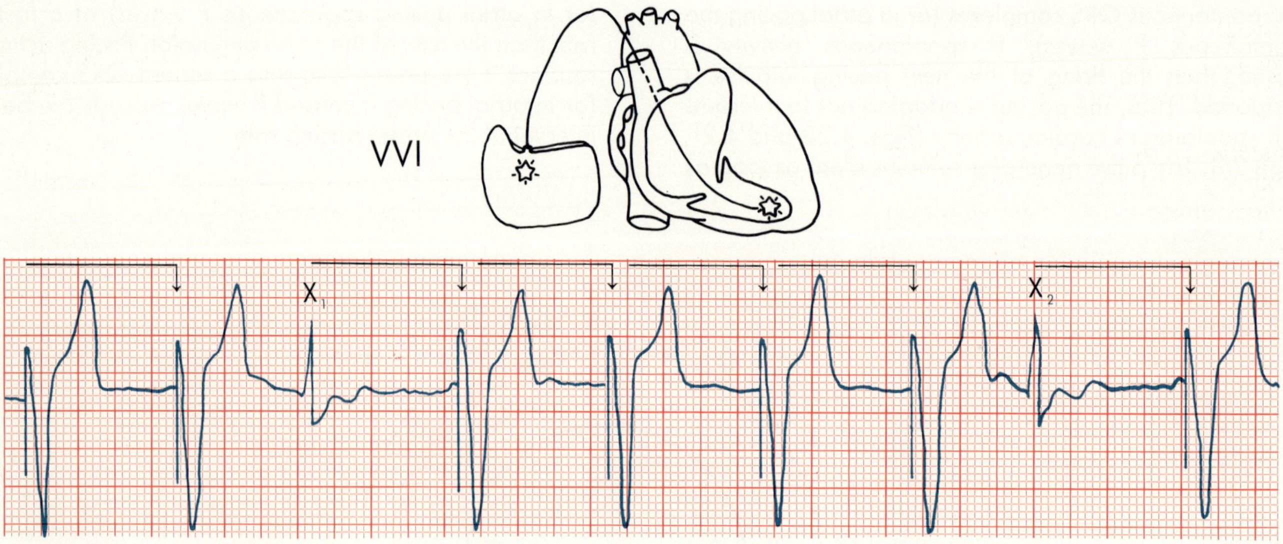

Fig. 4.20
Ventricular inhibited pacing. Inhibited pacing (VVI pacing). The technical features of the pulse generator are those stated in Fig. 4.19. The basic rate is 72/min, the basic interval 833 ms
The ECG shows that the otherwise steady paced rhythm is suspended by the appearance of spontaneous QRS complexes (X_1 – X_2) but resumes after a pause corresponding to the basic interval of the pulse generator

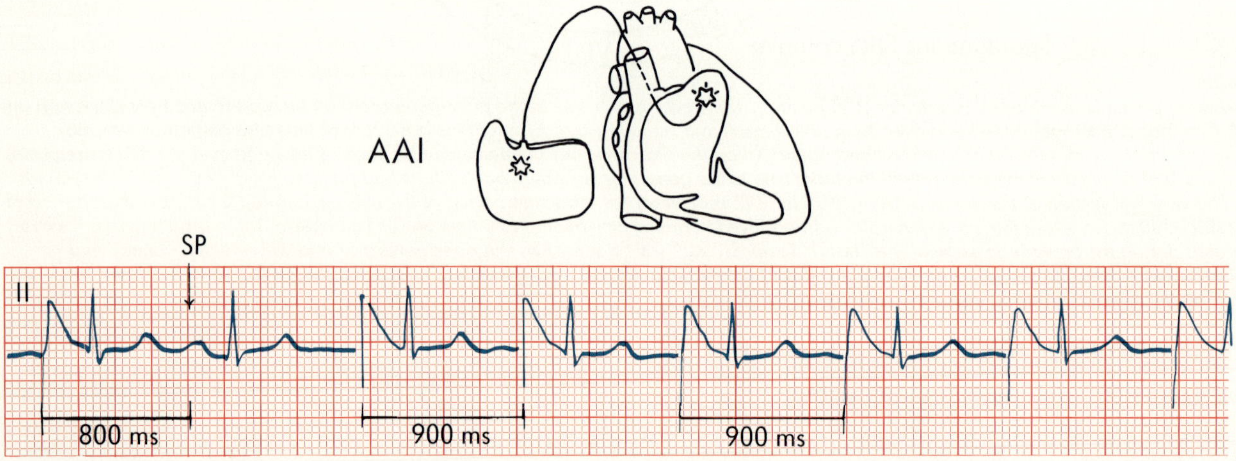

Fig. 4.21
Atrial inhibited pacing. Inhibited pacing (AAI pacing). A sinus P wave (SP) appears 800 ms after the recording of the former pacemaker spike and paced induced P wave. This is before the elapse of the basic interval of the pacemaker which is 900 ms. The pacemaker is inhibited but resumes its pacing activity after the elapse of a basic interval (900 ms) and continues to pace the basic rate. $\frac{60.000}{900}$ = 67/min uninterrupted by spontaneous cardiac activity

Pacemaker malfunction and the ECG [99, 100, 103–105]

Although technical developments and quality control have made pacemaker failure, *pacemaker malfunction,* rare occasional events do occur (Fig. 4.22).

Pacemaker malfunction is first and foremost diagnosed by changes in the pacemaker ECG. Significant ECG findings indicating pacemaker malfunction include exit block, undersensing and oversensing, which for the most common mode of pacing, ventricular inhibited pacing (VVI pacing), are explained and illustrated in Figs. 4.23–4.25, page 98/99. The functional state of the pacemaker can be assessed by the *magnet test* which is performed during ECG recording by placing a powerful magnet on the skin over the pacemaker pocket. The magnet changes inhibited pacing to fixed rate pacing which by its rate can signal battery drainage. Information on "pacemaker threshold", a complex parameter, which relates both to state of the batteries, the pacing electrodes and the myocardial threshold for pacing may also be obtained from the magnet test.

Atrial and ventricular pacemakers (AAI and VVI pacemakers) [99, 100, 106, 107]

Atrial pacing synchronizes atrial and ventricular activation. For this reason and others, the implantation of an atrial inhibited pacemaker (AAI pacemaker, Fig. 4.21) is to be preferred in the patient with sinoatrial block or sinus arrest and no complicating atrioventricular or intraventricular conduction defect.

Ventricular pacing, most often in the form of the implantation of a ventricular inhibited pacemaker (VVI pacemaker, Fig. 4.20) has been and still is the most commonly used treatment not only for AV block but also for sinoatrial block. The advantages of the VVI pacemaker include the simple and easy insertion of the electrode in the right ventricle and the comparatively inexpensive pulse generator. The major drawbacks of VVI pacing are:

– Lack of physiological heart rate response with exercise in the patient with third degree AV block (and in the rare case of slow sinus node response to exercise).

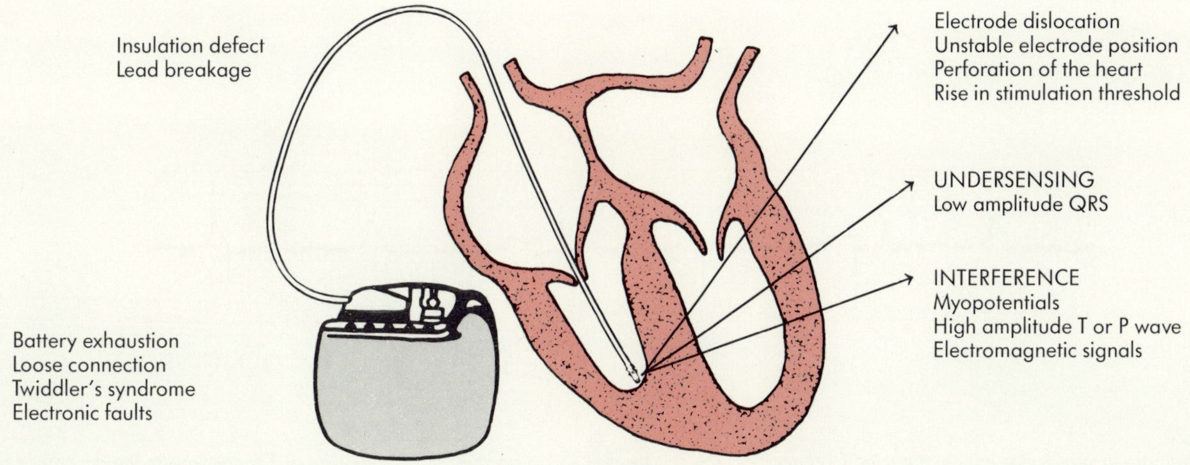

Fig. 4.22
Pacemaker malfunction. A survey of the great variety of complications which may cause pacemaker malfunction

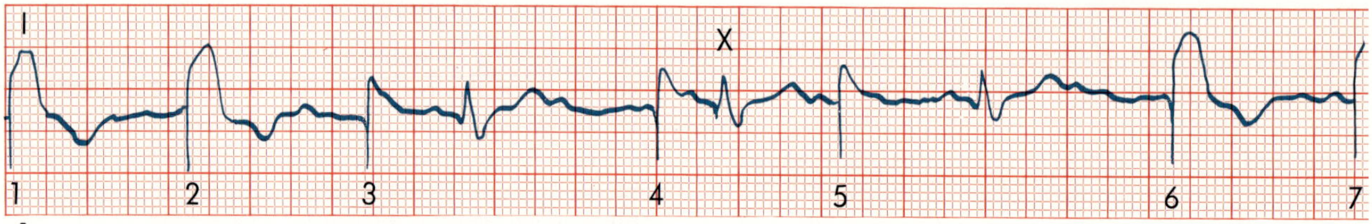

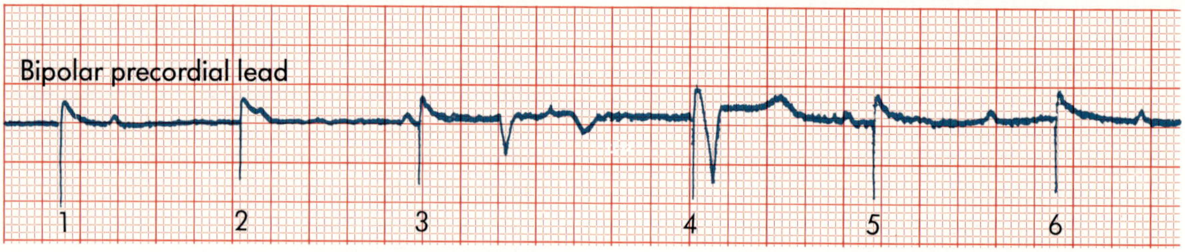

Fig. 4.23
Exit block in ventricular inhibited pacing (VVI pacing). The characteristic finding is a pacemaker spike not followed by any QRS complex despite the fact that the pacemaker spike falls within the non-refractory period of the ventricles (after the T wave and before the QRS complex)

A Intermittent exit block. While pacemaker spikes 1, 2, 6 and 7 are followed by paced QRS complexes, 3, 4 and 5 are not, though they all do fall outside the refractory period of the myocardium. One of the two recorded spontaneous QRS complexes is sensed by the pacemaker, since the distance to the following pacemaker spike (no. 4) correlates well with the basic interval of the pulse generator. The other spontaneous QRS complex (the one marked with an x) is not sensed because it falls within the refractory period of the pacemaker (see legend Fig. 4.19) known to be 350 ms. Thus, the sensing function of the pacemaker appears intact

B Intermittent exit block. There is exit block related to pacemaker spikes 1, 2, 3, 5 and 6 while pacemaker spike 4 is followed by a paced QRS complex. The spontaneous AV nodal escape complex appearing shortly after the fourth pacemaker spike induces a pause in pacing which is resumed one basic interval after the AV nodal escape complex. Thus, sensing function is preserved

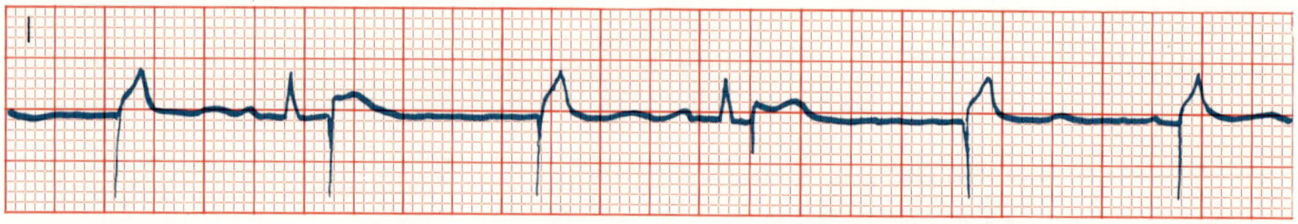

Fig. 4.24
Undersensing in ventricular inhibited pacing (VVI pacing). The pacemaker spikes appear at a steady rate of 72/min despite the occurence of two spontaneous sinus induced QRS complexes. Pacemaker spikes 2 and 4 fall on the ST segment of the sinus complexes (within the refractory period of the myocardium Fig. 4.13) which explains that they are not followed by paced QRS complexes. The cause of undersensing is a low amplitude QRS complex in the intracardiac electrogram.

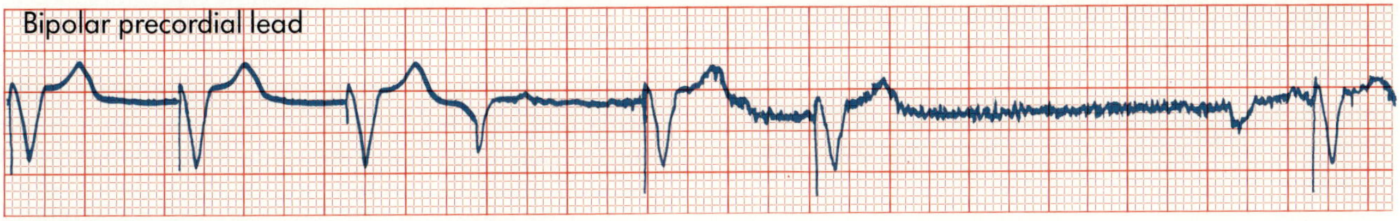

Fig. 4.25
Oversensing due to interference from myopotentials. To the right in the tracing there is a 2 second pause between two ventricular paced QRS complexes. Before and during the pause the baseline of the ECG is broad and irregular most likely due to interference from myopotentials. The patient could voluntarily elicit the pauses in the paced rhythm by contracting his pectoral muscle. To the left in the ECG there are three paced QRS complexes followed by a ventricular extrasystole which is properly sensed since the postextrasystolic pause before pacing is resumed equals the rate interval in the basic rhythm of the pacemaker

– Asynchrony of atrial and ventricular activation which in a few patients will cause troublesome effects in the form of the *pacemaker syndrome*. It is an ill defined complex of symptoms with distressing pulsations in the neck and chest, fatigue, dizziness or sometimes episodes of near fainting.

The lack of a physiological heart rate response to exercise may be overcome by the implantation of a rate responsive pacemaker or a dual chamber pacemaker.

AV synchrony can be restored by the implantation of an atrial pacemaker when appropriate, or the implantation of a dual chamber pacemaker.

The rate responsive (rate modulated) pacemaker [108, 109]

The lack of physiological heart rate regulation in the patient treated by ventricular pacing for third degree AV block, may be overcome by the implantation of a pulse generator offering so-called rate responsive or rate modulated pacing. This type of pulse generator is equipped with a sensor for one of the physiological parameters which vary with body activity. It can be a piezo crystal sensing body vibrations, or it can be a sensor which registers the respiratory rate, the body temperature, or the length of the QT interval (shortens with increasing activity). In response to the signal reflecting increased body activity the pulse generator increases the pacing rate.

Rate responsive pulse generators can also be used in atrial pacing to overcome a reduced sinus node response to exercise e.g. in the sick sinus syndrome (page 289).

The pacemaker code for rate responsiveness is an R placed in the fourth position of the letter code. Thus, the code for rate responsiveness in inhibited ventricular pacing will be VVI-R and for rate responsiveness in inhibited atrial pacing AAI-R.

The dual chamber pacemaker [110–112]

The dual chamber pacemaker offers the advantages of both physiological heart rate regulation and atrioventricular synchrony and is characterized by:

- Two pacing electrodes, an atrial and a ventricular electrode, with pacing and sensing via both electrodes.

- An inbuilt "AV logic" where the sensing of a P wave will "trigger" the firing of a ventricular pacing impulse but with a delay corresponding to a normal PR interval. At the same time the pacemaker will function as an atrial inhibited pacemaker with subsequent but "PR delayed" ventricular pacing.

- Both atrial and ventricular pacing will be suppressed for the period of a pacing cycle whenever a spontaneous QRS complex is sensed by the ventricular electrode.

ECGs of dual chamber pacing are illustrated and described in Figs. 4.26 and 4.27. The dual chamber pacemaker can have one particular and troublesome unwanted effect. It can function as the technical equivalent of an accessory AV connection in the WPW syndrome (Fig. 7.1, page 189) and cause a pacemaker mediated re-entry tachycardia (Fig. 4.28, page 102). An attack of re-entry tachycardia may be induced by a retrograde P wave related to retrograde (VA) conduction. Retrograde (VA) conduction of critically timed ventricular impulses occurs in most individuals with an intact AV

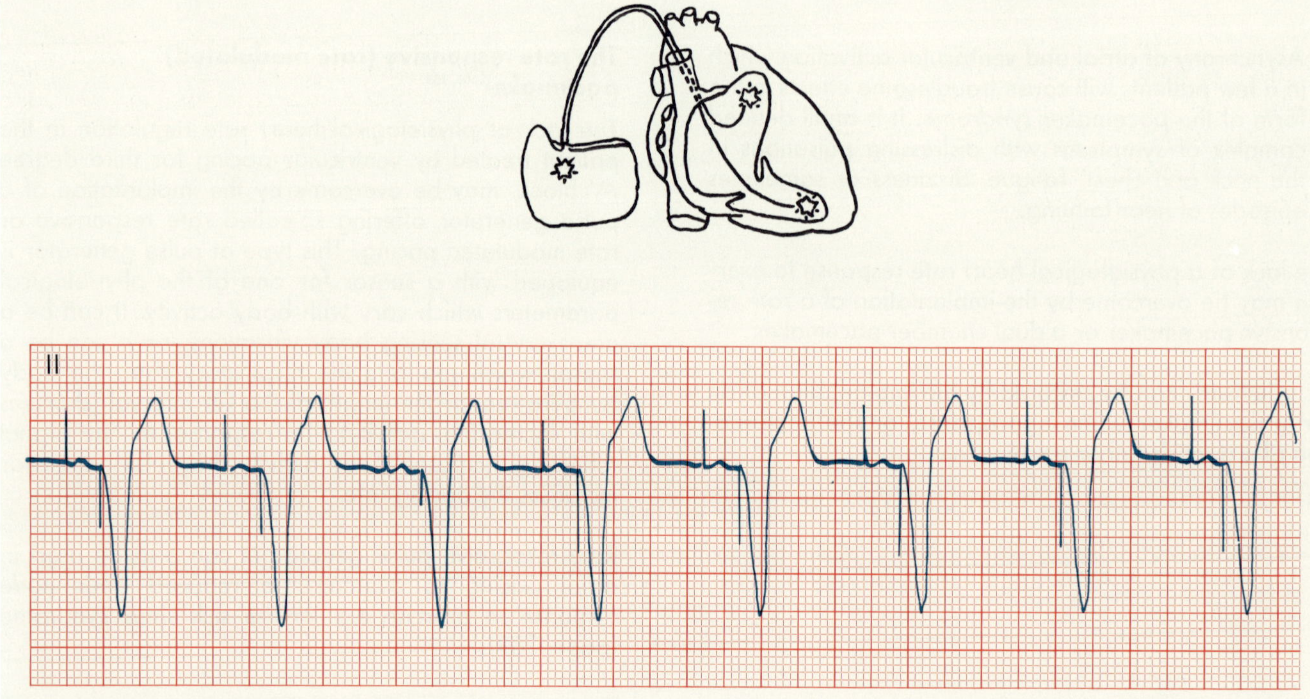

Fig. 4.26
Dual chamber pacing. The atrial pacemaker spike is followed by pacing induced P wave which again after a "PR interval" of 200 ms consistently is followed by a ventricular paced QRS complex

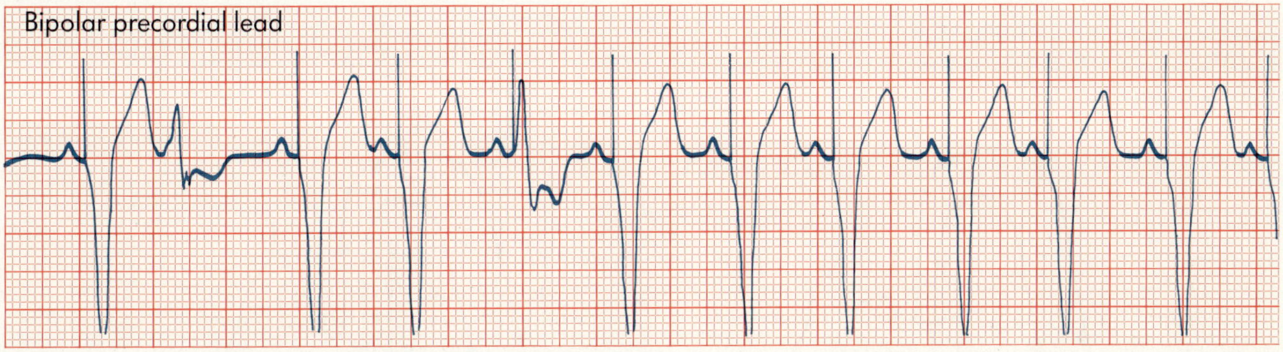

Fig. 4.27
Dual chamber pacing. Spontaneous P waves consistently sensed by the atrial electrode and followed by a ventricular paced QRS complex after a "PR interval" of 200 ms. Two ventricular extrasystoles break the regular P-QRS rhythm

conduction system and in a fair number of patients with AV block of both second and third degree. The retrograde P wave is sensed by the atrial electrode of the dual chamber pacemaker and is anterogradely AV conducted to the ventricles via the pacemaker, resulting in a paced QRS complex. The QRS paced complex may create a further retrograde P wave which is sensed – and so on. The anterograde (AV) conduction pathway of the re-entry circuit (Fig. 7.1) consists of the atrial lead, the pulse generator and the ventricular lead. The route of return for the impulse to the atria is the AV conduction system. Eventually the "endless loop tachycardia" is terminated by e.g. exhaustion of retrograde VA conduction with increasing degrees of VA block. Placing a magnet over the pacemaker will temporarily convert the pacing mode from synchronous to asynchronous pacing and is an effective and safe mode of terminating the tachycardia. Attacks of pacemaker mediated re-entry tachycardia can usually be prevented by reprogramming the pacemaker with a slight modification of its technical specifications (prolongation of the "refractory period" of atrial sensing).

With recent technical developments the dual chamber pulse generator (DDD type) has become a highly reliable device, and the implantation of the DDD pacemaker is now a routine procedure in most cardiological centres. DDD pacemaker implantation is used on a large scale in the treatment of Stokes-Adams' syndrome (page 262) and occasionally in the hypertensive carotid sinus syndrome (page 282) and in the sick sinus syndrome (page 286).

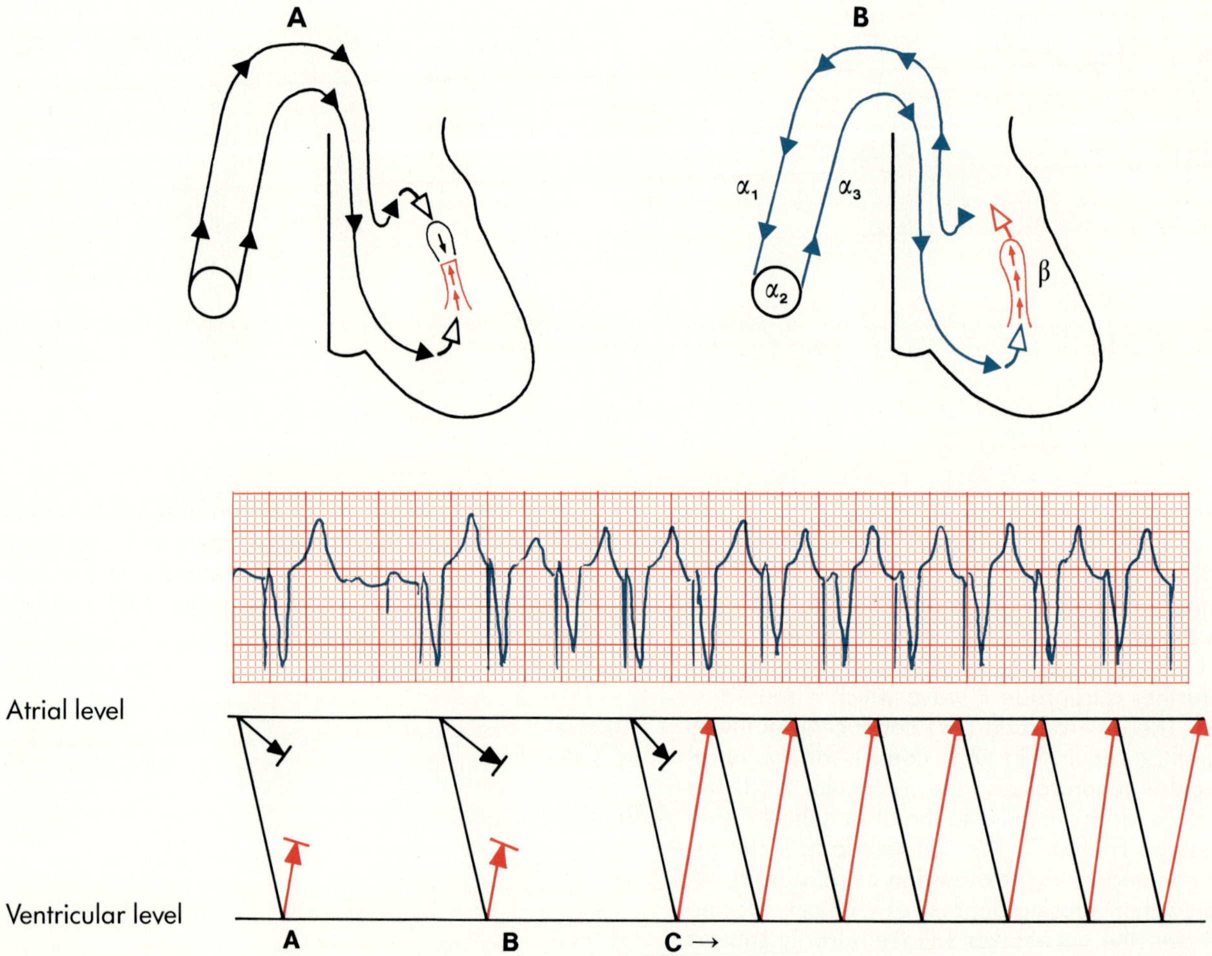

Fig. 4.28
Pacemaker mediated re-entry tachycardia (endless loop tachycardia)

A Normally there is no VA conduction of the ventricular impulse because either of AV dissociation with collision of the atrial and ventricular impulses in the AV node or of an organic but intermittent VA block

B A critically timed ventricular extrasystole (VE) may succeed in passing retrogradely through the AV conduction system and induce a retrograde P wave. The retrograde P wave is sensed by the pacemaker which after a delay paces the ventricle. The pace induced QRS complex may be VA conducted and result in another retrograde P wave which again is sensed triggering the pacemaker to pace the ventricle – and so on

1. Coumel P. The management of clinical arrhythmias. An overview on invasive versus non-invasive electrophysiology. Europ Heart J 1987; 8: 92–99.
2. Morganroth J, Horowitz LN. Antiarrhythmic drug therapy 1988: For whom, how and where? Am J Cardiol 1988; 62: 461–65.
3. Wasman MB, Waid RW, Sharma AD, et al. Vagal techniques for termination of paroxysmal supraventricular tachycardia. Am J Cardiol 1980; 46: 655–64.
4. Wellens HJJ. Wolff-Parkinson-White syndrome. Part II. Treatment. Mod Concepts Cardiovasc Dis 1983; 52: 57–59.
5. Mehta D, Ward DE, Wafa S, Camm AJ. Relative efficacy of various physical manoeuvres in the termination of junctional tachycardia. Lancet 1988; i: 1181–85
6. Vaughan Williams EM. A classification of antiarrhythmic actions reassessed after a decade of new drugs. J Clin Pharmacol 1984; 24: 129–47.
7. Singh BN, Opie LH, Harrison DC, et al. Antiarrhythmic drugs. In: Opie LH, ed. 2nd edition. Drugs for the heart. Orlando, New York, London, 1987; 54–90.
8. Woosley RL, Funck-Brentano C. Overview of the clinical pharmacology of antiarrhythmic drugs. Am J Cardiol 1988; 61: 61–69.
9. Crevasse L. Quinidine: An update on therapeutics, pharmacokinetics and serum concentration monitoring. Am J Cardiol 1988; 62: 22–23.
10. Koch-Weser J. Drug therapy. Dispyramide. New Engl J Med 1979; 300: 957–62.
11. Campbell RWF. Drug therapy. Mexiletine. New Engl J Med 1987; 316: 29–34.
12. Sandøe E, Julian DG, Bell JW, eds. Management of ventricular tachycardia: Role of mexiletine. Amsterdam: Excerpta Medica, 1978.
13. Johansson BW, Stavenow L, Hanson A. Long-term clinical experience with mexiletine. Am Heart J 1984; 107: 1099–1102.
14. Duff HJ, Roden D, Primm K, et al. Mexiletine in the treatment of resistant ventricular arrhythmias: Enhacement of efficacy and reduction of dose-related side effects by combination with quinidine. Circulation 1983; 67: 1124–28.
15. Halinen MO. Mexiletine for the management of ventricular arrhythmias in ischemic heart disease. Clin Prog Electrophysiol Pacing 1986; 4: 568.
16. Sheldon RS, Duff HJ, Brent Mitchell L, et al. Effect of oral combination therapy with mexiletine and quinidine on left and right ventricular function. Am Heart J 1986; 115: 1030–35.
17. Moak JP, Smith RT, Garson A. Mexiletine: An effective antiarrhythmic drug for treatment of ventricular arrhythmias in congenital heart disease. JACC 1987; 10: 817–24.
18. Harrison DC, ed. Cardiac arrhythmias. A decade of progress. Boston, Mass.: G.K. Hall Medical Publishers, 1981; 205–312.
19. Podrid PJ. Special symposium on propafenone. J Electrophysiol 1987; 1: 501–90.
20. Geibel A, Meinertz T, Zehender M, et al. Antiarrhythmic efficacy and tolerance of oral propafenone in patients with frequent ventricular arrhythmias: Experience of a multicentre study. Europ Heart J 1989; 10 (Suppl. E): 81–87.
21. Dressler F, et al. Die Behandlung von Herzrhythmusstörungen mit Propafenon bei Säuglingen und Kindern. Monatsschr Kinderheilkd 1985; 133: 154–57.
22. Anderson JL, Pritchett ELC. International symposium on supraventricular arrhythmias: Focus on flecainide. Am J Cardiol 1987; 62 (Suppl. D): 1–67.
23. Wren C, Campbell RWF. The response of paediatric arrhythmias to intravenous and oral flecainide. Br Heart J 1987; 57: 171–75.
24. Morganroth J, ed. A symposium: Use of beta blockers as antiarrhythmic agents. Am J Cardiol 1987; 60 (Suppl. D): 1–67.
25. Oates JA, Wood AJJ. Drug therapy. Amiodarone. New Engl J Med 1987; 316: 455–66.
26. Olsson SB, Edvardsson N. Delayed repolarization as antiarrhythmic action. Europ Heart J 1988; 9 (Suppl. B): 37.43.
27. Kopelman HA, Horowitz LN. Efficacy and toxicity of amiodarone for the treatment of supraventricular tachyarrhythmias. Prog Cardiovasc Dis 1089; 31: 355–66.
28. Greene HL. The efficacy of amiodarone in the treatment of ventricular tachycardia or ventricular fibrillation. Prog Cardiovasc Dis 1989; 31: 319–54.
29. McKenna WJ, Oakley CM, Krikler DM, et al. Improved survival with amiodarone in patients with hypertrophic cardiomyopathy and ventricular tachycardia. Br Heart J 1985; 53: 412–16.
30. Singh BN, Deedwania P, Nademanee K, et al. Sotalol. A review of its pharmacodynamic and pharmacokinetic properties, and therapeutic use.
31. Murtzam A, Campbell RWF. Specific drugs for specific ventricular arrbythmias. An evalation of current therapy and the role of propafenone. Europ Heart J 1989; 10 (Suppl. E): 41–47.
32. Storstein L. Role of digitalis in ventricular rate control in atrial fibrillation. In: Kulbertus HE, Olsson SB, Schlepper M, eds. Atrial fibrillation. Mölndal, Sweden: Astra Cardiovascular, 1982; 285–93.
33. Neuss H. Control of ventricular rate in atrial fibrillation: Role of verapamil. In: Kulbertus HE, Olsson SB, Schlepper M, eds. Atrial fibrillation. Mölndal, Sweden, 1982; 294–303.
34. Mølgaard H, Bjerregaard P, Jørgensen HS. 24-hour antiarrhythmic effect of conventional and slow-release verapamil in chronic atrial fibrillation. Europ J Clin Pharmacol 1987; 33: 447–53.
35. Steinberg JS, Katz RJ, Bren GB, et al. Efficacy of oral diltiazem to control ventricular response in chronic atrial fibrillation at rest and during exercise. JACC 1987; 9: 405–11.
36. James MA, Channer KS, Papouchado M, et al. Improved control of atrial fibrillation with combined pindolol and digoxin therapy. Europ Heart J 1989; 10: 83–90.
37. Rowland E, McKenna WJ, Harris L, et al. Amiodarone in the prophylaxis of atrial fibrillation. In: Kulbertus HE, Olsson SB, Schlepper M, eds. Mölndal, Sweden: Astra Cardio vascular, 1982; 262–71.
38. Roden DM. Role of the electrocardiogram in determining electrophysiologic end points of drug therapy. Am J Cardiol 1988; 62: 34–38.
39. Schlepper M. Cardiodepressive effects of antiarrhythmic drugs. Europ Heart J 1989; 10 (Suppl. E): 73–80.
40. Hoffmeister HM, Hepp A, Seipel L. Negative inotropic effect of class-I-antiarrhythmic drugs: Comparison of flecainide with disopyramide and quinidine. Europ Heart J 1987; 8: 1126–32.
41. Ravid S, Podrid PJ, Lampert S, et al. Congestive heart failure induced by six of the newer antiarrhythmic drugs. JACC 1989; 14: 1326–30.

42. Woosley RL. Pharmacokinetics and pharmacodynamics of antiarrhythmic agents in patients with congestive heart failure. Am Heart J 1987; 114: 1280–91.
43. Bergfeldt L, Rosenqvist M, Vallin H, et al. Disopyramide induced second and third degree atrioventricular block in patients with bifascicular block. An acute stress test to predict atrioventricular block progression. Br Heart J 1985; 53: 328–34.
44. Alboni P, Cappato R, Paparella N, et al. Electrophysiological effects and mechanism of action of oral quninidine in patients with sinus bradycardia and first degree A-V nodal block. Europ Heart J 1987; 8: 1080–89.
45. Buss J, Neuss H, Bilgin Y, Schlepper M. Malignant ventricular tachyarrhythmias in association with propafenone treatment. Europ Heart J 1985; 6: 424–28.
46. Cowan JC, Bourke J, Campbell RWF. Arrhythmogenic effects of antiarrhythmic drugs. Europ Heart J 1986; 7 (Suppl. A): 133–36.
47. Creamer JE, Nathan AW, Cam AJ. The proarrhythmic effects of antiarrhythmic drugs. Am Heart J 1987; 114: 397–406.
48. Brugada P, Wellens HJJ. Arrhythmogenesis of antiarrhythmic drugs. Am J Cardiol 1988; 61: 1108–11.
49. Julian DG. The arrhythmogenic effects of antiarrhythmic drugs. Europ Heart J 1988; 9 (Suppl. B): 1–4.
50. Davy JM, Sirinelli A, Le Guludec D, et al. Mode of action of antiarrhythmic drugs and the implicated arrhythmogenic risk. Europ Heart J 1988; 9 (Suppl. B): 5–12.
51. Buchalter M, Campbell RWF. Arrhythmogenesis and programmed stimulation techniques. Europ Heart J 1988; 9 (Suppl. B): 13–17.
52. Rydén L. Noninvasive techniques in the evaluation of the arrhythmogenic effects. Europ Heart J 1988; 9 (Suppl. B): 19–23.
53. Furlanello F. Paradoxical proarrhythmic phenomena evaluated by non-invasive methods. Europ Heart J 1988; 9 (Suppl. B): 25.
54. Hohnloser SH, Meiertz T. Recorded sudden cardiac death: Relationship to antiarrhythmic therapy. Europ Heart J 1988; 9 (Suppl. B): 27–31.
55. Horowitz L. Proarrhythmia – taking the bad with the good. New Engl J Med 1988; 319: 304–05.
56. The Cardiac Arrhythmia Suppression Trial (CAST) In vestigators. Preliminary report: Effect of encainide and flecainide on mortality in a randomized trial of arrhythmia suppression after myocardial infaction. New Engl J Med 1989; 321: 406–12.
57. Editorial. Flecainide and CAST. Lancet 1989; 2: 481–82.
58. Podrid PJ. Aggravation of arrhythmia: A complication of antiarrhythmic drug therapy. Europ Heart J 1989; 10 (Suppl. E): 66–72.
59. Levine JH, Morganroth J, Kadish AH. Mechanisms and risk factors for proarrhythmia with type Ia compared with Ic antiarrhythmic drug therapy. Circulation 1989; 80: 1063–69.
60. Keren A, Tzivoni D, Gavish D, et al. Etiology, warning signs and therapy of torsade de pointes. A study of 10 patients. Circulation 1981; 64: 1167–74.
61. Webb CL, Dick M, Rocchini AP, et al. Quinidine syncope in children. JACC 1987; 9: 1031–71.
62. Brugada J, Sassine A, Escande D, et al. Effects of quinidine on ventricular repolarization. Europ Heart J 1987; 8: 1340–45.
63. Gössinger HD, Siostrzonek P, Schmoliner R, et al. Sotalol-induced torsades de pointes in a patient with pre-existent normal response to programmed ventricular stimulation. Europ Heart J 1987; 8: 1351–53.
64. Lery G, Laiat R, Barthelemy M, et al. Torsade de pointes during loading with amiodarone. Europ Heart J 1987; 8: 541–43.
65. Forfar JC, Gribbin B. Torsade de pointes after amiodarone withdrawal. Effects of mild hypokalemia on repolarization. Europ Heart J 1984; 5: 510–12.
66. Robertson CE, Miller HC. Extreme tachycardia complicating the use of disopyramide in atrial flutter. Br Heart J 1980; 44: 602–03.
67. Orning OM. The use of tocainide, encainide, lorcainide and flecainide for supraventricular arrhythmias. Europ Heart J 1984; 5 (Suppl. B): 81–6.
68. Nathan AW, Hellestrand KJ, Bexton RS, et al. Proarrhythmic effects of the new antiarrhythmic agent flecainide acetate. Am Heart J 1984; 107: 222–28.
69. Danahy DT, Aronow WS. Licocaine-induced cardiac rate changes in atrial fibrillation and atrial flutter. Am Heart J 1978; 95: 474–82.
70. Vrobel TR, Miller PE, Mostow ND, et al. A general overview of amiodarone toxicity: Its prevention, detectio, and management. Prog Cardiovasc Dise 1989; 31: 393–426.
71. Nademanee K, Piwonka RW, Singh BN, et al. Amiodarone and thyroid function. Prog Cardiovasc Dis 1989; 31: 427–37.
72. Dunn M, Glassroth J. Pulmonary complications of amiodarone toxicity. Prog Cardiovasc Dis 1989; 31: 447–53.
73. Horowitz LN. Detection of amiodarone pulmonary toxicity: To screen or not to screen, that is the question! JACC 1988; 12: 789–90.
74. Jaillon P. Antiarrhythmic drug interactions: Are they im portant? Europ Heart J 1987; 8 (Suppl. A): 127–32.
75. Stohler JL, Kowey PR, Marinchak RA. Drug interactions with propafenone. J Electrophysiol 1987; 6: 568–74.
76. Marcus FI, Opie LH, Sonnenblick EH. Digitalis, sympathometics, and inotropic-dilators. In: Opie LH, ed. Drugs for the heart. Orlando, New York, London: Grune & Stratton, Inc., 1987; 91–110.
77. Smith TW. Digitalis: Mechanisms of action and clinical use. New Engl J Med 1988; 318: 358–65.
78. Ideker RE, Chen P-S, Shibata N, et al. Current concepts of the mechanisms of ventricular defibrillation. In: Breithardt G, Borggrefe M, Zipes DP, eds. Nonpharmacological therapy of tachyarrhythmias. Mount Kisco, New York: Futura Publishing Co., 1987.
79. Resnekov L. High-energy electrical current in the management of cardiac dysrhythmias. In: Mandel WJ, ed. 2nd edition. Cardiac arrhythmias. Their mechanism, diagnosis, and management. Philadelphia, London, New York: J.B. Lippincott Co., 1987; 738–53.
80. Standards and guidelines for cardiopulmonary resuscitation and emergency cardiac care. JAMA 1986; 255: 2942–43 and 2967–68.
81. Nordlander R. Anticoagulation in atrial fibrillation cardioversion. In: Kulbertus HE, Olsson SB, Schlepper M, eds. Mölndal, Sweden: Astra cardiovascular, 1982; 256–57.
82. Orko R. Anaesthesia for cardioversion: A comparison of diazepam, thiopentone and propanidid. Br J Anaesth 1976; 48; 257–62.
83. Hagemeijer F, Van Mechelen R, Smalbraak DWT. Fentanyletomi date anaesthsia for cardioversion. Europ Heart J 1982; 3: 155–58.

84. Mann DL, Maisel AS, Atwood JE, et al. Absence of cardioversion-induced ventricular arrhythmias in patients with therapeutic digoxin levels. JACC 1985; 5: 882.
85. Levine PA, Barold SS, Fletcher RD, et al. Adverse acute and chronic effects of electrical defibrillation and cardioversion on implanted unipolar cardiac pacing systems JACC 1983; 1: 1413.
86. Adgey AAJ, Patton JN, Campbell NPS, et al. Ventricular defibrillation: Appropriate energy levels. Circulation 1979; 60: 219–22.
87. Gutgesell HP, Tacker WA, Geddes LA, et al. Energy dose for ventricular defibrillation of children. Pediatrics 1976; 58: 898–901.
88. Ward DE, Camm AJ. Clinical electrophysiology of the heart. London: Edward Arnold, 1987.
89. Brugada P, Wellens HJJJ, eds. Cardiac arrhythmias: Where to go from here? Mount Kisco, New York: Futura Publishing Co., 1987.
90. Breithardt G, Borggrefe M, Zipes DP, eds. Nonpharmacological therapy of tachyarrhythmias. Mount Kisco, New York: Futura Publishing Co., 1987.
91. Gallagher JJ, Selle JG, Svenson, et al. Surgical treatment of arrhythmias. Am J Cardiol 1988; 61: 27–44.
92. Fontaine G, Sheinman MM, eds. Ablation in cardiac arrhythmias. Mount Kisco, New York: Futura Publishing Co., 1987.
93. Editorial. Automatic defibrillators. Lancet 1988; i: 1199–1201.
94. Furman S. AICD benefit. Pace 1989; 399–400.
95. Lau CP, Cornu E, Camm AJ. Fatal and nonfatal cardiac arrest in patients with an implanted antitachycardia device for the treatment of supraventricular tachycardia. Am J Cardiol 1988; 61: 919–21.
96. Møller M, Simonsen E, Arnsbo P, et al. Long-term efficacy of automatic scanning antitachycardia pacemaker. Pace 1989; 12: 425–30.
97. Furman S. Combined automatic implantable cardioverter-defibrillator and pacemaker systems. JACC 1989; 13: 132–33.
98. Parsonnet V, Furman S, Smyth NPD, et al. Optimal resources for implantable cardiac pacemakers. Pacemaker Study Group. Circulation 1983; 68: 227–44.
99. Barold SS, ed. Modern cardiac pacing. Mount Kisco, New York: Futura Publishing Co., 1985.
100. Furman S, Hayes D, Holmes D. A practice of cardiac pacing. Mount Kisco, New York: Futura Publishing Co., 1986.
101. Madsen JK, Meibom J, Videbæk R, et al. Transcutaneous pacing: Experience with the Zoll noninvasive termporary pacemaker. Am Heart J 1988; 116: 7–10.
102. Berstein AD, Camm AJ, Fletcher RD, et al. The NASPE/BPEG generic code for antibradyarrhythmia and adaptive-rate pacing and antitachyarrhythmia devices. Pace 1987; 10: 794–99.
103. Schüller H, Fåhraeus T. Pacemaker electrocardiograms – An introduction to practical analysis. Solna, Sweden: Siemens-Elema, 1983.
104. Fåhraeus T, Schüller H. Pacemaker electrocardiography. In: Macfarlane PW, Veitch Lawrie TD, eds. Comprehebnsive electrocardiology. Theory and practice in health and disease. New York, Oxford: Pergamon Press, 1989; 1177–97.
105. Parsonnet V, Bernstein AD, Lindsay B. Pacemaker-implantation complication rates: An analysis of some con tributing factors. JACC 1989; 13: 917–21.
106. Rosenqvist M, Brandt J, Schueller H. Long-term pacing in sinus node disease: Effects of stimulation mode on cardiovascular morbidity and mortality. Am Heart J 1988; 116: 16–22.
107. Ausubel K, Furman S. The pacemaker syndrome. Ann Intern Med 1985: 420–29.
108. Rydén L. The future of single chamber pacing. Pace 1986; 9: 1131–35.
109. Camm AJ, Garratt C, Paul V. Single-chamber rate adaptive pacing. J Electrophysiol 1989; 3: 181–89.
110. Kristensson B-E, Arnman K, Smedgård, et al. Physiological versus single-rate ventricular pacing. A double-blind cross-over study. Pace 1985; 8: 73–84.
111. Harthorne JW, Eisenhauser AC, Steinhaus DM. Pacemaker-mediated tachycardias: An unresolved problem. Pace 1984; 7: 1140–47.
112. Serge Barold S, Falkoff MD, Ong LS, et al. Pacemaker endless loop tachycardia: Termination by simple techniques other than magnet application. Am J Med 1988; 85: 817–22.

Chapter 5
Extrasystole, escape and parasystole

Extrasystole, escape and parasystole [1, 2, 5]

Extrasystoles [1–3]

An extrasystole is a premature impulse which usually shows a fixed and probably causal relationship to the preceding complex in the basic cardiac rhythm. Thus, in an ECG tracing with repeated recordings of an extrasystole over a period of time the distance from the extrasystole to the preceding complex, the coupling interval of the extrasystole (I-coup, Fig. 5.1) is constant from one extrasystole to the next. Current hypotheses on the mechanism of this fixed coupling focus on triggered activity and re-entry (Fig. 3.4, page 41). Since the extrasystole is ectopic in origin and premature in appearance it is often named an ectopic or a premature beat, complex or depolarization (abbreviated PB, PC and PD). However, these commonly used synonyms have been classified as "non-preferred terms" by the ISFC/WHO task force on definition and classification of cardiac arrhythmias.

ECG diagnosis

The complexes marked Ex in Fig. 5.1 are extrasystoles as they arrive early (I-coup < I-n). The upper tracing (A) shows a supraventricular extrasystole with a narrow QRS complex (QRS < 0.12 s), the lower tracing (B) a ventricular extrasystole with a widened QRS complex (QRS ≥ 0.12 s). Nothing can be said about fixed coupling since each ECG tracing contains only one extrasystole.

Differential diagnosis: Escape and parasystole

Fig. 5.2 shows a late ectopic impulse arriving after the time for the next anticipated complex of the basic cardiac rhythm. It is not an extrasystole related to increased pacemaker activity but its functional antagonist, an *escape*. It occurs as a substitute for the normal complex, a rescue mechanism precipitated by a delay in impulse formation or conduction allowing a subsidiary ectopic pacemaker (Fig. 1.6, page 5) to "escape" at its own slow inherent rate. The upper tracing (A) shows a supraventricular escape (QRS < 0.12 s) secondary to SA block, the lower tracing (B) a ventricular escape (QRS ≥ 0.12 s).

Parasystole (see end of the Chapter, Fig. 5.15, page 120) may be misdiagnosed as an extrasystole but occurs independently of the basic cardiac rhythm with a continually varying "coupling interval" contrasting with the fixed coupling interval of the extrasystole.

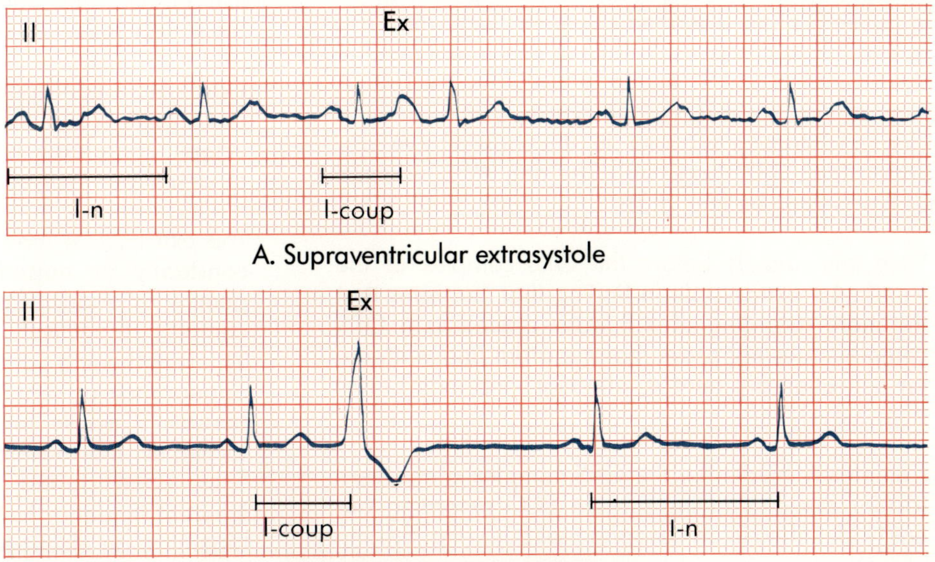

A. Supraventricular extrasystole

B. Ventricular extrasystole

Fig. 5.1
Extrasystole (Ex)

I-n = normal cardiac cycle
I-coup = coupling interval

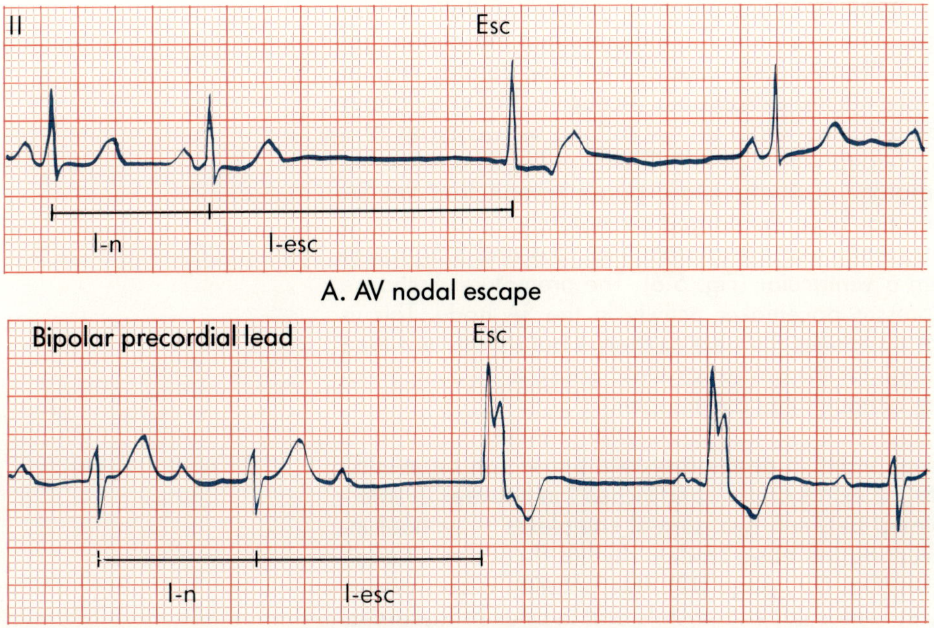

A. AV nodal escape

B. Ventricular escape

Fig. 5.2
Escape (Esc)

I-n = normal cardiac cycle
I-Esc = escape interval

The postextrasystolic pause [2]

The pause following the extrasystole, the *postextrasystolic pause* (I-pEx), is termed *compensatory* when it is long enough to compensate for the prematurity of the postextrasystolic pause (I-coup + I-pEx = 2 x I-n). A compensatory postextrasystolic pause is the common finding in ventricular extrasystole. It is caused by AV dissociation (Fig. 3.17, page 50). The non AV conducted sinus P wave can be (Fig. 5.3):

A Seen immediately before the QRS complex of the ventricular extrasystole (a finding that illustrates that the mere recording of a P wave preceding a QRS complex does not prove that the atrial and ventricular activation are related, although this may be so) (Fig. 5.3 A).

B Completely hidden by the QRS complex of the ventricular complex in the surface ECG recording but easily identified in an oesophageal ECG (Fig. 5.3 B).

C Discernible in the ST segment of the extrasystole immediately after the QRS complex (Fig. 5.3 C).

The term *non-compensatory* postextrasystolic pause (Figs. 5.4–5.6, page 112) indicates that the interval between the two complexes of the basic cardiac rhythm containing the extrasystole (I-coup + I-pEx) is longer than a normal cycle but not as long as two cycles (2 x I-n > I-coup + I-pEx > I-n). The recording of a non-compensatory postextrasystolic pause reveals that the SA node has been discharged prematurely, usually from a supraventricular extrasystole (Figs. 5.4 and 5.5), rarely from a ventricular (Fig. 5.6). The premature discharge depresses pacemaker activity in the SA node. This in turn postpones the next discharge but usually not long enough for the postextrasystolic pause to be compensatory, although that can happen.

Occasionally, a postextrasystolic pause can be missing with the extrasystole "sandwiched" in between – *interpolated* between two normal complexes – without interrupting the basic cardiac rhythm (I-coup + "I-pEx" = I-n)(Fig. 5.7, page 112). Interpolation occurs primarily in ventricular extrasystole and in sinus bradycardia. The PR interval of the sinus complex following the interpolated extrasystole is often prolonged most likely due to retrograde conduction of the ventricular impulse into the lower part of the AV node with corresponding relative refractoriness and prolonged AV conduction time of the shortly following sinus impulse.

Extrasystole can appear singly (Fig. 5.14, 1, page 118) or in pairs (couplets) (Fig. 5.14, 4 A); three or more ectopic complexes in rapid succession over 100/min is, by definition, *tachycardia* (Fig. 5.14, 4 B, page 119).

The extrasystole may come and go randomly, or can constantly or episodically appear as bigeminy, trigeminy or quadrigeminy, every second, third or fourth complex respectively being an extrasystole (Fig. 5.14, 2). Lengthening of the cardiac cycle favours the appearance of ventricular extrasystole; the long compensatory pause following a ventricular extrasystole facilitates the development of another extrasystole. Thus, once started, ventricular extrasystole has an inherent tendency to be selfperpetuating as ventricular bigeminy, an electrophysiological pattern of behaviour often termed *the rule of bigeminy*.

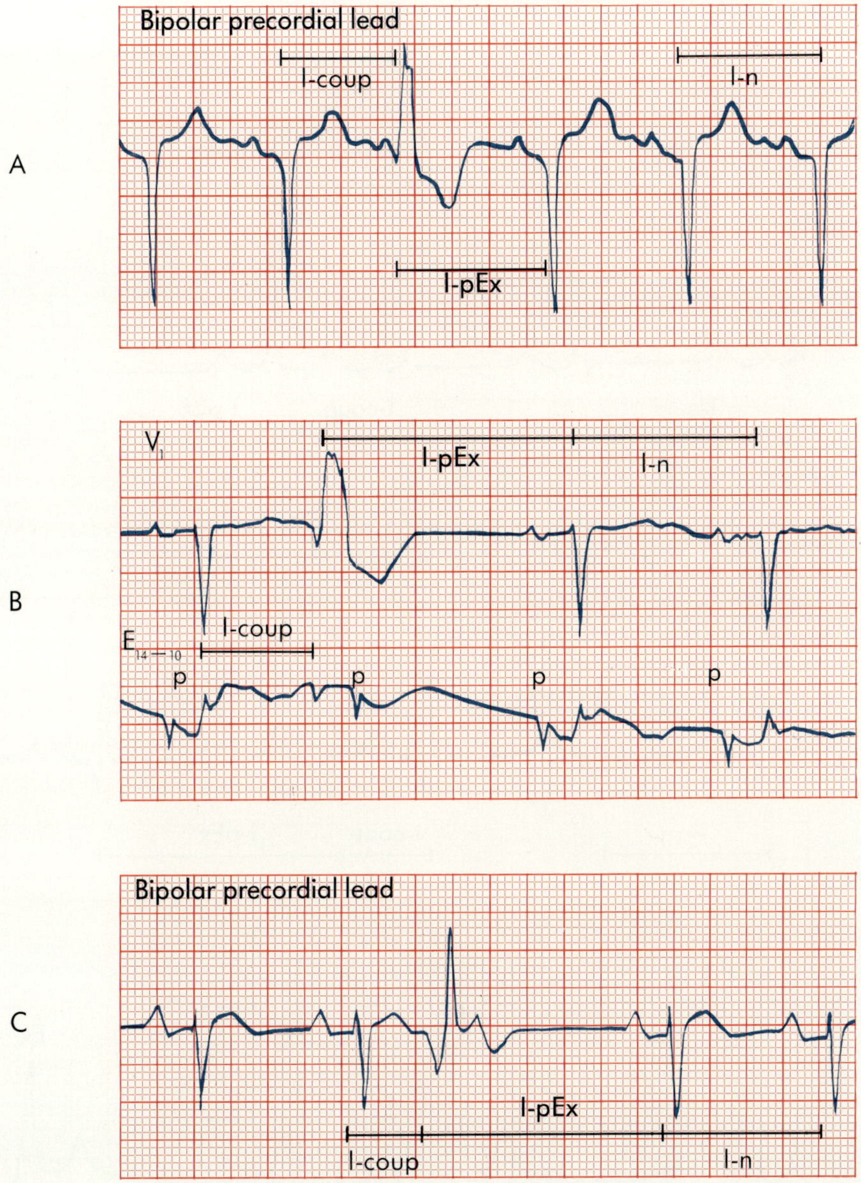

Fig. 5.3
Postextrasystolic compensatory pause and AV dissociation in ventricular extrasystole. I-coup = coupling interval; I-n = normal cardiac cycle. I-pEx = postextrasystolic pause. E_{14-10} = oesophageal lead. For explanation see text

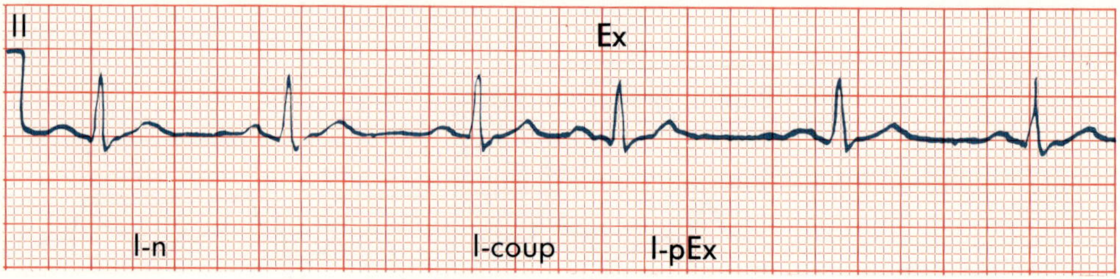

Fig. 5.4
Atrial extrasystole
QRS complex < 0.12 s wide preceded by an upright P wave; non-compensatory postextra-systolic pause

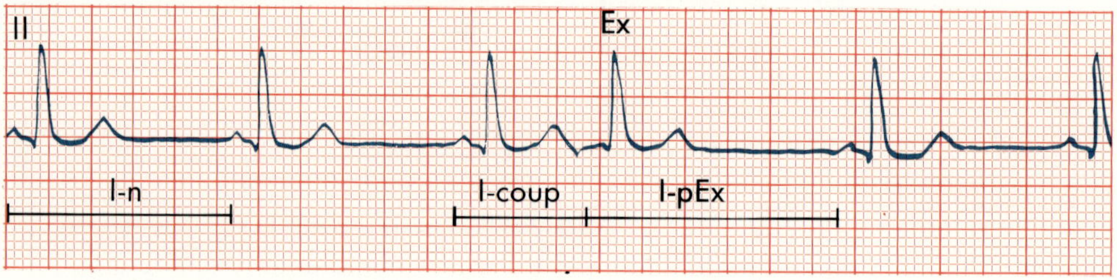

Fig. 5.5
AV nodal extrasystole
QRS complex < 0.12 s preceded by a retrograde P wave, non-compensatory postextra-systolic pause

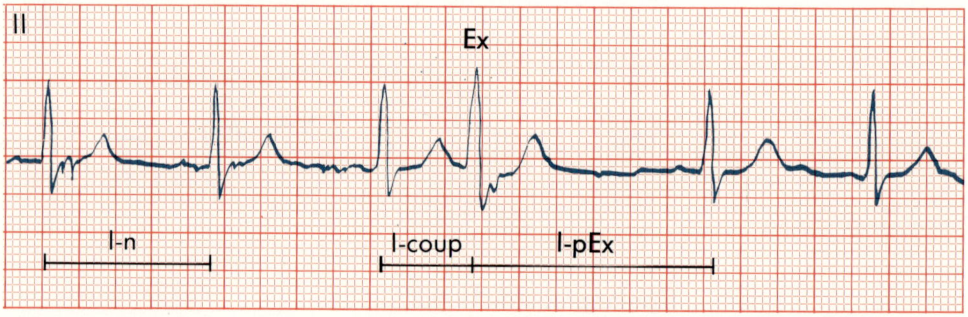

Fig. 5.6
Ventricular extrasystole with non-compensatory postextra-systolic pause. A retrogradely conducted P wave is seen in the latter part of the ST segment of the ventricular extrasystole. It resets the SA node, thus explaining the exceptional finding of a non-compensatory postextrasystolic pause in ventricular extrasystole

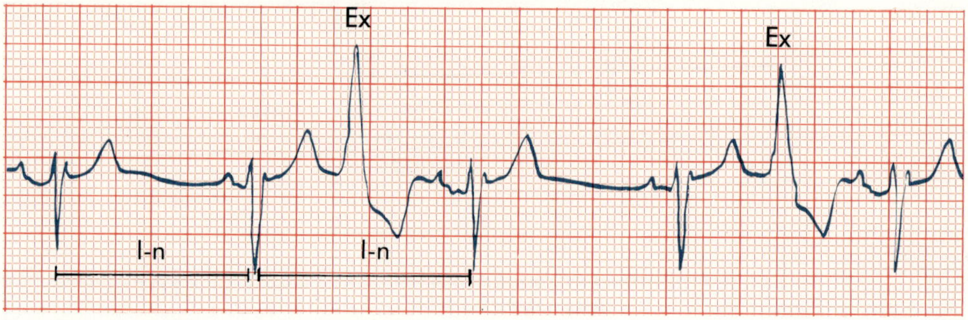

Fig. 5.7
Interpolation in ventricular extrasystole. Sinus bradycardia (56/min) and modest PR interval prolongation in the sinus complex following the inter-polated extrasystole

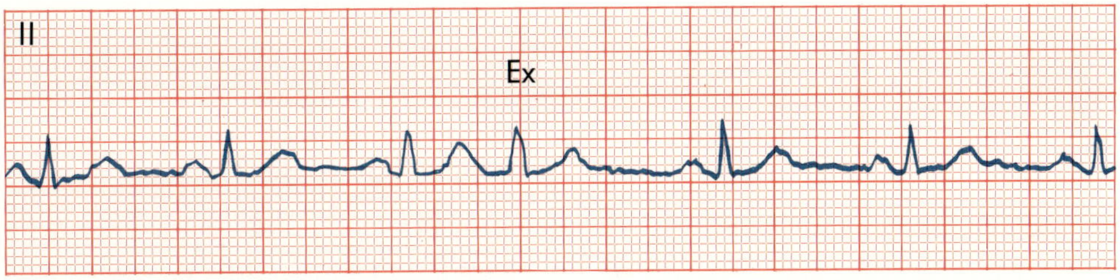

Fig. 5.8
Atrial extrasystole. Narrow QRS (< 0.12 s), preceded by premature upright P in lead II; PR prolonged (0.28 s), non-compensatory postextrasystolic pause

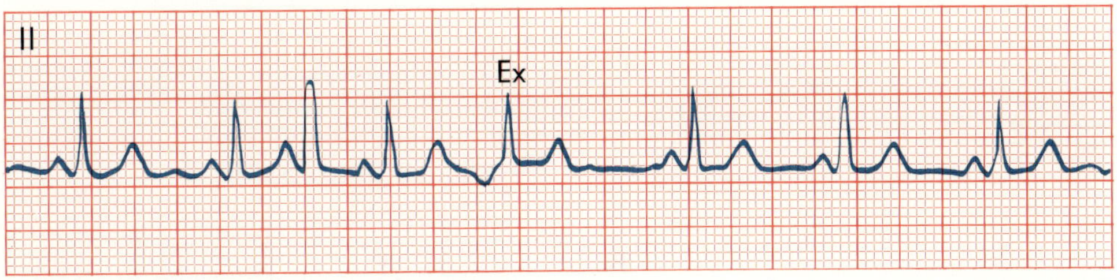

Fig. 5.9
AV nodal extrasystole. Narrow QRS (< 0.12 s) preceded by a premature negative P wave in lead II, non-compensatory postextrasystolic pause

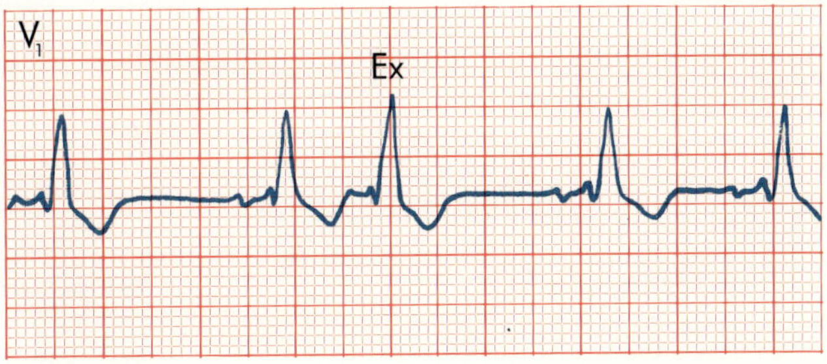

Fig. 5.10
Supraventricular extrasystole (Ex) in a patient with right bundle branch block. The extrasystole is supraventricular as the premature QRS complex is identical to that seen in sinus rhythm i. e. a right bundle branch block pattern. The postextrasystolic pause is non-compensatory. The diagnosis of right bundle branch block is made on the premise: rR′ pattern in lead V_1, QRS complex width 0.13 s ≥ 0.12 s (Fig. 9.4, p. 228)

Supraventricular extrasystoles

ECG diagnosis[2, 4–8]

The common hallmarks in the diagnosis of supraventricular extrasystole are:

1 A premature QRS complex similar to that seen in sinus rhythm which usually means a narrow QRS complex (< 0.12 s) (Figs. 5.1 A, 5.4, 5.5, 5.8, 5.9). A widened QRS complex (≥ 0.12 s) can be seen in the patient with bundle branch block (Fig. 5.10) or, occasionally due to aberrant ventricular conduction (see 4 C below).

2 A premature P wave which can be difficult or impossible to identify because it may be superimposed on the previous T wave or buried in the premature QRS complex. When the P wave is visible, a distinction can be made between atrial and AV nodal extrasystole by the polarity of the P wave and its time relationship to the QRS complex (Fig. 5.4, 5.5, 5.8, 5.9). Occasionally the P wave may be the one and only ECG manifestation of the extrasystole (see 4 A below).

3 A non-compensatory postextrasystolic pause.

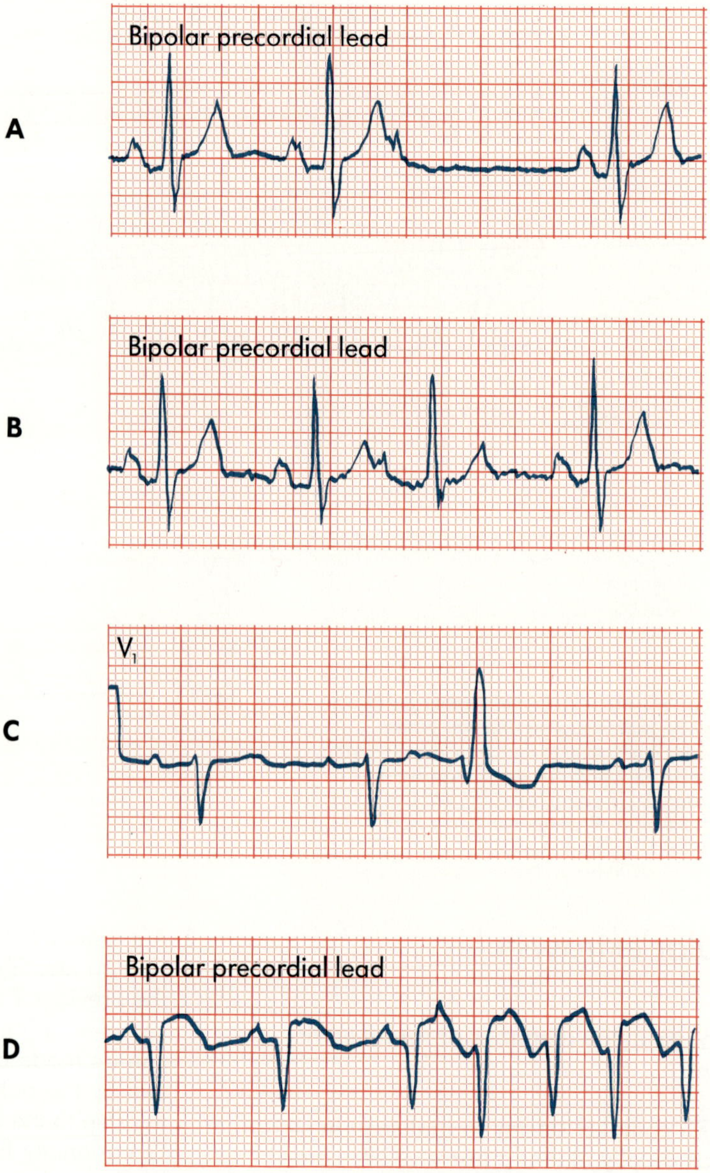

Fig. 5.11
Short coupling interval in supraventricular extrasystole. For explanation see text

4 A short coupling interval can modify the appearance of the supraventricular extrasystole by reason of (Fig. 5.11)

A The absolute refractory period of the AV node (Fig. 3.14 A, page 49). The extrasystole is not AV conducted and thus manifest only as a P wave (Fig. 5.11 A).

B The relative refractory period of the AV node (Fig. 3.14 B). The supraventricular impulse is AV conducted but with a prolonged PR interval (Fig. 5.11 B).

C The refractory period of one but not the other of the two bundle branches (Fig. 3.11, page 46). Because of aberrant ventricular conduction the QRS complex is widened (> 0.12 s) with a bundle branch block pattern, most often a right bundle branch block pattern (Fig. 5.11 C).

D The *vulnerable phase of the atria* (Fig. 3.9, page 44). The premature supraventricular impulse may precipitate atrial fibrillation (Fig. 5.11 D).

Differential diagnosis [2, 4–7]

The differential diagnosis between a supraventricular extrasystole with aberrant ventricular conduction and a ventricular extrasystole can be difficult. The recording of a typical bundle branch block pattern, an only moderate QRS widening to 0.12–0.14 s and a non compensatory postextrasystolic pause (Fig. 5.11 C) are in favour of a supraventricular extrasystole.

The postextrasystolic pause following a non-AV conducted supraventricular extrasystole (Fig. 5.11 A) can be mistaken for SA block (Fig. 11.2, page 281).

Symptoms

Supraventricular extrasystoles most often cause no symptoms but they can be the source of "extrasystolic sensations", described as the heart turning cartwheels, standing still for a moment, or occasionally beating very hard. Some patients can feel even an isolated extrasystole, while others can have many without any sense of discomfort. Moreover, sensitivity to extrasystoles in the same patient can vary greatly from day to day.

Aetiology [9, 10]

Population studies with 24-hour ambulatory ECG monitoring have shown a fairly high incidence of supraventricular extrasystoles in normal individuals. Above the age of forty years up to 200 supraventricular extrasystoles per 24 hours is a common finding.

Slight digitalis overdosage is often associated with supraventricular extrasystoles.

Prognosis

Supraventricular extrasystoles are of no prognostic significance but in patients with paroxysmal atrial fibrillation, attacks may be preceded by increasing numbers of supraventricular extrasystoles.

Management

Symptomatic patients should be reassured about the benign nature of the pulse irregularity. They might be advised against excessive consumption of tobacco, tea, coffee and chocolate which can worsen the tendency for extrasystole. Treatment with beta blocking agents or verapamil might be considered, but is rarely necessary.

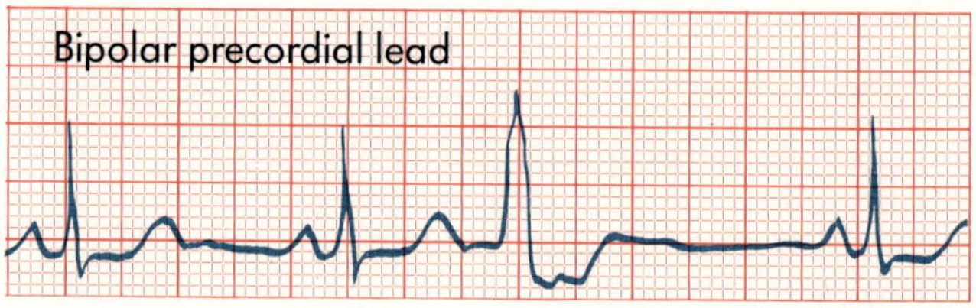

Fig. 5.12
Ventricular extrasystole. Arrives prematurely, the wide QRS complex differs completely from the narrow complex in sinus rhythm, compensatory postextrasystolic pause

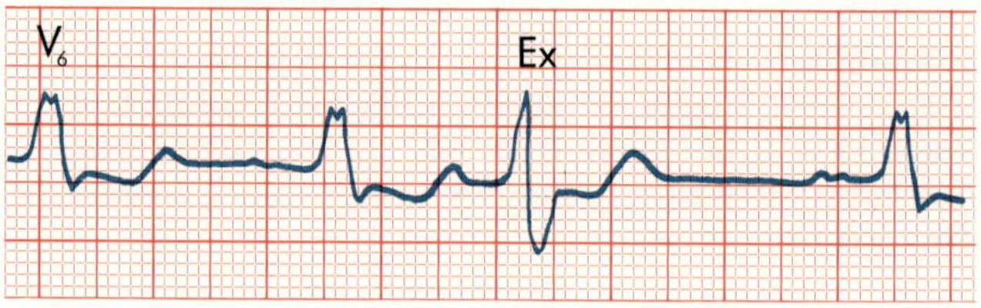

Fig. 5.13
Ventricular extrasystole in a patient with left bundle branch block. The extrasystole is ventricular as the width, axis and pattern of the QRS complex differ completely from that seen in sinus rhythm. The postextrasystolic pause is compensatory. The diagnosis of left bundle branch block is based on the premise: rR′ pattern in leads V_{5-6} and QRS complex width that is ≥ 0.12 s (Chapter 9)

Ventricular extrasystoles

ECG diagnosis [2]

The simple diagnostic hallmarks of ventricular extrasystoles are:

1 A premature, wide, bizarre QRS complex with fixed coupling interval to the preceding QRS complex of the basic cardiac rhythm (Fig. 5.12). In the case of bundle branch block with QRS widening in sinus rhythm the ventricular origin of an extrasystole will be disclosed by a change in QRS configuration and usually also in width (Fig. 5.13).

2 A subsequent compensatory extrasystolic pause (Figs. 5.3, page 111, 5.12, 5.13) or interpolation of the premature QRS complex between two sinus complexes (Fig. 5.7, page 112). Rarely a non-compensatory pause can be seen due to retrograde atrial activation (Fig. 5.6, page 112).

Based on frequency and complexity ventricular extrasystoles are often classified in five degrees according to the criteria proposed by Bernard Lown (Fig. 5.14, page 118).

Differential diagnosis [4–8]

The diagnosis of ventricular extrasystoles is usually very easy, but the following conditions may present differential diagnostic problems:

– Supraventricular extrasystoles with aberrant ventricular conduction (Fig. 5.11 C, page 114)

– Atrial fibrillation and flutter with intermittent aberrant ventricular conduction (Figs. 6.23, page 149 and 6.24, page 150)

– Ventricular parasystole (Fig. 5.15, page 120)

Symptoms

Many patients do not feel the extrasystoles, however frequent they may be; others suffer "extrasystolic sensations" (see supraventricular extrasystoles).

The haemodynamic consequences of ventricular extrasystoles are usually minor if any. Bigeminy may reduce the pulse rate by 50 % due to incomplete diastolic filling of the ventricles prior to the premature ventricular contraction. The reduced pulse rate is well tolerated in the individual with a well preserved myocardium, but may worsen the circulatory condition of the patient who prior to onset of the bigeminy is in congestive heart failure or shock.

Aetiology [9–16]

Ventricular extrasystoles are a common finding in the healthy individual if the cardiac rhythm is followed by 24-hour ambulatory ECG monitoring. The number of extrasystoles increases with age. As a rough guide, an upper limit of "normal" of 100 ventricular extrasystoles may apply until the age of forty and of 200 above this age. Repetitive (paired) and multiform ventricular extrasystole may also be seen in normal individuals. The more frequent and complex the extrasystoles become, however, the more likely is underlying heart disease e.g. acute myocardial infarction, chronic ischaemic heart disease or cardiomyopathy. Ventricular extrasystole, often as bigeminy, is a common sign of digitalis overdosage (Chapter 12, page 292). Ventricular extrasystoles can be induced by treatment with Class I antiarrhythmic drugs, particularly Class IA drugs (quinidine, disopyramide, procainamide) and Class IC drugs (propafenone, flecainide). Hypokalaemia can play a role in the genesis of ventricular extrasystole.

Additional investigations

24 hour ambulatory ECG monitoring by portable tape recorders help assess frequency and complexity of ventricular extrasystole. Exercise ECG is indicated if there is suspicion about ischaemic heart disease and/or complaints of palpitations or tendency for fainting in relation to physical strain. Echocardiography is worthwhile if there is suspicion of underlying cardiomyopathy.

Prognosis [12–17]

This relates to the type and severity of underlying heart disease. In the *otherwise healthy individual* without heart disease and with no history suggesting paroxysms of ventricular tachycardia e.g. no fainting, the prognosis is not significantly different from normal. In the *early stage of acute myocardial infarction* ventricular extrasystole is very common. It has been assumed that the recording of ventricular extrasystoles of Lown grade 3–5 (Fig. 5.14, page 118) could forewarn of paroxysms of ventricular fibrillation but the correlation is poor. In the *survivor of acute myocardial infarction* the risk of death within the first 2 years after discharge from hospital is significantly higher in the group of patients who on ambulatory ECG monitoring 2 to 4 weeks after infarction have ventricular extrasystoles of more than three per hour and/or in runs of three or more (by definition ventricular tachycardia). Many of these patients will also have impaired left ventricular function but the recording of "complex" ventricular arrhythmias contains significant, independent prognostic information.

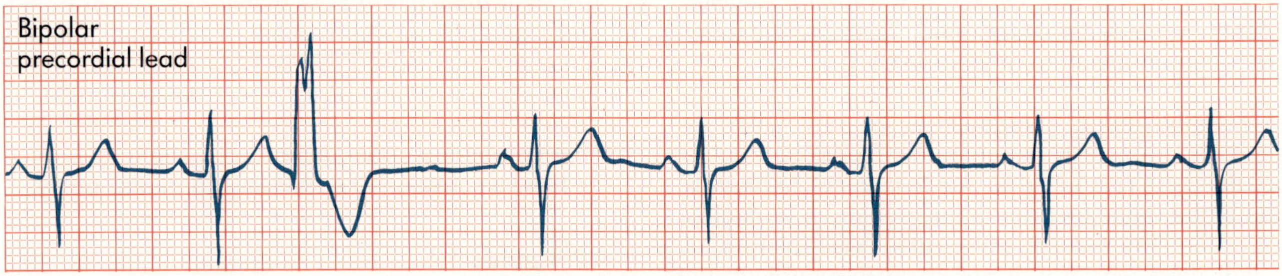

Grade 1: Occasional unifocal ventricular extrasystole

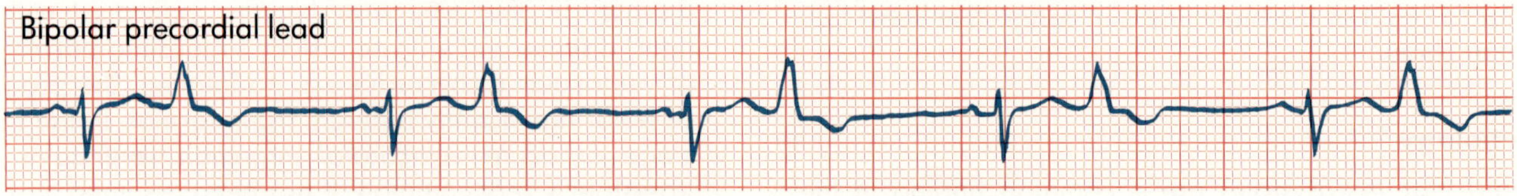

Grade 2: Frequent unifocal ventricular extrasystole in the form of bigeminy (every second complex is an extrasystole)

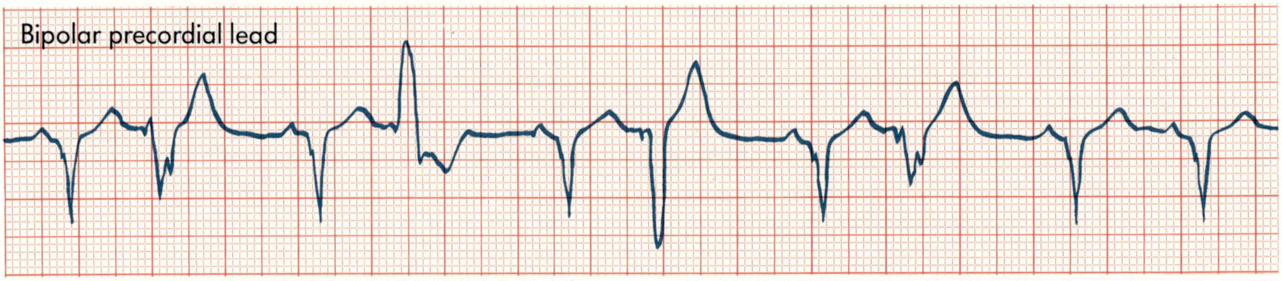

Grade 3: Multifocal ventricular extrasystole with three or four foci involved

Fig. 5.14
Lown's criteria (1975) for a grading system of ventricular extrasystole

Management

Ventricular extrasystoles in the apparently healthy individual

The discomfort from the extrasystolic sensations is often lessened following explanation of the benign nature of the sensations. A reduced consumption of tobacco, coffee, tea and chocolate may reduce the number of extrasystoles. A short-term treatment with a tranquillizer may prove helpful in suppressing symptoms. Antiarrhythmic drug treatment if required is along the lines stated for long-term prophylaxis in paroxysmal ventricular tachycardia. The drug of first choice might be a beta blocking agent; next, a Class IB drug (mexiletine, tocainide) or the combination of a Class IB drug and a beta blocking agent. Class IA drugs (quinidine, disopyramide, procainamide) and Class IC drugs (propafenone, flecainide) should be given only to patients with severe complaints of extrasystolic sensations, due to the risk of proarrhythmic side effects.

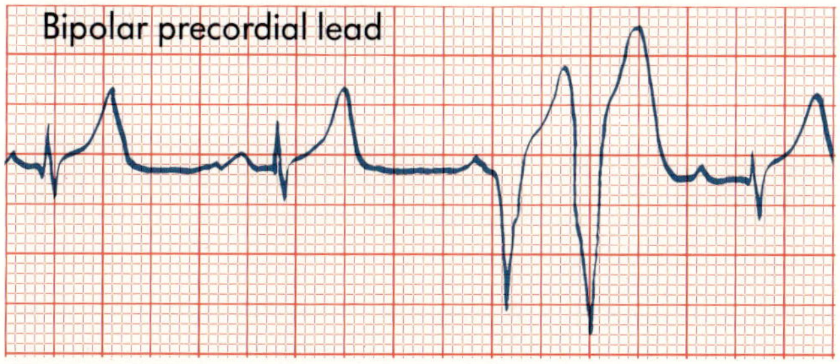

Grade 4: Repetitive ventricular extrasystole
A. Pairs (couplets) of ventricular extrasystoles

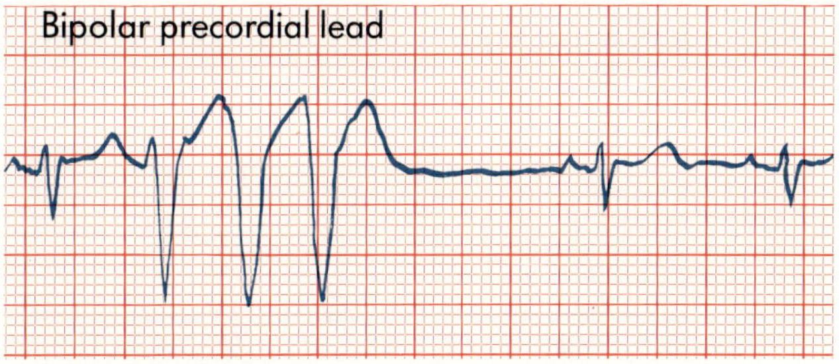

B. Salvos of three ventricular extrasystoles (a brief episode of ventricular tachycardia)

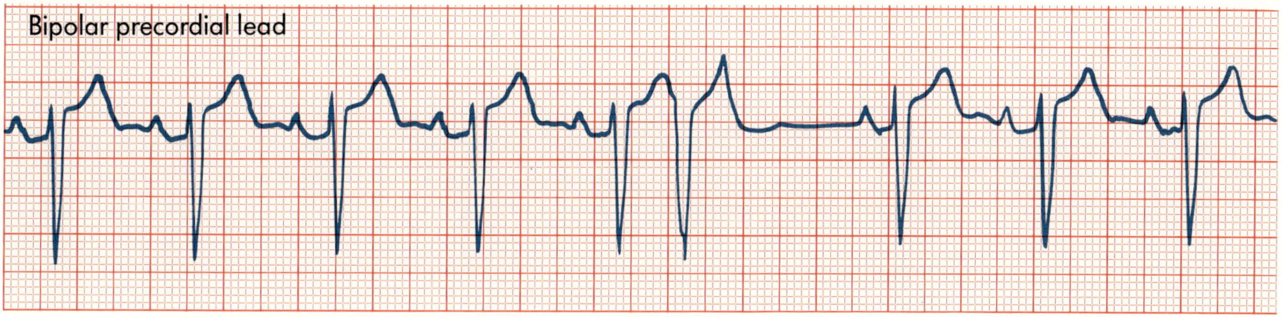

Grade 5: R-on-T phenomenon. Because of the shor coupling interval, the ventricular extrasystole hits the preceding complex within the initial four fifths of the T wave
Fig. 5.14 (continued)

Ventricular extrasystoles in acute myocardial infarction [12]

There is usually no urgency and on the whole few indications for treating ventricular extrasystole in acute myocardial infarction. If for one reason or another (e.g. reduced pulse rate caused by bigeminy) it is found desirable to treat, then lignocaine administered intravenously is often highly effective.

Ventricular extrasystoles in chronic coronary artery disease [13–22]

It has been widely assumed that the suppressive effect of antiarrhythmic drug therapy on the frequency and complexity of ventricular extrasystoles on 24-hour ambulatory ECG monitoring would be reflected by reduction of patients with lethal attacks of ventricular tachycardia and fibrillation in coronary artery disease. However, in several long-term trials with various Class I antiarrhythmic drugs (aprindine, mexiletine and tocainide), all drugs proved effective in reducing the average frequency of ventricular extrasystoles, yet in no trial was the reduction in ventricular extrasystoles associated with a significant reduction in sudden death mortality. In a recent published series of survivors of acute myocardial infarction with a high incidence of complex ventricular arrhythmias (CAST study) treated on a

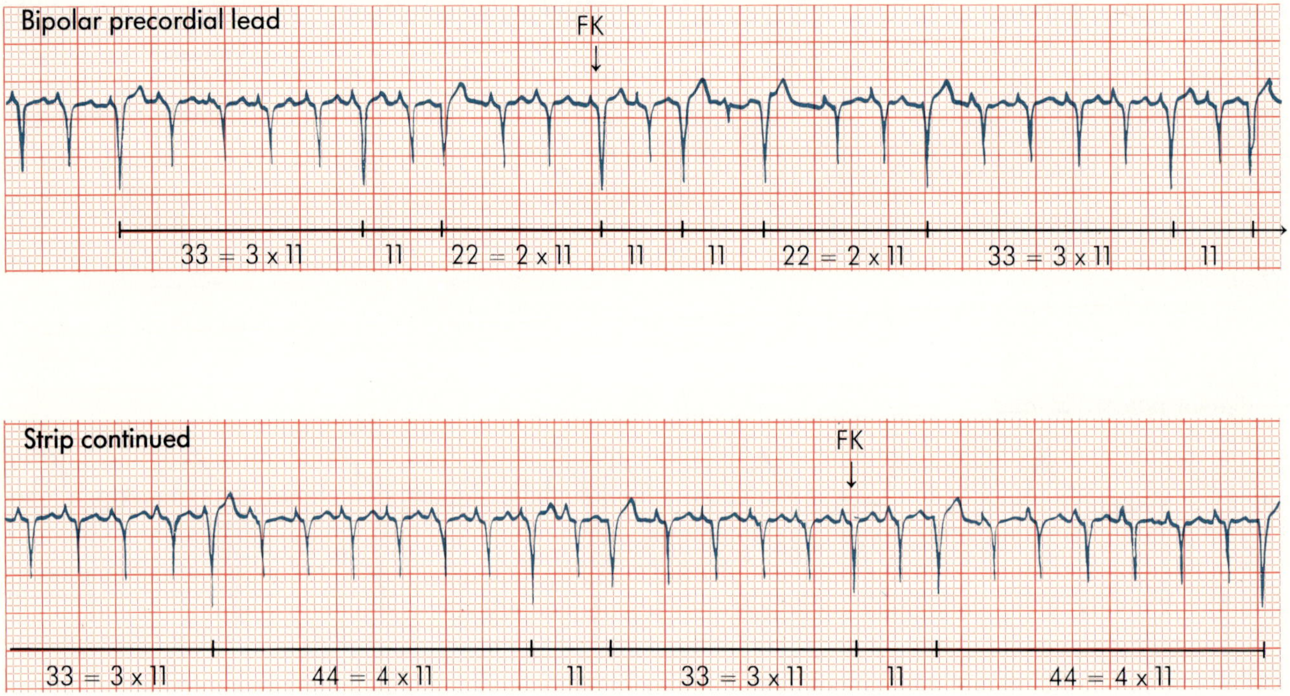

Fig. 5.15
Ventricular parasystole. Paper speed = 10 mm/s. There are a number of ventricular complexes with a distance from the preceding sinus complex varying between 0.60 – 0.80 s. The interectopic interval is a multiple of 1.10 s. The QRS complexes marked FC are fusion complexes since they arrive at the expected time of an ectopic complex are preceded by a sinus P and have a configuration intermediate between that of the normal sinus complex and the ectopic complex

long-term basis (24 months) with the two Class IC agents, flecainide and encainide, mortality was double in the treated group compared to the control series (5.1 % versus 2.3 %).

By contrast, long-term treatment with beta blocking agents has been reported to significantly lower mortality in survivors of acute myocardial infarction over a 2-year period. Patients with and without ventricular extrasystole seemed to benefit equally. Thus, at present long-term prophylaxis with a beta blocking agent appears the treatment of choice in the high risk post infarction patient whether with or without ventricular extrasystoles.

In mild to moderate heart failure, frequency and complexity of ventricular extrasystoles may be significantly reduced by the treatment with angiotensin converting enzyme inhibitors (ACE inhibitors). There is no evidence that treatment with ACE inhibitors increases survival in mild to moderate heart failure, but this has been proven for patients with severe heart failure (NYHA Class III-IV).

Parasystole [2, 6, 23, 24]

Parasystole is a rhythm consisting of dual activation of a single cardiac chamber by two pacemakers (two impulse generating foci). One of the two pacemakers is often the heart's normal pacemaker, the SA node; the other, the *parasystolic pacemaker* is usually a ventricular pacemaker or more rarely an AV nodal pacemaker. The parasystolic pacemaker is protected from being continuously discharged and reset by the normally faster discharging pacemaker of the SA node by *entrance block* located in the vicinity of the parasystolic pacemaker. Entrance block is a *unidirectional* block which prevents impulse penetration from the surrounding myocardium to the pacemaker but does not interfere with impulse propagation in the opposite direction from the pacemaker to the surroundings. The parasystolic pacemaker will thus pace the heart at its own rate and only fail to do so when the myocardium is refractory, e.g. following activation by the SA node, just as the SA node fails to pace the heart after prior activation by the parasystolic pacemaker. Discharge of the SA node and the parasystolic pacemaker will occasionally coincide, in which case the two pacemakers will activate their respective parts of the ventricular myocardium before the two activation waves meet and stop further impulse propagation. Such an event is designated a *fusion complex* and is manifested on the ECG by a QRS complex the configuration of which is intermediate between that of the normal sinus and that of the parasystolic ventricular complex. Similar fusion complexes can be seen in artificial pacing of the heart (Fig. 4.18 B, page 94) and in ventricular tachycardia (Fig. 6.28, page 158).

ECG diagnosis

The following features are characteristic of parasystole (Fig. 5.15):

1 Identical ectopic complexes appearing at varying distances from the preceding normal beat, a phenomenon often described as a "varying coupling interval". The term is easy to remember but admittedly inappropriate, as the "variability" indicates that the ectopic pacemaker is in fact unrelated to the basic cardiac rhythm. Parasystole should be suspected whenever the interval between the ectopic complex and the preceding complex of basic cardiac rhythm varies by more than 0.06 s.

2 The *interectopic intervals* are simple multiples of the same integer, which equal the discharge rate in the parasysto lic pacemaker and can be measured in the ECG as the shortest interectopic interval. However, a precisely constant parasystolic discharge rate is rare; the majority of cases will show variations in the shortest interectopic interval of 0.04 to 0.12 s.

3 *Fusion complexes* (FC) caused by simultaneous activation of the two pacemakers of the ventricular or rarely the atrial myocardium. The fusion complexes have a configuration inter mediate between that of the normal QRS complex and that of the parasystolic QRS complex.

Aetiology, prognosis, management

Parasystole can occur in otherwise healthy individuals but is more often seen in relation to severe organic heart disease. It is usually transient but can persist for years. It is usually of little clinical significance and antiarrhythmic treatment is rarely warranted.

References Chapter 5

1. WHO/ISFC Task Force. Definition of terms related to cardiac rhythm. Europ J Cardiol 1978; 8: 127–44.
2. Scherf D, Schott A. Extrasystoles and allied arrhythmias. London: William Heinemann, 1973; Introduction VII–IX, 45–255, 269–328 and 361–82.
3. Schamroth L. The physiological basis of ectropic ventricular rhythm: A unifying concept. In: Sandøe E, Julian DG, Bell JW, eds. Management of ventricular tachycardia – role of mexiletine. Amsterdam: Excerpta Medica, 1978; 83–128.
4. Blondeau M. Aberrant ventricular conduction. (Functional, paradoxical and intermittent bundle branch block). In: Puech P, Siama R, eds. The cardiac arrhythmias by the arryhthmia working group of the French Cardiac Society. Paris: Corbière and Roussel, 1979; 127–38.
5. Pick A, Langendorf R. Interpretation of complex arrhythmias. Philadelphia: Lea & Febiger, 1979; 3–5 and 367–90.
6. Marriott HJL, Conover MH. Advanced concepts in arrhythmias. Aberrant ventricular conduction: 244–67. Phase 3 and phase 4 block: 155–66. St. Louis: The C.V. Mosby Co., 1983.
7. Schamroth L. Aberrant ventricular conduction. Ingelheim am Rhein: Boehringer Ingelheim Postgraduate Medical Services, 1983.
8. Kennedy RJ. The onset of atrial fibrillation in man. Am Heart J 1971; 82: 429–30.
9. Bjerregaard P. Premature beats in healthy subjects 40–79 years of age. Europ Heart J 1982; 3: 493–503.
10. Ingerslev J, Bjerregaard P. Prevalence and prognostic significance of cardiac arrhythmias detected by ambulatory electrocardiography in subjects 85 years of age. Europ Heart J 1986; 7: 570–75.
11. Campbell RWF. Ventricular ectopic activity and its relevance to aircrew licensing. Europ Heart J 1984; 5 (Suppl. A): 95–98.
12. Campbell RWF, Murray A, Julian DG. Ventricular arrhythmias in first 12 hours of acute myocardial infarction. Natural history study. Br Heart J 1981; 46: 351–57.
13. Møller M. Reliability of serial 24-hour ambulatory electrocardiography in predicting cardiac death after myocardial infarction. Europ Heart J 1982; 3: 67–74.
14. Thayssen P, Møller M, Haghfelt T, et al. Ventricular arrhythmias in relation to coronary artery stenosis and left ventricular performance. Europ Heart J 1982; 3: 35–41.
15. Panidis I, Morganroth J. Sudden death in hospitalized patients: Cardiac rhythm disturbances detected by ambulatory electrocardiographic monitoring. JACC 1983; 2: 798–805.
16. Bigger JT, Jr, Fleiss JL, Kleiger R, et al. For the Multicenter Post-Infarction Group. The relationship between ventricular arrhythmias, left ventricular dysfunction, and mortality in the 2 years after myocardial infarction. Circulation 1984; 69: 250–58.
17. Trappe H-J, Klein H, Wenzlaff P, et al. Arryhthmia profile and sudden death after myocardial infarction and cardiac arrest. J Electrophysiol 1988; 2: 37–45.
18. The Cardiac Arrhythmia Suppression Trial (CAST) In vestigators. Preliminary report: Effect of encainide and flecainide on mortality in a randomized trial of arrhythmia suppression after myocardial infarction. New Engl J Med 1989; 321: 406–12.
19. Julian DG. The arrhythmogenic effects of antiarrhythmic drugs. Europ Heart J 1988; 9 (Suppl. B): 1–4.
20. The Norwegian Multicenter Study Group. Timolol-induced reduction in mortality and reinfarction in patients surviving acute myocardial infarction. New Engl J Med 1981; 304: 801–07.
21. Beta Blocker Heart Attack Study Group. The beta blocker heart attack trial. JAMA 1981; 246: 2073–80.
22. Morganroth J, Lichstein E, Byington R, for the Beta-Blocker Heart Attack Trial Study Group. Beta-blocker heart attack trial: Impact of propranolol therapy on ventricular arrhythmias. Prev Med 1985; 14: 346–57.

22.A Captopril-Digoxin Multicenter Research Group: Comparative effects of therapy with captopril and digoxin in patients with mild to moderate heart failure. JAMA 1988; 259: 539–44

23. Davidenko JM, Nau GJ. Parasystole. In: Zipes DP, Rowlands DJ, eds. Progress in cardiology. Philadelphia: Lea & Febiger, 1988; 171–86.
24. Marriott HJL, Conover MH. Advanced concepts in arrhythmias. Parasystole. St. Louis: The C.V. Mosby Co., 1983; 211–29.

Chapter 6
Tachycardia

Tachycardia [1]

Tachycardia – rapid heart rate – is defined as three or more consecutive impulses at a rate exceeding 100/min. Higher rate limits apply in children with a rate limit of 150–200/min in infancy. The tachycardia is termed *sustained* if it lasts for more than 30 s, and non-sustained if it is of shorter duration.

Based on mode of onset and duration tachycardias are classified as:

1 *Paroxysmal tachycardia* has a sudden onset and offset. Paroxysmal tachycardia often occurs as a chronic intermittent condition with repeated attacks at varying time intervals over a long period of time, years. Used without further qualification the term "paroxysmal tachycardia" relates to this chronic intermittent condition.

2 *Non-paroxysmal tachycardia* starts with a gradual increase in heart rate (almost a physiological heart rate increase). This type of tachycardia is unusual. One rare example is non paroxysmal AV nodal tachycardia associated with digitalis intoxication.

3 *Chronic tachycardia* in which the tachycardia can continue for months or years. A well-known example is chronic atrial fibrillation.

4 *Repetitive tachycardia* which continuously alternates between episodes of tachycardia and sinus rhythm (Figs. 6.12, page 137 and 6.39, page 176).

Supraventricular tachycardia [2–8]

In supraventricular tachycardias impulse formation may emanate from sinus, atrial or AV junctional pacemakers located above the bifurcation of the bundle of His (Fig. 3.10, page 45) or it may be related to atrial flutter (Fig. 6.15, page 141), atrial fibrillation (Fig. 6.21, page 147) or pre-excitation (Fig. 7.1, page 189).

1 *Rate:* The basic diagnostic criterion for supraventricular tachycardia is the recording of three or more consecutive QRS complexes of supraventricular origin at a rate of more than 100/min.

2 *QRS complex:* The characteristic ECG feature in supraventricular tachycardia is a QRS complex similar to that recorded in sinus rhythm. Although closely similar there are commonly minor differences between complexes in tachycardia and those in sinus rhythm. The QRS complex in tachycardia may be slightly wider (but still less than 0.12 s wide), the initial upstroke (or downstroke) may be slurred, the QRS axis somewhat changed and the QRS amplitude increased or decreased. The ST segment may be depressed and the T wave inverted.

The characteristic finding is a slender QRS complex (< 0.12 s wide)(Figs. 3.10, page 45 and 6.1). However, a QRS complex of 0.12 s or more will be recorded in patients who have pre-existing QRS widening due to bundle branch block (Fig. 6.2, page 127). Occasionally, the QRS complex becomes significantly broader with the onset of the tachycardia due to aberrant ventricular conduction (Fig. 6.3, page 128/129).

Aberrant ventricular conduction can occur in any type of supraventricular tachycardia when, at a critical rate, the AV conducted impulse arrives at the bifurcation of the bundle of His just when one bundle branch has recovered and the other is still refractory (Fig. 3.11, page 46). The QRS complex broadens, usually in the range of 0.12–0.14 s. A right bundle branch block pattern, an rR′ pattern in leads V_{1-2} with a small r′ followed by a tall R (often nicknamed "little right, tall left, rabbit ear"), (Fig. 6.3), is recorded in approximately two thirds of the patients. A QRS pattern similar to that recorded in sinus rhythm, but broader, is seen in quite a number of patients. A left bundle branch block pattern with an rR′ pattern in leads V_{5-6} is found in few patients. Aberrant conduction may continue unchanged from the onset of the tachycardia (Fig. 6.3 A). Often, however, aberration will be present only in the first beat (Fig. 6.3 B) – or it can continue for one, two or several beats and then disappear. In supraventricular tachycardias with an irregular rhythm, primarily atrial fibrillation, aberrant ventricular conduction will

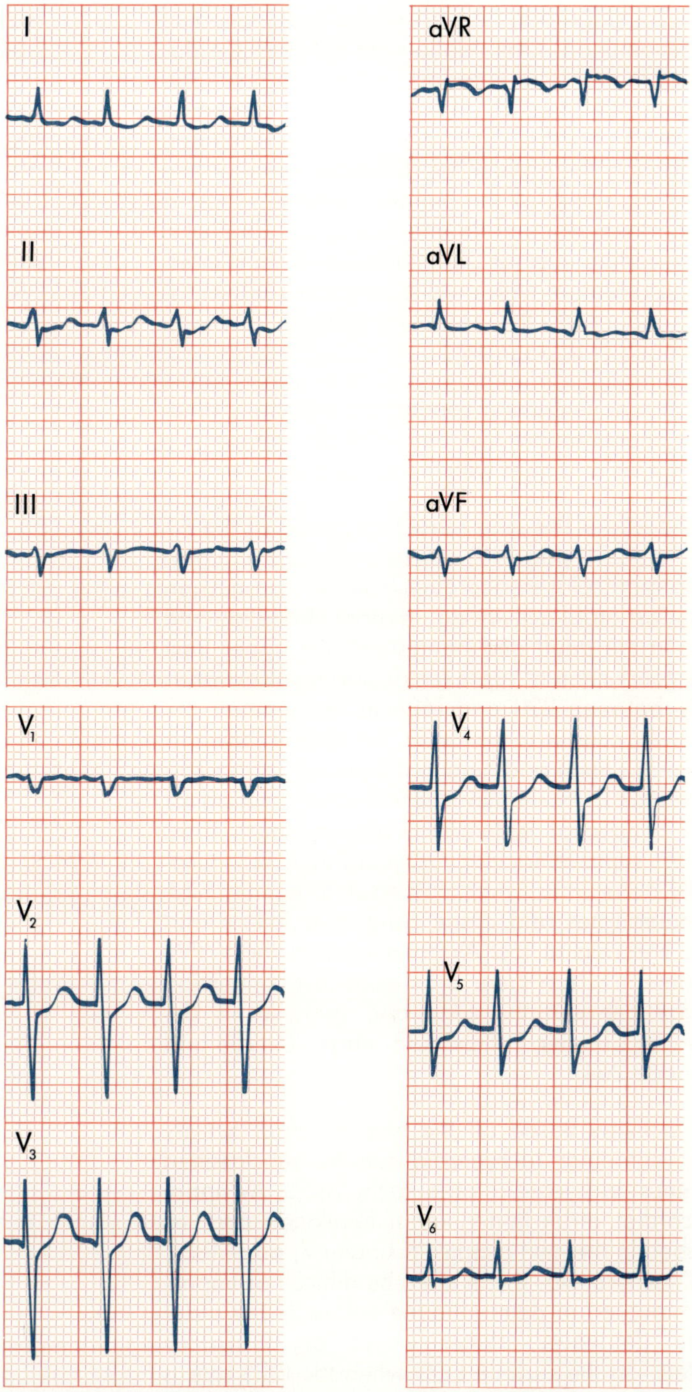

Fig. 6.1
Supraventricular tachycardia (QRS rate 190/min). Narrow QRS (< 0.12 s wide) is the common ECG finding in supraventricular tachycardia. As the tachycardia is regular, atrial fibrillation can be excluded. Further classification of supraventricular tachycardia can be made only after oesophageal ECG recording as atrial activity in this patient is not visible on the surface recording (see also Fig. 6.10, p. 135).

usually be intermittent and irregular in appearance (Fig. 6.23, page 149). A part of the explanation of the phenomenon is the relationship between the duration of the refractory period and the length of the preceding RR interval. The longer the preceding cycle, the longer the refractory period that follows, and, possibly the greater the difference between the refractory periods of the bundle branches. Thus, a long-short sequence of RR intervals in the form of a long preceding interval (X) followed by a short interval (Y) is a feature which will favour aberrant ventricular conduction, the so-called Ashman phenomenon (Fig. 3.11 B, page 46).

The aberrant ventricular conduction is a purely functional phenomenon without clinical significance which comes and goes with the tachycardia.

3 *AV conduction:* The long refractory period of the AV node (Fig. 3.14, page 49) acts as a safeguard to protect the ventricular myocardium from AV transmission of very fast atrial activity e.g. in atrial fibrillation and flutter. In the adult and adolescent, the upper limit for AV conduction of supraventricular impulses varies usually between 220 and 160/min. In general, the limit for AV conduction is low in the elderly (down to 100 impulses/min) and high in the young (up to 250 impulses/min). In infancy the refractory period of the AV conduction system may be very short. Thus, very fast supraventricular tachycardias which occasionally occur in in fancy may result in equally high ventricular rates and cause congestive failure and shock. The risks of fast AV conduction in the WPW syndrome in which there is an extra fast conduction pathway between the atria and ventricles is described in Chapter 7 (Figs. 7.13, page 202/203 and 7.14, page 204).

4 *Atrial activity:* Based on the type of atrial activity supra ventricular tachycardia can be subclassified into: Sinus tachycardia, atrial tachycardia, AV nodal tachycardia, atrial flutter, atrial fibrillation and, as described in the next chapter (Chapter 7, page 188), WPW tachycardia. It can often be difficult or impossible, however, to determine the nature of the atrial activity (P waves, flutter waves or fibrillatory wavelets) on the surface ECG when the QRS rate is fast and the QRST complexes are tightly packed. Thus, in the ECG recordings shown in Fig. 6.1 no P waves are visible in any of the 12 leads of the surface ECG.

Without the additional information given by recordings from an oesophageal or intra-atrial lead, the final diagnosis is "supraventricular tachycardia of unspecified type". Atrial fibrillation can be excluded because of the regularity of the rhythm, which is incompatible with a fibrillatory process (Fig. 3.7, page 44).

A The QRS complex is wide (0.16 s) with a positive, monophasic slightly blurred deflection, a nearby rR′ pattern in lead V_6 and a left bundle branch block pattern (Fig. 9.4, p. 228). If the patient were admitted during an attack of tachycardia, the likely diagnosis, based solely on the QRS complex during tachycardia, would be that of ventricular tachycardia

B When, however, the QRS pattern of (left) bundle branch block remains unchanged after conversion to sinus rhythm as in the present case, the identity of the QRS patterns in tachycardia and sinus rhythm confirms a diagnosis of supraventricular tachycardia

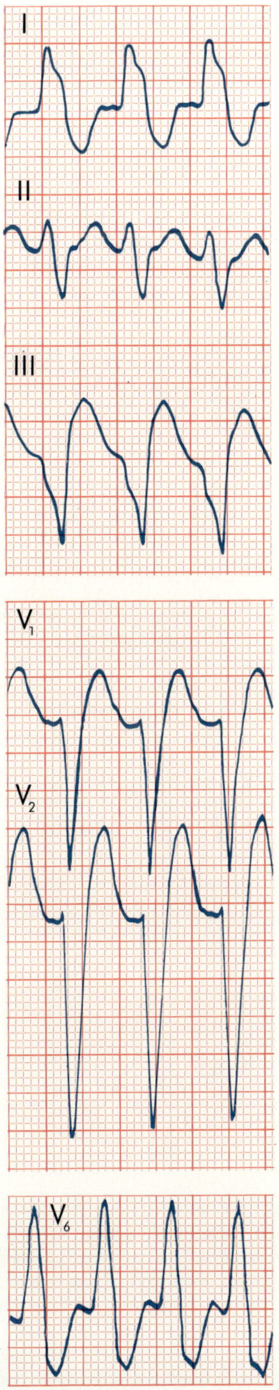

A

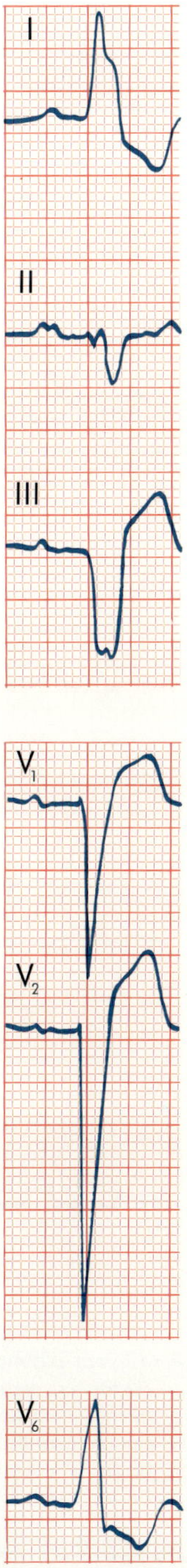

B

Fig. 6.2
Supraventricular tachycardia in a patient with bundle branch block

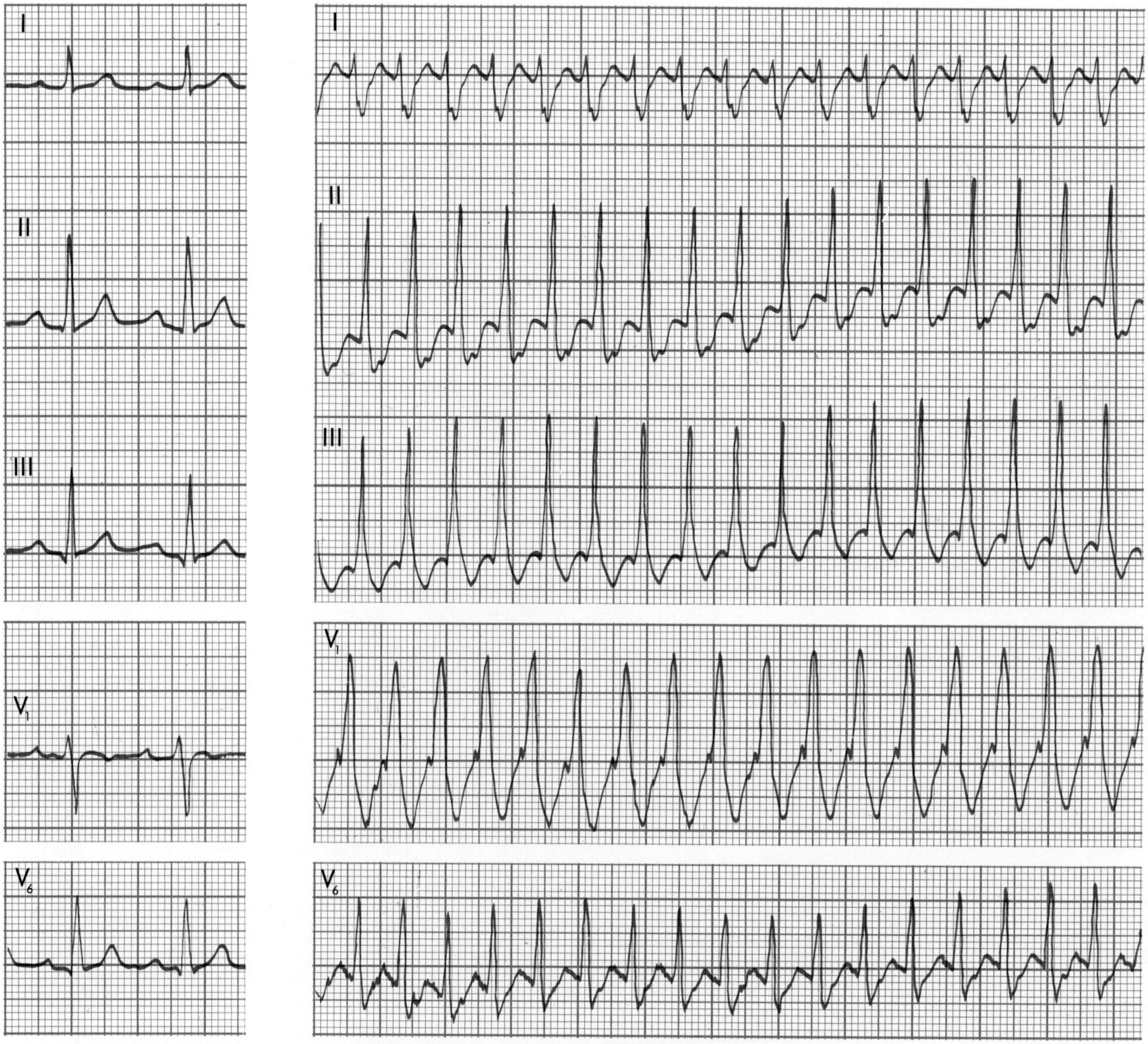

A 35-year-old man with paroxysms of tachycardia since the age of fifteen years. No signs of organic heart disease. To the left: ECG in sinus rhythm is normal. To the right: Tachycardia with regular rhythm and rate of 224/min. The QRS in tachycardia is quite different from the narrow complex recorded in sinus rhythm. The complex is wide (0.14 s) with an rR′ pattern, a right bundle branch block pattern. The right bundle branch block pattern suggests a diagnosis of supraventricular tachycardia but does not countermand a tachycardia of ventricular origin. An electrophysical study confirms a diagnosis of AV nodal tachycardia with aberrant ventricular conduction and a retrograde P wave buried in the QRS complex.

Fig. 6.3: Supraventricular tachycardia with aberrant ventricular conduction

Differential diagnosis

A QRS pattern similar to that of supraventricular tachycardia with aberrant ventricular conduction is produced by ventricular tachycardia. A whole spectrum of additional features characteristic of ventricular tachycardia can in this situation, however, assist in the differential diagnosis (see section on ventricular tachycardia and Figs. 6.25–6.31, page 155 – page 161). Circumstantial evidence in favour of a diagnosis of supraventricular tachycardia with abberant ventricular conduction would be:

- A QRS width of "only" 0.12–0.14 s, and
- A right bundle branch block pattern, *or*
- A QRS configuration similar to that in sinus rhythm.

During ECG monitoring in the CCU and perhaps more so during ambulatory ECG monitoring, artifacts can cause serious differential diagnostic problems for instance the artifact induced by teeth brushing (Fig. 6.4, page 130).

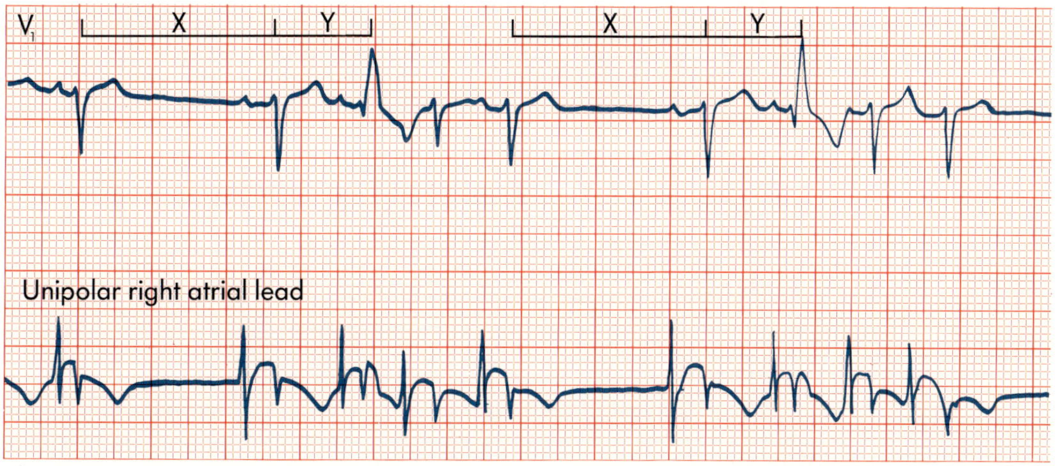

B Repetitive supraventricular (atrial) tachycardia with aberrant ventricular conduction in the first complex of the tachycardia. The first QRS complex in the two short episodes of supraventricular tachycardia, each consisting of three complexes, is widened to 0.12 s. The widening is explained by aberrant ventricular conduction since:

- *The widened complex follows a long-short RR sequence (X-Y) (Ashman phenomenon)*
- *A P wave is visible between the widened QRS complex and the T wave of the preceding sinus complex*
- *The widened complex presents with an rR′ pattern in lead V_1 i. e. a right bundle branch block pattern (Fig. 9.3 and 9.4, p. 227/228)*

Fig. 6.3

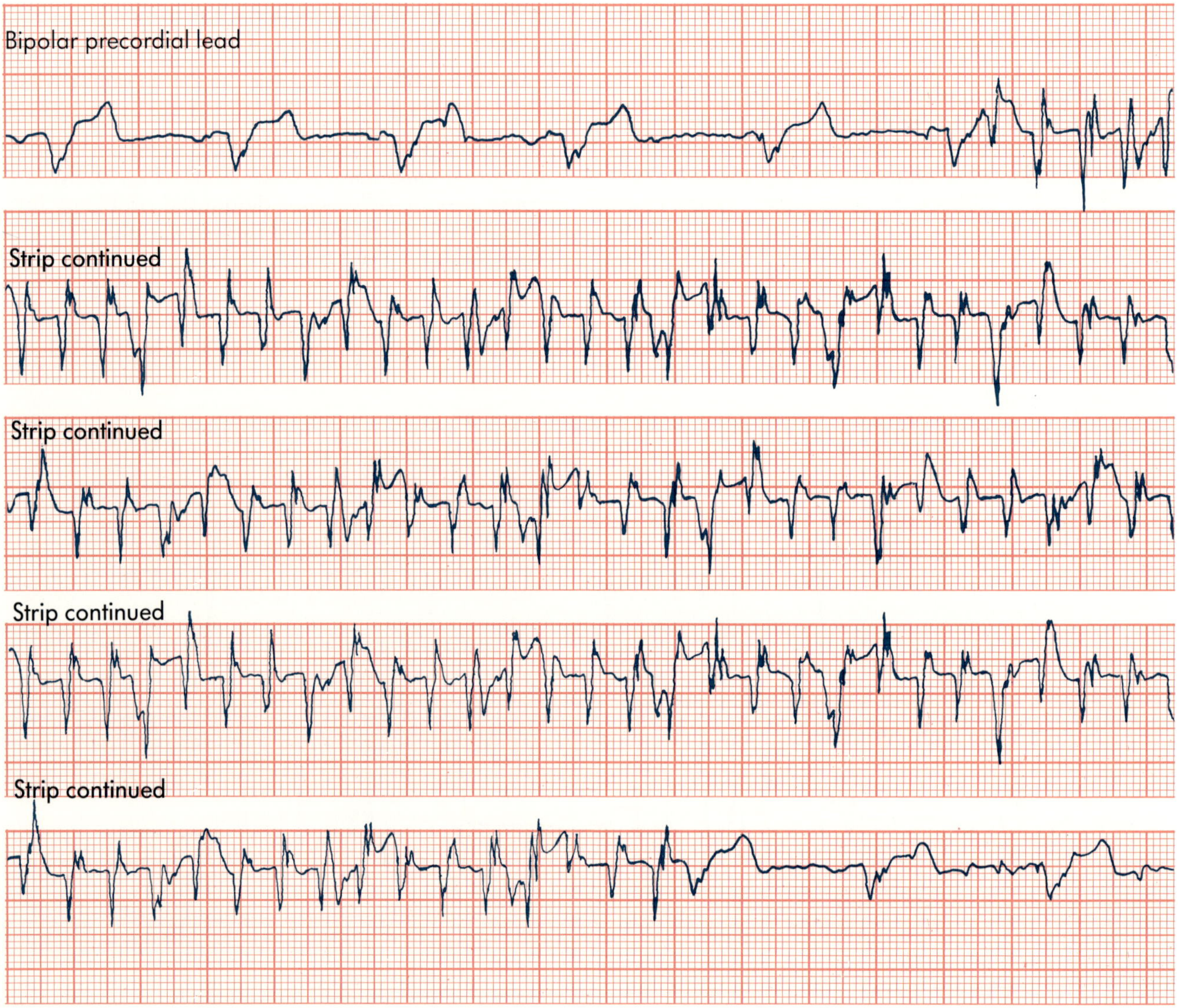

Fig. 6.4
Artifact supraventricular tachycardia induced by teeth-brushing. 25-year-old woman admitted to hospital due to fainting of unknown aetiology. The ECG strip was recorded by telemetry in the early morning. The patient felt no discomfort of any type during the recording. She was peacefully brushing her teeth at a brushing movement rate which assessed from the ECG was 255/min. Such ECG artefacts simulating fast supraventricular tachycardia are frequent during teeth brushing. The artifactual nature of the phenomenon appears from the "cast" of the original QRS complex which with some imagination can be recognized as appearing at an unchanged regular rhythm and rate throughout the episode of "tachycardia".

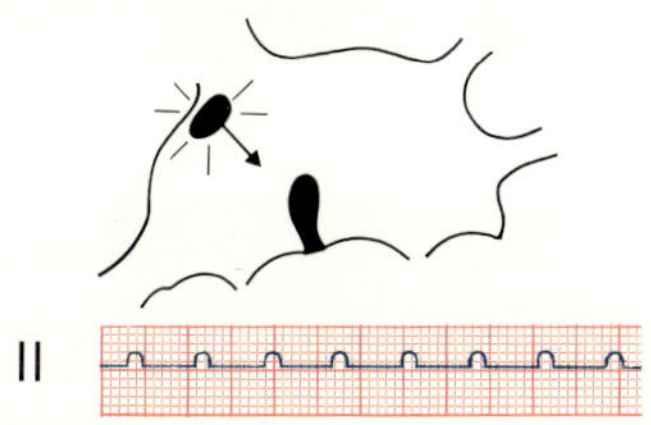

Fig. 6.5
P waves in sinus tachycardia

Sinus tachycardia [2, 3]

The pacemaker impulses emanate from the SA node (Fig. 6.5). The increased discharge rate is usually due to enhanced automaticity. A rare form of sinus tachycardia, repetitive sinus tachycardia is due to micro re-entry in the region of the SA node.

ECG diagnosis

The P wave is visible ahead of the QRS complex with a PR interval appropriate for the heart rate. The P wave is identical to that recorded in normal sinus rhythm with positive polarity in leads I, II and V_6 and usually also in III and aVF (Fig. 6.6). The atrial rate is 100–130–(140)/min, seldom faster.

Symptoms

These relate to the underlying disease or condition.

Aetiology

Sinus tachycardia usually occurs as a physiological response to shock, fever, anxiety, thyrotoxicosis, heart failure, acute myocardial infarction etc. Sinus tachycardia can be provoked or accelerated by parasympatholytic agents (atropine, ipratropium bromide, disopyramide) or sympathomimetic drugs (adrenaline, isoprenaline).

Additional investigations

X-ray of the chest, laboratory tests (haemoglobin, plasma T_3 and T_4) etc.

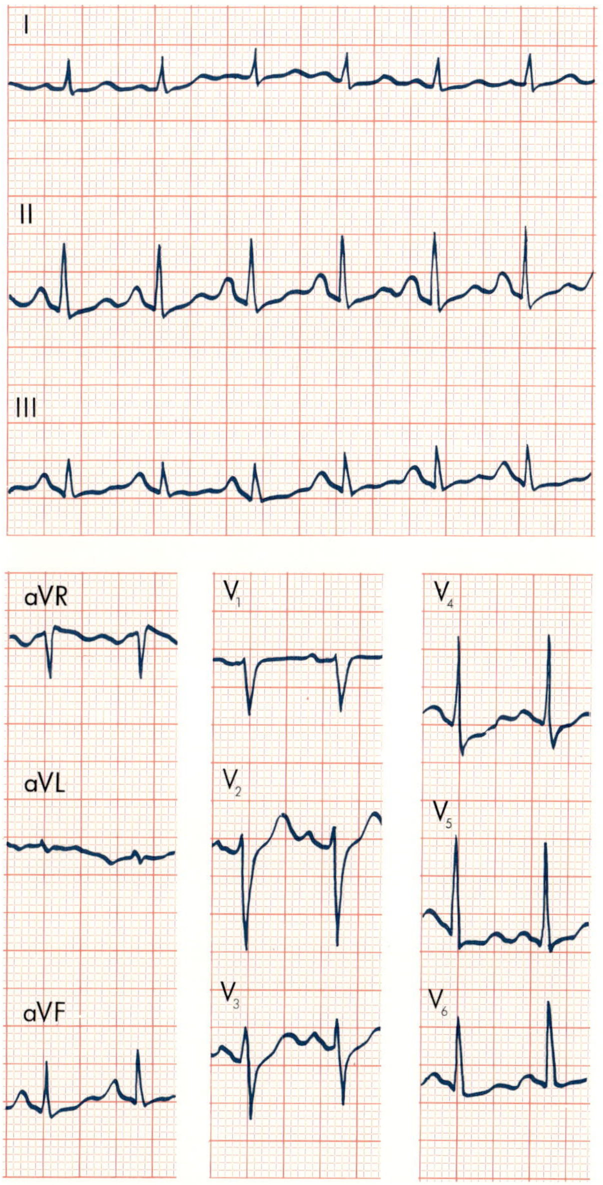

Fig. 6.6
Sinus tachycardia. Upright P waves in leads I, II, aVF, V_{5-6} of the same configuration as sinus P waves. QRS rate 117/min

Management

Diagnosis and treatment of the underlying disease is usually the only form of management which is required. In the symptomatic patient beta blocking agents might be considered.

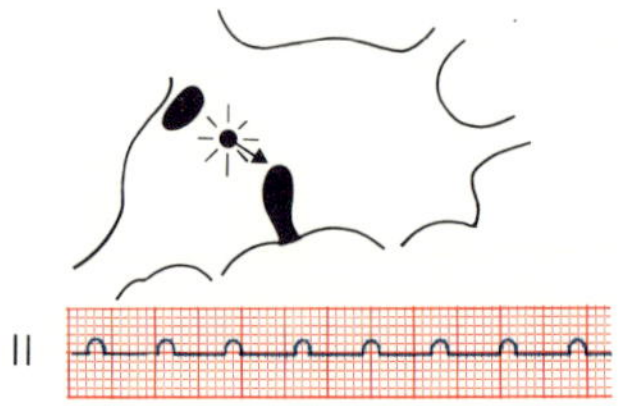

Fig. 6.7
P waves in atrial tachycardia

Atrial tachycardia [2–5, 9–13]

Atrial tachycardia is a rare type of supraventricular tachycardia. The pacemaker usually is located in the upper part of the right atrium (Fig. 6.7), sometimes in the lower part, rarely in the left atrium.

ECG diagnosis

P waves are recorded ahead of the QRS complex with a PR interval appropriate for the heart rate, or, not infrequently, prolonged. The P waves are different in configuration to the sinus P waves. When the pacemaker site is in the upper part of the right atrium (Fig. 6.7) they will be of the same polarity: positive in leads I, II, V_6 and usually also in III and aVF. When the pacemaker site is in the lower part of the atrium there is retrograde activation of the atria with negative polarity P waves in leads II, III and aVF. The P wave can be superimposed on the preceding T wave and thus difficult to identify (Fig. 6.8 A). When P waves are visible they are distinct from each other with an intervening isoelectric segment – the characteristic "isoelectric shelf" (Fig. 6.8 B). A common finding is an AV conduction ratio of 1:1 (Fig. 6.8 A) but a 2:1 ratio may sometimes be seen or an irregular alternation between a 1:1 and 2:1 ratio, often accompanied by changes in the length of the PR interval (Fig. 6.8 B) and termed *paroxysmal atrial tachycardia with block.*

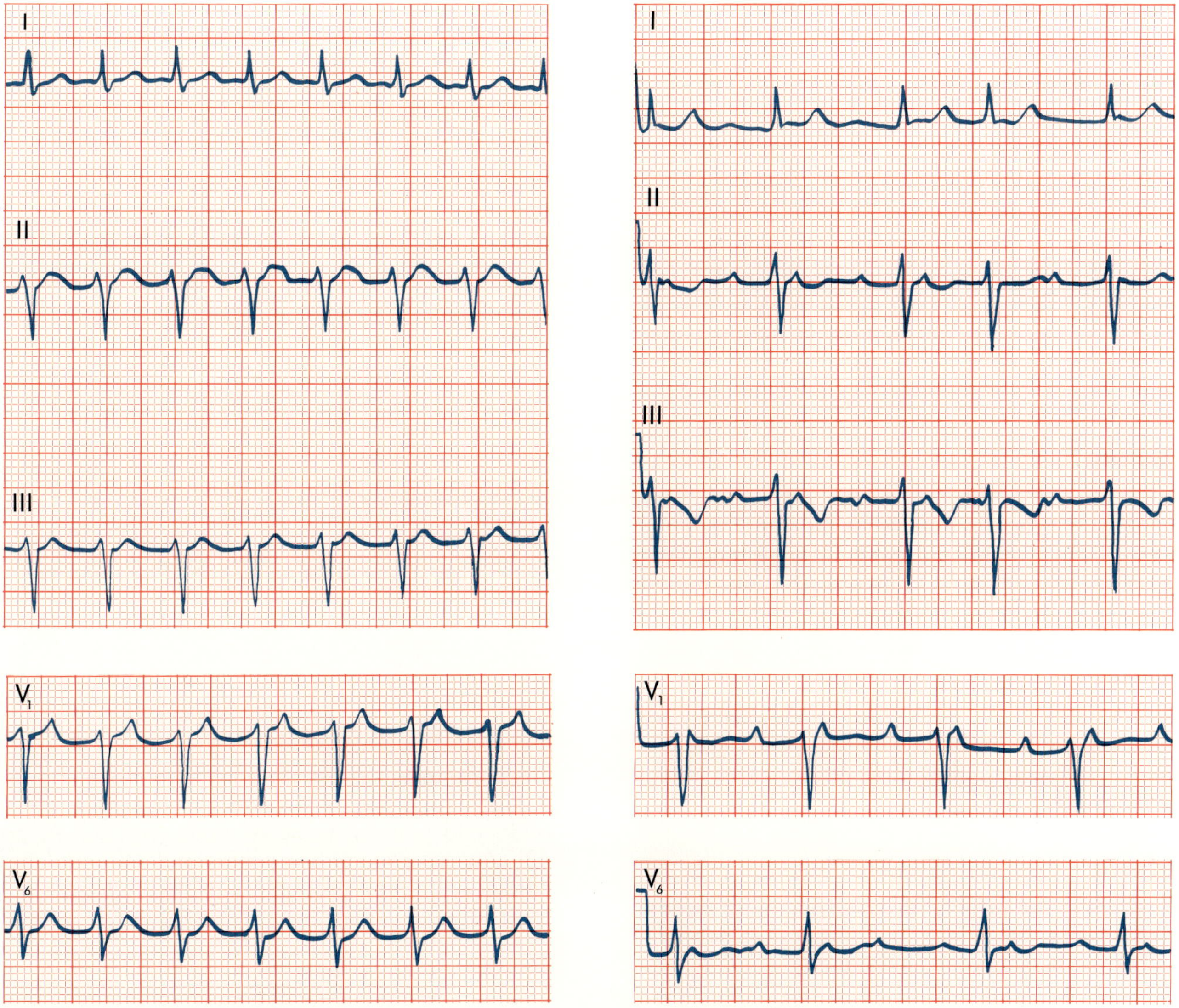

A Atrial and ventricular rate 140/min, AV conduction ratio: 1:1, PR interval: 0.24 s

B Atrial rate 150/min, ventricular rate 90/min, AV conduction ratio: 2:1 and 3:1, PR interval: 0.22–0.34 s

Fig. 6.8
Atrial tachycardia. P waves upright in lead II with an intervening isoelectric shelf. ECG from a 42-year-old male with leukemia (autopsy showed leukemic infiltration of the atrial and ventricular myocardium).

Differential diagnosis

The following differential diagnoses should be considered:

- *Sinus tachycardia*: P wave rate > 150/min is against sinus tachycardia
- *AV nodal tachycardia* and *WPW tachycardia:* In these the P wave reflects retrograde atrial activation (negative in lead II) with a typical time relationship to the QRST complex (Fig. 6.11, page 136)
- *Atrial flutter:* Flutter waves may be seen. They are continuous with one flutter wave merging into the next (Fig. 6.16, page 141) contrasting with the distinct P waves separated by an "isoelectric shelf" which is typical for atrial tachycardia (Fig. 6.8 B, page 133).

Symptoms

These relate to the tachycardia rate and to the severity of underlying heart disease. Unless the rate is very high (above 200/min) individuals without underlying heart disease can tolerate atrial tachycardia for long periods of time with only minor symptoms.

Aetiology

Similar to that of AV nodal tachycardia. Paroxysmal atrial tachycardia with block may occur with digitalis intoxication but is more often observed unrelated to digitalis therapy (Fig. 6.8 B).

Prognosis

This relates to the severity of underlying heart disease. The recurrence rate is high, but prognosis is normal in an otherwise healthy young individual.

Additional investigations

Drug refractory paroxysmal atrial tachycardia should be referred to a cardiological center for electrophysiologic studies.

Management

As for AV nodal tachycardia.

AV nodal tachycardia [2–5, 12, 14, 15]

The pacemaker site usually is in the AV node (Fig. 6.9). A high proportion of AV nodal tachycardias are secondary to re-entry in the AV node (Fig. 3.5 A, page 42). An exception is non-paroxysmal AV nodal tachycardia which most probably is related to triggered automaticity.

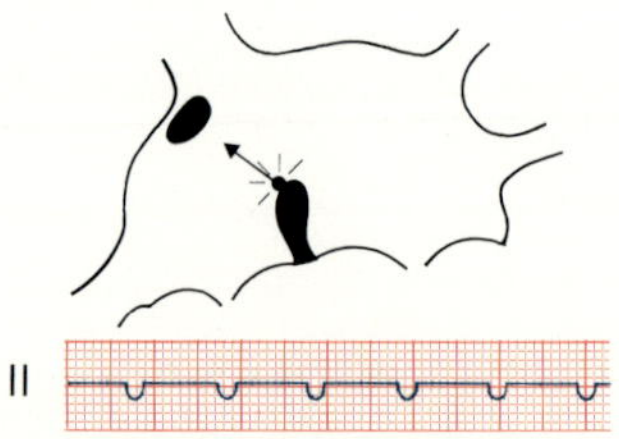

Fig. 6.9
Retrograde P waves in AV nodal tachycardia

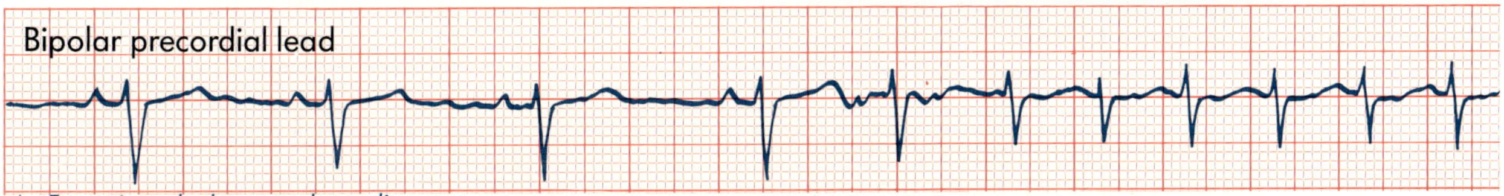

A From sinus rhythm to tachycardia

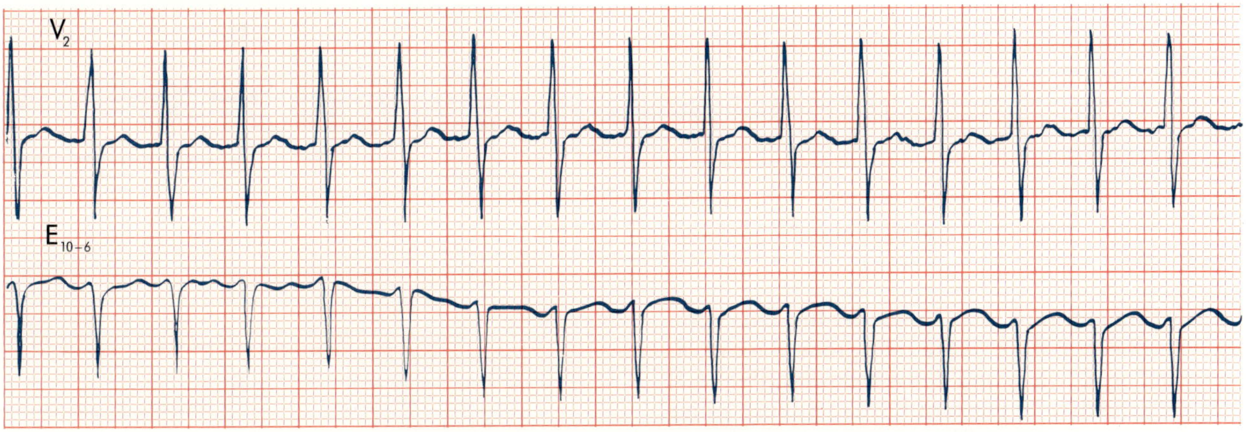

B Oesophageal ECG recording (E_{10-6}) reveals one P wave hidden in every QRS complex, suggesting a diagnosis of AV nodal tachycardia

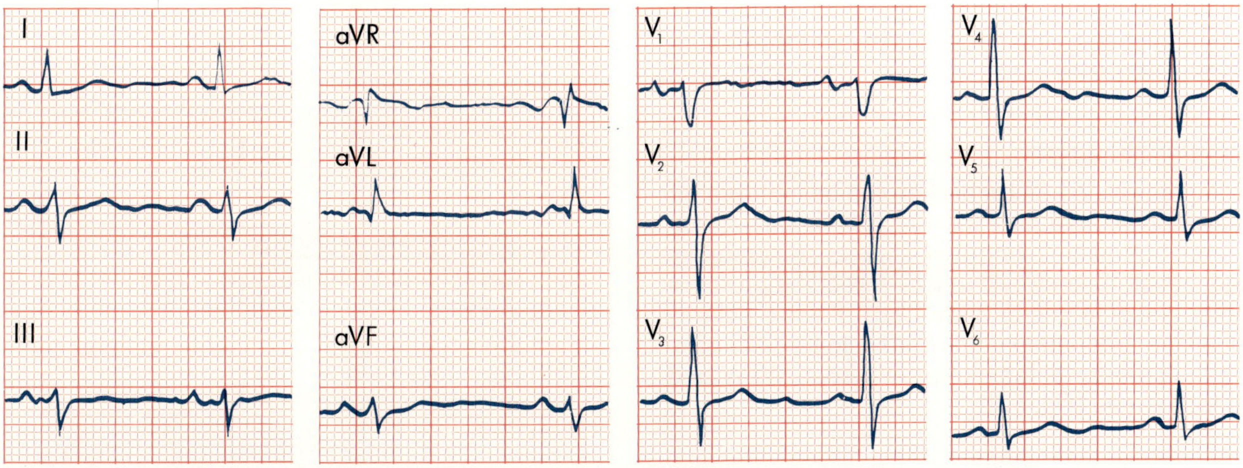

C A 12-lead ECG during sinus rhythm. The diagnosis of supraventricular tachycardia was confirmed by electrophysiological studies in the cardiac laboratory demonstrating that the tachycardia could be precipitated by critically timed impulses applied to the septum in the inflow tract of the right ventricle

Fig. 6.10
AV nodal re-entry tachycardia (Fig. 6.1, p. 125 from the same patient). ECG during tachycardia shows narrow QRS complexes at a regular rhythm rate of 150/min but no P waves. Oesophageal ECG shows a P buried in the QRS suggesting a diagnosis of AV nodal re-entry tachycardia, a diagnosis later confirmed by electrophysiologic studies.

ECG diagnosis

When visible the P waves reflect retrograde activation of the atria (opposite in polarity to sinus P) so they are negative in lead II and usually also in leads aVF and III. Because they often coincide with the QRS (see below), the P waves usually cannot be seen on the surface ECG. The time relationship between the P wave and the QRS complex varies as follows (Figs. 6.11 and 3.13, page 48):

A About two thirds of the patients with AV nodal re-entry tachycardia have simultaneous atrial and ventricular activation and on the ECG the P wave is buried in the QRS complex (Fig. 6.11 A).

B The majority of the remaining patients have an inverted P wave immediately after the QRS complex (Fig. 6.11 B).

C In a few patients the P wave precedes the QRS complex with $R_1P' > P'R_2$ (P' is the retrograde P wave, R_1 the preceding R wave and R_2 the following)(Fig. 6.11 E). Most patients with this rare P wave pattern suffer from incessant repetitive AV nodal re-entry tachycardia (Fig. 6.12).

The atrial rate is most often 140–180/min but rates up to 250/min may occur.

Differential diagnosis

Atrial flutter with 2:1 AV conduction can be mistaken for AV nodal tachycardia since the trough between two flutter waves can mimic retrograde P waves. A careful inspection of all 12 leads will usually reveal the presence of flutter waves in one or more leads. P wave polarity and the time relationship of the P wave to the QRS complex is the basis for differentating AV nodal, WPW and atrial tachycardia (Fig. 6.11).

Symptoms

These relate to the duration of attack, the heart rate and the severity of underlying heart disease. In an otherwise healthy young individual the paroxysm of tachycardia usually is associated with a feeling of palpitations or fluttering in the chest. Some patients do not recognize the rapid heart rate at all, complaining only

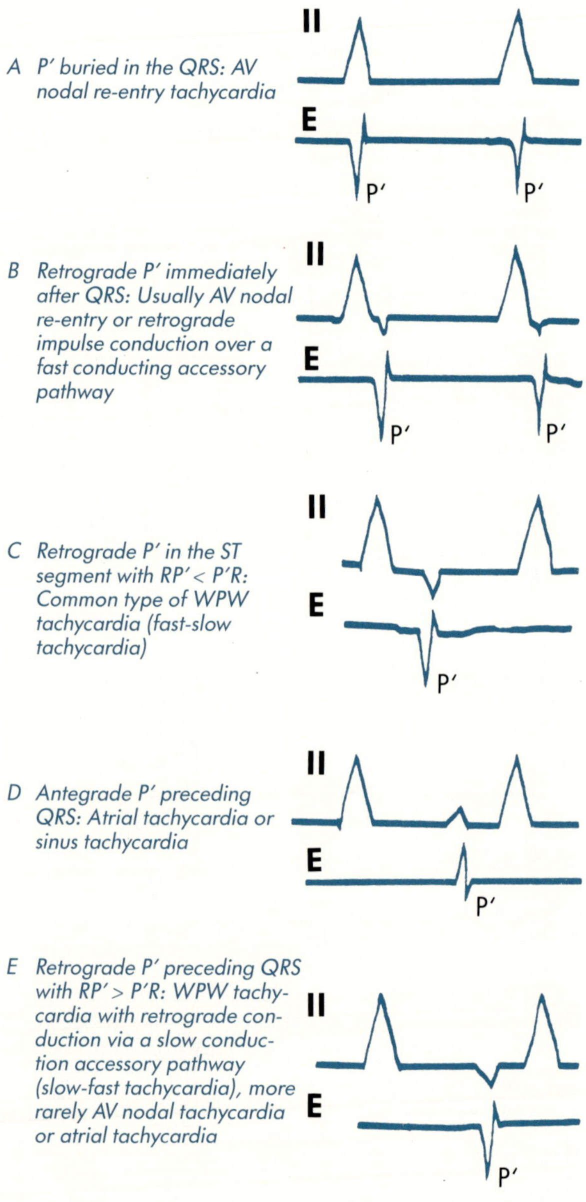

Fig. 6.11
Differential diagnosis of supraventricular tachycardias (QRS < 0.12 s) from timing and polarity of the P wave. ECG recorded in a bipolar standard lead (II) and an oesophageal lead (E).

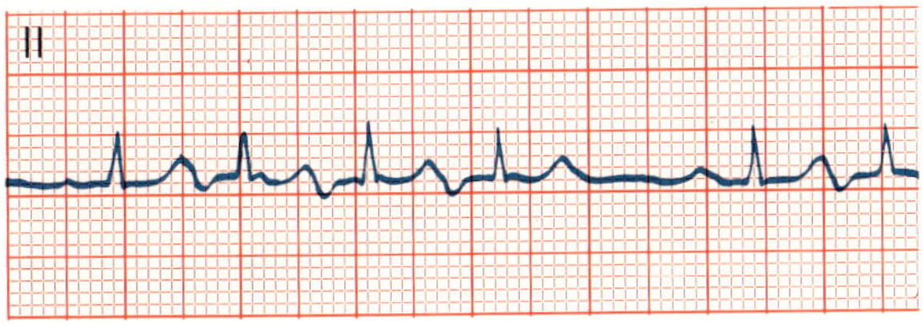

Fig. 6.12
Repetetive AV nodal re-entry tachycardia of the incessant type. 26-year-old woman with a consistent heart rate of 130-150/min most likely since birth. Normal functional capacity, no symptoms. Slight dilatation of the left ventricle at echocardiography, otherwise no sign of heart disease. Two sequences of tachycardia with an intervening sinus PQRST complex. The tachycardia is most likely AV nodal as the P waves are retrograde and the QRS complexes are narrow and identical to the sinus complex. QRS rate in tachycardia 150–180/min.

of more vague symptoms such as anxiety, breathlessness, fatigue or dizziness. The paroxysms are often followed or sometimes accompained by frequent micturation (urina spastica).

Aetiology

Isolated episodes of AV nodal tachycardia can be precipitated by infection (primarily pneumonia) and acute cardiac conditions such as acute myocardial infarction and pulmonary embolism. Usually, the attack of tachycardia starts suddenly but another form, traditionally called *"non-paroxysmal AV nodal tachycardia"* is characterized by a gradual rate increase from 60/min up to, but usually to not more than 130/min over the course of hours or days. This form is related to digitalis intoxication (Chapter 12, page 292). Paroxysmal AV nodal tachycardia with recurrent attacks over a long period of time, weeks, months or years occurs in a great variety of chronic cardiac diseases including chronic ischaemic heart disease, cardiomyopathy and valvular disease.

In an otherwise healthy young individual with paroxysmal supraventricular tachycardia, AV nodal re-entry tachycardia counts for more than half the cases (WPW tachycardia for an additional 40 % and atrial tachycardia for a few percentage). The paroxysms of AV nodal re-entry tachycardia can start in childhood, adolescence or adulthood, but once experienced, the arrhythmic recurrence rate is high but varies greatly with unpredictable arrhythmic free intervals of from days to years.

Prognosis

This relates to underlying heart disease. Prognosis in an otherwise healthy young individual with paroxysmal AV nodal re-entry tachycardia is most likely normal.

Management

Acute attack

1 *Search/treat for precipitating cause:* E.g. digitalis intoxication, infection, pneumonia.

2 *Try vagal manoeuvres:* Carotid massage, the Valasalva manoeuvre, squatting, "finger down the throat" etc.

3 *Intravenous therapy:* Verapamil, or a class IC drug (ajmaline, propafenone, flecainide) or a class IA drug (procainamide, disopyramide, quinidine).

4 If tachycardia continues or haemodynamic unstability prevails, *cardioversion* with an initial shock of 50 J.

Long term management

No therapy is indicated for the asymptomatic individual, for the patient with infrequent and well tolerated attacks or for patients who can readily terminate attacks with a vagal manoeuvre. Vagal manoeuvres are "cheap" and "free from unwanted effects". Patients should be encouraged to try the whole spectrum of vagal manoeuvres to identify by trial and error which manoeuvre or combination of manoeuvres is ideal for them.

Intermittent oral therapy is appropriate for the patient with infrequent but sustained attacks of tachycardia. Therapy is given as an oral loading bolus at the onset of palpitations followed by subsequent lesser doses at 4 or 6 hour intervals. The tachycardia will terminate when an adequate plasma level of the medication has been achieved.

Long-term pharmacologic prophylaxis is the most common form of treatment for the patient with frequent and sustained attacks. Alternatives for drugs of "first choice" include verapamil, Class IC drugs (propafenone, flecainide), Class IA drugs (quinidine, procainamide, disopyramide) and beta blocking agents. If not effective when given alone, a Class I drug may be given in combination with a beta blocking agent. Amiodarone often will be effective where other drugs have failed, but because of its potentially serious side effects it should (in the opinion of authors) be reserved for refractory patients.

Depending on the clinical situation and the available technical facilities and expertise, either empiric drug testing by the trial and error method or serial electrophysiological drug testing are used to select the optimal medication. In a young individual with frequent attacks of AV nodal re-entry tachycardia, antitachycardia surgery (Chapter 4, page 84) has become a promising alternative to life long antiarrhythmic drug therapy. An antitachycardia pacemaker may also be considered but reported success rates here vary considerably.

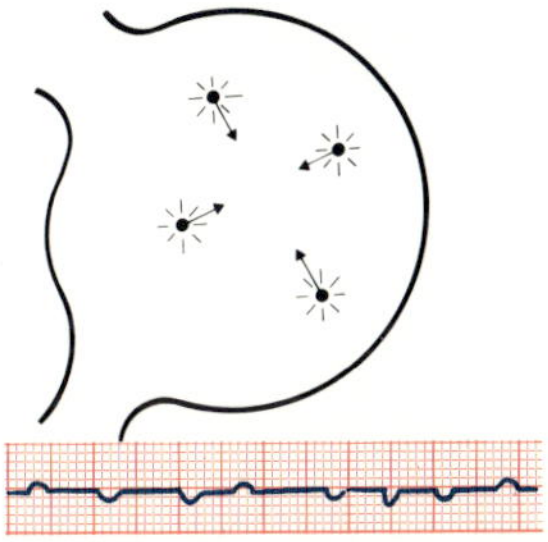

Fig. 6.13
Atrial activity in multifocal supraventricular tachycardia

Multifocal supraventricular tachycardia [16]

In multifocal supraventricular tachycardias the pacemaker site alters continuously between a multitude of ectopic atrial pacemakers and the AV node (Fig. 6.13).

ECG diagnosis

The diagnostic features of multifocal supraventricular tachycardia are (Fig. 6.14, page 140):

- P waves of varying configuration in an irregular rhythm at a rate of 100–250/min
- Isoelectric intervals (isoelectric "shelves") between the P waves
- Supraventricular QRS complexes in an irregular rhythm at the same or a lower rate than the P waves.

Differential diagnosis

The ventricular rate is irregular, as in atrial fibrillation, but P waves (although of varying configuration) are present with an intervening isoelectric interval.

Aetiology

It is most often seen in severe cardiac disease with congestive failure, as in chronic cor pulmonale or severe coronary artery disease and often related to alcohol abuse.

Prognosis

Due to the severity of the underlying cardiac disease the mortality rate is high regardless of treatment.

Management

The prognosis usually is poor. Drug treatment usually is ineffective. Digitalis can be tried but cautiously.

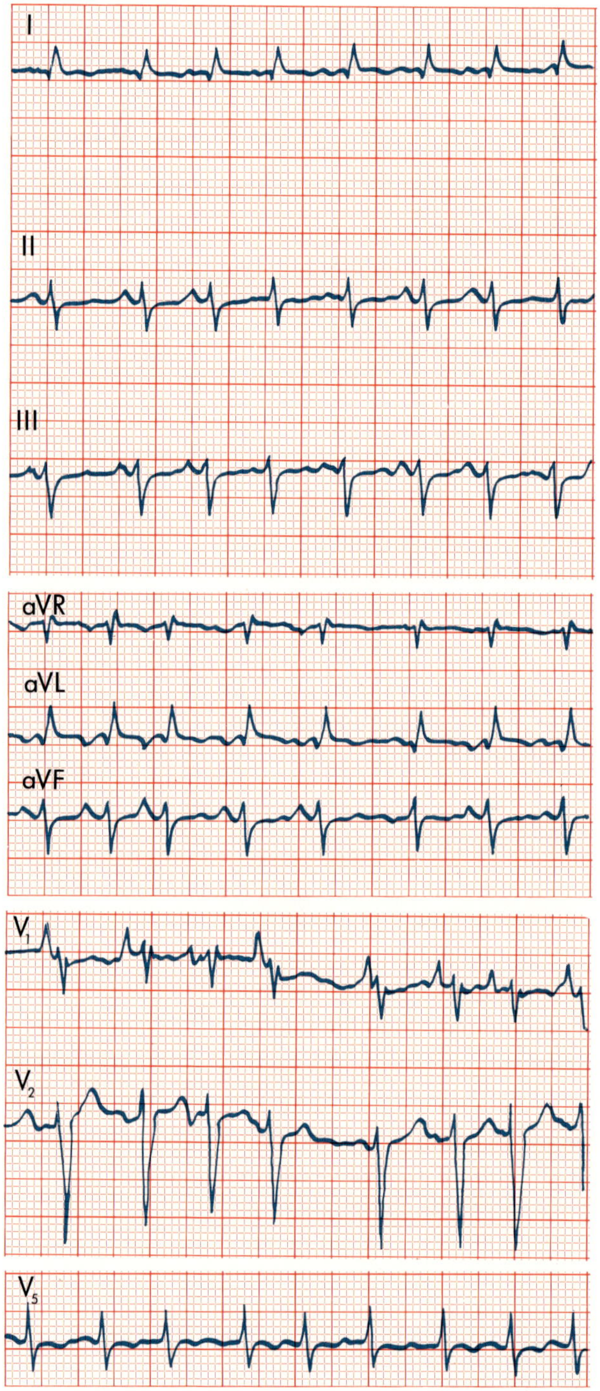

Fig. 6.14
Multifocal supraventricular tachycardia. ECG from patient in the terminal stage of mitral stenosis. P waves of varying configuration and polarity, rate 150–165/min, irregular. AV conduction ratio 1:1. Narrow QRS complexes (< 0.12 s wide)

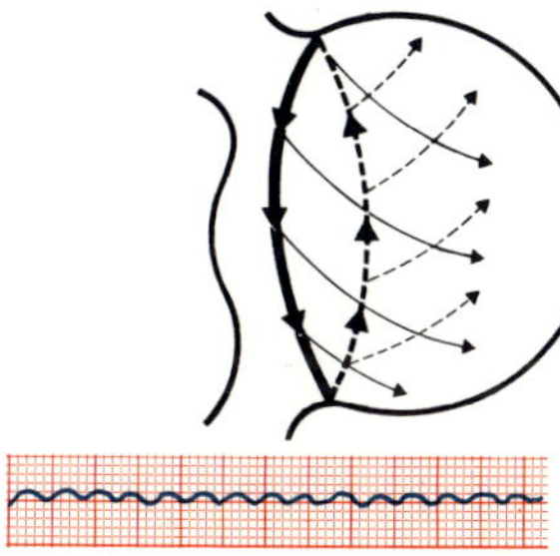

Fig. 6.15
Atrial flutter waves

Atrial flutter[17–24]

Atrial activation is by a circus movement of an impulse in the right atrium – a large circuit with a circumference usually of several centimeters (Fig. 6.15); rarely a group of rapidly discharging pacemaker cells somewhere in the atria is the mechanism of flutter.

ECG diagnosis

1 *Flutter waves:* Atrial activity is represented by repetitive broad P waves called *flutter* waves which have a regular and rapid rate above 200 and usually between 250 and 350/min. The flutter waves show a *sawtooth* or *picket fence* appearance with one flutter wave merging into the next without an intervening isoelectric shelf. The appearance of the flutter is not consistent from one patient to another but the characteristic feature is the continuity of the flutter (Fig.

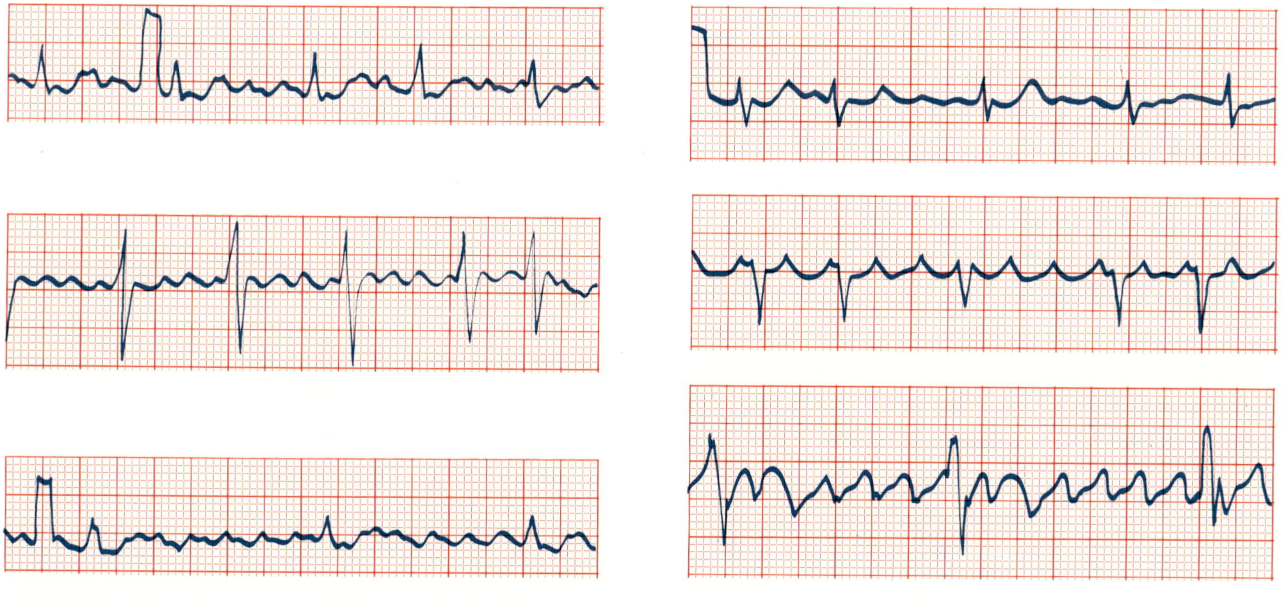

Fig. 6.16
Flutter waves in atrial flutter. ECG recordings from six different patients with atrial flutter. The appearance of the flutter varies, but a consistent and characteristic feature is the continuity of the flutter; the downstroke of one flutter wave is followed by the immediate upstroke of the next wave without any intervening isoelectric interval. The rate of the flutter waves vary between 300 and 400/min, the AV conduction ratio between 2:1 and 6:1, the QRS complex is narrow (< 0.12 s wide). The QRS rhythm in one recording is regular, while in others irregular, but with an RR interval that is a multiple of the length of the flutter wave

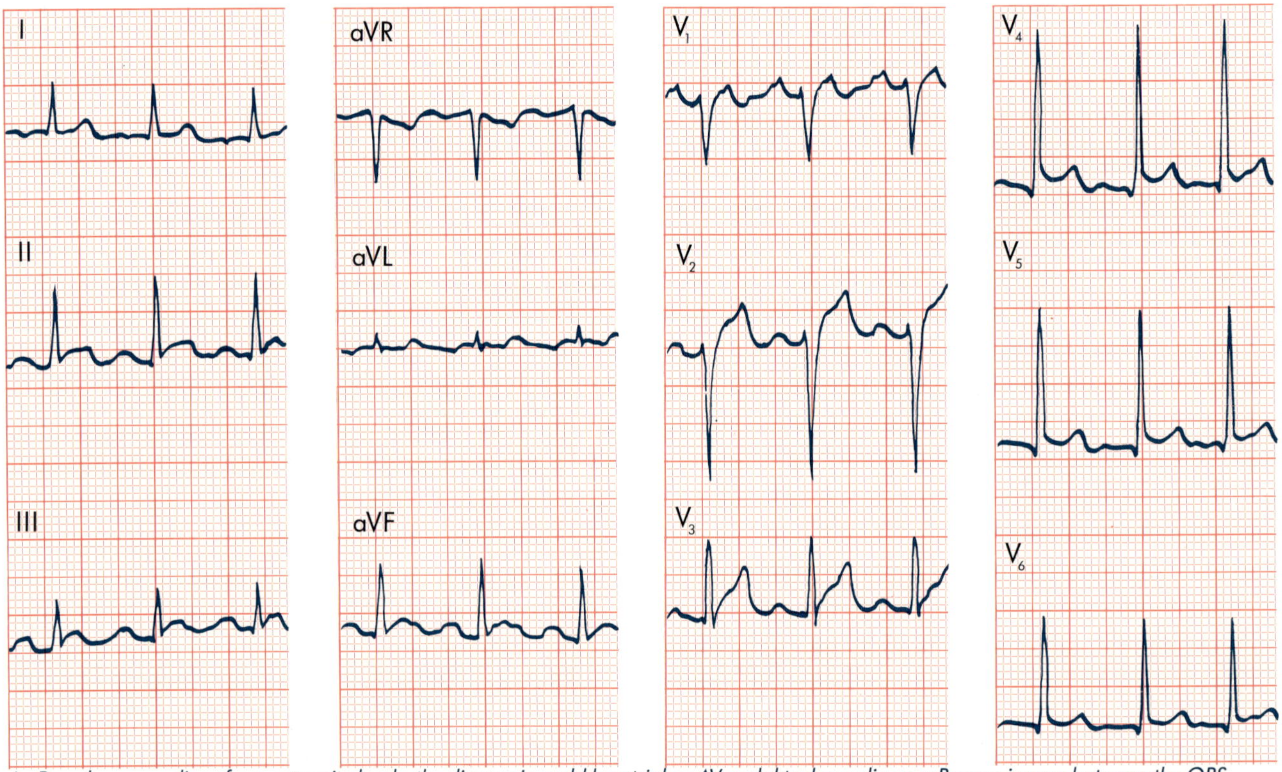

A Based on recordings from extremity leads, the diagnosis could be atrial or AV nodal tachycardia as a P wave is seen between the QRS complexes

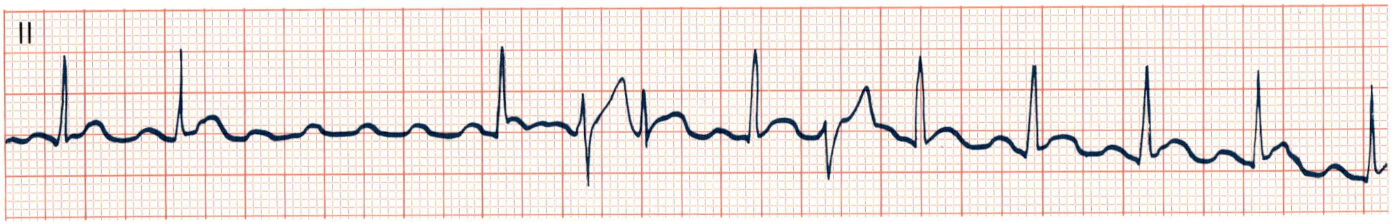

B The diagnosis of atrial flutter with a 2:1 conduction is confirmed during monitoring when the AV conduction ratio spontaneously is increased and the flutter waves previously hidden by the QRS complexes become distinct

Fig. 6.17
Atrial flutter with a 2:1 AV conduction ratio

6.16, page 141). Thus, a diagnosis of atrial flutter is confirmed by the recording of *flutter activity* in one or more leads, (or the recording of atrial deflections, P waves, at a regular rate *above* 250/min).

2 *AV conduction:* The AV conduction ratio (denominator in ratio is the number of flutter waves; numerator – the ones that elicit a QRS complex) may or may not be constant, to produce either a regular or an irregular ventricular rhythm. When the rhythm is irregular the interval between the QRS complexes is a multiple of the flutter wave cycle length (minor additional irregularities are due to a modest variation in AV conduction time). A constant 2:1 AV conduction ratio with a regular ventricular rate of about 150/min is the common finding in the untreated patient (Fig. 6.17 A). An alternating AV conduction ratio from 3:1 to 4:1 and a corresponding irregular ventricular rhythm is the common pattern when the heart rate slows with therapy (Fig. 6.16). Alternatively there may be a slow regular ventricular rhythm due to a consistent 3:1 or 4:1 AV conduction ratio (Figs. 6.18 A and B, page 144).

An AV conduction ratio of 1:1 with a catastrophic high ventricular rate of 200–250/min or more can occur:

- In the WPW syndrome (Fig. 7.14, page 204), or
- As a complication of treatment with Class I drugs in particular Class IA and IC drugs (Fig. 4.7, page 78), or
- Rarely, with unknown electrophysiologic background (Fig. 6.18 D).

3 *Supraventricular QRS complexes:* The QRS complex usually is narrow (< 0.12 s) (Figs. 6.16–6.18) but wide QRS complexes (≥ 0.12 s) may be due to bundle branch block, aberrant ventricular conduction (Fig. 6.19, page 146), ventricular extrasystole (Fig. 6.20, page 146) or the WPW syndrome (Fig. 7.14).

Differential diagnosis

Atrial flutter with 2:1 AV conduction and every second flutter wave concealed by a QRS complex may be misdiagnosed as sinus, atrial or AV nodal tachycardia, depending on the polarity of the flutter wave visible between QRST complexes (Fig. 6.17 A). Vagal manoeuvres may increase the AV conduction ratio and reveal a part of the sawtooth flutter, or a spontanous rise in vagal tone during long-term ECG monitoring can result in a transient glimpse of the flutter (Fig. 6.17 B). The mere recording of an atrial rate (P wave rate) of 250/min or above by itself confirms the diagnosis of atrial flutter, whereas an atrial rate of 200–250/min would be consistent with both atrial flutter and atrial tachycardia. The critical diagnostic feature in this context is the recording of flutter activity in one or several leads, or in atrial tachycardia recognizing a consistent isoelectric shelf between the P waves (Fig. 6.8, page 133).

Prognosis

This relates to the severity of the underlying heart disease. As with atrial fibrillation there is a risk of arterial embolism.

Additional investigations

Underlying mitral stenosis and thyrotoxicosis may be overlooked. Auscultation should be thorough and supplemented if necessary by echocardiography. Thyroid function (plasma T_3 and T_4) should be routinely checked in patients without known underlying heart disease.

Symptoms

The haemodynamic consequences of atrial flutter vary with the ventricular rate and the functional state of the heart. Atrioventricular conduction usually is less stable than in atrial fibrillation. Medication (digitalis, verapamil or beta blockade, see later) often can slow the initial fast ventricular rate and render the patient symptom free at rest. Exercise and straining, however, may still provoke sudden increases in heart rate (Fig. 6.18) causing palpitations, shortness of breath and restricting functional capacity. Episodes of 1:1 AV conduction (Fig. 6.18 D) may result in syncope.

Aetiology

As for atrial fibrillation but it is a less common arrhythmia. Atrial flutter with fairly slow ventricular rate, seen in the elderly usually is benign and may not require treatment.

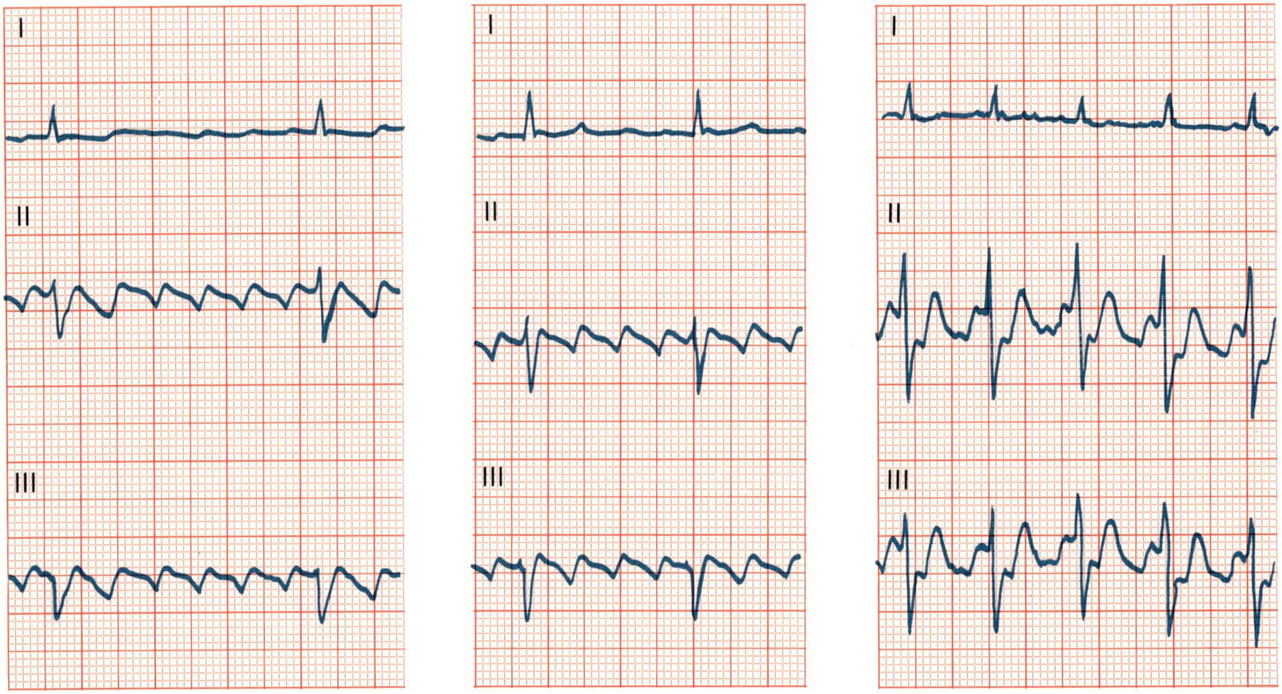

A Sleep
ECG during sleep. AV–CR: 6:1 and ventricular rate (VR) 41/min

B Rest
Awake but reclining. AV–CR 4:1, VR 64/min

C 50 W – 2 min
After work load with 50 watts for 2 minutes on bicycle ergometer. AV–CR 2:1, VR 128/min

Fig. 6.18
Atrial flutter with an AV conduction ratio (AV–CR) at sleep and rest of 6:1 or 4:1 decreasing to 2:1 and 1:1 during exercise on a bicycle ergometer with a corresponding stepwise increase in heart rate from 41/min to 64, 128 and 236/min.

Management

Acute attack

1 *I.v. digitalis* or *verapamil:* Both drugs reduce heart rate and may restore sinus rhythm. The most immediate effect is achieved by verapamil, which is the preferred drug for the patient without congestive failure.

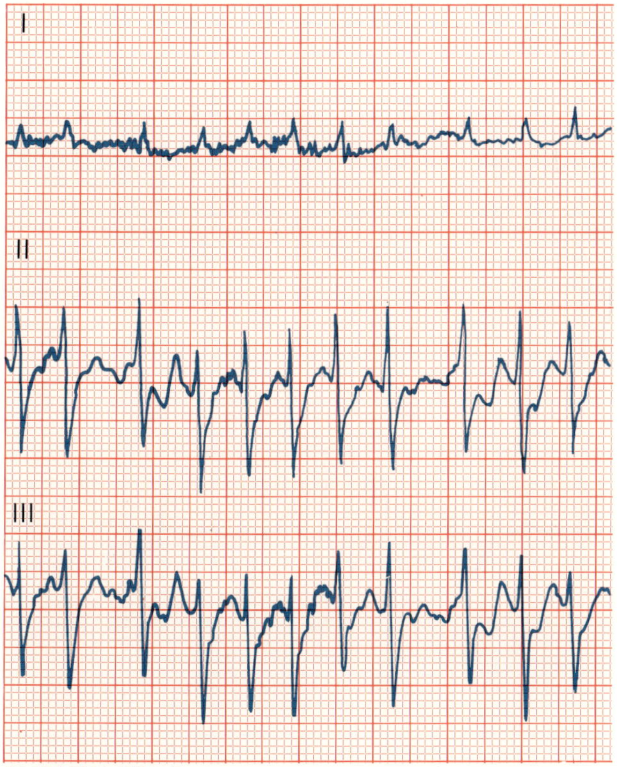

D 100 W – 1/2 min
AV–CR: 1:1, VR 236/min

Fig. 6.18 (continued)

2 In the critically ill patient with acute myocardial infarction, congestive failure and/or shock early *cardioversion* should be undertaken. Atrial flutter is very sensitive to this form of treatment and often responds to a DC countershock of only 25 J with conversion to sinus rhythm or occasionally atrial fibrillation.

3 *Overdrive atrial pacing* at a high rate (350–400/min) often is used to control atrial flutter in the postoperative period after cardiac surgery. Before closure of the chest the surgeon may temporarily fix pacing electrodes on the atrium. These can be pulled out when no longer needed. If an attack of atrial flutter occurs in the postoperative period, high rate pacing (above the flutter rate) is started. In about 50 % of patients when the pacemaker rate is gradually slowed after this overdrive, sinus rhythm will be restored.

Long-term prophylaxis of paroxysmal atrial flutter

Digitalis usually is administered with the primary aim of reducing the ventricular rate should an attack occur. Supplementary treatment with an antiarrhythmic agent is mandatory for prophylaxis of attacks. First choice drugs for combination with digitalis are the Class IA agents (quinidine or disopyramide), the Class IC agents (propafenone, flecainide), verapamil (alternatively diltiazem) or a beta blocking agent. The drug of second or third choice is amiodarone which often is effective but which is limited by its side effects. In the drug refractory patient, His bundle ablation may be considered (Fig. 4.10, page 85). His bundle ablation, however, makes the patient pacemaker dependent, so pacemaker failure (happily a rare event due to modern pacemaker technology) carries a risk of sudden death.

Treatment of chronic atrial flutter

The ventricular rate usually can be slowed to 60–80/min by digitalization and/or a beta blocking agent, verapamil (alternatively diltiazem) or amiodarone. Despite drug control of the ventricular rate at rest, physical and/or emotional stress will often still induce increases in the ventricular rate related to sudden changes in the AV conduction ratio from for instance 3–6:1 down to 2:1 or even 1:1 with a corresponding rise in ventricular rate from 50–80 to 120 and

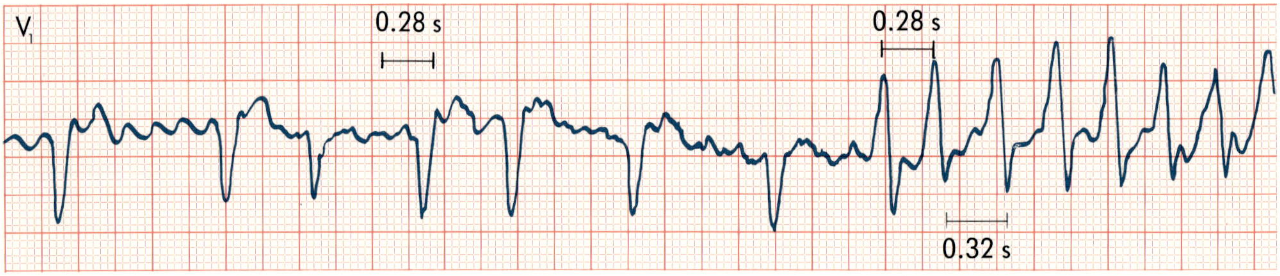

Fig. 6.19
Atrial flutter with episodes of aberrant ventricular conduction. First a period with distinct flutter waves and supraventricular QRS complexes with a width of 0.11 s. The AV conduction ratio varies between 3:1 and 4:1. The QRS rate is approximately 90/min and irregular.

Next a period with a QRS of 200/min and QRS complexes widened to 0.20 s. The high and wide monophasic QRS complexes which cover the baseline completely give an impression of ventricular tachycardia, but the RR interval in these periods of very fast tachycardia is 0.28–0.32 s i. e. the length of two flutter waves. Thus, the intermittent QRS widening seems to be due to aberrant ventricular conduction induced by an episodic decrease in the AV conduction ratio to 2:1 and a corresponding rise in the ventricular rate.

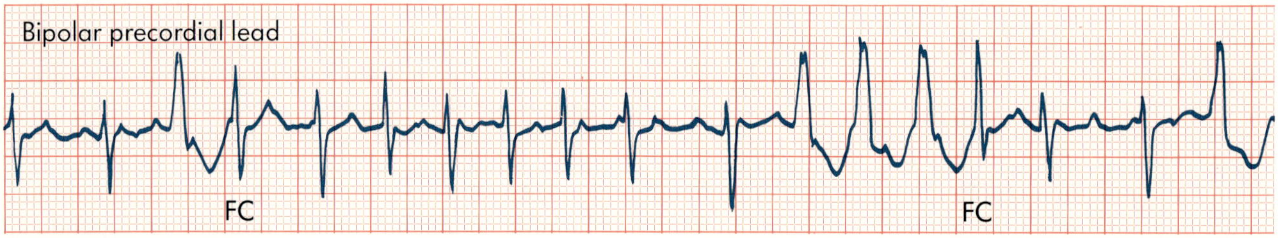

Fig. 6.20
Atrial flutter, ventricular extrasystole and ventricular tachycardia. Atrial flutter with narrow QRS complexes, < 0.12 s wide, and flutter waves which become visible when the AV conduction ratio falls from the prevailing 2:1 to 3:1. Moreover, the recording shows three episodes with from two to four widened monophasic QRS complexes, most likely ventricular extrasystole and tachycardia since:

- *The coupling interval is fixed.*
- *The RR intervals in the runs of widened complexes are 0.32, which cannot be converted into a multiple of the flutter wave length (0.21 s)*
- *The QRS complexes are of large amplitude, monophasic and the last complex in each sequence is an intermediate, a fusion complex (FC), between the widened QRS complex and the normal narrow QRS complex.*

The moderate QRS complex widening to only 0.12 s and the lack of compensatory postextrasystolic pauses are features favouring a diagnosis of aberrant ventricular conduction, but they do not outweigh the stronger ECG evidence in favour of ventricular extrasystole listed above

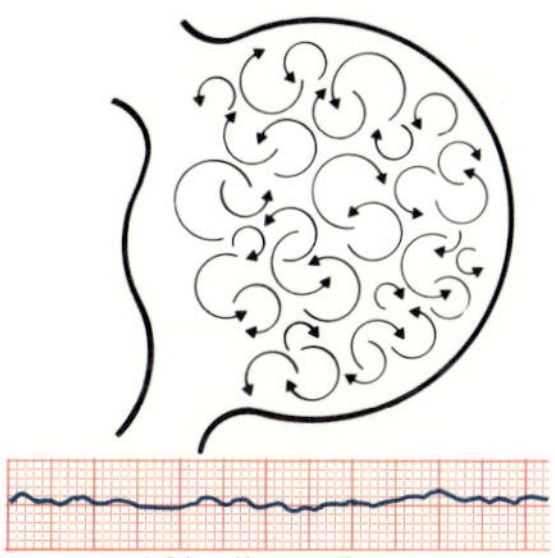

Fig. 6.21
Fibrillatory wavelets (f waves in atrial fibrillation)

240/min (Fig. 6.18, page 144/145). For this reason DC cardioversion to restore sinus rhythm or to convert to atrial fibrillation which is easier regulated by medication flutter may be worth undertaking. The risk of recurrence of flutter following restoration of sinus rhythm can be reduced by the same prophylactic drug regime as used for paroxysmal atrial flutter.

Atrial fibrillation [18,19,25–39]

Next to sinus tachycardia atrial fibrillation is the most common form of tachycardia. It reflects turbulent activation of atrial myocardium (Figs. 3.7, page 44 and 6.21). Atrial fibrillation in the WPW syndrome is a specific electrophysiological and clinical problem which is discussed separately (Chapter 7, page 197).

ECG diagnosis

1 *Fibrillatory activity:* P waves are absent and the baseline consists of irregular waves, fibrillatory wavelets (f-waves) which continuously change in shape, duration, amplitude and direction (Fig. 6.21). Fibrillation may be coarse with large deflections but more often is fine with deflections that are sometimes so small that they cannot be recognized with certainty on the surface ECG.

2 *Irregular ventricular rhythm:* AV conduction is totally irregular, as is the ventricular rate (irregularly irregular rhythm). In the untreated patient, the ventricular rate usually is between 150 and 200/min. This varies greatly, however, and rates in the range of 50–100/min are not uncommon in the elderly. Digitalis may reduce the ventricular rate from 160/min in the previously untreated patient (Fig. 6.22 A, page 148) and to 60–80/min in the fully digitalized patient (Fig. 6.22 B). The absence of P waves and the completely irregular rhythm are the essential diagnostic criteria without which the diagnosis of atrial fibrillation should not be made.

3 *Supraventricular QRS complexes:* The QRS complex is usually narrow (< 0.12 s) but intermittent QRS widening may occur due to aberrant ventricular conduction (Fig. 6.23, page 149) ventricular extrasystoles (Fig. 6.24, page 150) and in the WPW syndrome (Figs. 7.12, page 201 and 7.13, page 202/203).

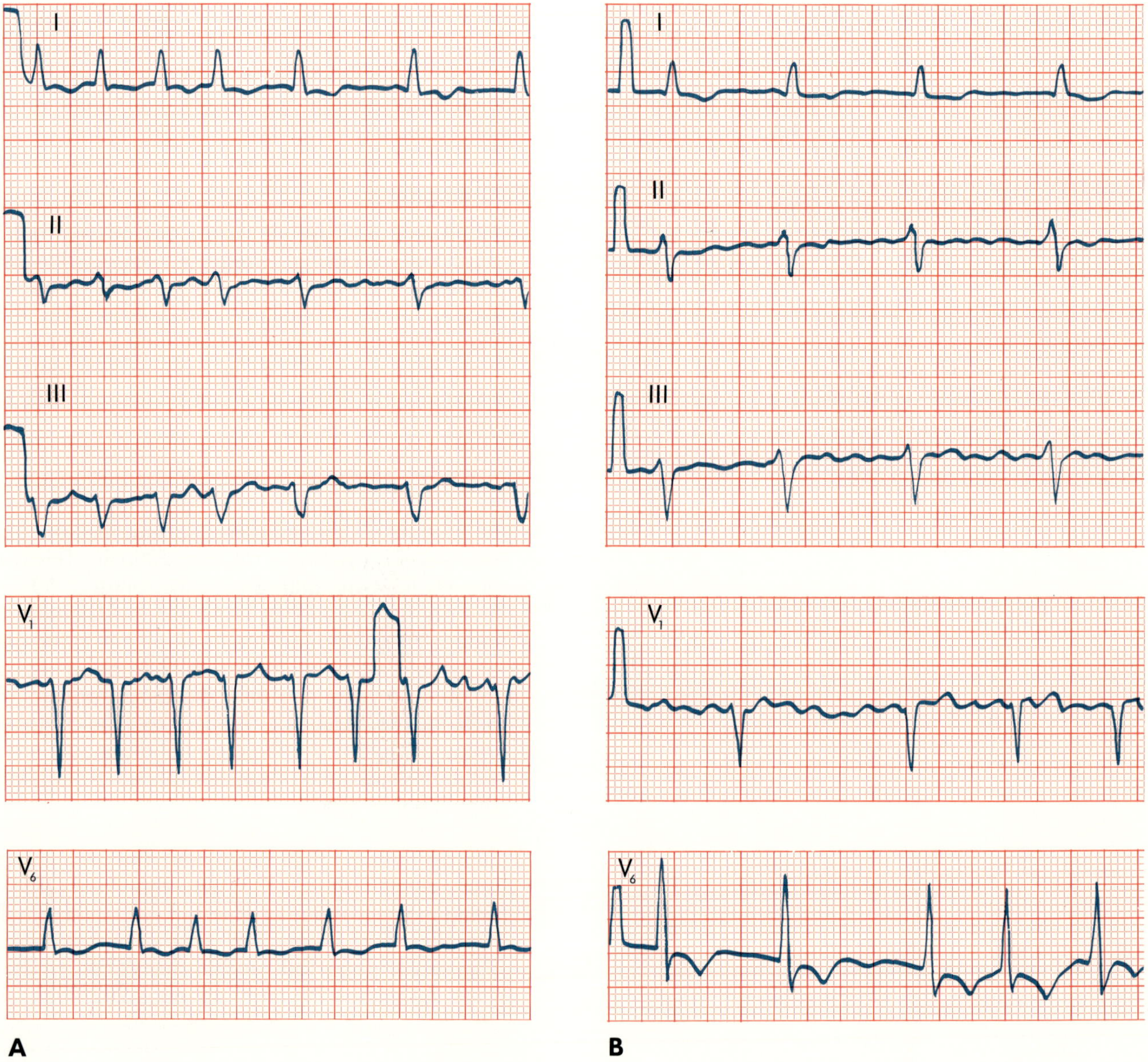

Fig. 6.22
Atrial fibrillation (A) untreated and (B) after digitalis. In both cases, atrial fibrillatory wavelets, supraventricular QRS complexes and perpetual irregular QRS rhythm can be seen. QRS frequency is 150/min and 80/min respectively. Changes in the T wave can be seen from A to B (especially pronounced in lead V_6), and can be attributed to digitalis.

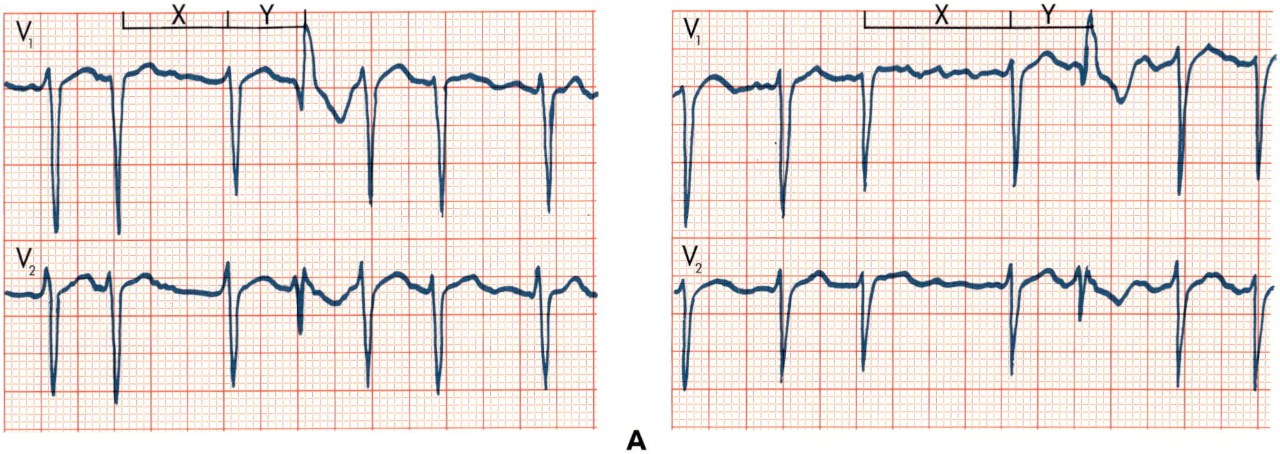

A

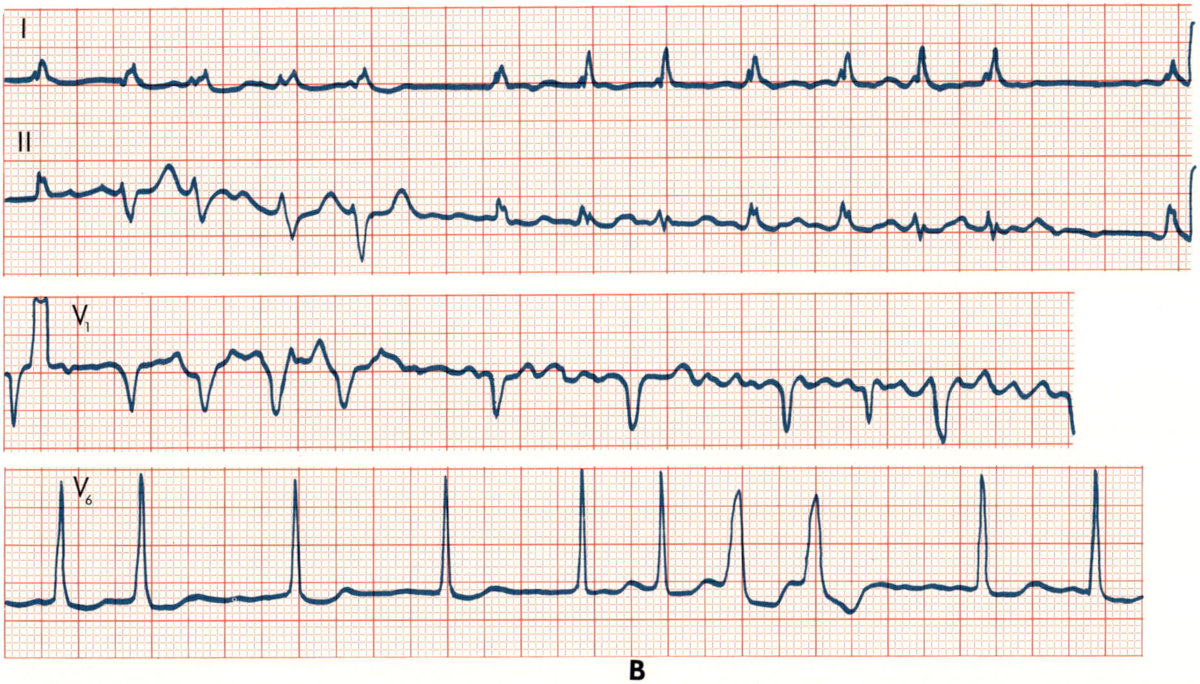

B

Fig. 6.23
Atrial fibrillation with intermittent complex widening due to aberrant ventricular conduction. The diagnosis of atrial fibrillation is in both recordings related to the absence of P waves, a fibrillatory baseline and QRS complexes in a totally irregular rhythm. Factors suggesting aberrant ventricular conduction as the cause of the QRS complex widening are:

A QRS complex width of only 0.12 s. rR′ pattern in lead V_1 (right bundle branch block pattern). The widened QRS complexes following long (X)-short (Y) sequences in the RR intervals (the Ashman phenomenon, Chapter 3, p. 46). No specific long RR interval following the widened QRS complex (no compensatory postextrasystolic pause)

B Gradual changes in the QRS widening. QRS width of 0.14 s at its greatest. No definite change in the form of the QRS complex, it simply becomes broader

Symptoms

The haemodynamic consequences of atrial fibrillation depend on the functional state of the heart, and the ventricular rate. Whereas a paroxysm of atrial fibrillation in a patient with severe mitral stenosis or coronary artery disease may provoke pulmonary oedema if the ventricular rate is 130–150/min, atrial fibrillation in an otherwise healthy individual rarely causes circulatory problems even with significantly higher ventricular rates.

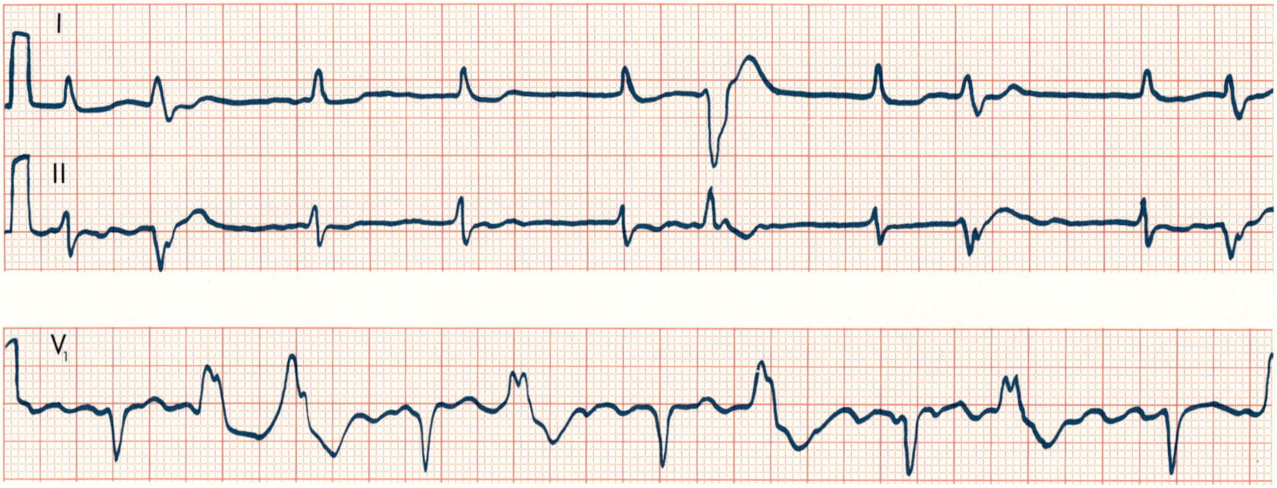

Fig. 6.24
Atrial fibrillation and ventricular extrasystole. The basic arrhythmia is atrial fibrillation with an absence of P waves, a fibrillatory baseline and supraventricular QRS complexes (< 0.12 s wide) in a totally irregular rhythm. A few widened QRS complexes are recorded, most likely ventricular extrasystole since:

- *The coupling interval is fixed*
- *The QRS complex is very wide 0.18–0.20 s, with an Rr′ pattern in V_1*

A marked compensatory postextrasystolic pause is seen in the standard leads but not in the recording from lead V_1. The QRS complex of the ventricular extrasystole varies considerably in form, most likely due to a varying degree of fusion with activation of the ventricular myocardium, partly from the ectopic ventricular pacemaker, partly from AV conducted supraventricular impulses

Aetiology

Single isolated episodes of atrial fibrillation are associated with a variety of conditions: Acute infections (particularly those which affect the lungs), acute myocardial infarction, pulmonary embolism, acute alcohol overindulgence and iatrogenic interventions such as gastroscopy, bronchoscopy or cardiac catherization.

Paroxysmal and chronic atrial fibrillation can be due to:

- *Cardiac disease.* This is the situation in the great majority of patients. Particular forms of cardiac disease are those with elevated left atrial pressures and associated left atrial dilatation. The most common aetiologies are ischaemic heart disease, hypertensive heart disease and dilated cardiomyopathy. Atrial fibrillation is frequent in mitral disease, particularly mitral stenosis, where it often occurs as the first and for a time the only clinical manifestation of the valvular disease
- *WPW syndome.* (Figs. 7.12, page 201 and 7.13, page 202/203) and *sick sinus syndrome* (Fig. 11.7, page 287)
- *Thyrotoxicosis* is an uncommon but curable cause of atrial fibrillation. In older patients particularly clinical signs of thyrotoxicosis may be absent and atrial fibrillation may exist as the only clinical manifestation of the endocrine disorder
- Possibly *alcohol abuse.*

Paroxysmal and, sometimes chronic atrial fibrillation can develop in otherwise completely healthy individuals, so-called *lone atrial fibrillation.* The attack rate in lone atrial fibrillation often changes in a highly unpredictable way and during periods when there are prolonged and/or frequent attacks, the qualitiy of life can be severely impaired. Over years paroxysmal atrial fibrillation may become chronic. In patients whose symptoms start after the age of 60 years their arrhythmia features may merge with the "sick sinus syndrome" with alternating paroxysms of atrial fibrillation and SA block causing syncope or presyncope (Fig. 11.7).

In many patients with paroxysmal atrial fibrillation their attacks are related to psychological stress or strenuous exercise, seemingly in relation to *increased sympathetic nervous tone.* Others experience attacks during the night or while resting or relaxing during the day. The latter, probably *vagally mediated* attacks, may be preceded by a slowing of the heart rate.

Prognosis

The prognosis is primarily related to the severity of the underlying heart disease. There is an additional risk of embolic complications, however, with a five-fold risk of stroke (compared to the sinus rhythm patient) when atrial fibrillation is chronic. The risk for the patient with paroxysmal atrial fibrillation is minor.

Survival in lone atrial fibrillation is near normal but with an increased risk of embolism and stroke.

Additional investigations

Underlying mitral stenosis and thyrotoxicosis may be overlooked. Careful auscultation should be supplemented if there is any doubt by echocardiography. Thyroid function (plasma T_3 and T_4) should be checked routinely in the patient without underlying heart disease. A history of alcohol abuse which may have an aetiological role in the development of "lone" atrial fibrillation should be sought.

Management

Acute attack

1 *Search/treat underlying cause/disease:* E.g. pneumonia, acute myocardial infarction, pulmonary embolism, shock etc.

2 *Medication:* Digitalis is the primary treatment of atrial fibrillation with a rapid ventricular rate. In the acutely ill patient it should be given intravenously, in less urgent situations, by mouth. Over the 12–24 hours of digitalization sinus rhythm may be reestablished but more often atrial fibrillation continues with a slower stable ventricular rate of around 100/min. A further reduction in ventricular rate to a level of 60–80/min usually occurs in the course of the following days. If digitalization does not yield an adequate effect it can be supplemented by verapamil or by a beta blocking agent. This will further inhibit AV conduction and thus reduce the ventricular rate or sometimes restore sinus rhythm. A beta blocking agent is the drug of choice for slowing the ventricular rate in patients with thyrotoxicosis. Drugs used in combination with digitalization to restore sinus rhythm are the Class IA drugs (quinidine, and disopyramide) and the Class IC drugs (ajmaline, propafenone or flecainide).

3 *Cardioversion* usually will restore sinus rhythm but the recurrence rate is high particularly in patients with enlarged hearts and/or congestive failure.

Long-term prophylaxis in paroxysmal atrial fibrillation

Paroxysmal atrial fibrillation is difficult to treat. Digitalis usually is the drug of first choice. It can reduce the frequency and/or duration of the attacks and it can limit the ventricular rate during future attacks. Alternative drugs include verapamil or diltiazem, a beta blocking agent, a Class IA agent (quinidine or disopyramide) or a Class IC agent (propafenone or flecainide). The most effective drug in preventing atrial fibrillation is amiodarone but as in atrial flutter, its unwanted effects limit its use. Refractory patients with frequent attacks despite prophylactic drug treatment or who have intolerable side effects are candidates for His bundle ablation (Fig. 4.10, page 85).

Long-term control of ventricular rate in chronic atrial fibrillation

In almost all patients with chronic atrial fibrillation digitalization will decrease the ventricular rate to a *stable* level in the range of 60–90/min. Supplementary treatment with verapamil or diltiazem or with a beta blocking agent may be necessary to control the ventricular rate in a few patients. Amiodarone is often effective when other drugs have failed. In the rare patient in whom the ventricular rate cannot be controlled by drugs His bundle ablation should be considered (Fig. 4.10, page 85).

Cardioversion for chronic atrial fibrillation

The decision to cardiovert a patient with chronic atrial fibrillation should be based on the likelihood of maintaining the reestablished sinus rhythm for a reasonably long period of time. Candidates for defibrillation are those whose atrial fibrillation has persisted after cure of their thyrotoxicosis, younger patients without obvious heart disorders and those in whom the onset of atrial fibrillation is recent.

The recurrence rate after cardioversion is high in mitral stenosis, in patients with significantly enlarged hearts and when atrial fibrillation has been of more than 6 months duration. There is no consensus on the virtue of cardioverting the older patient whose atrial fibrillation is well controlled by digitalization and who has a normal heart size. Many clinicians including the authors follow a conservative approach avoiding cardioversion.

The patient is prepared for cardioversion by:

- *Anticoagulant therapy* with a vitamin K antagonist to minimize the risk of peripheral embolism.
- *Medication* with a Class IA drug (quinidine, disopyramide or procainamide), or with a Class IC drug (propafenone or flecainide), usually started 1 or 2 days prior to DC cardioversion. In about one third of the patients the antiarrhythmic drug regime will restore sinus rhythm. In the remainder it may help maintain sinus rhythm in the first hours after cardioversion.

– *Digitalization* can be continued up to the day of cardioversion. Digitalis intoxication, however, carries a risk of serious arrhythmic complications at cardioversion and for the following 24 hours.

Following successful cardioversion, digitalization should be continued for at least a period of time to ensure control of ventricular rate should fibrillation recur. There is debate whether long-term treatment with antiarrhythmic drugs can reduce the relapse rate after an initially successful cardioversion. Drugs claimed to have value for this indication include Class IA drugs (quinidine, disopyramide and procainamide), Class IC drugs (propafenone and flecainide), verapamil and amiodarone.

Anticoagulant therapy in atrial fibrillation

Long-term anticoagulation should be considered in patients with chronic atrial fibrillation. The decision on whether to start a long-term (life long) anticoagulant treatment with its cost and inconvenience has to be based on the individual risk-benefit ratio relating to age, patient compliance and bleeding risk.

Ventricular tachycardia [40–50]

The pacemaker site is most often re-entry in the Purkinje fibers (Fig. 3.4, page 41).

ECG diagnosis [40–42]

1 *Rate:* The basic diagnostic criterion is the recording of three or more consecutive QRS complexes of ventricular origin at a rate of more than 100/min. The tachycardia is named sustained if it continues for more than 30 s and non-sustained if it lasts less than 30 s.

2 *QRS complex:* The QRS complex can vary in width and form from a relatively narrow complex of 0.12–0.14 s with a "typical bundle branch pattern" (right or left) to a wide complex in the range of 0.15–0.24 s with a bizarre configuration and ST deviation and abnormal T waves. In the great majority of cases the complex will have one or more of the following features which are characteristic of a tachycardia of ventricular origin:

- QRS duration ≥ 0.16 s (Figs. 6.27–6.31, page 157–161)
- A monophasic tall R wave in V_1 or more commonly an Rr′ pattern in V_1 with a tall R wave followed by a smaller r′ nicknamed the "tall right, small left, rabbit ear pattern" (Fig. 6.25 A)
- A QS pattern or an rS pattern with a deep and broad S wave in V_6 (Fig. 6.25 B)
- A concordant positive or negative QRS pattern in the precordial leads V_1–V_6 (positive concordance and negative concordance) (Fig. 6.26)
- Left axis deviation (Fig. 6.31 A).

QRS complexes originating from the free wall of the right ventricle usually have a net positive QRS area in leads V_{5-6} and I (QRS polarity similar to left bundle branch block). QRS complexes originating from the free wall of the left ventricle have a net positive QRS area in leads V_{1-2} (QRS polarity similar to right bundle branch block) (Fig. 3.16, page 50); whereas QRS complexes originating in the septal or apical regions may have either QRS polarity.

3 *Atrial activity:* In ventricular tachycardia there is usually AV dissociation. Thus the SA node continues activating the atria at a normal or near normal rate independent of the rapid ventricular activation. In a small but not insignificant group of patients (30–40 %) the ventricular impulses are conducted retrogradely through the His bundle and the AV node to the atria, resulting in retrograde atrial activation.

AV dissociation: By careful inspection of the tightly packed QRS complexes, P waves sometimes can be discerned on the surface ECG (Fig. 6.27 A) or can be visualized by recording from an oesophageal or intra-atrial lead (Figs. 6.27 B, 6.28). The P waves usually occur regularly at a normal rate of 60–100/min in contrast to the rapid rate of the QRS complexes. An atrial impulse occasionally succeeds in traversing the AV conduction system to the ventricular level to initiate a QRS complex – a *ventricular capture* (the ventricles are captured by an impulse originating in the atria) (Fig. 6.28). In complete ventricular capture all parts of the ventricles are activated by the sinus impulse. In incomplete capture only a part is activated by the sinus impulse, while the remainder is activated by the ectopic ventricular pacemaker. *Complete ventricular capture* is characterized by a slender QRS complex identical to that seen in sinus rhythm. *Incomplete ventricular capture* produces a "fusion complex", intermediate in form and width between the slender complex of sinus rhythm and the broad complex of the tachycardia.

Retrograde atrial activation: Retrograde atrial activation produces retrograde P waves which are time related to the QRS complexes. The ventriculo-atrial (VA) conduction ratio may be 1:1, 2:1 or 3:1, the latter situations producing a P wave rate equal to one half or to one third of the ventriclar rate. The VA conduction ratio may be constant or alternating (Fig. 6.29). Occasionally, VA transmission is of second degree type I (Wenckebach).

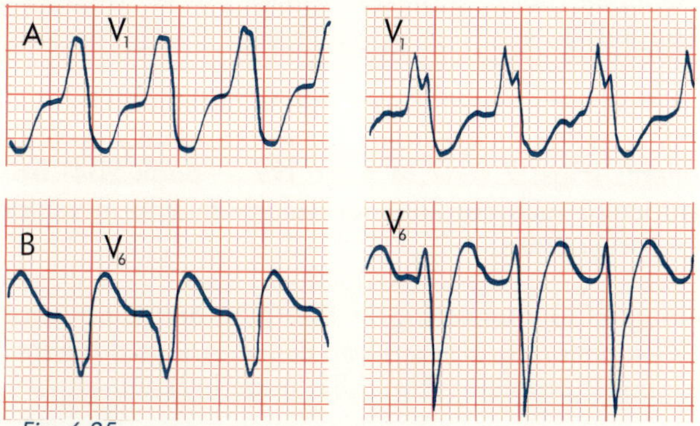

Fig. 6.25
Characteristic QRS pattern in ventricular tachycardia
A R′ or Rr′ in V_1
B QS or rS in V_6

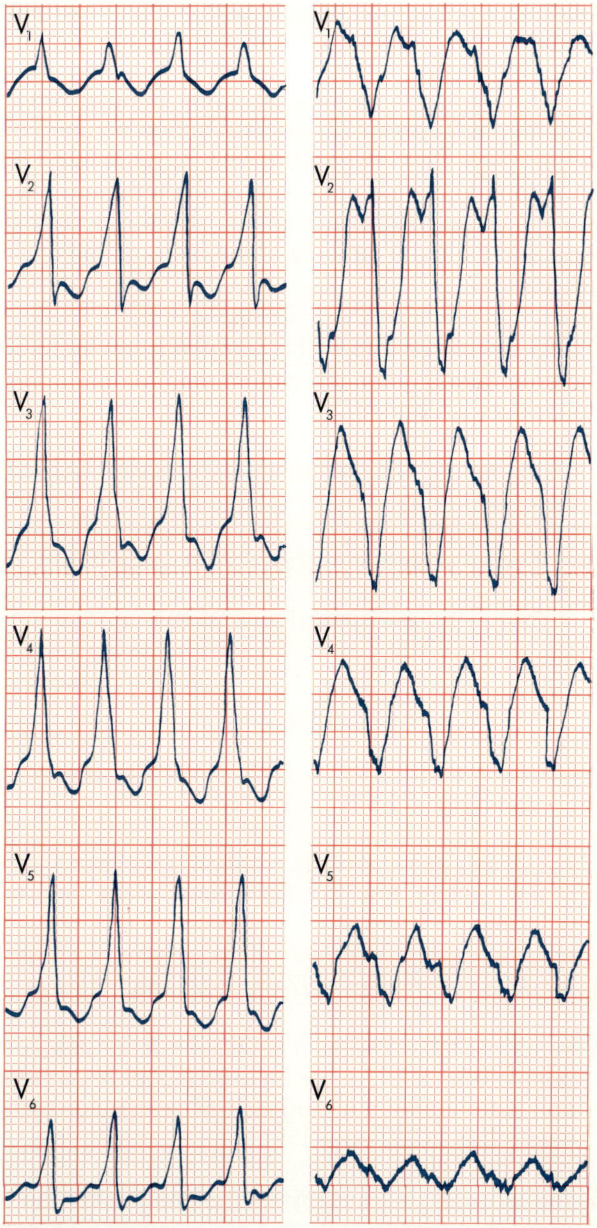

A B

Fig. 6.26
Concordant QRS patterns in ventricular tachycardia
A Positive concordans
B Negative concordans

Differential diagnosis[6–8, 40–42]

Confronted with a regular wide QRS complex tachycardia (QRS ≥ 0.12 s) the chance of a ventricular origin is approximately 80 %. The major differential diagnosis is a supraventricular tachycardia with bundle branch block (Fig. 6.2, page 127) or aberrant ventricular conduction (Figs. 3.11, page 46 and 6.3, page 128/129). The recording of one or several of the following "ventricular" characteristics will help to make a correct diagnosis in the great majority of the cases of ventricular tachycardia:

1 *QRS duration ≥ 0.16 s* (This criterion is not useful for differentiating when the patient has bundle branch block in sinus rythm).

2 *Characteristic QRS patterns* of ventricular tachycardia:

  - R or Rr′ pattern in V_1 (Fig. 6.25 A, page 155)
  - QS or rS pattern in V_6 (Fig. 6.25 B)
  - Concordant positive QRS pattern in precordial leads (Fig. 6.26 A, page 155)
  - Concordant negative QRS pattern in precordial leads (Fig. 6.26 B)
  - Left axis deviation (This criterion is not useful when the patient has bundle branch block in sinus rhythm).

3 *AV dissociation* (Figs. 6.27 and 6.28, page 158).

4 *Retrograde P waves with a QRS-P relationship compatible with a 2:1, 3:1 or an even higher VA conduction ratio* supports a diagnosis of ventricular tachycardia (Fig. 6.29, page 159).

5 The recording in sinus rhythm (before or after the attack) of a *ventricular extrasystole with a QRS complex identical to the complex in tachycardia* favours a common origin of the extrasystole and the tachycardia from the same ventricular pacemaker (Figs. 6.30, page 160 and 6.31, page 161). A ventricular origin of the extrasystole is confirmed by the presence of a compensatory postextrasystolic pause (Fig. 5.3, page 111).

A difficult differential diagnosis is to distinguish the wide QRS complex tachycardias seen occasionally in WPW patients (Figs. 7.11–7.14 page 199 – page 204) from ventricular tachycardias, particularly multiform ventricular tachycardia.

During ECG monitoring in the CCU and ambulatory ECG monitoring artifacts can cause serious differential diagnostic problems (Fig. 6.32, page 162).

Symptoms

Most often ventricular tachycardia develops in a patient with severely damaged myocardium and the rate of the tachycardia usually is high, 180–200/min. In this setting ventricular tachycardia may cause or aggravate heart failure and shock. When ventricular tachycardia develops in a patient with a fairly well preserved myocardium, however, or if the rate of the tachycardia is not more than 120–150/min, the patient may be only slightly affected if at all. As a substantial number of patients with supraventricular tachycardia may develop cardiac failure or shock, the diagnosis of a tachycardia as ventricular or supraventricular always requires the recording of an ECG and cannot be inferred from the haemodynamic effects.

Aetiology

Ventricular tachycardia often implies severe organic heart disease. The common causes are *acute myocardial infarction*, chronic ischaemic heart disease and cardiomyopathy. Occasionally, paroxysmal ventricular tachycardia occurs in otherwise healthy young people without evidence of organic heart disease (see specific ventricular tachycardias).

Antiarrhythmic drug treatment, in particular treatment with the Class IC agents, encainide and flecainide, may induce attacks of ventricular tachycardia or aggravate a preexisting tachycardia (Chapter 4 page 71).

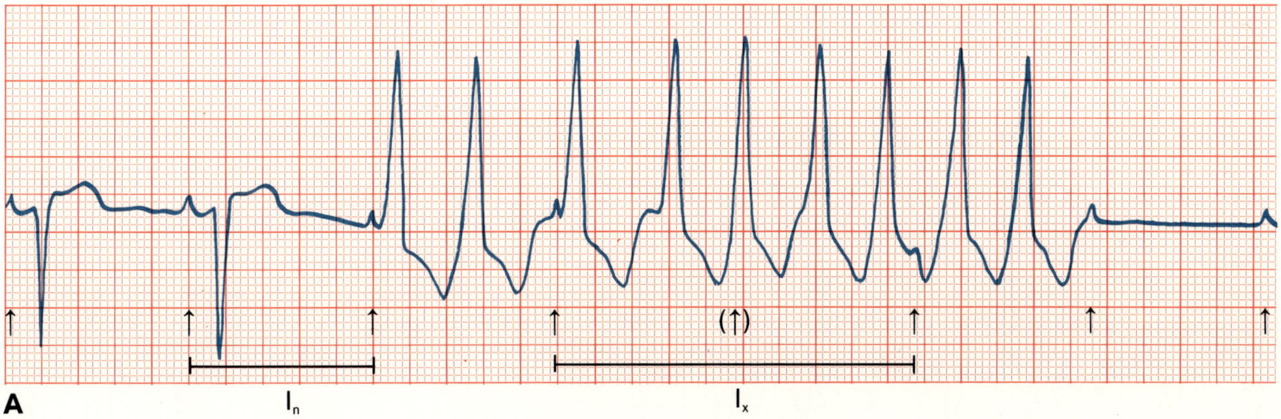

A

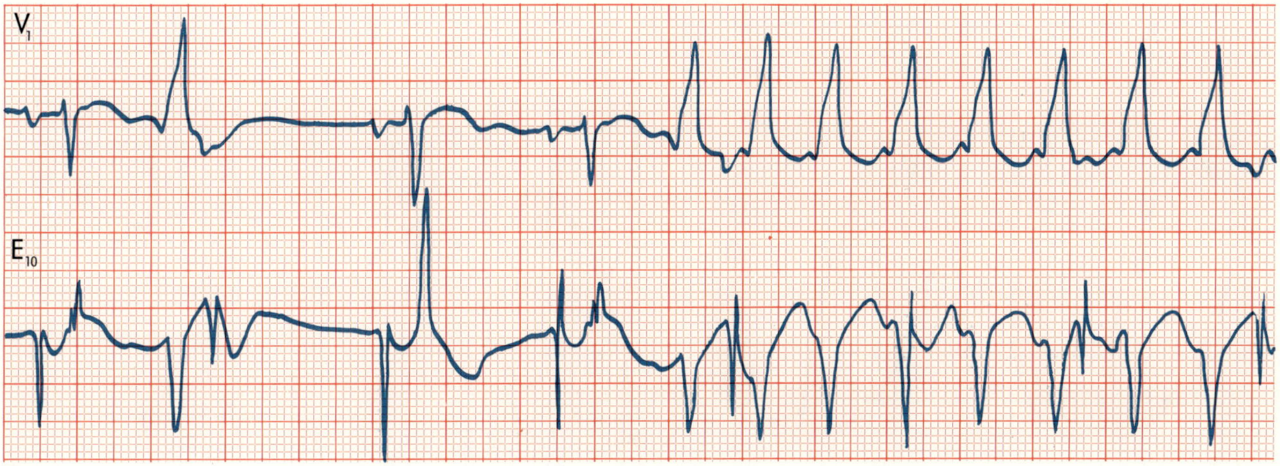

B

Fig. 6.27
Ventricular tachycardia with AV dissociation. The ventricular origin of the tachycardia is suggested by the wide, monophasic QRS complexes and confirmed by the presence of AV dissociation.

A Sinus P waves at an unchanged rate are visible just before some of the QRS complexes as a deflection in the ST segment of just after the T wave. The arrow within brackets marks the position of a sinus P wave falling on and hidden by a QRS complex ($I_x = 2 \times I_n$). QRS rate in tachycardia 130–160/min. Sinus P wave rate 62/min.

B The P waves are not clearly visible in the surface lead (V_1) but distinctly recorded in the oesophageal lead (E_{10}). The QRS rate in tachycardia is 149/min, the sinus P wave rate is 64/min. The attack of tachycardia is preceded by a ventricular extrasystole with a QRS complex of the same type as the QRS complex in tachycardia. It appears from the oesophageal lead that the background of the compensatory postextrasystolic pause is also AV dissociation.

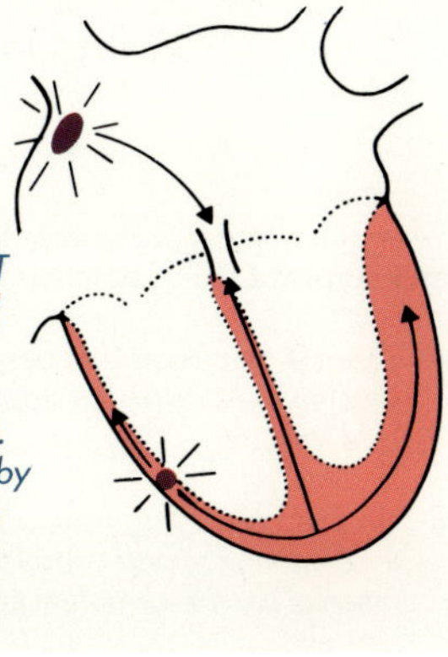

Additional investigations

An acute attack of sustained ventricular tachycardia is a life threatening condition which requires emergency admission to a Coronary Care Unit for ECG monitoring and management. Recurrent paroxysmal ventricular tachycardia should be referred to a cardiological unit with facilities for electrophysiologic studies to optimize selection of long-term antiarrhythmic drug prophylaxis or to explore non-pharmacologic antitachycardia alternatives.

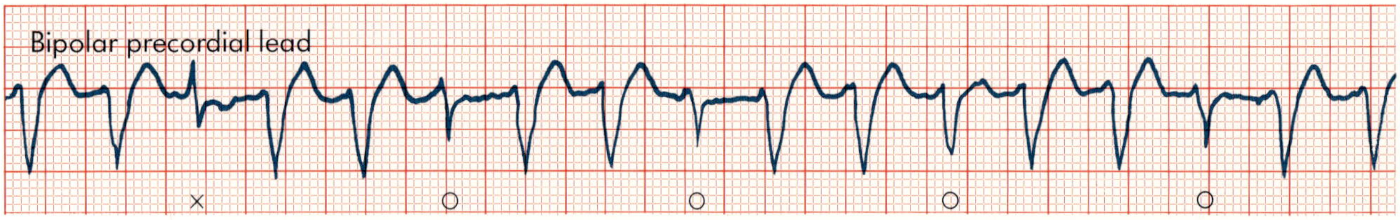

A

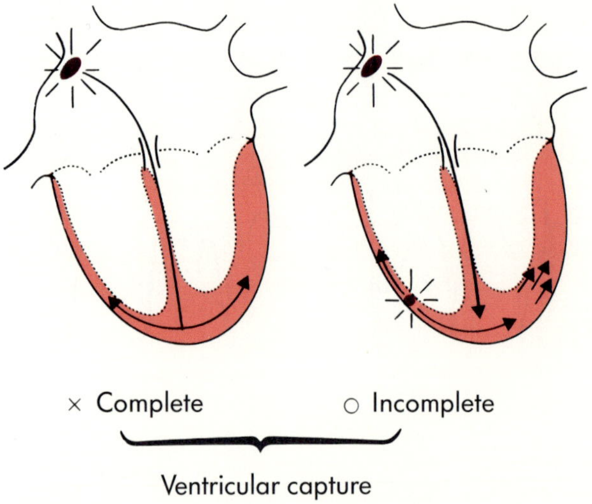

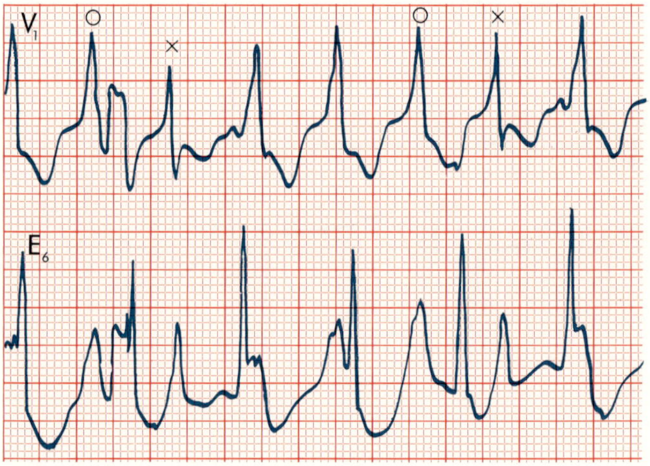

B

Fig. 6.28
Ventricular tachycardia with AV dissociation and ventricular captures. The ventricular origin of the tachycardia is suggested by the wide, monophasic QRS complexes and confirmed by the presence of ventricular captures and underlying AV dissociation.

A *There is an alternation between wide ventricular complexes, narrower QRS complexes most likely representing different degrees of incomplete ventricular capture (o) and a very narrow QRS complex most likely representing a complete capture (x), QRS rate: 140–150/min and irregular.*

B *An ECG recording from another patient. The surface recording (V_1) shows differences in QRS complex width most likely caused by incomplete (o) and complete (x) ventricular captures. The oesophageal ECG recording confirms the presence of AV dissociation. The PR interval for the complete captures is 0.20 s, within the range of normal AV conduction time. QRS rate: 140, sinus P wave rate 99–100/min.*

Prognosis

Paroxysmal ventricular tachycardia which degenerates to ventricular fibrillation after a period of seconds or minutes is the common cause of sudden death in chronic ischaemic heart disease and cardiomyopathy (Fig. 6.44, page 183).

Management

Acute attack [12]

1 *Search/treat for precipitating factors:* Electrolyte derangements, myocardial ischaemia, shock, arrhythmogenic side effects of antiarrhythmic drugs, digitalis overdosage etc.

2 *Intravenous medication:* The treatment of first choice is the intravenous injection of a bolus dose of lignocaine (100 + 100 mg). To maintain restored sinus rhythm a continous intravenous infusion of lignocaine is appropriate. During transport to hospital the i.v. infusion of lignocaine can be supplanted by an intramuscular injection (300 mg lignocaine i.m.).

Drug alternatives of second choice are the intravenous injection of a beta blocking agent, a Class IA drug (disopyramide or procainamide), a Class IB drug (mexiletine or tocainide) or a Class IC drug (ajmaline, propafenone or flecainide). Intravenously administered amiodarone may be effective in some patients where other drugs fail. Only two or a maxi-

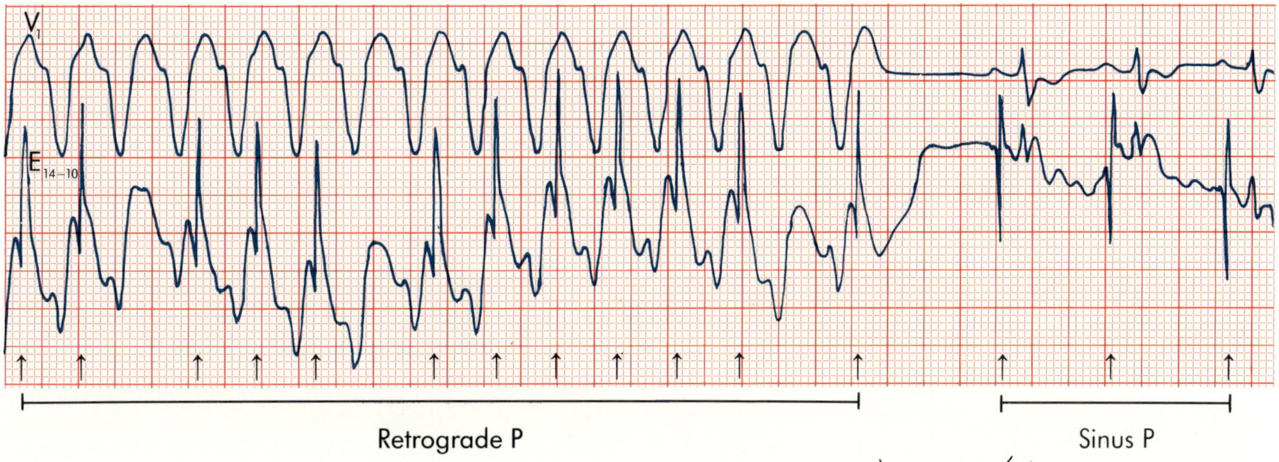

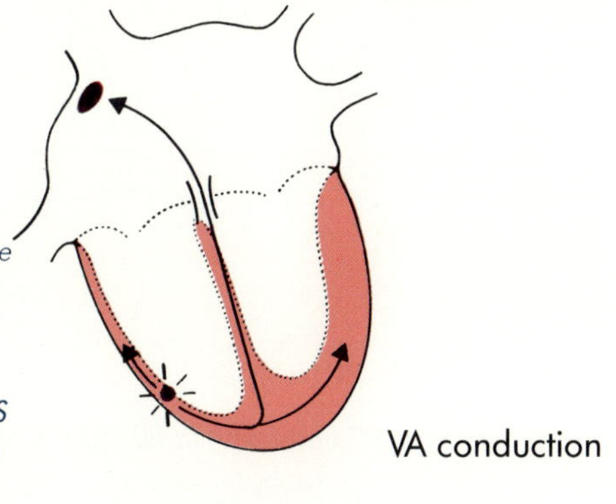

Fig. 6.29
Ventricular tachycardia and ventriculo-atrial (VA) conduction. The ventricular origin of the tachycardia is suggested by the wide, monophasic QRS complexes (0.18 s) quite different from the QRS complexes in sinus rhythm. The diagnosis is confirmed by the intermittent recording of 2:1 VA conduction. Atrial activity is not visible in the surface lead, but retrograde P waves (P waves quite opposite polarity of sinus P waves) are distinct in the oesophageal ECG recording Y(E_{14-10}). The P waves are chronologically related to the QRS complexes which are VA conducted, with the VA conduction ratio alternating between 1:1 and 2:1.

mum of three preparations should be given in refractory situations.

3 *Cardioversion:* Cardioversion is the treatment of choice if there is no prompt effect of intravenous lignocaine. An initial shock of 100 J should be followed by 200 + 200 + 360 J. Each fresh drug intervention should be followed by a repeated attempt at cardioversion.

Antiarrhythmic drugs for the long-term prophylaxis of ventricular tachycardia [12, 38, 44–46, 48–50]

1 *Single drug treatment:* This is best provided by a class IB antiarrhythmic drug (mexiletine, tocainide), which has the least arrhythmogenic effect, followed if required by a Class IA drug (quinidine, disopyramide, procainamide) or a Class IC drug (propafenone, flecainide). Recent reports have stressed the risk of an arrhythmogenic effect (sudden death) with the two Class IC drugs flecainide and encainide when used for long-term medication in patients with chronic ischaemic heart disease.

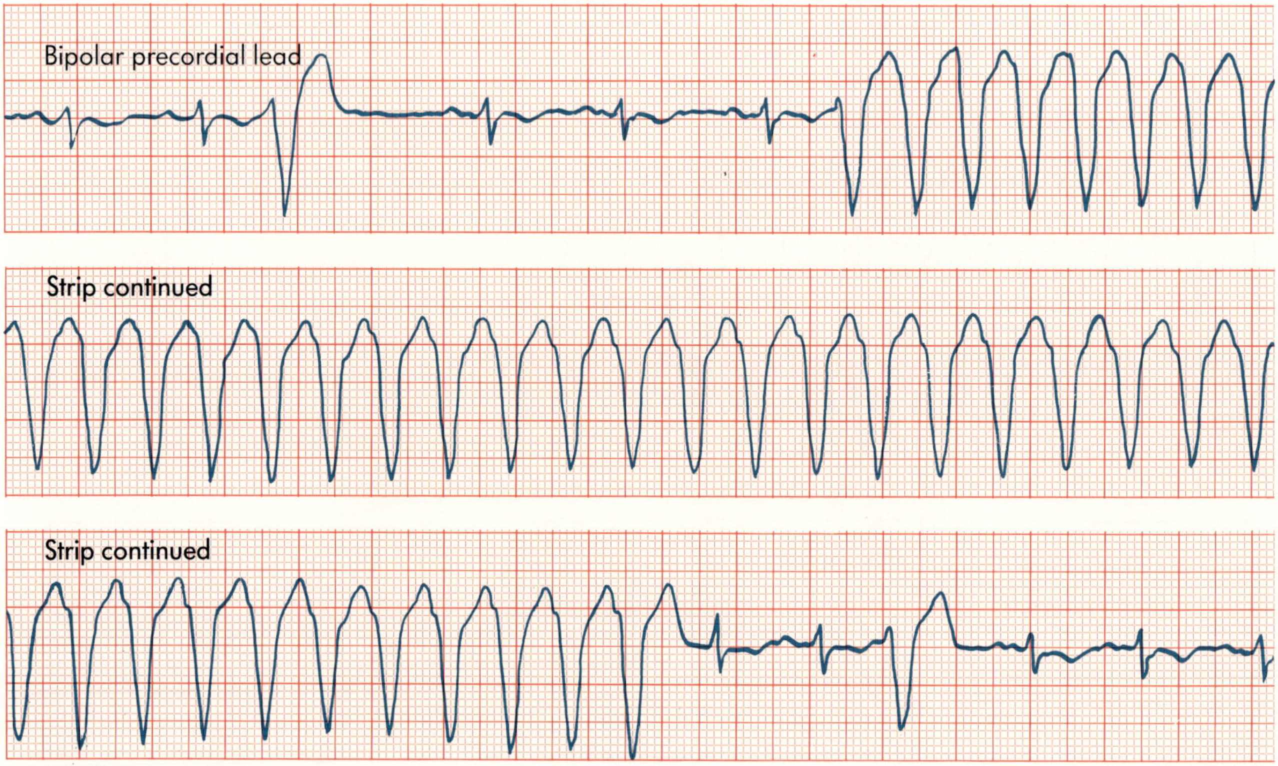

Fig. 6.30
Ventricular tachycardia and the diagnostic significance of ventricular extrasystole. The diagnosis of ventricular tachycardia is suggested by the recording of a wide (0.20 s) monophasic QRS complex in tachycardia, quite different from the narrow QRS complex seen in sinus rhythm. Ventricular origin of the tachycardia is finally confirmed by the recording of ventricular extrasystole before and after tachycardia with the same QRS configuration as the one seen in tachycardia. It appears from the compensatory postextrasystolic pause that the extrasystole is most likely of ventricular origin.

2 *Combination of a Class I drug with a beta blocking agent:* For example a Class IB drug (mexiletine or tocainide) combined with a beta blocking agent. With the exception of effort induced ventricular tachycardia and the long QT syndrome, beta blocking agents given alone rarely are effective in preventing attacks of ventricular tachycardia.

3 *Amiodarone:* This usually is administered as a single drug but may be combined with a beta blocking agent, or more exceptionally with a Class I drug (its combination with a Class IA drug is associated with an increased risk of inducing torsade de pointes ventricular tachycardia). Despite its many side effects amiodarone is highly effective and should be the drug of first choice for ventricular tachycardia complicating cardiomyopathy, particularly hypertrophic cardiomyopathy. It is also used by many cardiologists as first medication in paroxysmal ventricular tachycardia complicating chronic ischaemic heart disease.

Since attacks of ventricular tachycardia often occur with time intervals of weeks to months or even years, and as the attacks usually are life threatening, the efficacy of the recommended antiarrhythmic drug should be tested as far as possible before the patient leaves hospital.

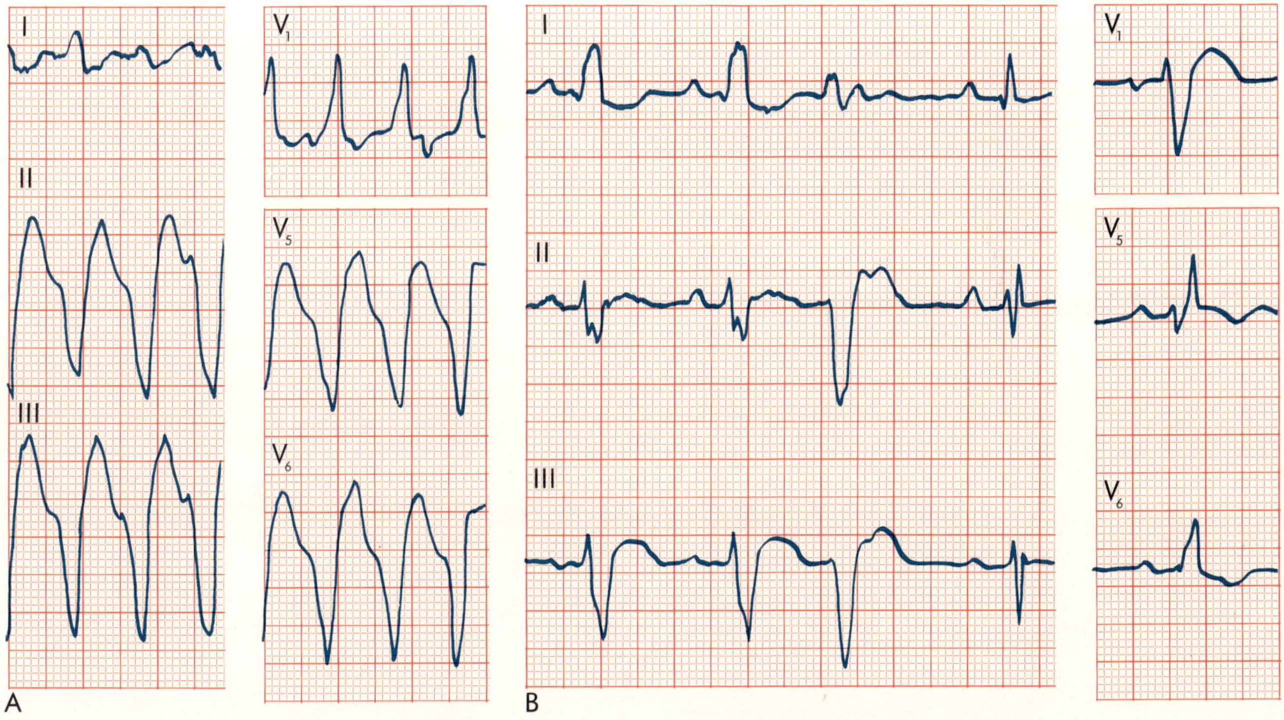

Fig. 6.31
Ventricular tachycardia, bundle branch block and ventricular extrasystole. QRS complex widening is seen in both tachycardia and sinus rhythm; but the QRS complex configuration is quite different. The QRS complex in sinus rhythm shows a left bundle branch block (rR′ pattern in leads V_{5-6}) shows a positive monophasic deflection in lead V_1 resembling a right bundle branch block pattern. The ventricular origin of the tachycardia is confirmed by the recording of ventricular extrasystole in sinus rhythm and a QRS complex identical to the one recorded during tachycardia. The ventricular origin of the extrasystole is confirmed by the recording of a compensatory postextrasystolic pause.

There are two approaches which may be used, singly or in combination:

- *Programmed electrical pacing:* When a ventricular tachyarrhythmia is no longer inducible at programmed electrical stimulation or when inducibility is rendered more difficult by an antiarrhythmic drug, the rate of recurrence is low (below 10 %) Non-inducibility, however, occurs in only 10 to 30 % of patients. By contrast, in 40 to 60 % of those patients in whom the ventricular tachyarrhythmia remains inducible despite antiarrhythmic therapy arrhythmia recurrence or sudden death will occur. For amiodarone conflicting data exists.

- *Long term ECG monitoring by telemetry in the hospital (in a setting with rescucitation facilities):* If, during the observation period, the drug suppresses not only the attacks of sustained ventricular tachycardia but also complex ventricular arrhythmias (e.g. high frequency ventricular extrasystoles, pairs of ventricular extrasystoles and non-sustained ventricular tachycardia), then the prospects for a successful long-term suppression of the tachycardia are good. Carefully selected and tested antiarrhythmic medication can improve prognosis for patients with chronic ischaemic heart disease and paroxysmal ventricular tachycardia. In a great number of patients, however, no effective antiarrhythmic drug therapy can be found.

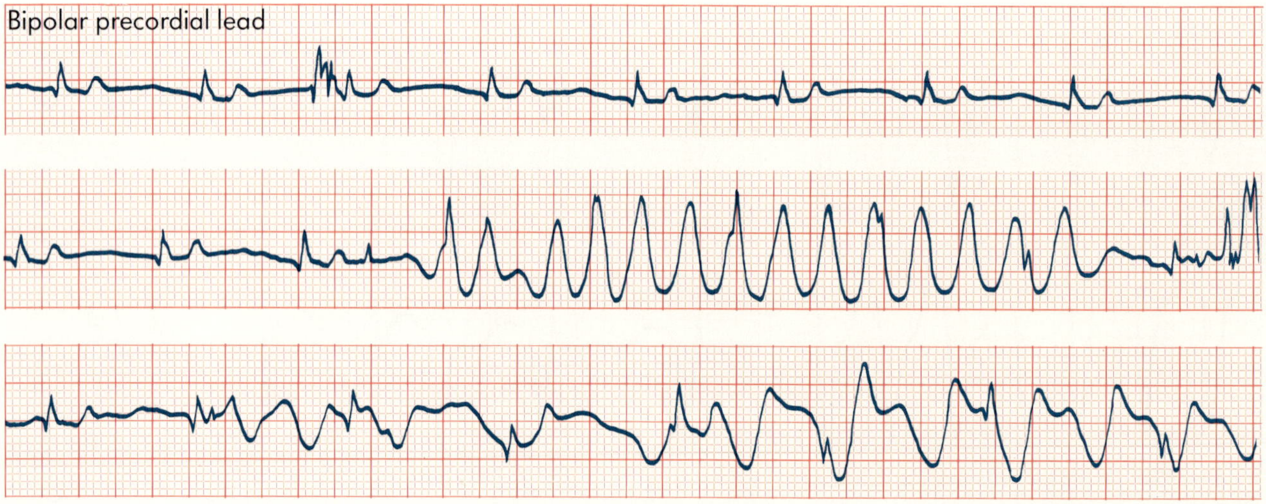

Fig. 6.32
Artifact ventricular tachycardia

Strip from the ECG monitoring of a 50-year-old man admitted with acute myocardial infaction. At first glance diagnosis might be ventricular tachycardia. However, the suspicion of an artifact is aroused by the recorded "noise" in both the upper and middle strip and confirmed by the finding that the regular heart rhythm can be followed through the episode of "tachycardia" in the form of the peak of the R wave intermittently superimposed on the fake QRS complexes of the artifact tachycardia.

This subset of patients is characterized by a persistance of complex and frequent ventricular extrasystoles or by a lack of change in the pacing inducibility of the ventricular tachycardia. They are candidates for non-pharmacologic interventions including antitachycardia surgery or the implantation of an automatic implantable cardioverter/defibrillator (AICD).

Antitachycardia surgery [43–47]

In chronic ischaemic heart disease with paroxysmal ventricular tachycardia optimal candidates for surgery are patients with a circumscribed ventricular aneurysm and paroxysms of monomorphic ventricular tachycardia. Endocardial resection of ventricular myocardium is guided by electrophysiologic mapping, and the surgeon usually will perform an aneurysmectomy and myocardial revascularization by coronary artery bypass grafting.

In patients with diffuse left ventricular dysfunction, surgical measures are limited by a high intraoperative and postoperative mortality, and the recurrence rate of tachycardia is high. Furthermore, *in patients with unstable ventricular tachycardia that rapidly degenerates into ventricular fibrillation,* presently available mapping techniques are unsatisfactory. Performed as the only surgical intervention, myocardial revascularization by coronary artery bypass grafting usually is inefficient for controlling paroxysmal ventricular tachycardia related to coronary artery disease. An exception is when attacks of ventricular tachycardia appear in conjunction with documented episodes of myocardial ischaemia (Fig. 14.22, page 336/337).

Implantation of an AICD unit [43, 45–47]

Implantation of an AICD unit (Fig. 4.11, page 86) should be considered in patients who have infrequent but life threatening attacks. The patient may have a completely refractory arrhythmia or be someone in whom antiarrhythmic drug treatment reduces but does not eliminate the paroxysms of ventricular tachycardia.

Specific forms of ventricular tachycardia

Within the group of ventricular tachycardia there are specific forms which are characterized by a specific ECG pattern and/or clinical features and management needs e.g.:

- Torsade de pointes ventricular tachycardia
- Multiform ventricular tachycardia
- Bidirectional ventricular tachycardia
- Paroxysmal ventricular tachycardia of right ventricular dysplasia
- Paroxysmal ventricular tachycardia in the otherwise healthy young individual.

Torsade de pointes ventricular tachycardia [51–66]

In a clinical context torsade de pointes ventricular tachycardia has two or three diagnostic elements. The diagnosis is initially suggested by the ECG of a tachycardia with a "torsade de pointes" pattern (see below). The diagnosis, however, requires additional support from a between-attack ECG showing AV block or QT prolongation. Last but not least the diagnosis is confirmed by a positive therapeutic response to pacing and/or beta blockade.

ECG diagnosis

1 *ECG in tachycardia:* Torsade de pointes is French for "turning or twisting around a point", and reflects the characteristic ECG feature of the tachycardia: A continous undulation of the QRS axis around the isoelectric line with a 360° rotation over a sequence of 5–20 complexes. The progressive QRS axis shift is best seen by a simultaneous three-lead ECG recording (Fig. 6.33, page 164) but is also seen, though less reliably on single-lead ECG monitoring (Figs. 6.34 C,

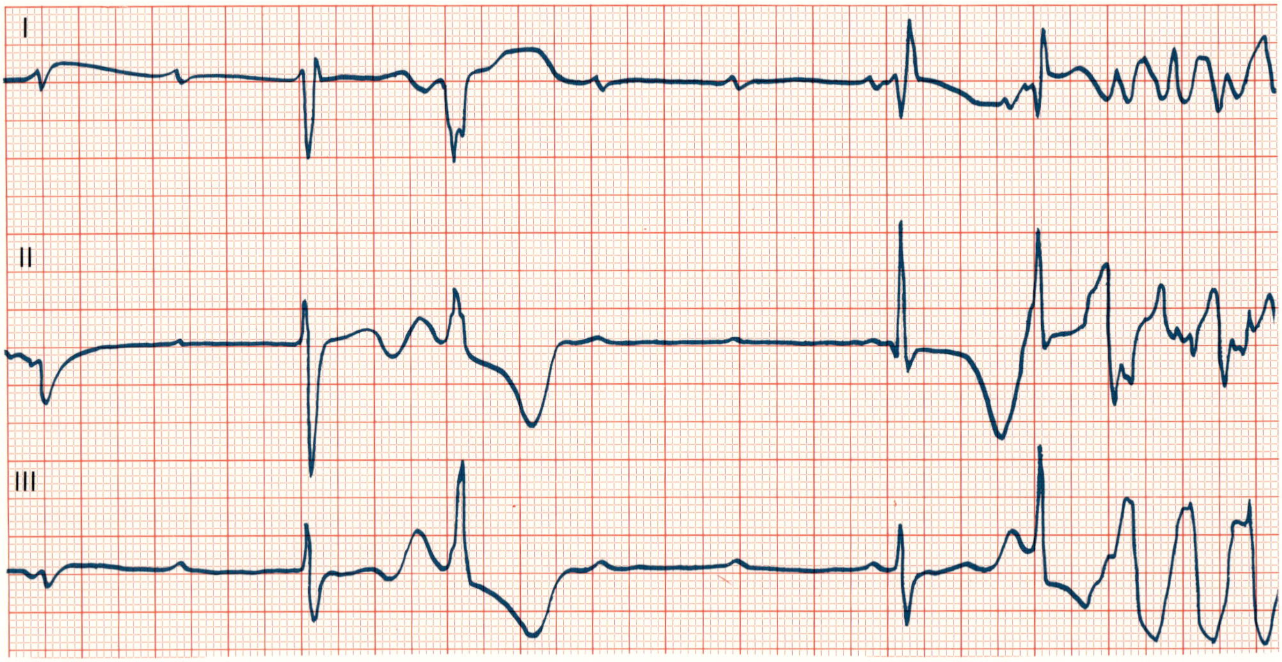

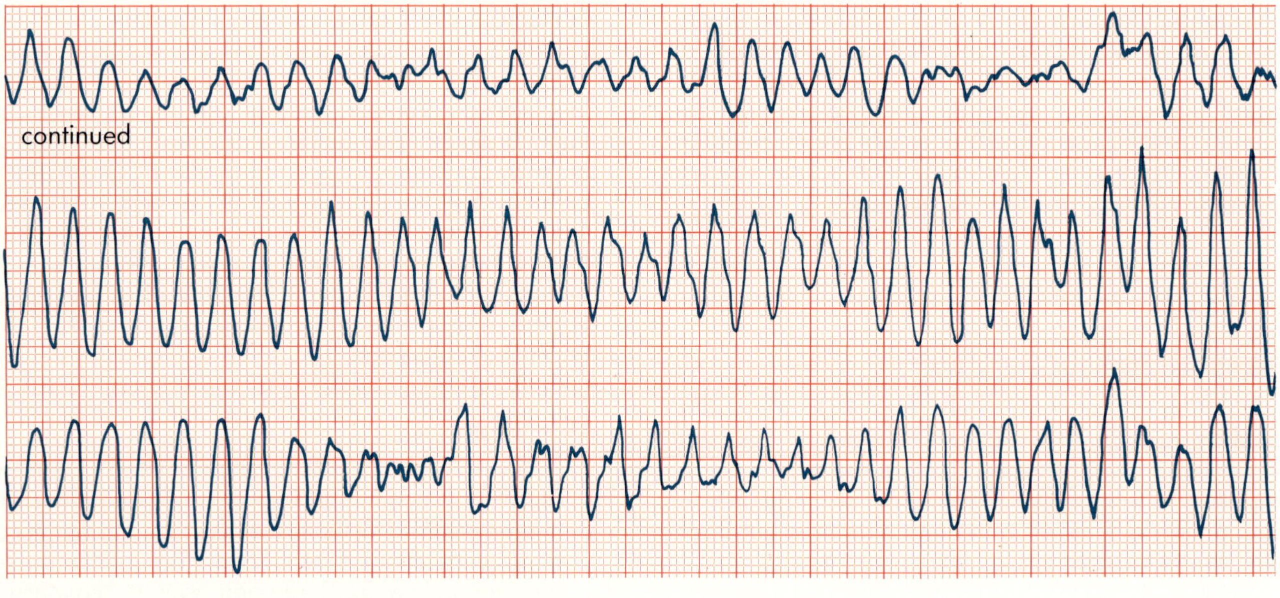

Fig. 6.33
Torsade de pointes ventricular tachycardia in third degree AV block. ECG from an 80-year-old male suffering from syncope during the preceding 2 weeks. No sign of acute myocardial infarction. Serum potassium 3.8mmol/l. Syncope during ECG recording. Cessation of fainting spells and tachycardia after implantation of pacemaker.

page 167 and 6.35 B, page 169). From a dominant QRS deflection in one direction there is a gradual change to the opposite direction and back again. In some patients the shifting QRS axis may be interrupted by runs of uniform QRS complexes with a stable axis, which means that if the ECG recording is not long enough the tachycardia may be misclassified as an "ordinary" ventricular tachycardia and not torsade de pointes. Initiation of torsade de pointes usually is by a ventricular extrasystole occurring late, on the downslope of the T wave, or thereafter on the U wave (Figs. 6.33, 6.34 C, 6.35 B).

2 *Between-attack ECG:* Of major diagnostic importance is to document between attacks AV block (Fig. 6.33), QT prolongation and/or T/U wave abnormalities (Figs. 6.34 and 6.35) on the standard ECG. The T waves may be broad and often are notched, peaked, biphasic or inverted.

  High amplitude U waves opposite in polarity to that of the T wave often are recorded. In the congenital long QT syndromes (see later) the length of the QT interval may vary with time in the same individual, and may be normal or near normal on any single tracing.

Differential diagnosis

ECG recognition of torsade de pointes is based more on pattern recognition than on definite criteria. Apart from the classical case there are arrhythmias of torsade type which are difficult or impossible to differentiate from multiform ventricular tachycardia (see next section). A suspected diagnosis of torsade de pointes ventricular tachycardia should be confirmed by a between-attack ECG recording of AV block or QT prolongation often associated with T/U wave abnormalities. Additional but circumstantial evidence supporting a diagnosis of torsade de pointes ventricular tachycardia would be a history of taking a medication which prolongs the QT interval; a family history of deafness, fainting and/or sudden death at a young age suggesting a congenital long QT syndrome (see later); or severe hypokalaemia (see later). Negative findings in all these respects suggest a diagnosis of multiform ventricular tachycardia and so too does a negative effect of both pacing and beta blockade.

QT prolongation which does not predispose to torsade de pointes occurs in:

- The WPW syndrome and bundle branch block. When WPW syndrome (PR $\leq$ 0.12 s) or bundle branch block (QRS $\geq$ 0.12 s) are present the QT will be prolonged

- Hypocalcaemia. QT prolongation in this condition is due to a prolongation of the ST segment and is not associated with T/U abnormalities

- Ventricular rhythms.

Symptoms

Torsade de pointes usually lasts for only a period of 20–60 s before it either reverts to a normal rhythm or it degenerates to ventricular fibrillation. With the onset of the tachycardia, cardiac output falls rapidly towards zero. The major symptoms of torsade de pointes are presyncope, syncope and sudden death.

Aetiology

Paroxyms of torsade de pointes occur in AV block (1), the acquired long QT syndromes (2) and the congenital long QT syndromes (3).

1 *AV block:* Torsade de pointes occurs as a sudden and unexpected complication of third degree AV block (Fig. 6.33) and advanced AV block (Fig. 10.11, page 265). A precipitating factor in these conditions might be hypokalaemia induced by diuretic treatment or perhaps hypomagnaesemia.

2 *Acquired long QT syndromes:* QT prolongation with a documented risk of torsade de pointes may be due to:

  - *Antiarrhythmic drugs:* QT prolongation of varying degree occurs with the Class I A drugs (quinidine, procainamide, disopyramide), the beta blocking agent sotalol and with amiodarone. Torsade de pointes is a common complication of intoxication with these drugs but can occur also with therpeutic dosages. The prolongation of the QT interval is, however, a consistent accompaniment to the antiarrhythmic action of these drugs but a relationship between the risk of torsade de pointes ventricular tachycardia and some critical QT value or increment in the QT value has not been established. Over and above QT prolongation per se, quinidine syncope has been associated with the development of prominent and abnormal U waves (though again without a clear definition of a high risk threshold.

A few cases of torsade de pointes have been described related to sotalol. Amiodarone often is associated with significant QT prolongation yet very few cases of torsade de pointes have been reported.

- *Psychotropic drugs:* Intoxication with the tricyclic antidepressants and the benzodiazepine thioridazine may cause significant QT prolongation with a risk of sudden life threatening attacks of torsade de pointes (Fig. 6.34).

- *Severe hypokalaemia, subarachnoid bleeding and myxoedema* can cause QT prolongation which in *rare cases* may be complicated by attacks of torsade de pointes.

Chronic ischaemic heart disease and/or ventricular hypertrophy can cause QT prolongation which may or may not be associated with paroxysmal ventricular tachycardia but not especially with ventricular tachycardia of the torsade de pointes type.

3 *Congenital long QT syndromes (Jervell-Lange-Nielsen and Romano-Ward syndromes):* There are two congenital syndromes characterized by QT prolongation, near fainting and a risk of sudden death. In one, the Jervell-Lange-Nielsen syndrome (the Surdo-cardiac syndrome), there is associated deafness. In the other, the Romano-Ward syndrome, hearing is normal. Both syndromes are hereditary. Fainting spells usually begin in childhood, sometimes in infancy, although the onset may be as late as the second or third decade, particularly in the Romano-Ward syndrome. The frequency of attacks varies from several times a day to less than once every several years. There is a tendency for the frequency to decrease with age. Some members of a family with QT prolongation may have frequent attacks, while other family members with the same degree of QT prolongation may have few if any attacks and be symptom free for life. Some patients faint in relation to fear or anxiety. Others respond to a specific irritant such as being awakened in the early morning by the sound of an alarm clock (Fig. 6.35, page 168/169). Often the attacks occur in a completely unpredictable way, although there is a tendency for a higher frequency in the early morning hours. Most patients tolerate physical exercise well.

ECG screening of relatives of symptomatic patients with the long QT syndrome will reveal a number of *asymptomatic individuals* who have definite ECG abnormalities with QT prolongation and T/U wave changes.

The time interval between attacks may vary from weeks to months up to years. Between attacks the ECG usually shows sinus rhythm, often a sinus bradycardia at a rate of 50–60/min. Thus, long-term ECG monitoring is of little if any help in the diagnosis.

Prognosis

Torsade de pointes carries a risk of degeneration to ventricular fibrillation and thereby a risk of sudden death.

In the congenital long QT syndromes, the mortality rate in the untreated *symptomatic patient* is significant, possibly as high as 30–50 % over a period of some years. However, some patients may survive for 50 or 60 years, despite repeated attacks. Treatment with beta blockade (see next section) offers an excellent prognosis both for suppression of attacks and for survival. The prognosis in the *asymptomatic individual with QT prolongation* is unpredictable. While many will live a normal life, others will develop symptoms. It is, however, *uncommon* for such patients to die at the first attack, although this is not unknown.

continued page 170

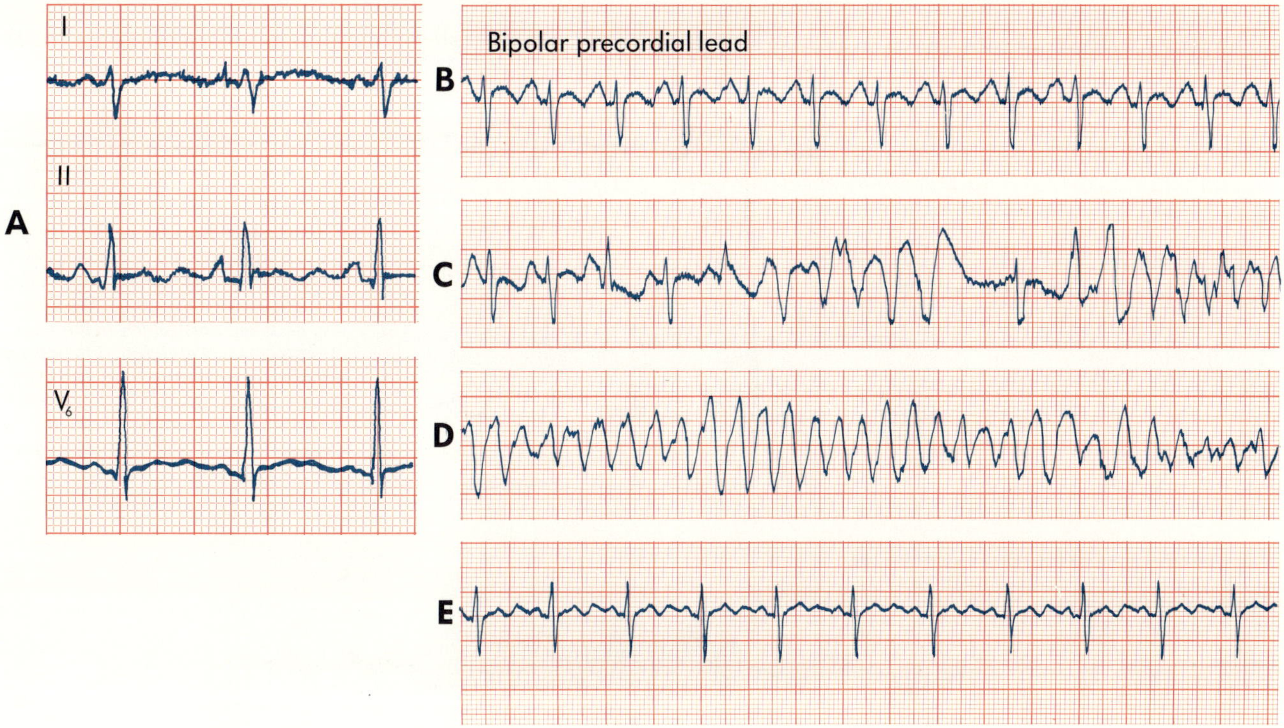

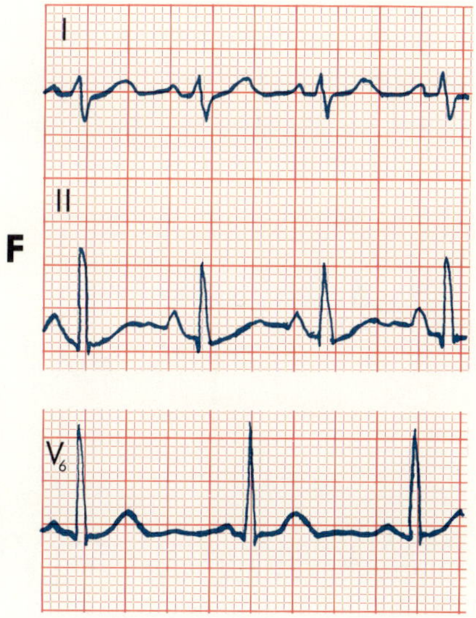

Fig. 6.34
Acquired long QT syndrome
25-year-old woman admitted after the intake of 1000 mg (100 tablets) of thioridazine with suicidal intent

A ECG 3 hours after admission, QT 0.52 which is far above normal (max normal QT at the actual heart rate of 85/min is 0.40 s, Table 2.1, p. 31)

B ECG strip from first 8 hours of ECG monitoring. Stable sinus rhythm

C ECG strip recorded shortly after B shows short episode of torsade de pointes ventricular tachycardia and the sudden start of a longer episode

D Continuation of C shows uninterrupted torsade de pointes ventricular tachycardia finally terminated by a DC countershock. Three hours later a new attack of torsade de pointes ventricular tachycardia which again had to be stopped by DC countershock. Hereafter sinus rhythm and an uneventful recovery

E Stable sinus rhythm after the second and final DC countershock

F ECG in third day, QT has normalized

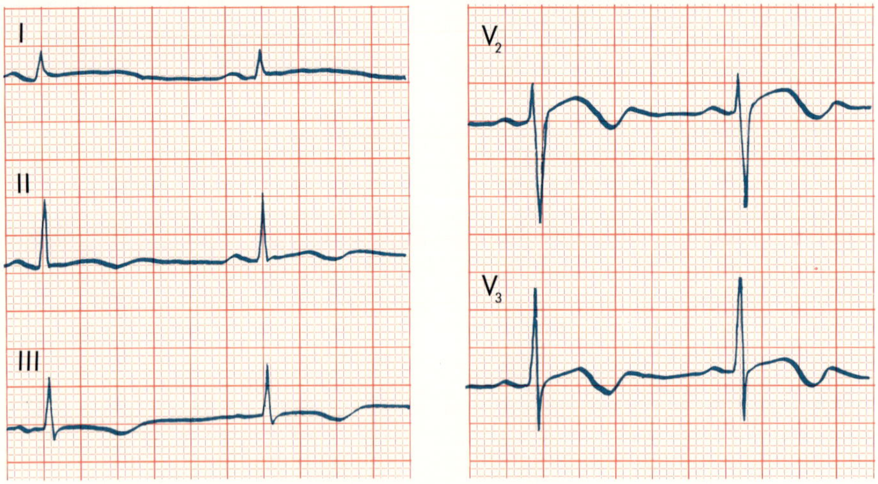

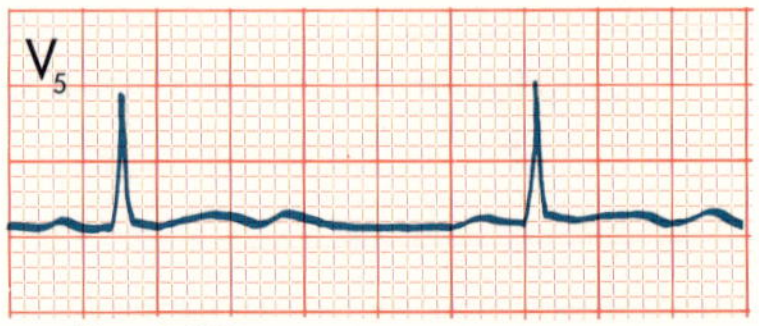

Fig. 6.35
Romano-Ward syndrome. ECG from a 13-year-old girl admitted due to repeated attacks of fainting, sometimes complicated with seizures. The fainting occurred particularly in the early morning, usually related to the abrupt jangling of an alarm clock. The ECG showed prolonged QT = 0.62 s (max normal at the actual heart rate 0.47 s) and abnormal T and U waves in the precordial leads.

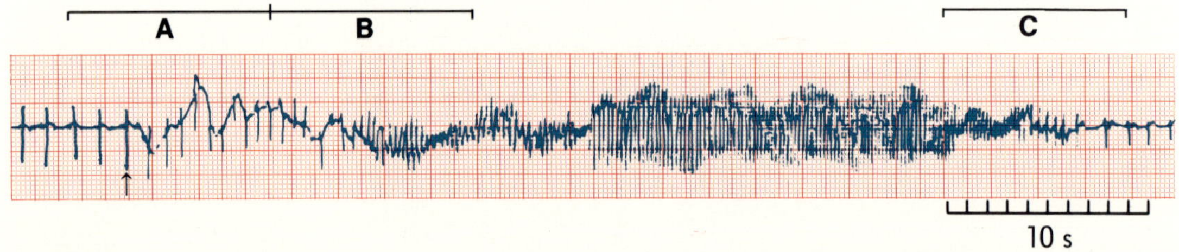

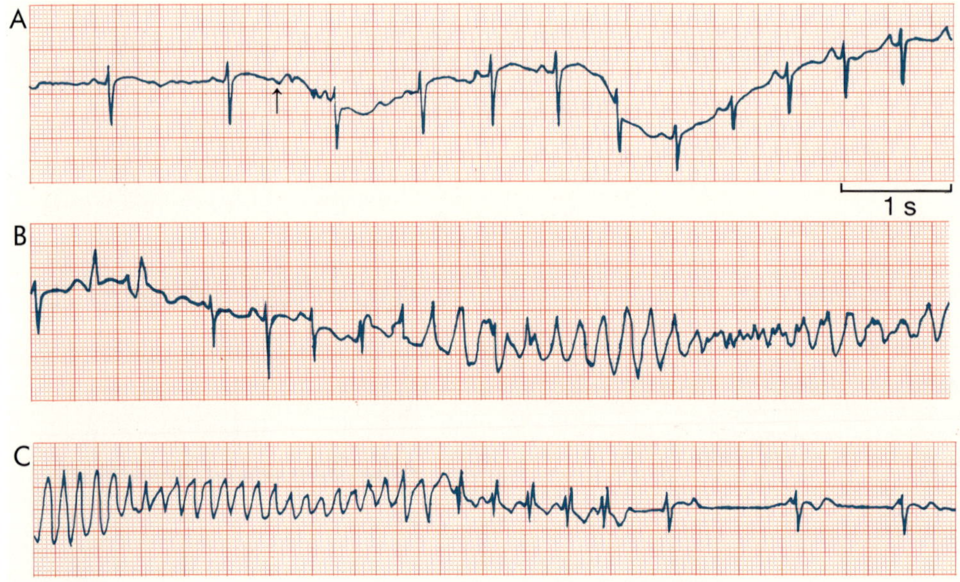

In relation to the abrupt awakening by the ringing of a brass bell in the early morning heart rate accellerated slightly over a period of 10 s (A) followed by the outbreak of torsade de pointes ventricular tachycardia (B) and spontaneous restoration of sinus rhythm 30 s later (C). Over the following 2 weeks the experiment with abrupt awakening in the morning was repeated five times each time with the same result (D–G): onset of torsade de pointes ventricular tachycardia after a latency period of 10–20 s. On one occasion the tachycardia deteriorated to ventricular fibrillation with immediate restoration of sinus rhythm following DC countershock. The patient was started on long-term prophylaxis with a betablocking agent and has had no new attacks over an 8 year follow-up.

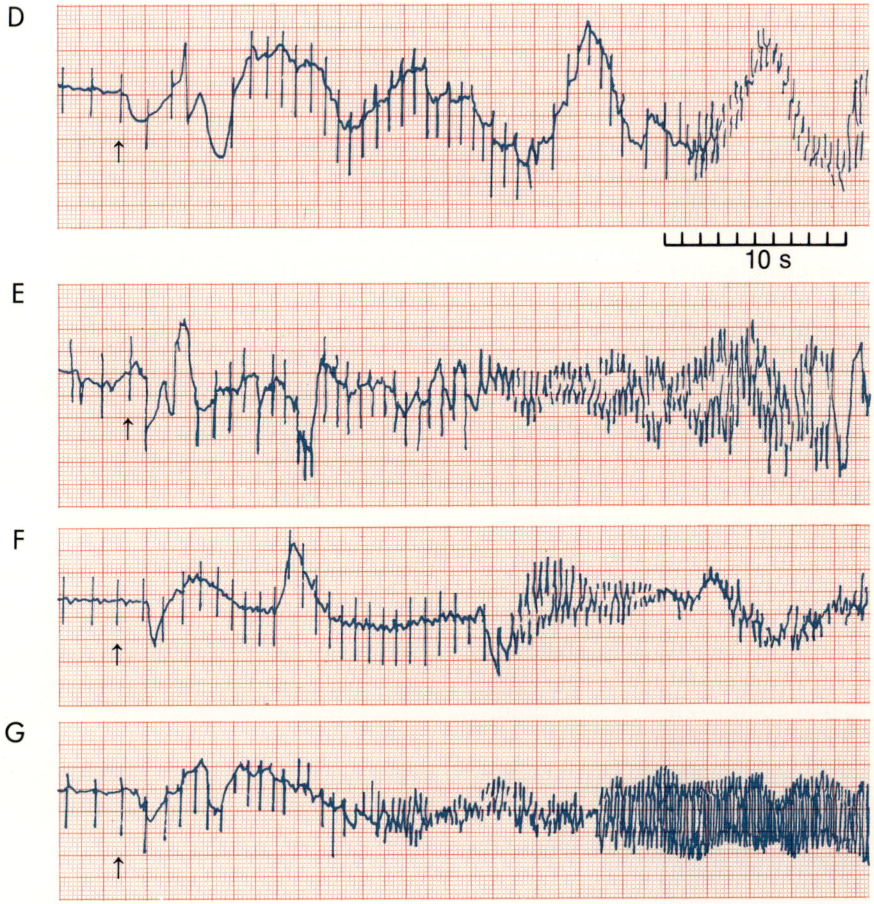

Fig. 6.35 (continued)

Management

A sustained attack of torsade de pointes usually can be stopped immediately by a DC countershock. Alternatively intravenous magnesium sulfate given as a bolus injection followed by an intravenous infusion has been recommended as an effective and safe procedure to stop the arrhythmia and prevent recurrences. Other options which might be considered are the intravenous bolus injection of adrenaline and/or isoprenaline infusion.

Prophylactic treatment should be based on the ECG and the aetiology of the condition:

1 If the torsade de pointes is *secondary to AV block,* artificial pacing at a rate of 80–100/min should be instituted. While this is being organized, the tachycardia may be controlled by an isoprenaline infusion. The serum potassium should be checked and hypokalaemia corrected.

2 Torsade de pointes induced by *antiarrhythmic drugs, tricyclic antidepressants* or *thioridazine* demands drug withdrawal, temporary transvenous pacing at a rate of 80–100/min, and if required supplementary treatment with beta blockade.

3 If the torsade de pointes is related to one of the *congenital long QT syndromes* (Jervell-Lange-Nielsen syndrome or Romano-Ward syndrome) life long treatment with a beta blocking agent is indicated. Rarely, supplementary treatment with artificial pacing may be required in some patients. Left stellate ganglionectomy has been tried with varying degrees of success in a number of drug resistant patients. The stellectomy may shorten the QT interval, but most often this is only for a short period of time after which the QT prolongation recurs. In the *asymptomatic* individual with QT prolongation in whom no ventricular arrhythmias are detected by long-term ECG monitoring, specific prophylactic drug therapy is not recommended.

If a tachycardia with torsades de pointe-like configuration develops and there is no concommitant bradycardia and/or QT prolongation then most likely it is not true torsades de pointes but multiform ventricular tachycardia which will respond to conventional antiarrhythmic treatment with lignocaine, another Class I drug, a beta blocking agent or amiodarone.

Multiform ventricular tachycardia [65–68]

In multiform ventricular tachycardia the ventricles are activated from two or more different pacemakers each characterized by its own typical form of QRS complex.

ECG diagnosis

The tachycardia is characterized by wide QRS complexes of varying configuration (Fig. 6.36). The variation in QRS configuration may be random or may show a repetitive pattern similar to or identical with the continuous undulation of the QRS axis seen in torsade de pointes ventricular tachycardia.

Differential diagnosis

As stated above, the ECG appearance during tachycardia may be similar or identical to the twisting QRS axis of torsade de pointes. Between attacks, however, there is no AV block, no QT prolongation, and no T/U wave anomalies. A difficult differential diagnosis can be that of atrial fibrillation and flutter complicating the WPW syndrome (Figs. 7.12–7.14, page 201 – page 204).

Aetiology

Often severe heart disease: Extensive acute myocardial infarction, chronic ischaemic heart disease or cardiomyopathy, and last but not least, Class I drugs, in particular the Class IC drugs, flecainide and encainide, followed by propafenone and the Class IA drugs, and,

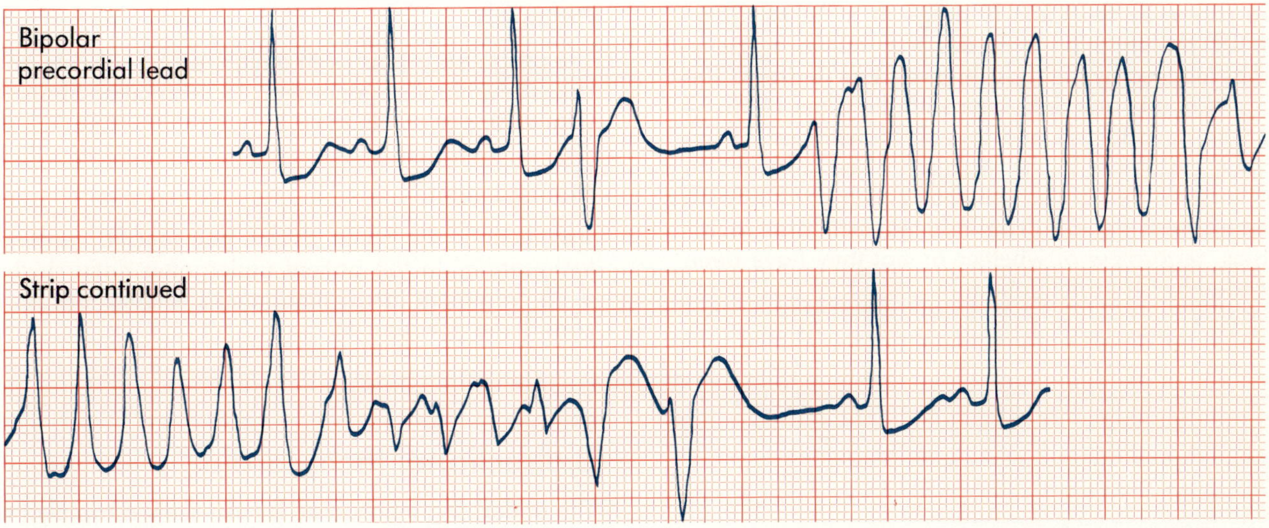

Fig. 6.36
Multiform ventricular tachycardia. ECG from a 48-year-old woman with former inferior wall infaction. Admitted in ventricular fibrillation after cardiac arrest on the sidewalk. No sign of new infarction but repeated episodes of self limiting multiform ventricular tachycardia during the following 1 week of ECG monitoring. Echocardiography shows normal left ventricle without aneurysm.

The ECG is similar in appearance to torsade de pointes ventricular tachycardia. However, ECG between attacks shows no AV block or QT prolongation, there is no hypokalaemia and the patient is not in treatment with antiarrhythmic or psycotropic drugs. Betablockade fails to prevent the paroxysms of tachycardia.

Following onset of amiodarone treatment no new attacks over a 3-year follow-up.

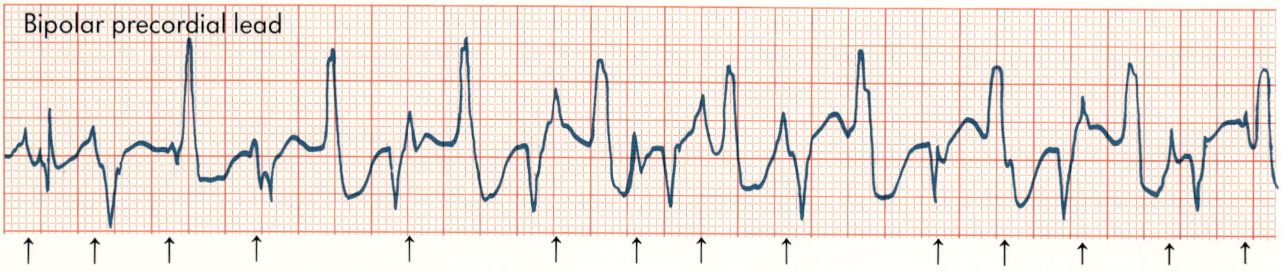

Fig. 6.37
Bidirectional ventricular tachycardia and double tachycardia in severe digoxin intoxication. ECG is from a 47-year-old male with mitral insufficiency and digoxin intoxication, with a serum digoxin level of 5.4 ng/ml. From the left, first a sinus complex with a bundle branch block pattern, next QRS complexes of alternating negative and positive polarity. The first two negatively directed QRS complexes are slightly different from the other of the same type, possibly an expression of partial ventricular capture (sinus P waves are observed immediately before the QRS complexes). There is AV dissociation during most of the recording period; P waves (arrows) are distinguishable through the ventricular rhythm. They come at intervals of 0.40 s or a multiple hereof, corresponding to an atrial rate of 150/min. The QRS rate is 170/min. The bidirectional tachycardia is initially irregular but finally regular.

more rarely, by the Class IB drugs. It is the exception that QT prolongation precedes the multiform tachycardias induced by the Class IC and Class IB drugs. This phenomenon is primarily seen with the Class IA drugs and with amiodarone and sotalol. Nonetheless, it has become customary in the literature of recent years to use "torsade de pointes ventricular tachycardia" as a common term for all drug induced multiform tachycardias, regardless of whether or not they have been preceded by QT prolongation.

Prognosis

The prognosis is poor with a high recurrence rate and a risk of eventual degeneration to ventricular fibrillation (Fig. 9.10, page 238/239).

Management

Treatment is the same as for non-specific ventricular tachycardia. In the patient undergoing antiarrhythmic drug treatment arrhythmogenesis should always be considered (Chapter 6).

Bidirectional tachycardia [69]

The underlying mechanism is most likely a rapidly firing pacemaker in the first undivided part of the left bundle branch with conduction to the left ventricle alternating between the anterior and posterior fascicles of the bundle (Fig. 9.2, page 225).

ECG diagnosis

The tachycardia usually occurs in short bursts. Successive ventricular complexes slow alternating axis deviation (Fig. 6.37).

Aetiology

Bidirectional tachycardia is a rare arrhythmia. It is most often related to digitalis overdosage in patients with advanced heart disease.

Management

Due to the risk of sudden death, immediate admission to a Coronary Care Unit for ECG monitoring is advised. Digitalis intoxication should be sought and if confirmed, treated as indicated in Chapter 12, page 292. The tachycardia itself can be treated with lignocaine, a beta blocking agent or amiodarone. DC cardioversion should be avoided if possible if digitalis intoxication is the aetiological basis of the arrhythmia.

Ventricular tachycardia due to arrhythmogenic right ventricular dysplasia [70–73]

Arrhythmogenic right ventricular dysplasia is a congenital cardiomyopathy with patchy fat infiltration and myocardial degeneration limited to the right ventricle. The major and usually only clinical manifestations are ventricular extrasystoles and attacks of fast ventricular tachycardia causing syncope and associated with a risk of sudden death. The attacks will often be induced by strenous attacks.

ECG diagnosis

Arrhythmogenic right ventricular dysplasia should be suspected in the young individual with ventricular extrasystoles and attacks of ventricular tachycardia showing a left bundle branch block morphology (positive QRS net area in V_{5-6}) suggesting a right ventricular origin of the ectopies. The ECG between attacks may show signs of a right ventricular disturbance such as right bundle branch block, incomplete right bundle branch block (Fig. 6.38, page 174) or ST segment depression and/or T wave inversion in leads V_{1-3}.

Differential diagnosis

Paroxysmal ventricular tachycardia with left bundle branch polarity can occur in young individuals without underlying heart disease (idiopatic right ventricular tachycardia).

Additional investigations

Usually the heart is normal clinically and radiographically. Echocardiography may reveal a slightly dilated right ventricle. Confirmation of the diagnosis may be obtained by right ventricular angiography which often will show a diffusely dilated right ventricle and/or deep fissuring ("pile of plates"), akinetic bulges or outpouchings particularly in the infundibular region, the apical region or in the diaphragmatic wall of the right ventricle under the tricuspid leaflet.

Management

Successful suppression of the attacks of tachycardia have been reported with sotalol in high dosage. Otherwise treatment of arrhythmogenic right ventricular dysplasia is broadly similar to that for non specific ventricular tachycardia. Surgical ablation of the arrhythmogenic focus in the right ventricle may be initially successful but there is a tendency for recurrences over a period of years.

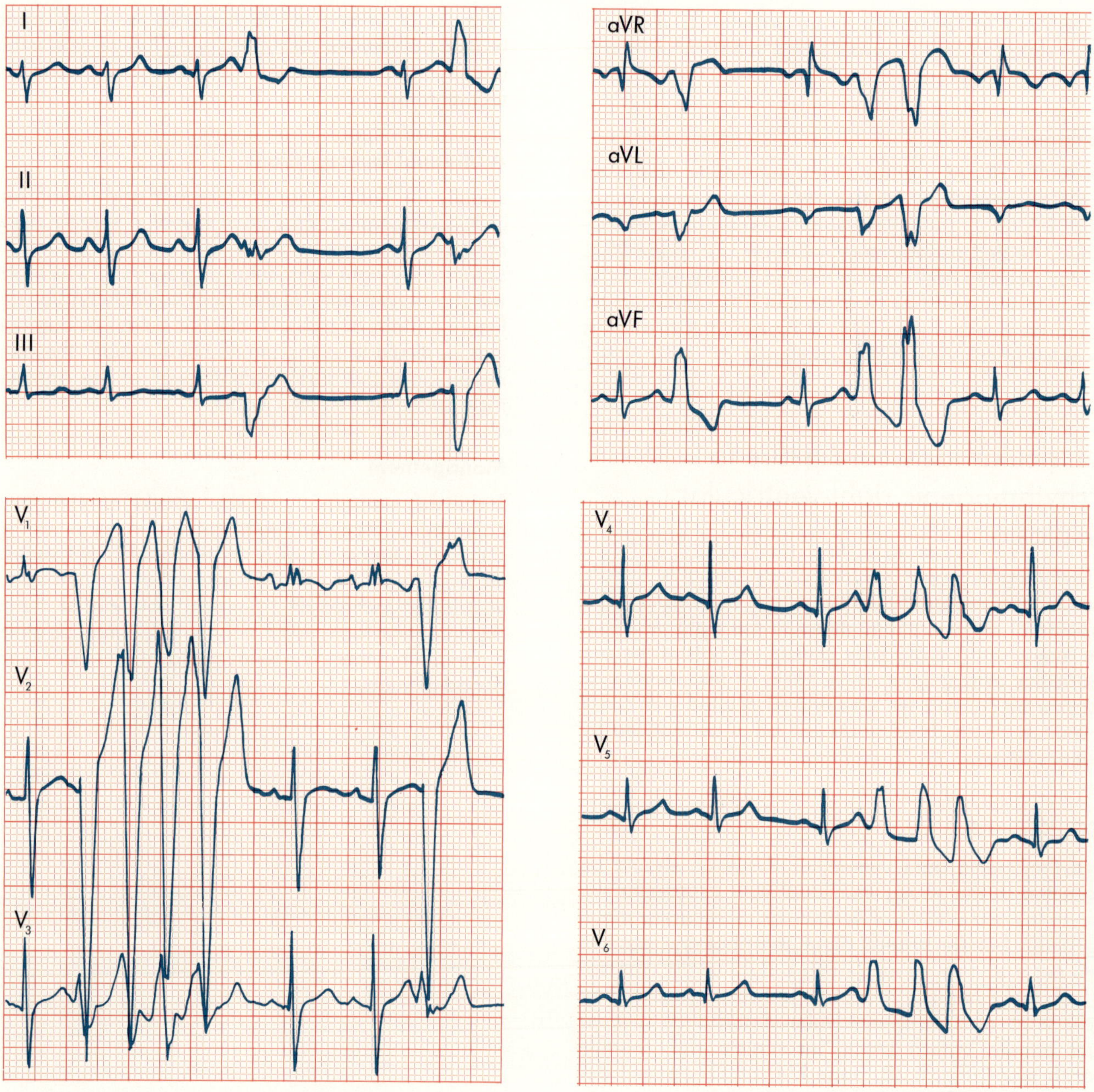

Fig. 6.38
Arrhythmogenic right ventricular dysplasia. A 6-year-old boy with fainting spells
A ECG at admission: Brief attacks of tachycardia with LBBB polarity

Ventricular tachycardia in the otherwise healthy young individual

Ventricular tachycardia without underlying heart disease is rare. Specific types with varying clinical and prognostic implications are:

- Repetitive monomorphic ventricular tachycardia (Gallavardin's tachycardia)
- Fascicular ventricular tachycardia, and
- Effort induced ventricular tachycardia.

Repetitive monomorphic ventricular tachycardia (Gallavardin's tachycardia)[74, 75]

This usually benign form of ventricular tachycardia is manifest by frequent runs of 3–10 ventricular complexes at a rate of usually not more than 130–140/min alternating with sinus rhythm. ECG monitoring may reveal periods of sustained ventricular tachycardia, but at a moderate rate (Fig. 6.39, page 176). The tachycardia is often present for years. It produces few if any symptoms, is not worsened by psychological or physical stress, and has not been associated with an increased mortality.

Management

This repetitive tachycardia is refractory to most antiarrhythmic medication. Verapamil has been reported to be effective but that has not been confirmed by the experience of the authors of this book.

continued page 180

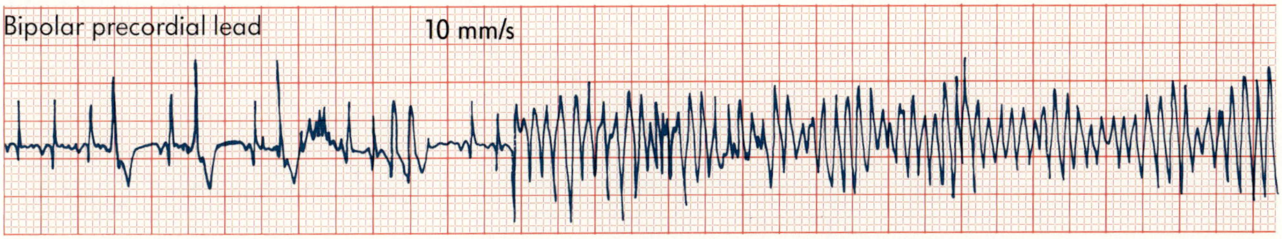

Fig. 6.38 (continued)
B ECG monitoring druing a fainting spell in hospital: Ventricular tachycardia degenerating into fibrillation. Sinus rhythm restored by DC countershock. Right ventricular angiocardiography showed minor changes in the infundibular region compatible with right ventricular dysplasia. Tachycardia tendency eventually controlled by combined treatment with amiodarone and flecainide.

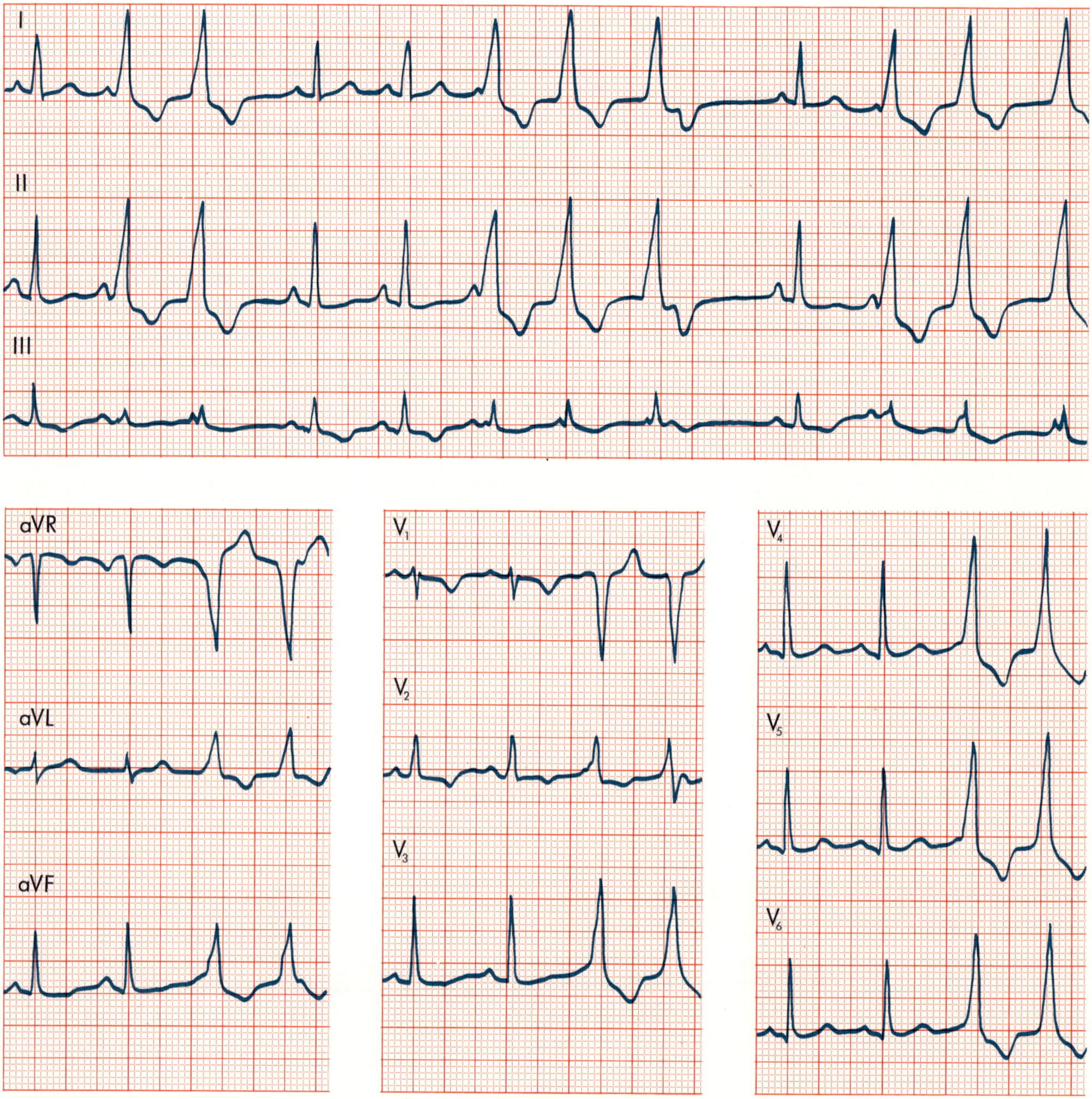

Fig. 6.39
Repetetive monomorph ventricular tachycardia in a 16-year-old otherwise healthy woman. There is an alternation between two to three ventricular complexes in a row at a rate of 100-140/min and one or two sinus beats. No response to antiarrhythmic medication (verapamil, betablocker, quinidine or flecainide). At a follow-up 3 years later at the age of 20 the tachycardia tendency was unchanged and the patient was symptom free with normal functional capacity.

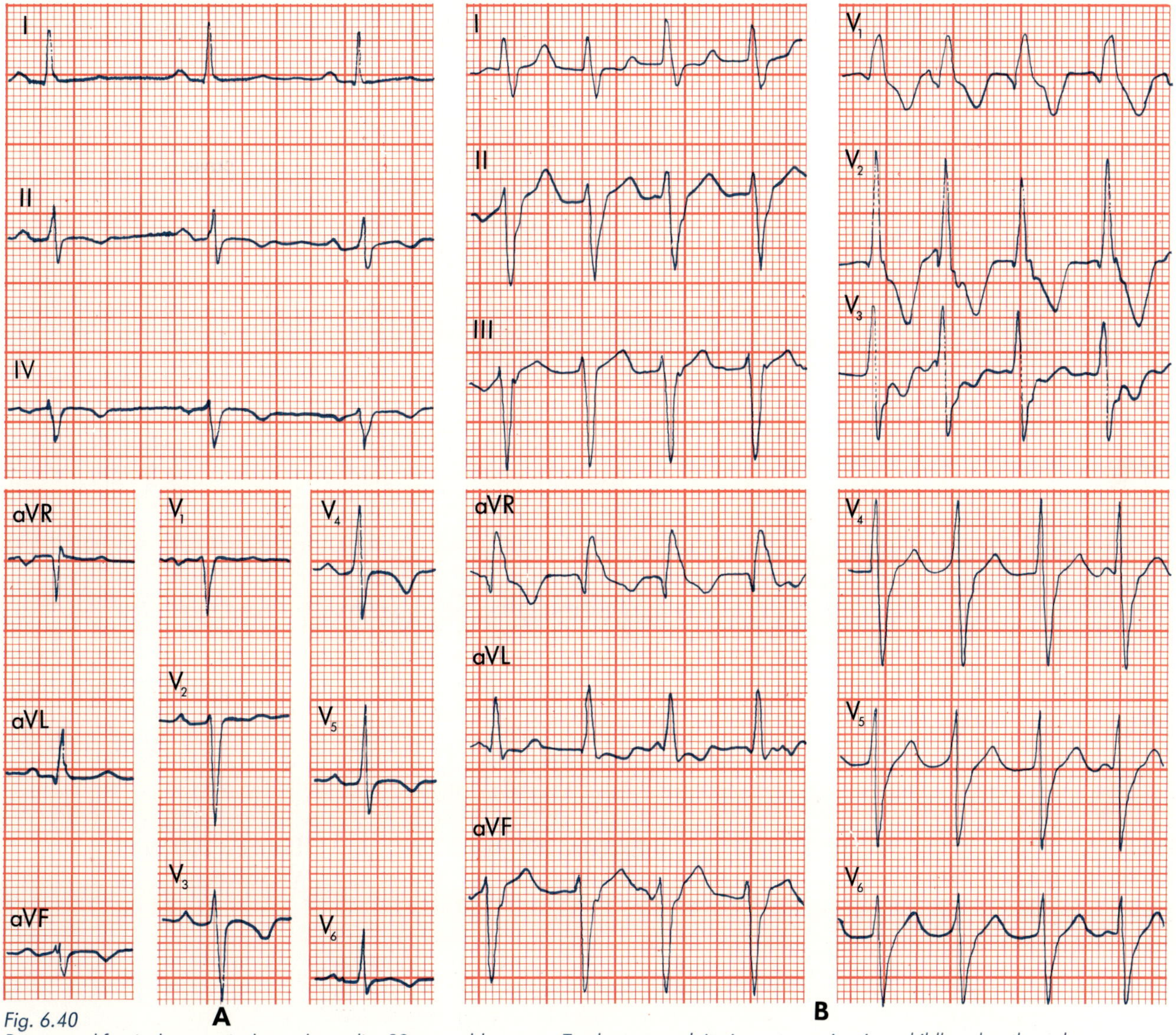

Fig. 6.40
Paroxysmal fascicular ventricular tachycardia. 32-year-old woman. Tendency to palpitations at exercise since childhood as the only cardiovascular complaint.

A ECG in sinus rhythm, negative T waves in V_3–V_6 possibly induced by preceding attack of ventricular tachycardia (Fig. 14.23, p. 339)

B ECG during an attack of tachycardia, QRS rate 130/min, QRS shows a right bundle branch configuration combinded with left anterior fascicular block

The diagnosis of fascicular ventricular tachycardia suggested by the ECG recording during the attack of tachycardia was later confirmed by an electrophysiologic study. The attacks of tachycardia could be terminated by verapamil administered intravenously. Few attacks on leng-term treatment with high dosage verapamil (300 mg of sustained release preparation daily).

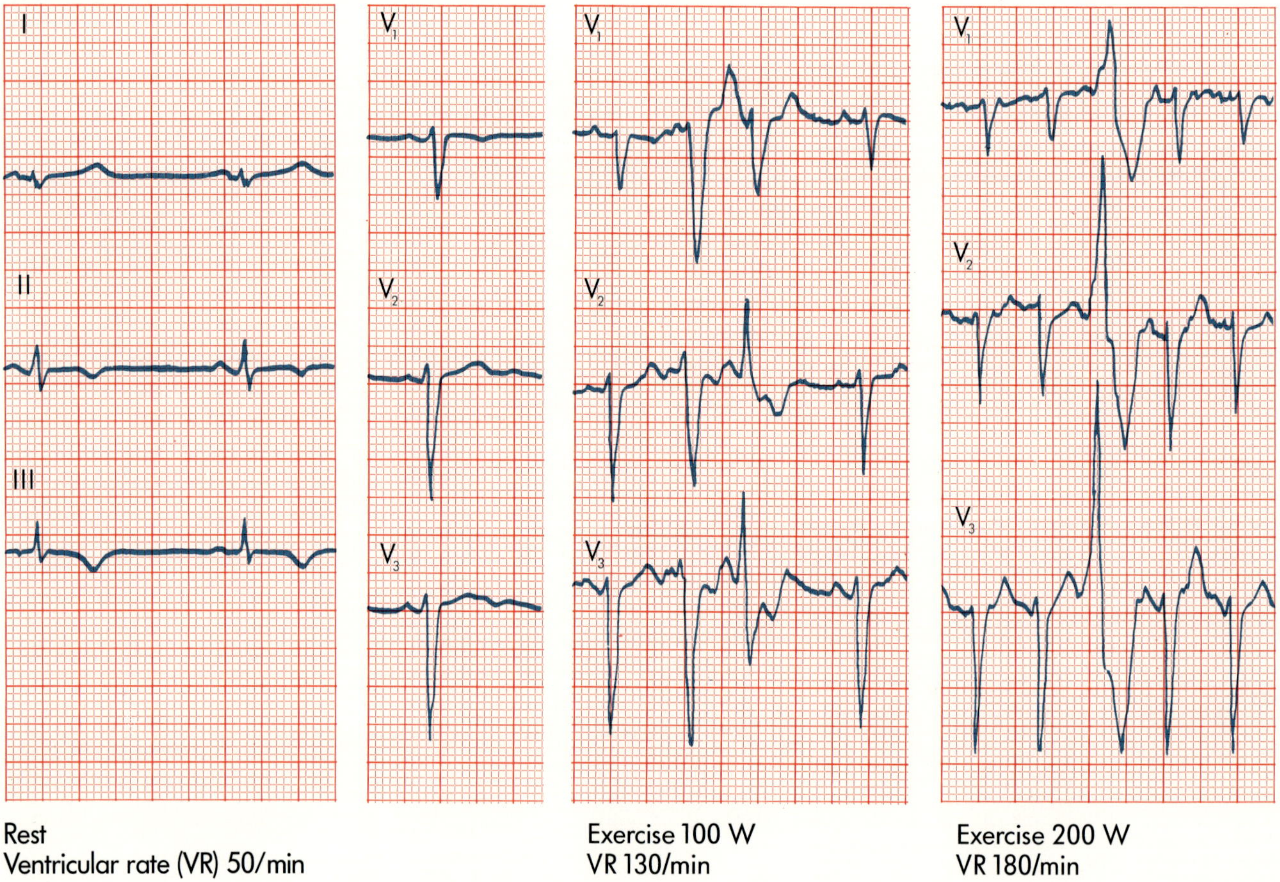

Fig. 6.41
Effort induced ventricular tachycardia. An ECG from a 19-year-old male who, for the past 3 months, suffered from attacks of syncope or dizziness during participation in sporting events. The ECG demonstrated abnormal T waves in several leads, but with a normal QT segment. Angiography revealed minor prolapse of the mitral valve. There was no sign of organic heart disease. The only abnormal finding during exercise on a bicycle ergometer was ventricular extrasystole which did not increase in intensity with increased stress. However, under heavy stress at 230 watts, ventricular tachycardia developed suddenly with a fast rate of 230, after which the patient fainted (see ECG next page). He recovered quickly after the disappearance of the tachycardia. Treatment with large doses of a beta-blocking agent (metoprolol 200 mg twice daily) was initiated. The patient was free from attacks for 2 years; but died suddenly presumably during a period where he neglected taking his medication.

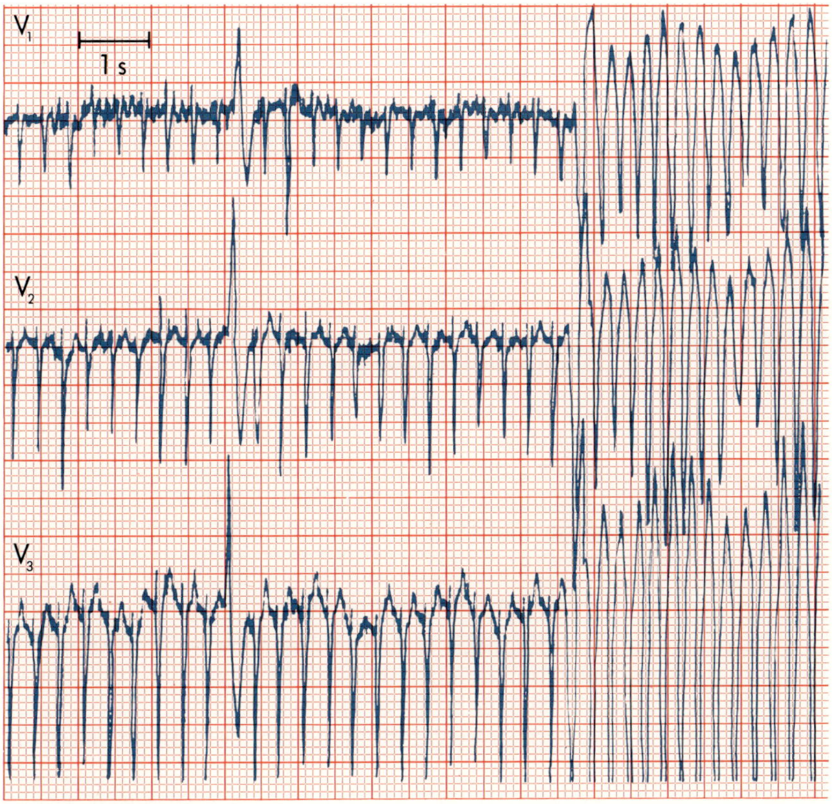

Exercise 230 W
VR 180/min – 230/min

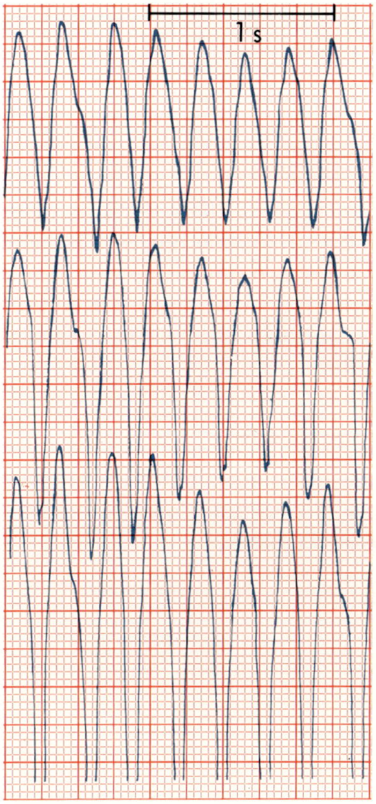

Fainting
VR 230/min

Fig. 6.41
(continued)

Paroxysmal fascicular ventricular tachycardia [76, 77]

This tachycardia originates in the posterior fascicle of the left bundle branch (Fig. 1.2, page 3).

ECG diagnosis

The tachycardia (Fig. 6.40 A, page 177) is characterized by a relatively narrow QRS complex (0.12–0.14 s) and a pattern similar to right bundle branch block with anterior fascicular block (RBBB + LAFB)(Fig. 9.7, page 231). Between attacks the ECG is usually normal (Fig. 6.40 B).

Management

An i.v. bolus injection of verapamil often terminates the attack. Long-term oral verapamil prophylaxis may prove successful.

Effort induced ventricular tachycardia [78–85]

ECG diagnosis

Effort induced ventricular tachycardia with syncope has been reported in otherwise healthy young individuals without underlying heart disease. The ECG of the tachycardia usually shows a net positive QRS area in V_{5-6} suggesting an origin in the right ventricle (Fig. 6.41, 178/179). ECGs between attacks often show repolarization (ST segment and/or T wave) anomalies.

Differential diagnosis

The differential diagnosis includes arrhythmogenic right ventricular dysplasia and effort induced ventricular tachycardia secondary to aortic stenosis, hypertrophic cardiomyopathy or ischaemic heart disease (Fig. 14.22, page 336/337).

Additional investigations

The diagnosis is corroborated by exercise testing (NB exercise testing is contraindicated in the patient with concommitant aortic stenosis as there is a risk of provoking ventricular fibrillation or circulatory collapse).

Management

The drug of first choice to detect effort induced ventricular tachycardia in the absence of heart disease is a beta blocking agent administered in submaximal dosage. When exercise induced ventricular tachycardia is found in an individual with evidence of ischaemic heart disease, myocardial revascularization by CABG or PTCA is the treatment of choice (Fig. 14.22).

Ventricular fibrillation [86–90]

During this arrhythmia there is chaotic activation of the ventricular myocardium (Figs. 3.6, page 43 and 3.8, page 44).

ECG diagnosis

Discrete QRST complexes are absent and are replaced by continuous very rapid, irregular deflections. The deflections can be relatively large, *coarse ventricular fibrillation,* or small, *fine ventricular fibrillation,* or, there may be an alternation between coarse and fine fibrillation (Fig. 6.42, page 182). The triggering event is a ventricular extrasystole which:

- Immediately or following a few rapidly occurring ventricular complexes, precipitates ventricular fibrillation (Fig. 6.43, page 182). This sequence of events is usually observed in the early stage of an acute myocardial infarction, when the extrasystole is often of R on T type. (Fig. 5.14-Grade 5, page 120).

- Precipitates ventricular tachycardia which subsequently degenerates to ventricular fibrillation after seconds or minutes or even longer (Fig. 6.44, page 183). This type of initiation is seen in the late stage of acute myocardial infarction and in many other conditions. The tachycardia initiating extrasystole usually falls after the T wave and may be late enough to coincide with or even to fall after the P wave of the following beat (the R on P phenomenon) (Fig. 6.44 A).

Occasionally, ventricular fibrillation develops by degeneration of torsade de pointes ventricular tachycardia.

Differential diagnosis

Fine fibrillation with small amplitude oscillations may be misdiagnosed as ventricular asystole. Likewise ventricular asystole with superimposed electrical noise or interference from myopotentials can be misdiagnosed as ventricular fibrillation.

Symptoms

In ventricular fibrillation there is a continuous wormlike twitching of the ventricular wall but no useful pumping activity of the heart. The result is a cardiac arrest. Loss of consciousness occurs within 8 to 10 s, and death follows if ventricular fibrillation continues for more than 3–5 min.

Aetiology

Ventricular fibrillation usually implies severe organic heart disease. It is the commonest cause of sudden death both in acute myocardial infarction and in chronic ischaemic heart disease. Moreover, ventricular fibrillation is the cause of sudden death in the WPW syndrome (Chapter 7, page 188), the long QT syndromes and effort induced ventricular tachycardia. Non-cardiac factors which may cause ventricular fibrillation include electrolyte derangements, drugs (in particular antiarrhythmic drugs) and a variety of electrical accidents e.g.:

- Lightning, accidental exposure to high voltage installations, or especially in children, to the ordinary household power supply.

- Pacing electrodes and intracardiac catheters can pass a weak "leakage current" when connected to faulty electrical equipment. This may trigger ventricular fibrillation.

- In acute myocardial infarction particularly inappropriate pacing (Fig. 10.9, page 261) in the first 4/5 of the T wave may induce ventricular fibrillation.

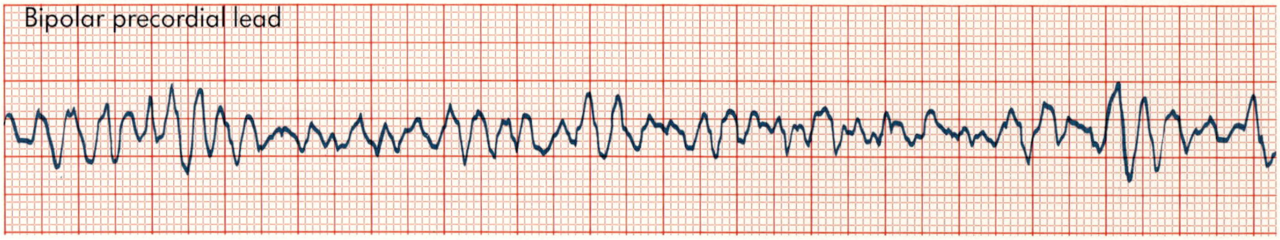

Fig. 6.42
Ventricular fibrillation. There is alternation between coarse and fine fibrillation.

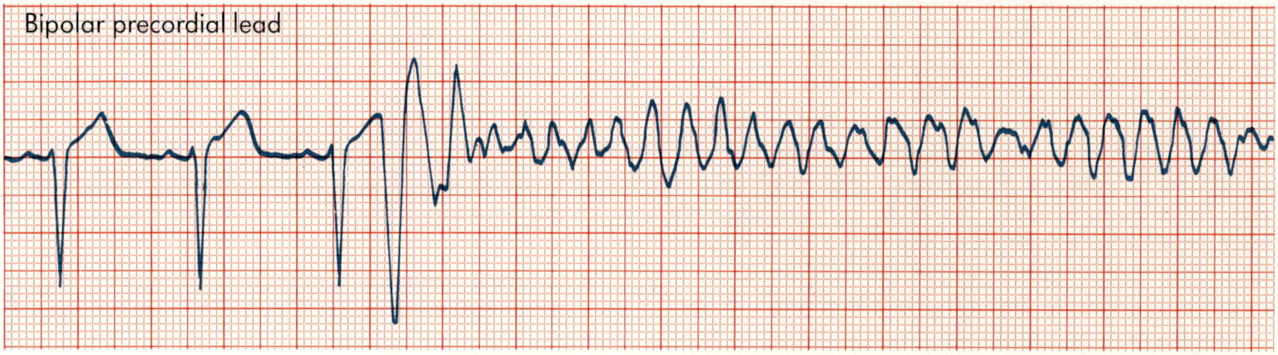

Fig. 6.43
Onset of ventricular fibrillation in the first hours of an acute myocardial infarction. Fibrillation is precipitated by the R on T phenomenon (a ventricular extrasystole which falls within the initial four fifths of the T wave of the preceding complex).

Prognosis

If untreated ventricular fibrillation will lead to irreversible cerebral death within a period of 3 to 5 min.

Long-term survival is good for survivors of ventricular fibrillation when it has occured in the early stage (first days) of acute myocardial infarction. Their 1 to 2 year survival is not significantly different from that of patients whose infarction was not complicated by ventricular fibrillation.

The risk of sudden death due to recurrence of ventricular fibrillation, however, is high (20 % or more over one year) in:

- Acute myocardial infarction with "late" ventricular fibrillation, (ventricular fibrillation in the second or third week after the infarction).
- Chronic ischaemic heart disease without evidence of acute myocardial infarction having precipitated the attack of ventricular fibrillation.

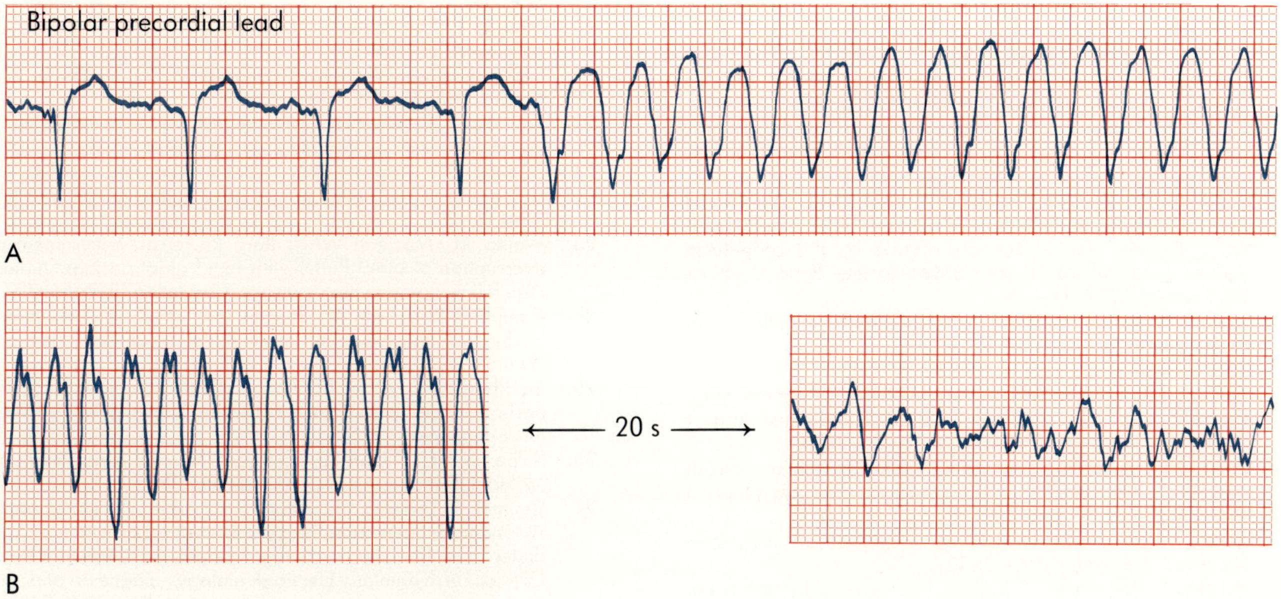

Fig. 6.44
Ventricular fibrillation in chronic ischaemic heart disease. Late ventricular extrasystole initiates ventricular tachycardia which after a period of time degenerates to ventricular fibrillation.

A Fast ventricular tachycardia (220/min) precipitated by a late ventricular extrasystole which arrives so late that it falls on or after the P wave ("the R on P phenomenon")

B Over the following minute accelleration of heart rate and subsequent degeneration to ventricular fibrillation

Management

Normal cardiac activity usually can be restored immediately by a DC countershock. If a shock cannot be applied immediately, resuscitation with cardiac massage and artificial ventilation should be started without delay and maintained while the following resuscitation procedures are performed.

The primary treatment is DC countershock (200 + 200 + 360 J). If unsuccessful the next line of treatment is either i.v. lignocaine or adrenaline, or both. Drugs of second choice might be a beta blocking agent, a Class IC or IA drug, or amiodarone or bretylium tosylate. Each drug bolus should be followed by a renewed series of DC countershocks.

Patients resuscitated from ventricular fibrillation in the late stage of acute myocardial infarction (second week) or with chronic ischaemic heart disease not complicated by acute myocardial infarction should be referred to a cardiological center with facilities for electrophysiological studies to determine the optimal approach for long-term prophylaxis (antiarrhythmic medication, antitachycardia surgery or an AICD implant).

References Chapter 6

1. WHO/ISFC Task Force. Definition of terms related to cardiac rhythm. Europ J Cardiol 1978; 8: 127–44.
2. Brugada P, Smeets JLRM, Wellens HJJJ. Spectrum of supraventricular tachycardias. Am J Cardiol 1988; 62: 4–7.
3. Gallagher JJ, Smith WM, Kasell J, et al. Use of the esophageal lead in the diagnosis of mechanisms of reciprocating supraventricular tachycardia. Pace 1980; 3: 440–51.
4. Bär FW, Brugada P, Dassen WRM, Wellens HJJ. Differential diagnosis of tachycardia with narrow QRS complex (shorter than 0.12 second). Am J Cardiol 1984; 54: 555–60.
5. Kuchar DL, Thorburn CW, Sammel NL, et al. Surface electrocardiographic manifestations of tachyarrhythmias: Clues to diagnosis and mechanism. Pace 1988; 11: 61–82.
6. Blondeau M. Aberrant ventricular conduction. (Functional parodoxical and intermittent bundle branch block.) In: Puech P, Slama R, eds. The cardiac arrhythmias by the arrhythmia working group of the French Cardiac Society. Paris: Corbière and Roussel, 1979; 127–38.
7. Schamroth L. Aberrant ventricular conduction. Ingelheim am Rhein: Boehringer Ingelheim Postgraduate Medical Services, 1983.
8. Marriott HJL, Conover MH. Advanced concepts in arrhythmias. Aberrant ventricular conduction: 244–67. Phase 3 and phase 4 block: 155–66. St. Louis: The C.V. Mosby Co., 1983.
8A. Gouaux JS, Ashman R. Auricular fibrillation with aberration simulating ventricular paroxysmal tachycardia. Am Heart J 1947; 34: 366.
9. Lown B, Wyatt NF, Levine HD. Paroxysmal atrial tachycardia with block. Circulation 1960; 21: 129.
10. Storstein O, Rasmussen K. Digitalis and atrial tachycardia with block. Br Heart J 1974; 36: 171–76.
11. Levine HD. The clinical diagnosis of PAT with block. In: Dreifus LS, Likoff W, Moyer JH, eds. Mechanisms and therapy of cardiac arrhythmias. The Fourteenth Hahnemann Symposium. New York, London: Grune & Stratton, 1966.
12. Singh BN, Opie LH, Harrison DC, et al. Antiarrhythmic agents. In: Opie LH, ed. Drugs for the heart. 2nd edition. Orlando, New York, London: Grune & Stratton, Inc. 1987; 54–90.
13. Huycke EC, Sung RJ. Atrial tachycardias. In: Zipes DP, Rowlands DJ, eds. Progress in cardiology. Philadelphia: Lea & Febiger, 1988; 313–25.
14. Sharma AD, Yee R, Guiraudon GM, et al. AV nodal reentry – Current concepts and surgical treatment. In: Zipes DP, Rowlands DJ, eds. Progress in cardiology. Philadelphia: Lea & Febiger, 1988; 129–45.
15. Ross DL, Johnson DC, Koo CC, et al. Surgical treatment of supraventricular tachycardia without the WPW syndrome: Current indications, techniques, and results. In: Brugada P, Wellens HJJ. Cardiac arrhythmias: Where to go from here? Mount Kisco, New York: Futura Publishing Co., 1987; 591–603.
16. Scher DL, Arsura EL. Multifocal atrial tachycardia: Mechanisms, clinical correlates, and treatment. Am Heart J 1989; 118: 574–80.
17. Waldo AL, Henthorn RW, Plumb VJ. Atrial flutter – Recent observations in man. In: Josephson ME, Wellens HJJ, eds. Tachycardias: Mechanisms, diagnosis, treatment. Philadelphia: Lea & Febiger, 1984.
18. Allessie MA, Lammers WJEP, Rensma PL, et al. Flutter and fibrillation in experimental models: What has been learned that can be applied to humans? In: Brugada P, Wellens HJJ. Cardiac arrhythmias: Where to go from here? Mount Kisco, New York: Futura Publishing Co., 1987; 63–83.
19. Olsson SB, Dohnal M. Is atrial fibrillation propencity linked to intrinsic AV-nodal function? New Trends Arrhythmias 1988; 4: 569–74.
20. Moleiro F, Mendoza IJ, Medin-Ravell V, et al. One to one atrioventricular conduction during atrial pacing at rates of 300/minute in absence of Wolff-Parkinson-White syndrome. Am J Cardiol 1981; 48: 789–96.
21. Robertson CE, Miller HC. Extreme tachycardia complicating the use of disopyramide in atrial flutter. Br Heart J 1980; 44: 602.
22. Danahy DT, Aronow WS. Lidocaine-induced cardiac rate changes in atrial fibrillation and atrial flutter. Am Heart J 1978; 95: 474–82.
23. Waldo AL, Maclean WAH, Karp RB, et al. Entrainment and interruption of atrial flutter with rapid atrial pacing: Studies in man following open heart surgery. Circulation 1977; 56: 737.
24. Campbell RM, Dick M, Jenkins JM, et al. Atrial overdrive pacing for conversion of atrial flutter in children. Pediatrics 1985; 75: 730.
25. Godtfredsen J. Atrial fibrillation. Etiology, course and prognosis. A follow-up study of 1 212 cases. Copenhagen: University of Copenhagen, 1975.
26. Kulbertus HE, Olsson SB, Schlepper M, eds. Atrial fibrillation. Mölndal, Sweden: Astra Cardiovascular, 1982.
27. Coumel P, Leclercq JF, Attuel P, Lavallee JP, Flammang D. Autonomic influences in the genesis of atrial arrhythmias: atrial flutter and fibrillation of vagal origin. In: Narula OS, ed. Cardiac arrhythmias. Electrophysiology, diagnosis and management. Baltimore, London: Williams & Wilkins, 1979:243–55.
28. Schlepper M. The autonomic nervous system and supraventricular rhythm disturbances (Einflüsse des autonomen Nerven systems bei supraventrikulären Rhythmusstörungen). Z Kardiol 1986; 75 (Suppl. 5): 35–40.
29. Brand FN, Abbott RD, Kannel WB, et al. Characteristics and prognosis of lone atrial fibrillation. 30-year follow-up in the Framingham study. JAMA 1985; 254: 3449–53.
30. Kopecky SL, Gersh BJ, McGoon MD, et al. The natural history of lone atrial fibrillation. A population-based study over three decades. New Engl J Med 1987; 317: 669–74.
31. Önundarson PT, Thorgeirsson G, Jonmundsson E, et al. Chronic atrial fibrillation – epidemiologic features and 14 year follow-up: A case control study. Europ Heart J 1987; 8: 521–27.
32. Greer GS, Wilkinson WE, McCarthy EA, et al. Random and nonrandom behaviour of symptomatic paroxysmal atrial fibrillation. Am J Cardiol 1989; 64: 339–42.
33. Petersen P. Thromboembolic complications in atrial fibrillation. Stroke 1990; 21: In press.
34. Storstein L. Role of digitalis in ventricular rate control in atrial fibrillation. In: Kulbertus HE, Olsson SB, Schlepper M, eds. Atrial fibrillation. Mölndal, Sweden: Astra Cardiovascular, 1982, 285–93.
35. Mølgaard H, Bjerregaard P, Jørgensen HS, et al. 24-hour antiarrhythmic effect of conventional and slow-release verapamil in chronic atrial fibrillation. Europ J Clin Pharma col 1987; 33: 447–53.
36. Steinberg JS, Katz RJ, Bren GB, et al. Efficacy of oral diltiazem to control ventricular response in chronic atrial fibrillation at rest and during exercise. JACC 1987; 9: 405–11.

37. James MA, Channer KS, Papouchado M, et al. Improved control of atrial fibrillation with combined pindolol and digoxin therapy. Europ Heart J 1989; 10: 83–90.
38. Rowland E, McKenna WJ, Harris L, et al. Amiodarone in the prophylaxis of atrial fibrillation. In: Kulbertus HE, Olsson SB, Schlepper M, eds. Mölndal, Sweden: Astra Cardio vascular, 1982; 262–71.
39. Petersen P, Godtfredsen J, Boysen G, et al. Placebo-controlled, randomised trial of warfarin and aspirin for prevention of thromboembolic complications in chronic atrial fibrillation. The Copenhagen AFASAK Study. Lancet 1989; i: 175–79.
40. Wellens HJJ, Brugada P. Diagnosis of ventricular tachycardia from the 12-lead electrocardiogram. Cardiol Clin 1987; 5: 511–25.
41. Akhtar M, Shenasa M, Jazayeri M, et al. Wide QRS complex tachycardia. Reappraisal of a common clinical problem. Ann Int Med 1988; 109: 905–12.
42. Dancy M, Camm AJ, Ward D. Misdiagnosis of chronic recurrent ventricular tachycardia. Lancet 1985; ii: 320–23.
43. Breithardt G, Borggrefe M, Zipes DP. Current aspects of pharmacological and nonpharmacological therapy of tachyarrhythmias. In: Breithardt G, Borggrefe M, Zipes DP, eds. Nonpharmacological therapy of tachyarrhythmias. Mount Kisco, New York: Futura Publishing Co., 1987; 1–14.
44. State-of-the-art consensus conference on electrophysiologic testing in the diagnosis and treatment of patients with cardiac arrhythmias. Circulation 1987; 75: 1–194.
45. Brugada P, Wellens HJJ, eds. Cardiac arrhythmias: Where to go from here? Mount Kisco, New York: Futura Publishing Co., 1987.
46. Ward DE, Camm AJ. Clinical electrophysiology of the heart. London: Edward Arnold, 1987.
47. Breithardt G, Borggrefe M, Zipes DP, eds. Nonpharmacological therapy of tachyarrhythmias. Mount Kisco, New York: Futura Publishing Co., 1987.
48. Horowitz LN, Borggrefe M. Many things are not found in books or journals ...but some things are! Value of electro physiologic testing in patients with malignant ventricular arrhythmias. Am J Cardiol 1988; 62: 1292–94.
49. Greenspon AJ, Volosin KJ, Greenberg RM, et al. Amiodarone therapy: Role of early and late electrophysiologic studies. JACC 1988; 11: 117–23.
50. Pratt CM, Thornton BC, Magro SA, et al. Spontaneous arrhythmia detected on ambulatory electrocardiographic recording lacks precision in predicting inducibility of ventricular tachycardia during electrophysiologic study. JACC 1987; 10: 97–104.
51. Dessertenne F. La tachycardie ventriculaire a deux foyers opposés variables. Arch Mal Coeur 1966; 2: 263–72.
52. Smith WM, Gallagher JJ. "Les torsades de pointes": An unusual ventricular arrhythmia. Ann Int Med 1980; 93: 578–84.
53. D'Alnoncourt CN, Zierhuet W, Lüderitz B. "Torsade de pointes" tachycardia – Reentry or focal activity? Br Heart J 1982; 48: 213–16.
54. Coumel P, Leclercq JF, Lucet V. Possible mechanisms of the arrhythmias in the long QT syndrome. Europ Heart J 1985; 6 (Suppl. D): 115–29.
55. Amlie JP, Kuo CS, Munakata K, et al. Effect of uniformly prolonged, and increased basic dispersion of repolarization on premature dispersion on ventricular surface in dogs: Role of action potential duration and activation time differences. Europ Heart J 1985; 6 (Suppl. D): 15–30.
56. Jervell A. The surdo-cardiac syndrome. Europ Heart J 1985; 6 (Suppl. D): 97–102.
57. Schwartz PJ, Locati E. The idiopathic long QT syndrome: Pathogenentic mechanisms and therapy. Europ Heart J 1985; 6 (Suppl. D): 103–14.
58. Stratmann HG, Kennedy HL. Torsades de pointes associated with drugs: Recognition and management. Am Heart J 1987; 113: 1470–82.
59. Fredlund B-O, Olsson SB. Long QT interval and ventricular tachycardia of "Torsade de Pointe" type in hypothyroidism. Acta med scand 1983; 213: 231–35.
60. Akiyama T, Batchelder J, Worsman J, et al. Hypocalcemic torsade de pointes. J Electrocardiol 1989; 22: 89–92.
61. Campbell RWF, Gardiner P, Amos PA, et al. Measurement of the QT interval. Europ Heart J 1985; 6 (Suppl. D): 81–83.
62. Puddu PE, Jouve R, Mariotti S, et al. Evaluation of 10 QT prediction formulas in 881 middle-aged men from the seven countries study: Emphasis on the cubic root Fridericia's equation. J Electrocardiol 1988; 21: 219–29.
63. Singh BN. When is QT prolongation antiarrhythmic and when is it proarrhythmic? Editorial. Am J Cardiol 1989; 63: 867–69.
64. Eldar M, Griffin JC, Abbott JA, et al. Permanent cardiac pacing in patients with the long QT syndrome. JACC 1987; 10: 600–07.
65. Zilcher H, Glogar D, Kaindl F. Torsades de pointes: Occurrence in myocardial ischaemia as a seperate entity. Multiform ventricular tachycardia or not? Europ Heart J 1980; 1: 63–71.
66. Tzivoni D, Keren A, Stern S. Torsades de pointes versus polymorphous ventricular tachycardia. Am J Cardiol 1983; 52: 639–40.
66A. Tzivoni D, Banai S, Schuger C, Benhorin J, Keren A, Gottnen S, Stern S. Treatment of Torsade de pointes with magnesium sulfate. Circulation 1988; 77: 392–97.
67. Josephson ME, Horowitz LN, Farshidi A, et al. Recurrent sustained ventricular tachycardia. 4. Pleomorphism. Circulation 1979; 59: 459.
68. Trappe H-J, Brugada P, Talajic M, et al. Value of induction of pleomorphic ventricular tachycardia during programmed stimulation. Europ Heart J 1989; 10: 133–41.
69. Lévy S, Aliot E. Bidirectional tachycardia: A new look on the mechanism. Pace 1989; 12: 827–34.
70. Rizzon P, Breithardt G, Chiddo A, eds. Arrhythmogenic right ventricle. Europ Heart J 1989; 10 (Suppl. D).
71. Rizzin P, Breithardt G, Chiddo A, eds. Arrhythmogenic right ventricle. Europ Heart J 1989; 10 (Suppl. D).
72. Blomström-Lundqvist C, Sabel K-G, Olsson SB. A long-term follow-up of 15 patients with arrhythmogenic right ventricular dysplasia. Br Heart J 1987; 58: 477–88.
73. Blomström-Lundqvist C, Selin K, Jonsson R, et al. Cardio angiographic findings in patients with arrhythmogenic right ventricular dysplasia. Br Heart J 1988; 59: 556–63.
74. Coumel P, Leclercq J-F, Slama R. Repetitive monomorphic idiopathic ventricular tachycardia. In: Zipes DP, Jalife J, eds. Cardiac electrophysiology and arrhythmias. Orlando, New York, London: Grune & Stratton, Inc., 1985; 457–68.
75. Slama R, Leclercq J-F, Coumel P. Paroxysmal ventricular tachycardia in patients with apparently normal hearts. In: Zipes DP, Jalife J, eds. Orlando, New York, London: Grune & Stratton, Inc., 1985; 545–51.
76. Ward DE, Nathan AW, Camm AJ. Fascicular tachycardia sensitive to calcium antagonists. Europ Heart J 1984; 5: 896–905.

77. Klein GF, Millman PJ, Yee R. Recurrent ventricular tachycardia responsive to verapamil. Pace 1984; 7: 938–48.
78. Wennevold A, Sandøe E. 6-14 years' beta-blockade in three children with paroxysmal ventricular fibrillation. In: Sandøe E, Julian DG, Bell JW, eds. Management of ventricular tachycardia – role of mexiletine. Amsterdam: Excerpta Medica, 1978; 429–32.
79. Palileo EV, Ashley WW, Swiryn S, et al. Exercise provocable right ventricular outflow tract tachycardia. Am Heart J 1982; 104: 185.
80. Sung RJ, Shen EN, Morady F, et al. Electrophysiologic mechanism of exercise-induced sustained ventricular tachycardia. Am J Cardiol 1983; 51: 525–30.
81. Wren C. Arrhythmias in children: The influence of exercise and the role of exercise testing. Europ Heart J 1987; 8 (Suppl. D): 25–28.
82. Epstien SE. Syncope and exercise in aortic stenosis. Am J Cardiol 1989; 24: 594–95.
83. Quyyumi AA, Crake T, Wright C, et al. The incidence and morphology of ischaemic ventricular tachycardia. Europ Heart J 1986; 7: 1037–44.
84. Rasmussen K, Lunde PI, Lie M. Coronary bypass surgery in exercise-induced ventricular tachycardia. Europ Heart J 1987; 8: 444–48.
85. Pedersen F, Pietersen A, Sandøe E. Silent myocardial ischaemia and life threatening ventricular arrhythmias. Ann Clin Res 1988; 20: 404–09.
86. Bayes de Luna A, Torner P, Guindo P, et al. ECG study of ambulatory sudden death. Review of 158 published cases. New Trends Arrhythmias 1985; I: 293–97.
87. Leclercq JF, Maisonblanche P, Cauchemez B, et al. Re spective role of sympathetic tone and of cardiac pauses in the genesis of 62 cases of ventricular fibrillation recorded during Holter monitoring. Europ Heart J 1988; 12: 1276–83.
88. Breithardt G, Borggrefe M, Martinez-Rubio A, et al. Patho physiological mechanisms of ventricular tachyarrhythmias. Europ Heart J 1989; 10 (Suppl. E): 9–18.
89. Lemery R, Brugada P, Della Bella P, et al. Ventricular fibrillation in six adults without overt heart disease. JACC 1989; 13: 911–16.
90. Standards and guidelines for cardiopulmonary resuscitation (CPR) and emergency cardiac care (ECC). JAMA 1986; 255: 2843–2982.

Chapter 7
Pre-excitation

Pre-excitation[1–3]

Pre-excitation (activation which is earlier than normal) is present when an impulse bypasses the normal delay in the AV node and is rapidly conducted from the atria to the ventricles (ventricular pre-excitation) or, from the ventricles to the atria (atrial pre-excitation). The rapid AV or, VA impulse transmission usually occurs via an extra AV conduction pathway, an *accessory AV connection*, in the form of a tiny band of myocardial fibres which bypass the AV node.

Electrocardiographically a distinction can be made between three types of pre-excitation syndromes (Fig. 7.1 upper part):

A *Wolff-Parkinson-White (WPW) syndrome* characterized by an accessory connection between the atria and ventricles which conducts in parallel with the AV node – His bundle but faster. The accessory AV connection can conduct impulses in both directions, from the atria to the ventricles and from the ventricles to the atria.

B *Concealed WPW syndrome* with an accessory AV connection which anatomically seems identical to the accessory AV connection of the WPW syndrome but which is functionally different since it is capable only of impulse conduction from the ventricles to the atria and not from the atria to the ventricles (it has a "built-in" unidirectional block for AV conduction).

C *Short PR syndrome* with a tract of atrial fibres that bypass the AV node and merge with the distal part of the AV node or His bundle.

A common feature of the pre-excitation syndromes is attacks of re-entry tachycardia (Fig. 7.1, lower part). During the tachycardia the normal AV conduction pathway (or part of it) functions as the one limb (α) and the accessory AV connection as the other limb (ß) of the re-entry circuit. Moreover, all three syndromes are associated with an increased incidence of paroxysms of atrial fibrillation. In two of the syndromes, the WPW syndrome (A) and the short PR syndrome (C), the potential for AV conduction over the accessory AV connection can result in a catastrophically rapid ventricular response with degeneration to ventricular fibrillation. Curiously, the loss of the normal timing of atrial and ventricular contraction which is a consistent feature of the two same syndromes causes no clinical symptoms.

The Wolff-Parkinson-White (WPW) syndrome[4–6]

The term WPW syndrome implies the ECG recording of signs of ventricular pre-excitation in the form of a WPW pattern (see below) associated with a history of paroxysms of tachycardia. However, not all individuals with a WPW pattern in the ECG have suffered or will eventually suffer from paroxysmal tachycardia. The incidence in the general population of ECG signs of ventricular pre-excitation in form of a *WPW pattern* (see below) has been estimated to be in the range of 0.1–0.2 %. The reported incidence of paroxysmal tachycardia varies with the selection criteria of the WPW population sample studied. In airline pilots with a WPW pattern recorded at a routine "check-up" the incidence of paroxysmal tachycardia is as low as 10–20 %, in the hospitalized patient as high as 40–80 %. Intermittently, attacks of atrial fibrillation occur in as many as 20–30 % of all patients with the WPW syndrome. Attacks of atrial flutter can occur but are rare.

The accessory AV connection bridges the AV ring at various sites: In the free wall of the left ventricle, anteriorly or posteriorly in the septal region or, in the free wall of the right ventricle Fig. 7.2, page 190). Multiple accessory AV connections may be present in the same patient.

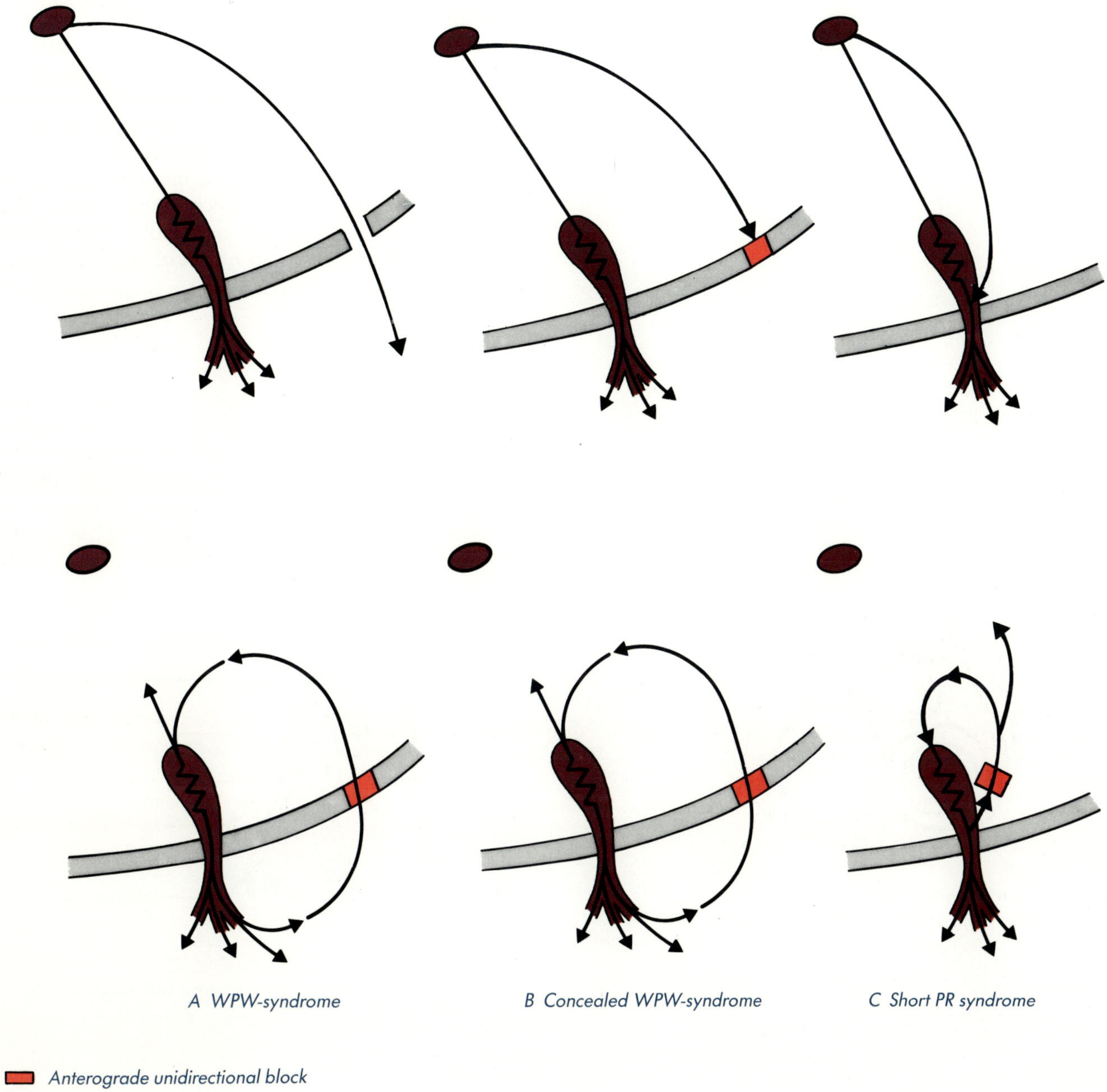

Fig. 7.1
Pre-excitation syndromes. AV conduction in sinus rhythm (above) and in re-entry tachycardia (below)

ECG diagnosis and differential diagnosis

Electrocardiographically the WPW syndrome is characterized by: a WPW pattern in sinus rhythm, paroxysms of re-entry tachycardia and, in some patients, paroxysms of atrial fibrillation or rarely atrial flutter.

WPW pattern (ECG diagnosis)[4–7]

The sinus impulse is conducted simultaneously down the accessory AV connection and the normal AV conduction system. The shorter conduction time over the accessory AV connection results in early activation of the ventricular wall adjacent to the ventricular end of the accessory AV connection. Impulse conduction through the normal AV conduction system takes slightly longer, but once it arrives at the ventricular level the impulse spreads very quickly through the bundle branches and Purkinje fibres to the various parts of the ventricular myocardium. Thus, the QRS complex is a fusion of two components (Fig. 7.3):

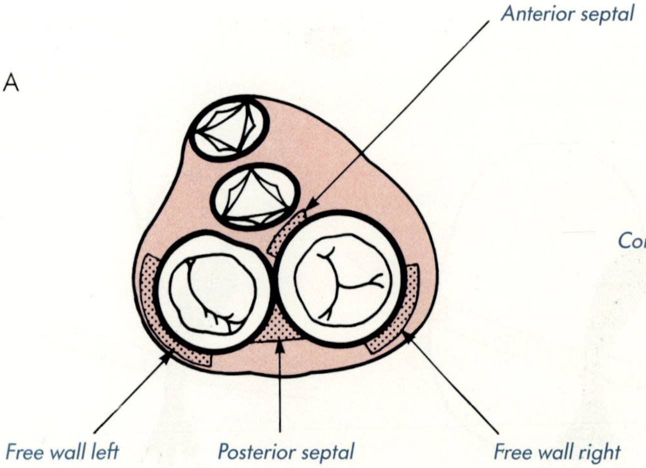

A A view of the heart from above showing the possible locations of the accessory AV connections

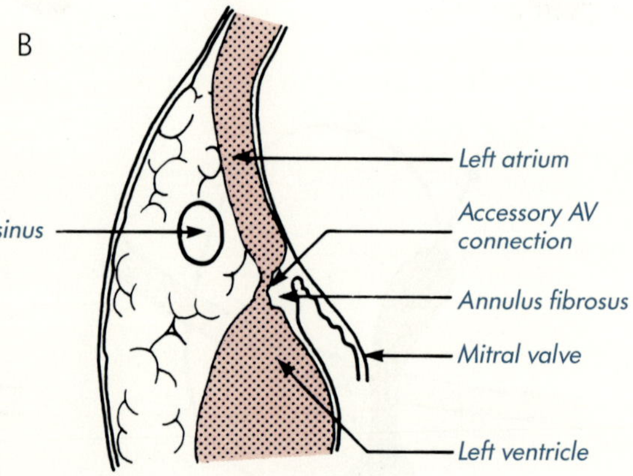

B A section through the left ventricular wall showing an accessory AV connection

Fig. 7.2
Predilection sites of the accessory AV connection in the WPW syndrome. The AV connections are very small, usually about 1 mm in diameter, the hatched areas in the drawing to the left indicate the zones in which the accessory AV connections are most often found

– An initial deflection, the *delta wave*, after the Greek letter delta (Δ) which it can resemble. The delta wave is produced by the fast impulse conduction over the accessory AV connection activating and pre-exciting part of the ventricular myocardium. The size of the delta wave depends primarily on the ratio between the conduction time through the accessory AV connection and the conduction time through the AV node and the bundle of His. The shorter the former or the longer the latter, the wider the delta wave (Fig. 7.4, page 192).

– A subsequent and usually the major part of the complex produced by impulse conduction through the AV node and the bundle of His. This portion resembles the normal QRS complex both in form and width. The altered sequence of ventricular activation is followed by secondary abnormalities in ventricular repolarization: ST segment displacement (depression or elevation) and a T wave polarity which is usually opposite to that of the delta wave.

The ECG characteristics of the WPW pattern comprise (Fig. 7.5, page 193):

– A *short PR interval* of 0.12 s or less (in the adult)

– A *delta wave* which appears as an initial slurring of the major deflection of the QRS complex (Fig. 7.5 A). A distinction is often made between *type A WPW* and *type B WPW* pattern. In type A the delta wave and the major part of the QRS complex in leads $V_{1-(2)}$ are positive, whereas in type B the delta wave and the major portion of the QRS complex in leads $V_{1-(2)}$ are negative (Fig. 7.5 B)

– A *wide QRS complex* varying in width from 0.10 s up to 0.20 s or more

– *ST segment displacement* (depression or elevation) and T *waves* opposite in direction to the delta wave.

The conduction capacity of the accessory AV connection often varies with time resulting in the recording of:

– An *alternating WPW pattern* (Fig. 7.6, page 194). The ECG recording shows abrupt alternations between a normal PQRS pattern and a typical WPW pattern.

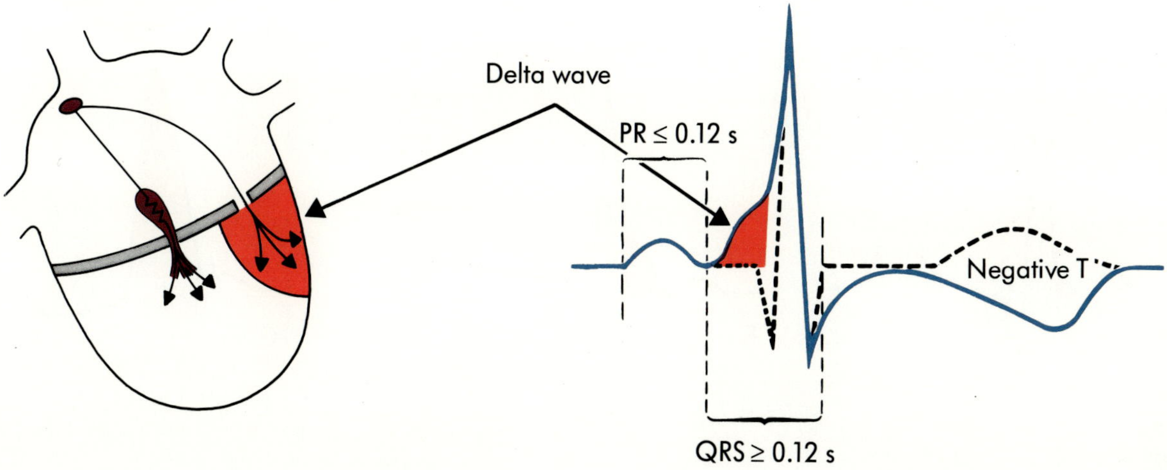

Fig. 7.3
The WPW pattern. The dotted line indicates normal AV conduction, the solid line concomitant AV conduction over the accessory and normal AV conduction pathway. Rapid conduction along the accessory pathway results in a short PR interval (0.12 s or less), a broadened QRS complex (0.12 s or more) with a delta wave and often abnormal T waves

– A *concertina effect* (Fig. 7.7, page 194). The delta wave changes gradually over a series of complexes from a typical WPW pattern with a short PR interval and a distinct delta wave to a normal PR interval followed by a narrow QRS complex without a delta wave. The process then reverses, the WPW pattern returns with gradual reappearance of the delta wave and shortening of the PR interval.

– *Episodic recordings of a WPW pattern (Fig. 7.8, page 195).* While some ECG recordings are normal, others show a typical WPW pattern.

The changes may occur from hour to hour or from day to day. Sometimes the accessory AV connection may remain electrophysiologically dormant for years before it suddenly starts conducting. The ECG will change from normal to one with a WPW pattern.

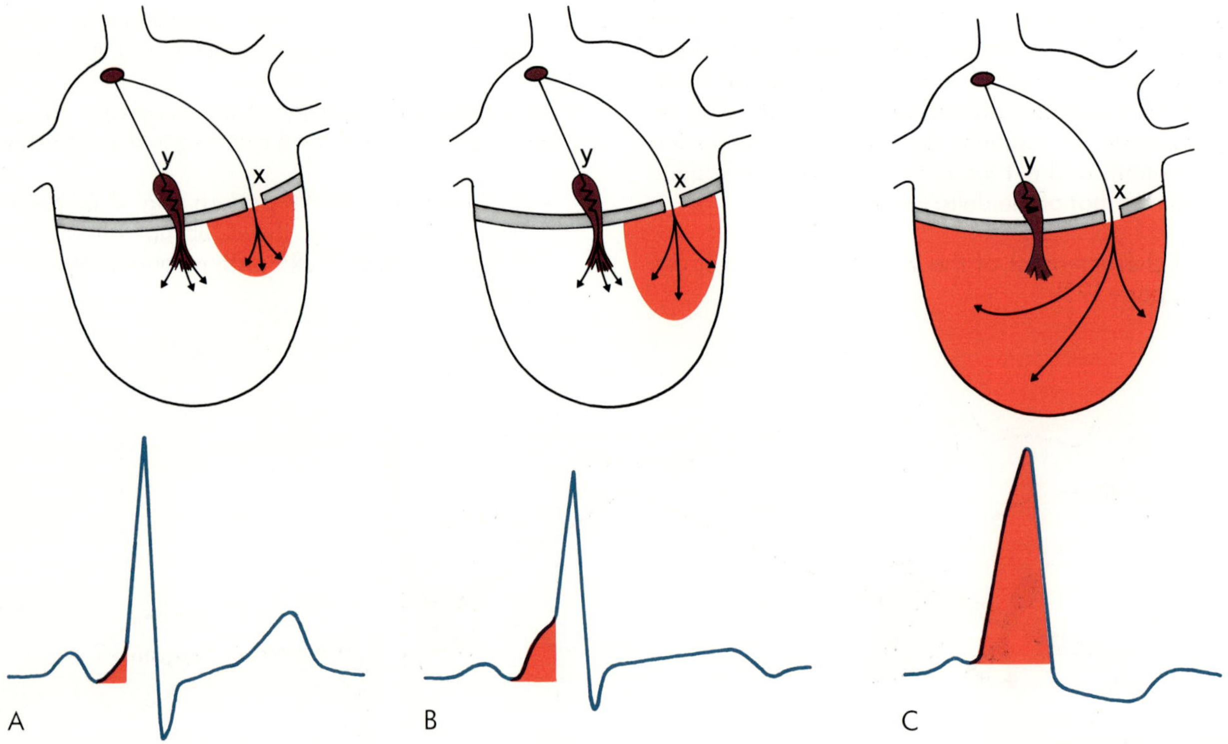

Fig. 7.4
The WPW pattern
The width of the delta wave depends on the ratio between the AV conduction time over the accessory AV connection (X) and over the AV node and bundle of His (Y)

A Small delta wave as X is only slightly shorter than Y
B Higher and broader delta wave due to a greater difference between X and Y
C Because of a very short X the QRS complex becomes one large delta wave

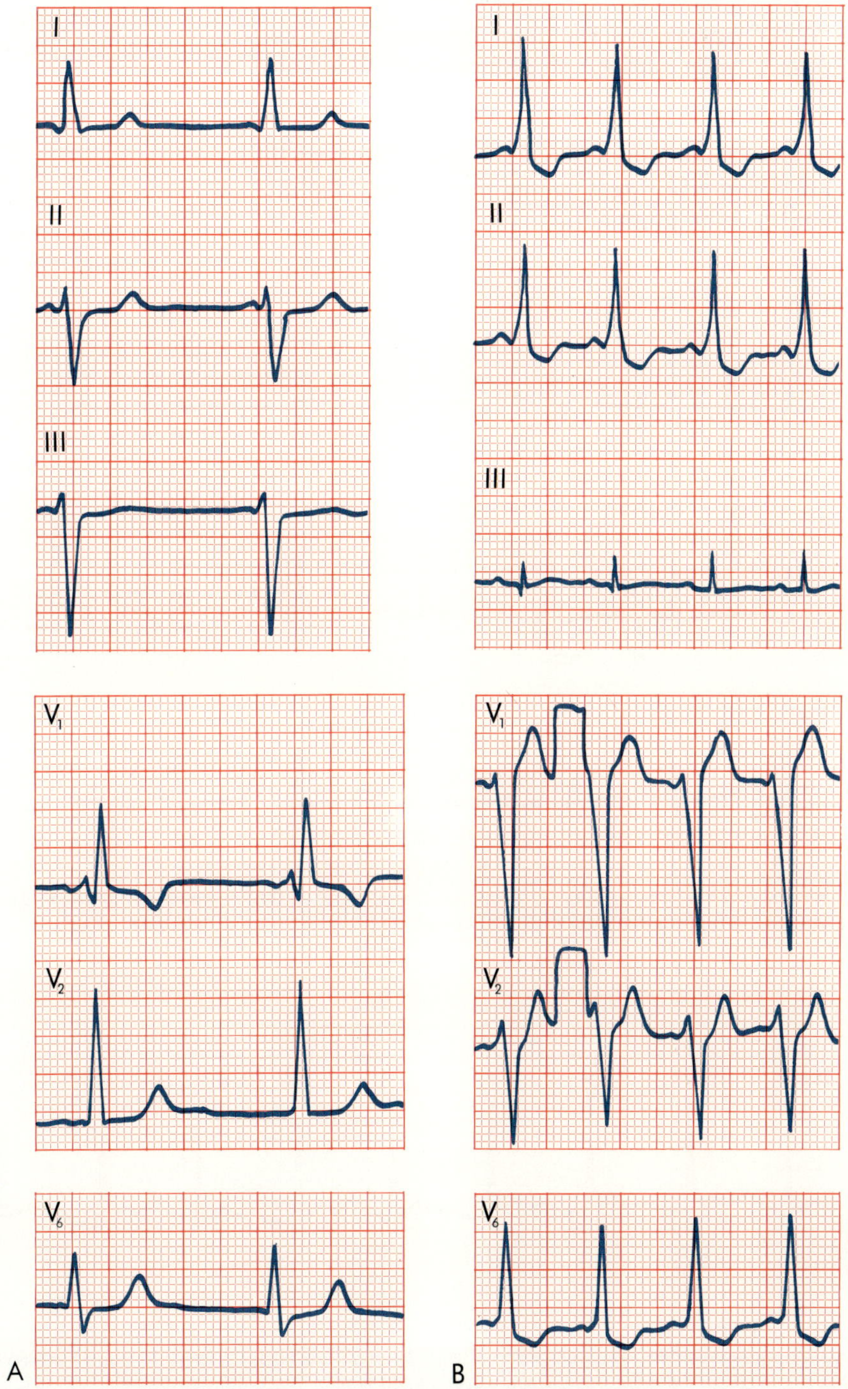

Fig. 7.5
Type A and type B WPW patterns

A Type A. The delta wave and the major part of the QRS complex in leads $V_{1-(2)}$ are positive. PR interval = 0.08 s, QRS complex = 0.16 s

B Type B. The major portion of the QRS complex in leads $V_{1-(2)}$ are negative. PR interval = 0.09 s, QRS complex = 0.12 s

WPW pattern (differential diagnosis)

The WPW pattern is "the great imposter" and can simulate a wide variety of pathological conditions. Thus:

- Negative delta waves (Fig. 7.10, page 198 lead III) may simulate Q waves caused by myocardial infarction (Fig. 14.6, page 316).
- The widened QRS complex (Fig. 7.8 lead III, V) may be mistaken for a bundle branch block pattern (Fig. 9.4, page 228).
- ST segment depression and T wave inversion can simulate myocardial ischaemia, (Fig. 14.16, page 327) and, as with changes related to myocardial ischaemia, they are exaggerated by exercise. These changes may also mimic left or right ventricular strain (Fig. 14.4, page 313).

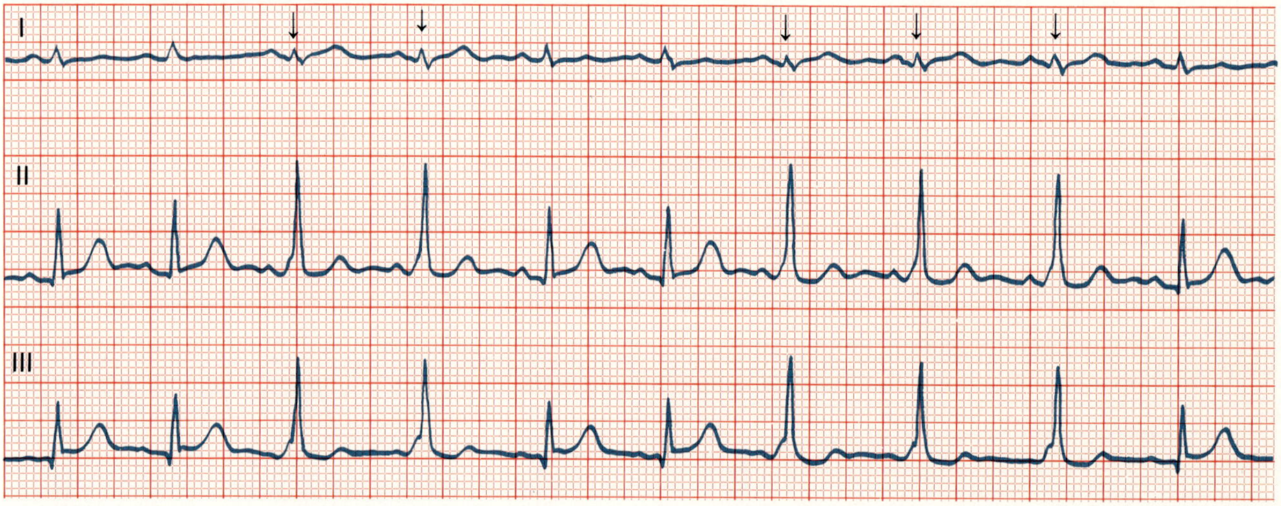

Fig. 7.6
Alternating WPW pattern. There is an anrupt change between QRS complexes with delta waves (arrow) and those without. Correspondingly, there is an abrupt change from wide QRS complexes (0.13 s) to normal complexes (0.08 s)

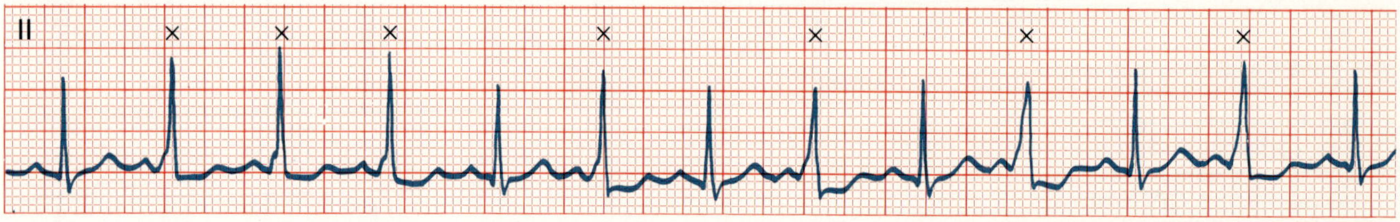

Fig. 7.7
WPW pattern with the concertina effect. The PR interval varies from 0.08–0.16 s and the QRS complex from 0.19–0.13 s, depending on the varying width of the delta wave. Delta waves can be seen in the complexes marked "x".

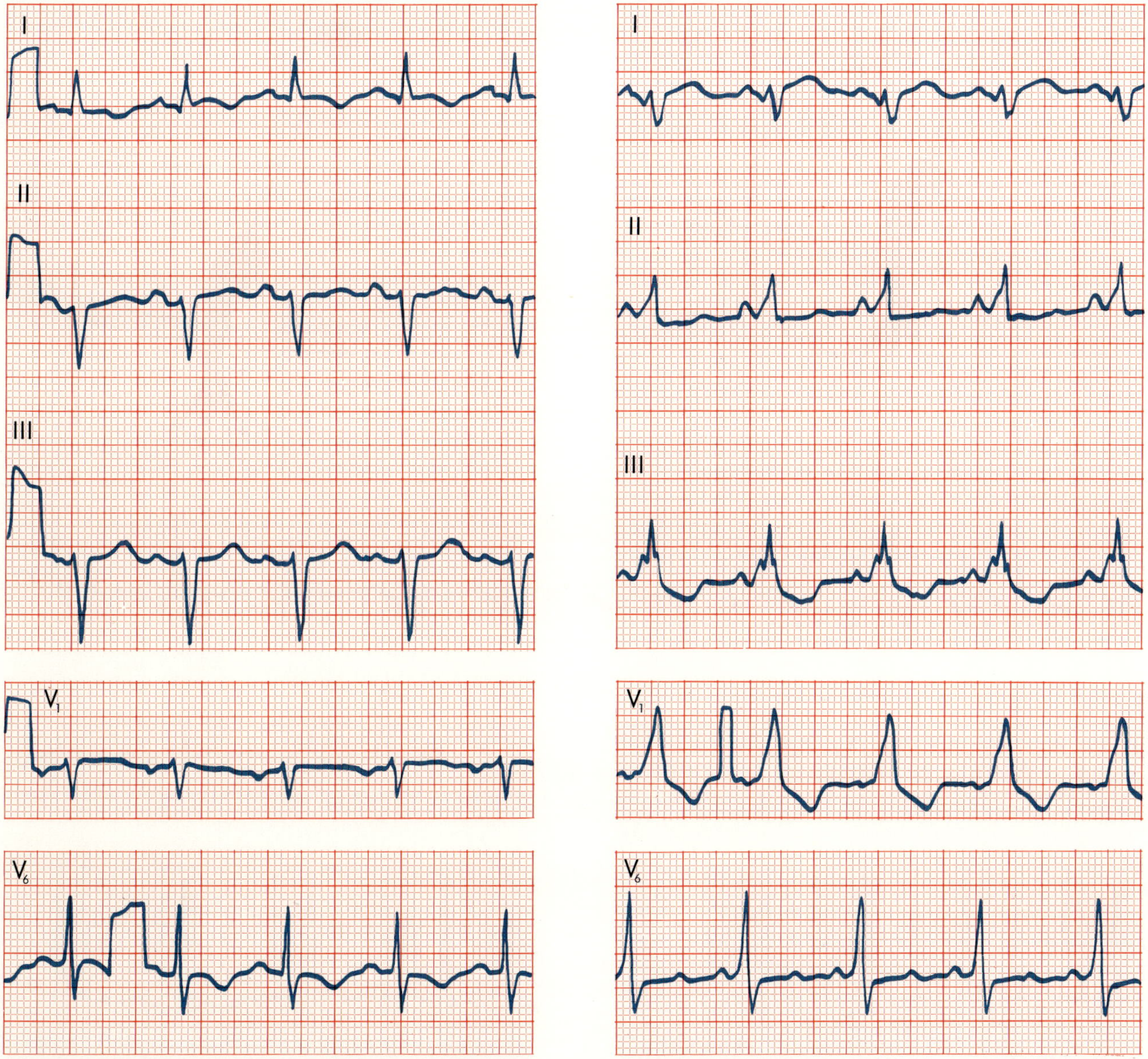

A ECG shows no sign of pre-excitation; PR interval = 0.21 s and QRS complex = 0.11 s. Left-sided axis deviation and negative T wave in leads I and V_6 are the only detectable abnormalities

B ECG recorded one month later reveals a constant WPW (type A) with distinct delta waves in leads II, III and V_1 as well as a short PR interval (0.11 s) and broadened QRS complex (0.20 s). A result of the merging of the delta wave with the QRS complex is a large positive deflection in lead V_1

Fig. 7.8
Intermittent WPW pattern

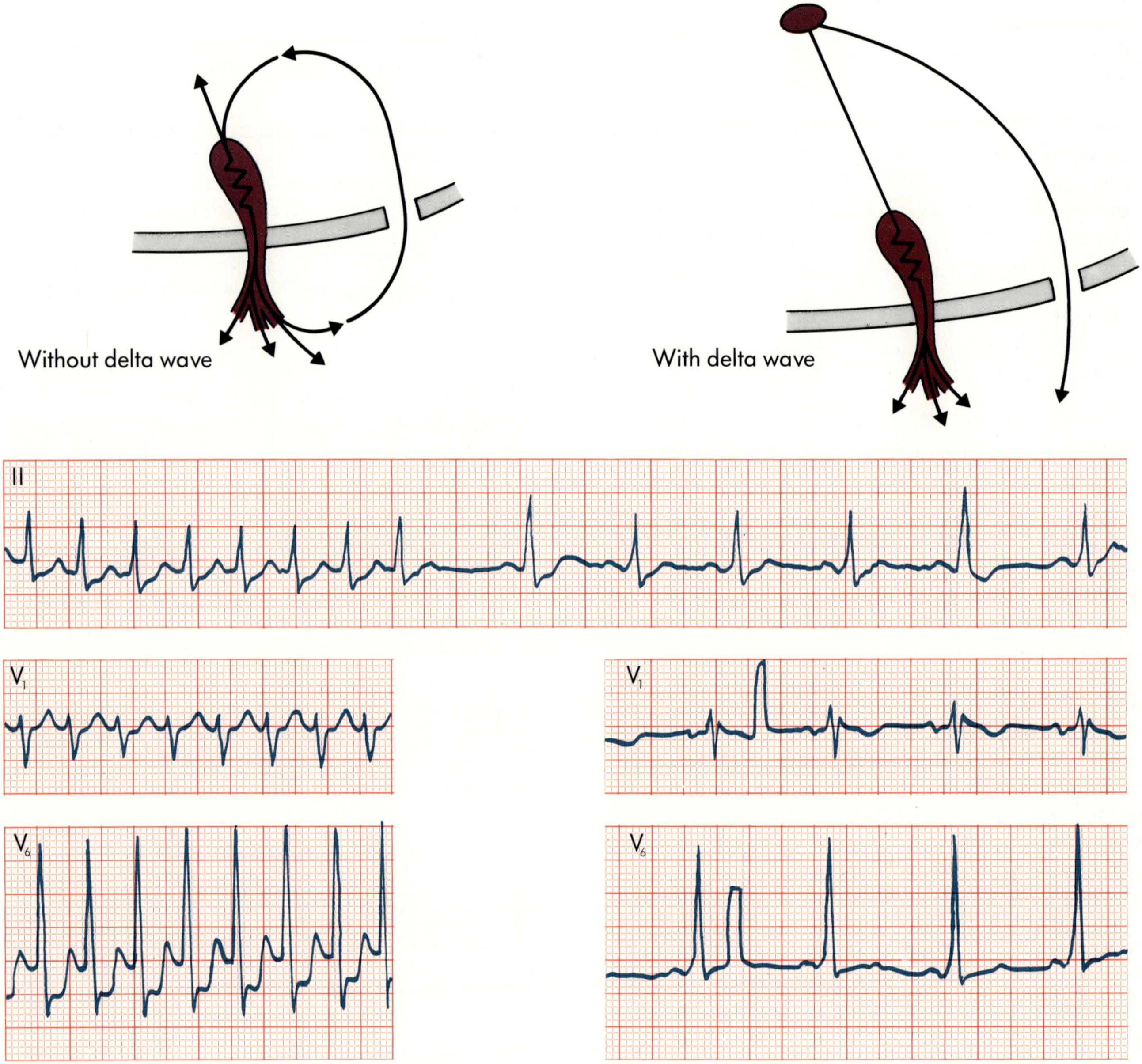

A In tachycardia narrow QRS complexes

B On return of sinus rhythm reappearance of the delta wave and a corresponding widening of the QRS complex

Fig. 7.9
The WPW syndrome

- QT interval prolongation may invite a misdiagnosis of long QT syndrome (Fig. 6.35, page 168/169).

A short PR interval is not unique to ventricular pre-excitation. It is seen in:

- Ventricular extrasystoles with a long coupling interval when the extrasystole falls after the next sinus P wave (Fig. 5.3 A, page 111). Although the sinus P wave and the QRS complex are not in fact electrophysiologically interdependent their timing may falsely convey this impression.

- AV nodal arrhythmia (Fig. 3.13 C, page 48). In this situation, the negative P wave in leads II, III and aVF will usually lead to the correct diagnosis.

WPW re-entry tachycardia (ECG diagnosis)[2,4–6]

During re-entry tachycardia AV conduction usually will be via the normal AV conduction pathway and VA conduction via the accessory AV connection. Thus, usually the QRS complex will be narrow during the tachycardia. A delta wave and a corresponding change to a broad QRS complex may be seen with resumption of sinus rhythm (Fig. 7.9). Often the rate is fast 180–250/min. The P wave (P′) is often discernible in the ST segment following the QRS complex with RP′ < P′R. The P wave may be better detected in this location by an oesophageal ECG. Atrial activation is retrograde – from below upwards, and if visible, the P wave will be negative in leads II, III and aVF (Fig. 7.10 B, page 198). Wide QRS complexes may be seen during the tachycardia; most often due to aberrant ventricular conduction, but sometimes due to reversal of the circus movement tachycardia with AV conduction through the accessory AV connection and VA conduction through the bundle of His and the AV node (Fig. 7.11 B, page 199).

WPW re-entry tachycardia (differential diagnosis)

The location of the P wave helps distinguish WPW re-entry tachycardia from AV nodal re-entry tachycardia (Fig. 6.11, page 136). WPW re-entry tachycardia with broad QRS complexes due either to aberrant ventricular conduction or to AV conduction via the accessory AV connection can be very difficult to differentiate from ventricular tachycardia without an electrophysiological study.

WPW atrial fibrillation and flutter (ECG diagnosis)[4–6,8]

The accessory AV connection has a potential for rapid AV conduction and during episodes of atrial fibrillation or flutter, the ventricular rate often is very high, ranging from 200 to 350/min. The QRS complexes are wide and bizarre and often show variable morphology. Last but not least, the rhythm is irregular in atrial fibrillation, but may be either regular or irregular in atrial flutter (Figs. 7.12–7.14, page 201 – page 204).

WPW atrial fibrillation and flutter (differential diagnosis)

During atrial fibrillation or atrial flutter in the WPW syndrome, when the ventricular rate exceeds 280/min, as it often does, the QRS complexes become more regular in form and the ECG pattern resembles that of fast ventricular tachycardia (Figs. 7.13 and 7.14). The marked irregularity of the ventricular response in atrial fibrillation, however, should minimize the risk of a misdiagnosis of multiform ventricular tachycardia.

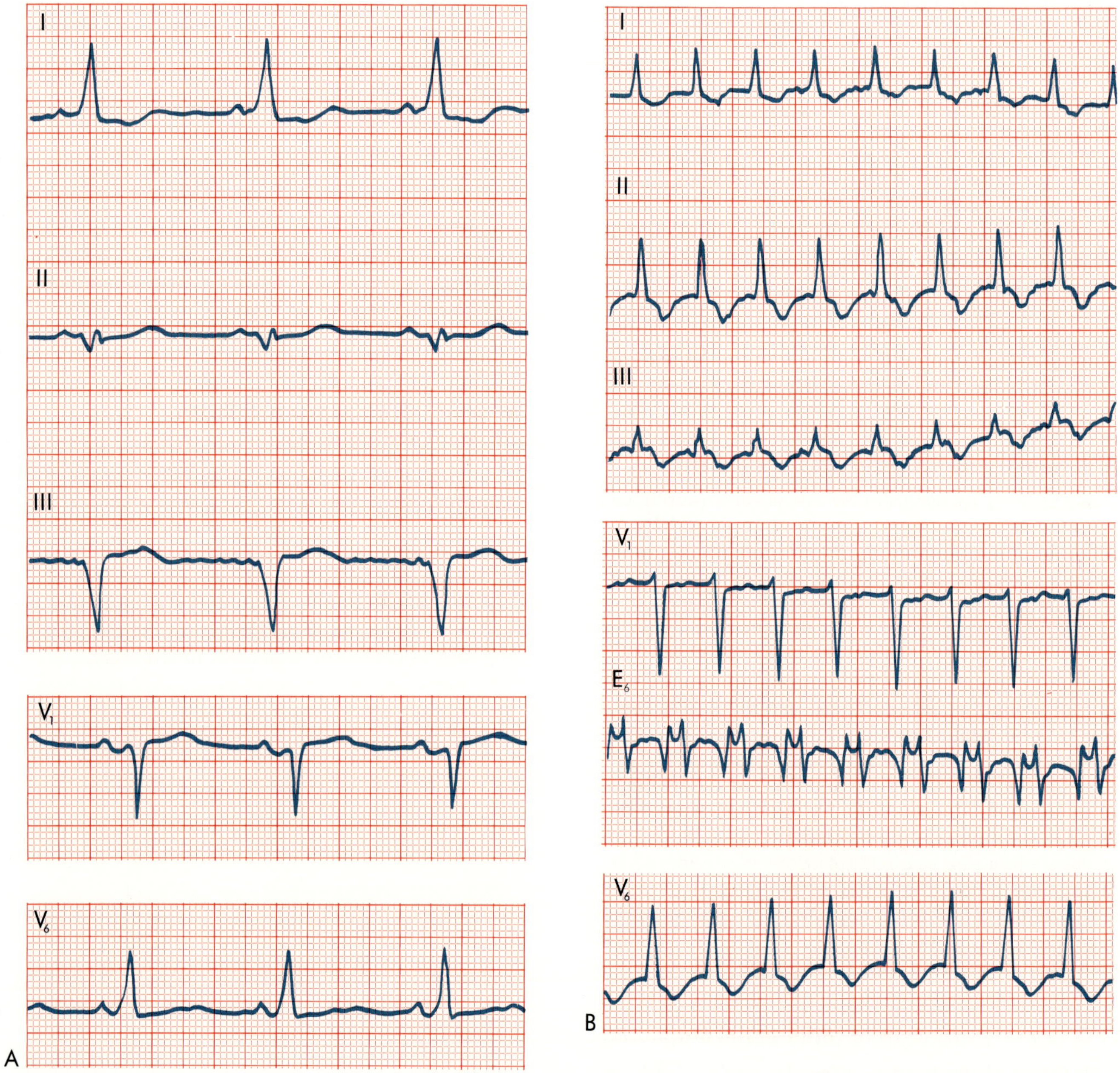

Fig. 7.10
WPW syndrome with WPW pattern in sinus rhythm (A) and paroxysm re-entry tachycardia (B)
A ECG in sinus rhythm. WPW pattern with short PR and delta wave (type B)
B Attack of re-entry tachycardia. The narrow QRS complexes occur at a regular rate of 160/min. Retrograde P waves are discernible in the ST segment in leads I, II, III and aVF (left-sided accessory AV connection). An oesophageal ECG (lead E) makes it evident that there is only one P wave sandwiched in between two QRS complexes

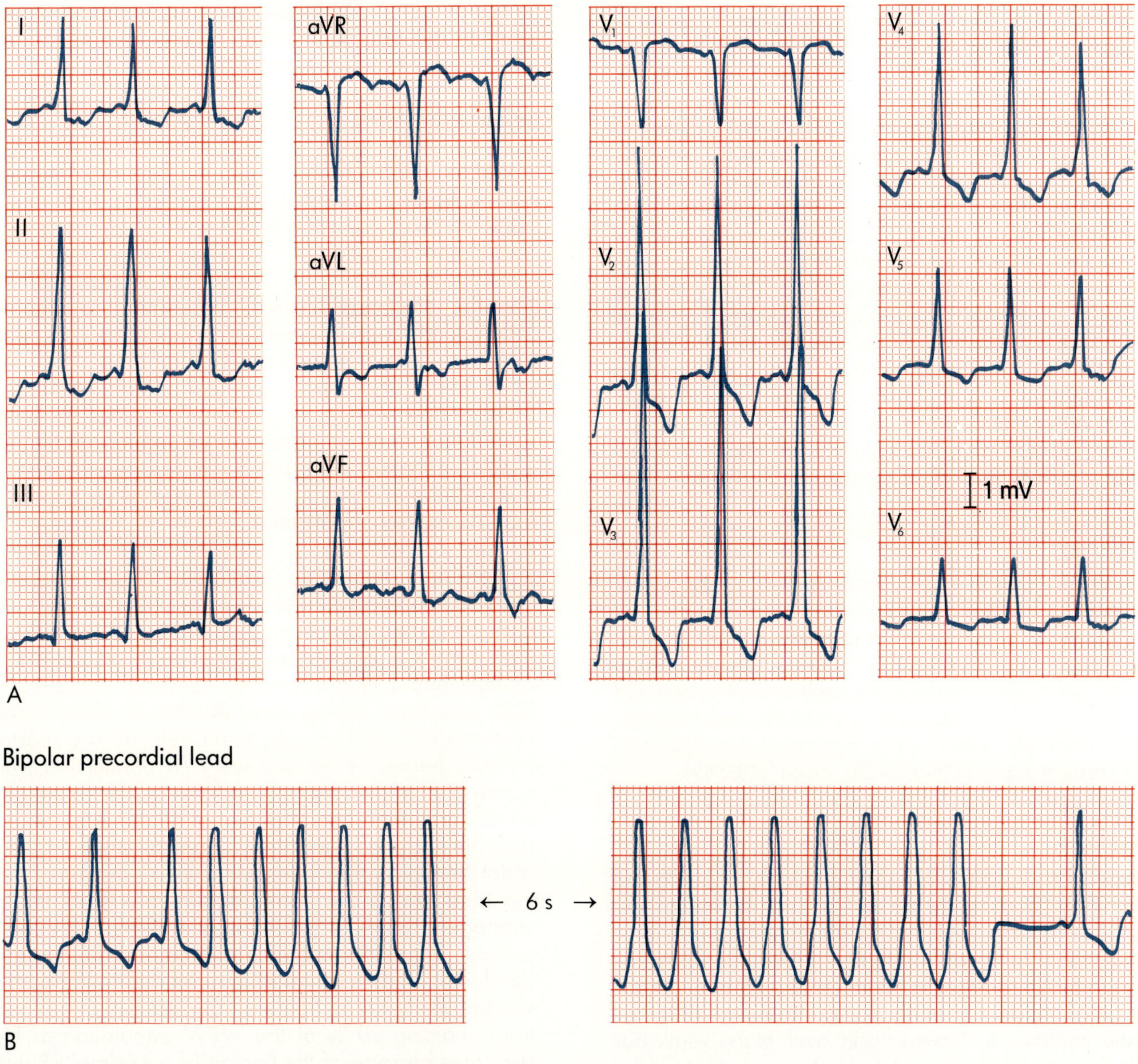

Fig. 7.11
WPW syndrome. In sinus rhythm (A) WPW pattern (type B). In tachycardia (B) wide QRS complexes of the same polarity as the delta wave and most likely due to an impulse caroussel with AV conduction via the accessory AV connection and VA conduction via the His bundle and the AV node; an alternative explanation might be QRS widening due to aberrant ventricular conduction

Symptoms [4–6]

Symptoms of paroxysmal re-entry tachycardia or atrial fibrillation or flutter are the only clinical manifestations of ventricular pre-excitation. The patient with a WPW pattern in the ECG and no attacks of tachycardia or fibrillation, thus, is asymptomatic. The great majority of patients who seek medical advice, however, have attacks of tachycardia at intervals of weeks or months. The attacks often are brief and stop spontaneously or can be terminated by vagal manoeuvres initiated by the patient himself. Some patients have frequent and sustained attacks which limit their work capacity and impair their quality of life. Other patients may have rare but severe episodes of fast re-entry tachycardia or atrial fibrillation causing syncope. Rarely, the first and only symptom in a formerly symptom free individual with a WPW pattern discovered at a routine investigation may be sudden death due to an attack of atrial fibrillation degenerating to ventricular fibrillation.

Aetiology [4–6]

The WPW pattern and syndrome is a congenital anomaly. A familial occurrence has been reported but is not the rule. The majority of patients, 80–90 %, with a WPW pattern on their ECG have otherwise normal hearts, although a variety of acquired and congenital cardiac defects are associated with WPW, including Ebstein's anomaly, mitral valve prolapse, and hypertrophic cardiomyopathy (Fig. 14.30, page 348/349).

Prognosis [4–6, 9–14]

Attacks of tachycardia can start in infancy or childhood or may first occur in the second or third decade of life, rarely later. Some children and adolescents reduce their frequency of tachycardias as they grow older, possibly due to fibrotic changes in the accessory AV connection. The great majority of patients with paroxysms of tachycardia continue to have attacks over many years but with unpredictable alternations between periods of infrequent and shortlasting attacks and periods of frequent and sustained attacks.

The great majority of the WPW population have a normal life expectancy. A few individuals, a small minority of the WPW population (accurate figures are unavailable) will die suddenly; in infancy, childhood, adolescence or later in life. Sudden cardiac death usually happens in the patient who has a history of paroxysmal tachycardia but can occur occasionally in the asymptomatic individual in whom a chance ECG recording prior to death has shown a WPW pattern.

From as *clinical point of view,* a history of syncope should be taken as indicating a former episode of very rapid tachycardia or fibrillation and so constitutes a sinister prognostic sign.

On the *electrocardiogram,* intermittent loss of the WPW pattern on a single recording (Fig. 7.6, page 194) or on serial recordings (Fig. 7.8, page 195) suggests a precarious accessory AV connection likely to have a slow ventricular response in atrial fibrillation and flutter and with little risk of sudden death. This simple and easily understood rule has its exceptions as evidenced by published case histories of sudden death in this category of patients.

A consistent finding in *electrophysiologic studies* of WPW patients who have been resuscitated from cardiac arrest or who have had repeated episodes of tachycardia associated with syncope, is an RR interval of less than 250 ms between consecutive pre-excited QRS complexes during atrial fibrillation. Thus, sudden cardiac death and syncope seems related to a short refractory period of the accessory AV connection which supports a correspondingly fast ventricular response to atrial fibrillation. The reliability of this finding makes it possible from an electrophysiological study in which atrial fibrillation has been induced by fast atrial pacing (this can be performed non-invasively by the oesophageal route) to classify about 80 % of all WPW patients as low risk with little chance of sudden cardiac death since their minimal RR interval in atrial fibrillation will be greater than 250 ms. Paradoxically, to classify the remaining 20 % of the WPW population as high risk cases because of the finding of a minimal RR interval (between delta wave QRS complexes) of less than 250 ms, however, would be wrong. The specificity of this feature is too low as a majority of patients with such a short refractory period of their accessory AV connection survive normally.

continued page 205

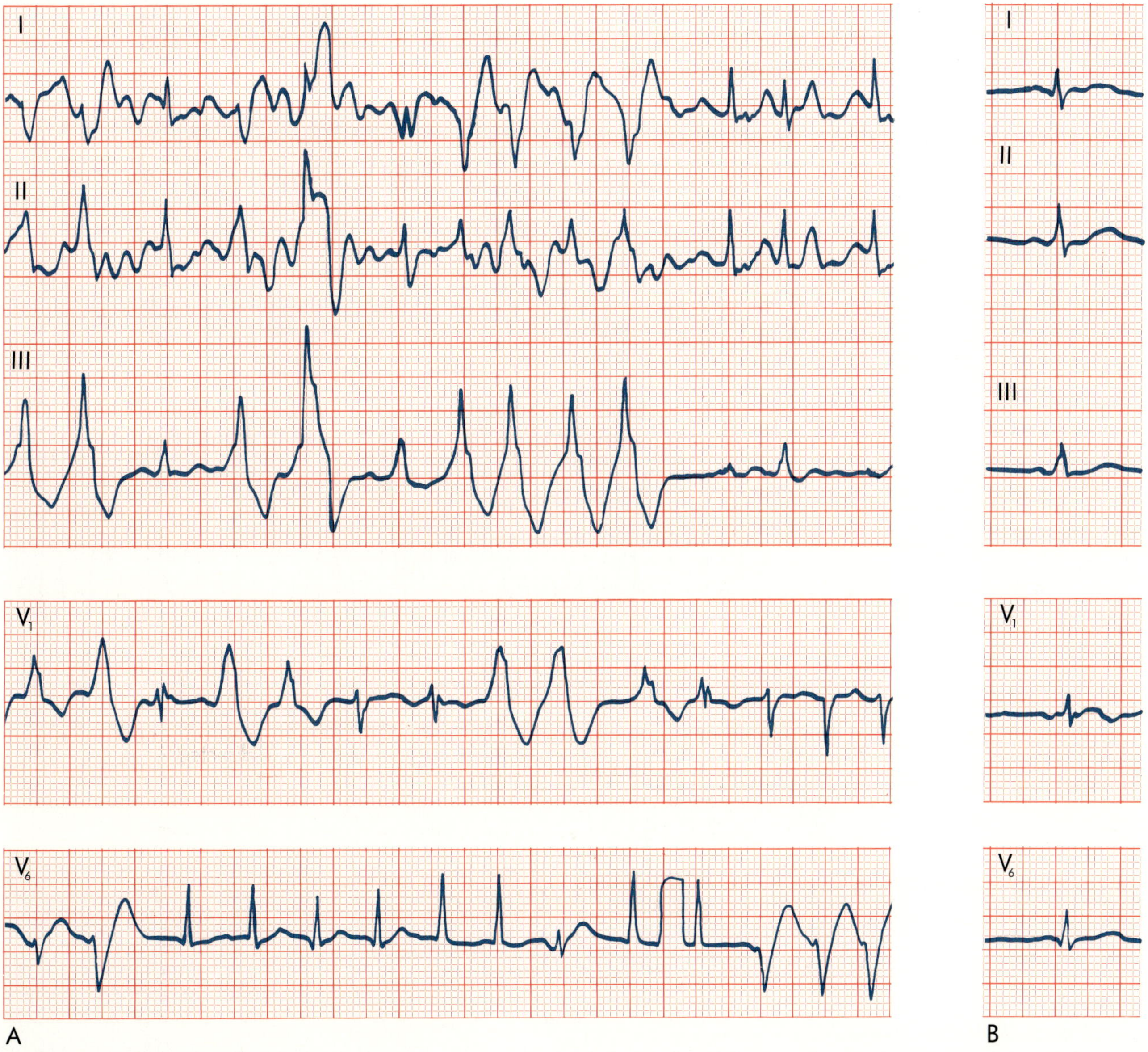

Fig. 7.12
Atrial fibrillation in the WPW syndrome
64-year-old female admitted in congestive heart failure

A ECG during the attack. "Bizarre" QRS complexes varying in form and width. The rhythm is totally irregular, rate 130/min. Atrial fibrillatory wavelets discernible in lead III

B ECG during sinus rhythm. A delta wave and short PR interval can clearly be seen in the extremity leads

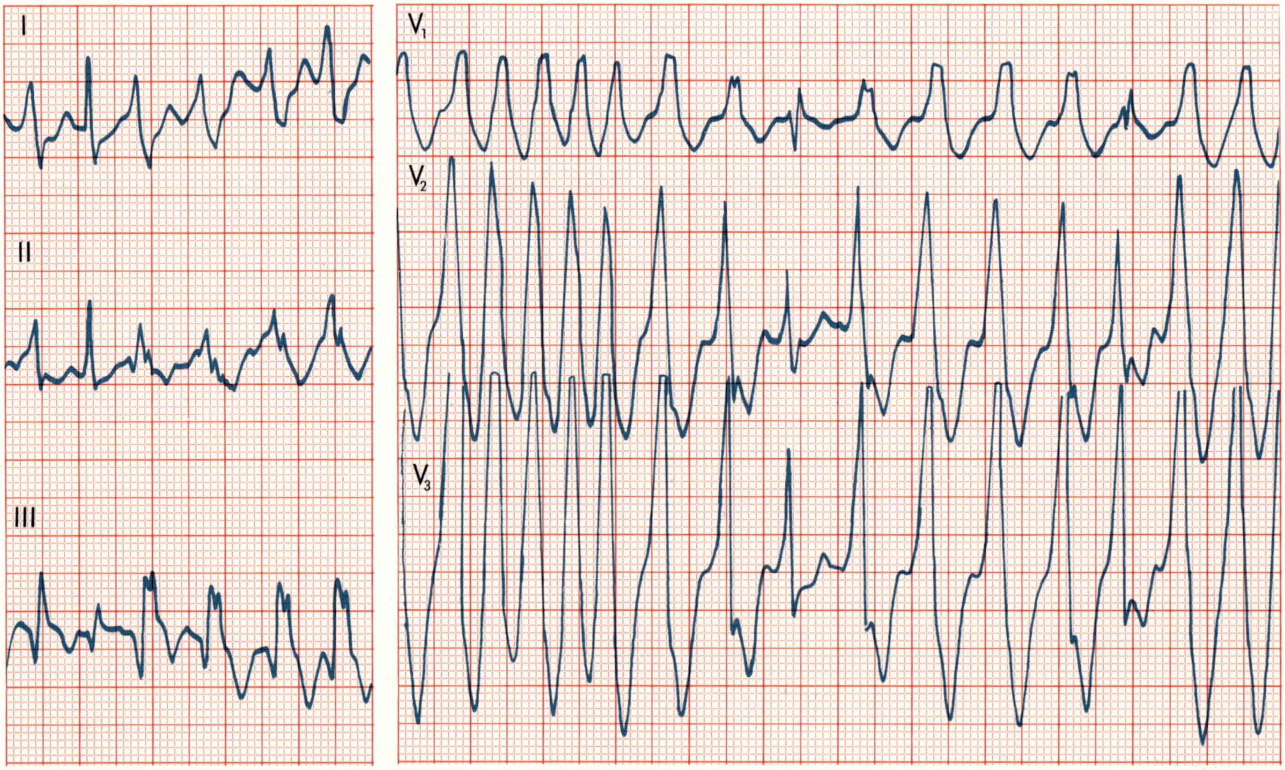

A

Fig. 7.13
Atrial fibrillation in the WPW syndrome
ECG-recording from a 20-year-old man admitted with palpitations and vertigo

A ECG at the time of admission revealed large diphasic broadened irregular (bizarre) QRS complexes. Rhythm totally irregular, rate 170–300/min, no visible atrial activity. Note the great variability in the QRS pattern and rate

B Spontaneous remission to sinus rhythm (short PR interval = 0.10 s), WPW pattern (type A) with delta wave in leads II, III and V_{1-2})

C ECG recorded later on the same day during re-entry tachycardia at a regular rate of 250/min with narrow QRS complexes. No P waves can be identified

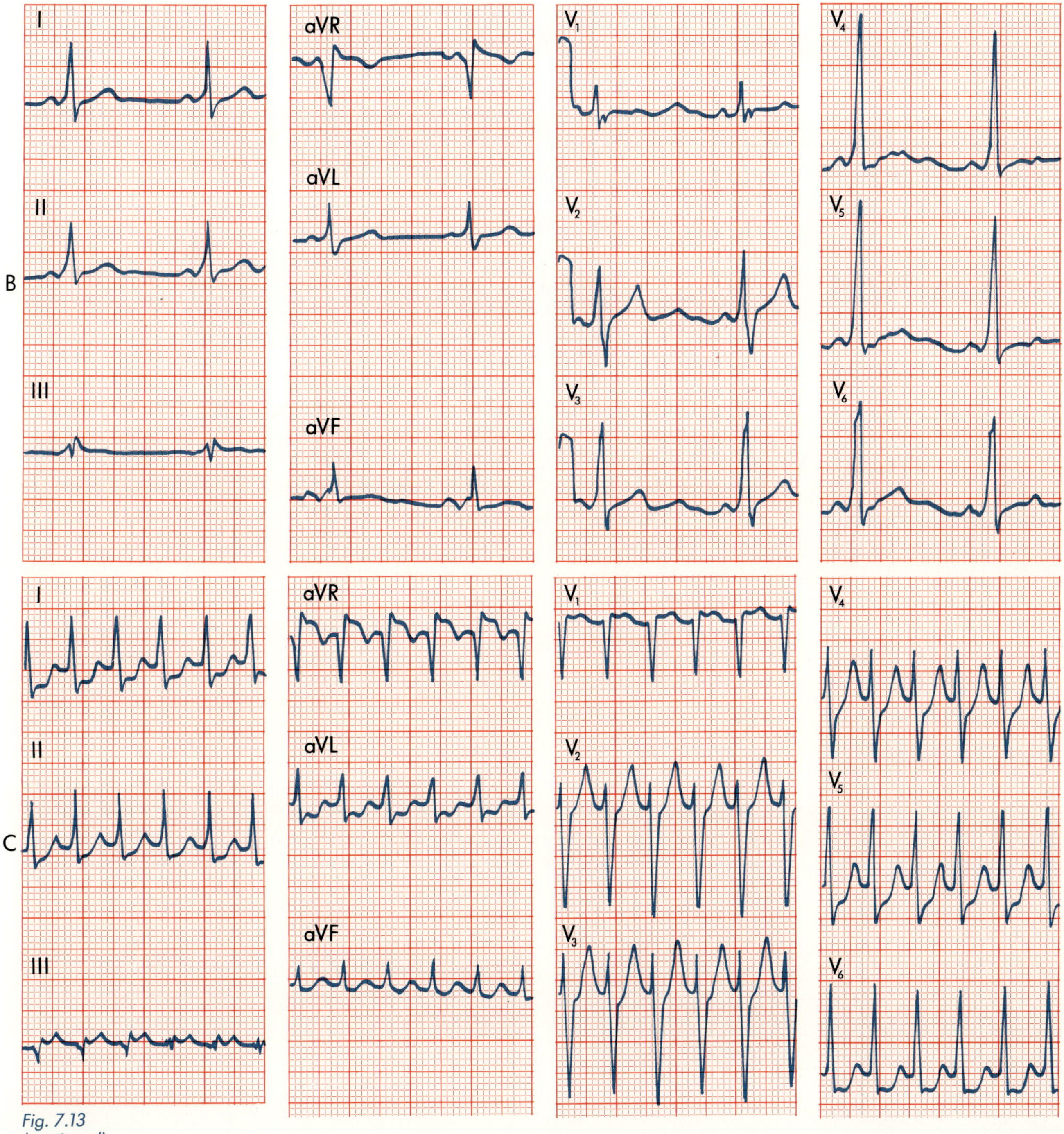

Fig. 7.13 (continued)

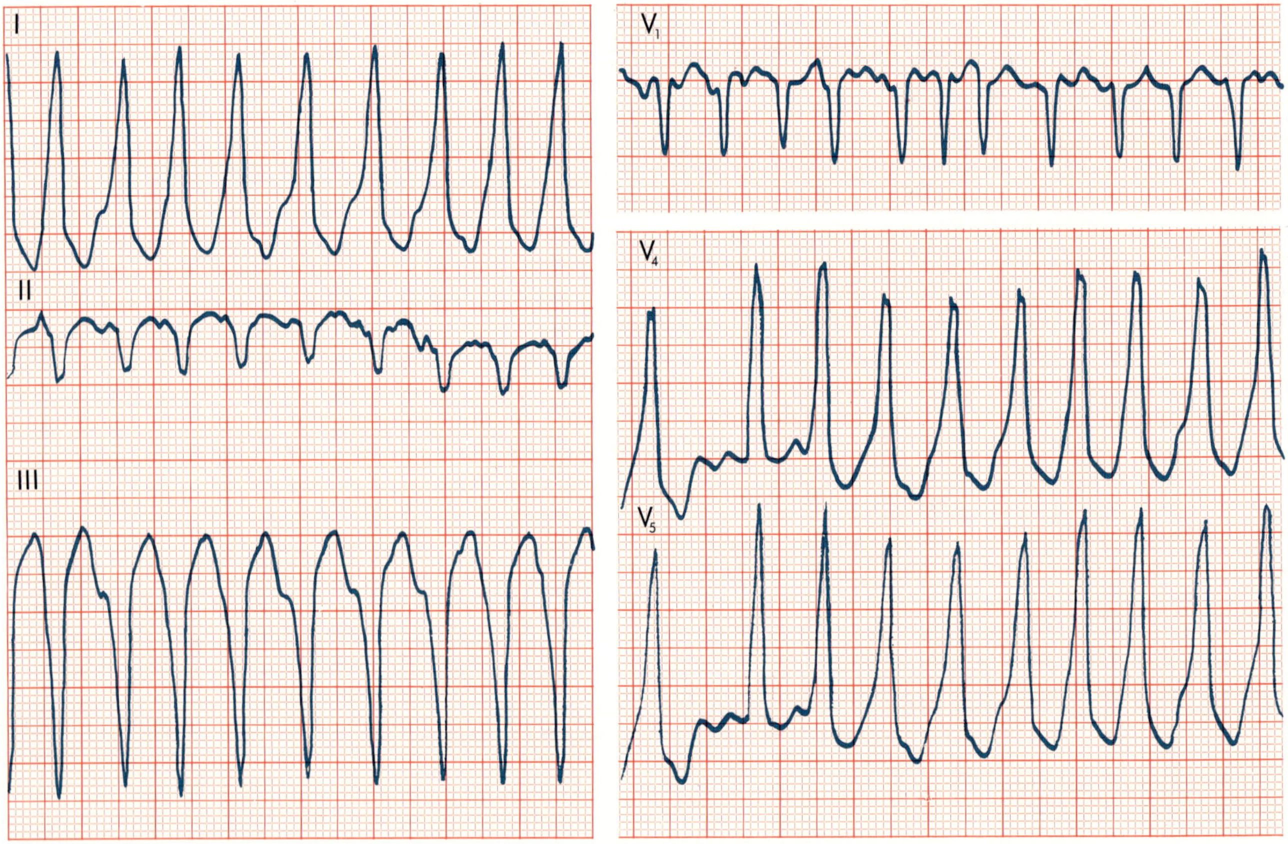

Fig. 7.14
Atrial flutter in the WPW syndrome. ECG recording from the same patient whose ECGs in sinus rhythm and re-entry tachycardia are shown in Fig. 7.10. However, in this recording the ECG shows wide monophasic QRS complexes which in the precordial leads vary considerably in width and appearance. Distinct flutter waves are recorded in leads V_1 and V_4; flutter rate is 300/min. The QRS complex rate varies from 180 to 220/min

Additional investigations [4–6, 15–17]

Natural history data on WPW "patients" with minor or no symptoms are so meager as to preclude identification of those who should be given therapy based on electrophysiologic observations. Electrophysiologic studies can be deferred in the asymptomatic individual and the patient with infrequent and well controlled attacks of tachycardia. The only exception to this rule might be the professional athlete, diver, train conductor or pilot who, if identified as "low risk" at an electrophysiologic study might be able to continue his profession. Thus, at present electrophysiologic studies should be reserved primarily for either patients who are considered candidates for surgery (see later) or for the patients with long time intervals between troublesome or for life threatening attacks of tachycardia (to help select and test a chosen drug treatment).

Management [4–6, 17]

Acute attack of WPW re-entry tachycardia

1 Try various vagal manoeuvers: Carotid sinus massage (Fig. 4.1, page 70), the Valsalva manoeuver, squatting, "finger down the throat", etc.

2 Intravenous antiarrhythmic therapy:

- A Class IC drug (ajmaline, propafenone, flecainide), or
- A Class IA drug (procainamide, disopyramide, quinidine)

3 If tachycardia continues or there is haemodynamic compromise, cardioversion with an initial shock of 50 J.

Acute attack of atrial fibrillation or flutter complicating WPW

1 Intravenous antiarrhythmic therapy:

- A Class IC drug (ajmaline, propafenone, flecainide) or,
- A Class IA drug (procainamide, disopyramide, quinidine) or,
- Amiodarone, which in the authors' opinion is the best drug for this situation.

2 DC cardioversion. In the haemodynamically unstable patient in shock or congestive failure this will be performed as an emergency procedure.

In WPW patients digoxin and verapamil have the potential to shorten the refractory period of the AV connection and so accelerate ventricular rate. Therefore without prior electrophysiologic assessment neither drug should be used in the treatment of an acute attack of atrial fibrillation or flutter. Indeed, neither should be used for WPW re-entry tachycardia as this may degenerate to atrial fibrillation. In infants, however, digoxin appears to be safe and useful (see later).

Long-term management

No therapy is indicated for the asymptomatic individuals, for patients with infrequent and well tolerated attacks or for patients who can terminate their tachycardias with a vagal manoeuver (Fig. 4.1, page 70). All patients should be instructed on the whole range of vagal manoeuvers such that by experimentation they may find the ideal manoeuver or combination of manoeuvres for themselves.

Intermittent oral therapy can be used for patients with infrequent but sustained attacks of tachycardia. This involves taking an oral bolus dose of an antiarrhythmic drug at the onset of palpitations followed by additional doses at 4 to 6 hour intervals. The tachycardia should terminate when an adequate plasma concentration of the medication has been achieved.

Long-term pharmacologic prophylaxis is the commonest treatment for patients with frequent and sustained attacks. Drugs of "first choice" include Class IC drugs (propafenone, flecainide), Class IA drugs (quinidine, procainamide, disopyramide) and beta blocking agents. If ineffective when given alone, the Class I drugs may be combined with a beta blocking agent.

Amiodarone is the most effective drug but because of its side effects it should be reserved for patients whose arrhythmias are refractory to other drugs and who, moreover, are not candidates for surgery. Administered cautiously amiodarone can be combined with a beta blocking agent or even a Class IC or IA drug, if required. Digitalis and possibly also verapamil should be avoided in older children and adults with WPW syndrome as there is a risk of accelerating the ventricular rate in the event of atrial fibrillation or flutter. In infancy, digitalis has been widely used successfully and safely, probably because infants very rarely develop atrial fibrillation.

Depending on the clinical situation, technical facilities and expertise, either empirical drug use tested by trial and error or drug selection by serial electrophysiological studies may be employed to select the optimal medication.

Antitachycardia surgery which interrupts the accessory AV connection offers a cure for the arrhythmia, eliminating not only the attacks of re-entry tachycardia but also attacks of atrial fibrillation and flutter.

Surgical treatment of the WPW syndrome in a centre with an experienced surgeon and electrophysiologist offers a high success rate and a low operative risk so widening the indications for surgical intervention.

The *indication for surgery* is clear in the patient:

- Resuscitated from sudden cardiac death, or
- With attacks of atrial fibrillation or flutter leading to syncope or presyncope despite appropriate drug treatment, or
- With frequent symptomatic attacks of tachycardia not controlled by drug therapy.

The best approach for young patients who can be controlled by medication but who face the prospect of a lifetime of drug therapy remains unclear. With the refinement of surgical techniques the trend is towards surgical treatment of this group of patients particularly if they have an RR interval in atrial fibrillation of less than 250 ms and/or amiodarone is required for control of the arrhythmias. When considering the appropriateness of surgery in a particular patient with the WPW syndrome, expected unoperated morbidity and mortality and the calculated operative morbidity and mortality should be compared.

Concealed WPW syndrome[2–6]

The basis of this syndrome is an accessory AV connection anatomically identical to that of the WPW syndrome but with unidirectional block for AV conduction and thus capable only of VA impulse transmission.

ECG diagnosis and differential diagnosis

The ECG in *sinus rhythm* is normal (Fig. 7.15, page 208 to the right) since AV impulse conduction occurs only via the normal AV conduction pathway (AV node and His bundle). The ECG appearance during *re-entry tachycardia* (Fig. 7.15 to the left) is identical to that of re-entry tachycardia in the WPW syndrome with usually a retrograde P wave (P′) in the ST segment and RP′ interval that is shorter than the P′R interval (Fig. 6.11 C, page 136). In a few patients the ventriculo-atrial conduction time over the accessory AV connection is long, longer than over the AV conduction time over the AV node-His-Purkinje pathway. The ensuing tachycardia shows an RP′ interval which is longer than the P′R interval (Fig. 6.11 E). Like the patients with the uncommon form of AV nodal re-entry tachycardia and similar RP′/P′R characteristics, these patients usually suffer from incessant repetitive paroxysms of tachycardia or permanent tachycardia.

The ECG in *atrial fibrillation and flutter* cannot be distinguished from non-WPW atrial fibrillation or flutter and the ventricular response is not unduly rapid since AV conduction occurs only via the normal AV conduction pathway.

Symptoms, aetiology and prognosis

These are similar to the WPW syndrome but as high frequency atrial activity during atrial fibrillation and flutter are not AV transmitted via the accessory AV connection, there is little risk of syncope and no risk of sudden death.

Additional investigations

Referral for electrophysiologic study is indicated when surgery is contemplated and might be considered for the selection and testing of antiarrhythmic drug treatment.

Management

Management is as for the WPW syndrome except that digitalis and verapamil can be used *without* the risk of accelerating the ventricular response to atrial fibrillation and flutter.

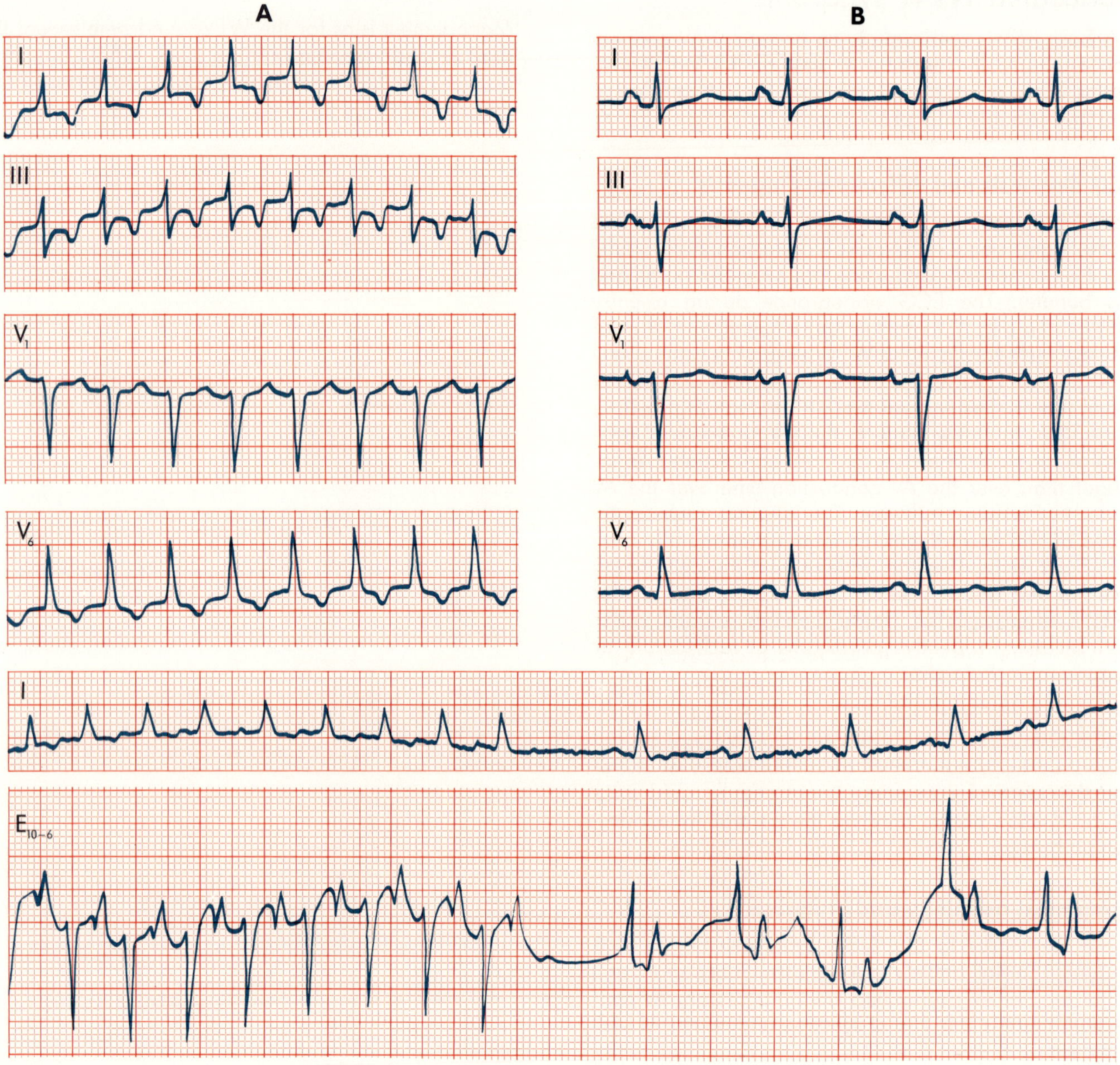

Fig. 7.15
Concealed WPW syndrome. Tachycardia ECG (to the left): QRS rhythm regular, QRS rate 150/min, QRS complex narrow (< 0.12 s), P waves visible in most leads superimposed on the T wave with RP' < P'R. Timing of the retrograde P wave in the RR interval suggests a diagnosis of WPW tachycardia which later has been confirmed in an electrophysiological study. Sinus rhythm (to the right): Normal without signs of preexcitation (PR 0.16 s, no delta wave)

Short PR syndrome [3, 18, 19]

In the short PR syndrome (formerly named the Lown-Ganong-Levine syndrome) the patient's ECG shows a short PR interval followed by a normal QRS complex (no delta wave) and there is an associated history of paroxysmal tachycardia. The basis of the PR shortening and the tachycardias are atrial fibres which bypass the conduction delay in the upper part of the AV node shortcircuiting the atrial myocardium to the distal part of the AV node or His bundle (Fig. 7.1 C, page 189).

ECG diagnosis

The diagnosis is based on (Fig. 7.16, page 210):

- A short PR interval of 0.12 s or less in the adult
- A normal QRS complex without either a delta wave or abnormal widening
- A history of paroxysmal tachycardia.

Differential diagnosis

A short PR interval may be due to AV nodal rhythm (Fig. 3.13 C, page 48). Thus, before making a diagnosis of the short PR interval syndrome, it should be ascertained that the P wave vector is normal – positive in leads I and II.

A PR interval shortened to about 0.12 s without any history of paroxysmal tachycardia is a not infrequent finding in otherwise healthy individuals. Its pathoanatomical basis is obscure and it is of no clinical or prognostic significance in the symptom free individual.

Symptoms, aetiology, prognosis, additional investigations

These are as for the WPW syndrome. The clinical significance is related to attacks of re-entry tachycardia and atrial fibrillation. Atrial fibrillation may be associated with a rapid ventricular rate and a risk of degeneration to ventricular fibrillation. Attacks of atrial flutter may be associated with 1:1 AV conduction and a ventricular rate in the range of 220–300/min.

Management

Management is as for the WPW syndrome.

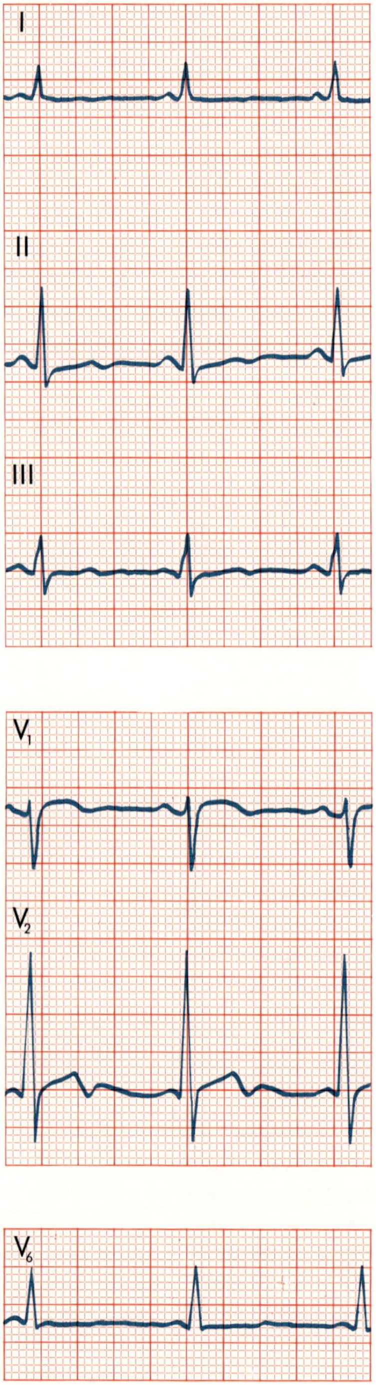

Fig. 7.16
Short PR interval syndrome. 69-year-old male with repeated attacks of supraventricular tachycardia over a period of several years. ECG in sinus rhythm shows a short PR interval (0.11 s), no delta wave and a normally narrow QRS complex (less than 0.12 s wide). ECG during tachycardia (not presented) showed supraventricular tachycardia at a regular rate of 190/min

1. Davies MJ, Andersopn RH, Becker AE. The conduction system of the heart. London, Boston: Butterworths, 1983.
2. Wellens HJJ, Brugada P. Mechanisms of supraventricular tachycardia. Am J Cardiol 1988; 62: 10–15.
3. Gallagher JJ. Variants of preexcitation. Update 1984. In: Zipes DP, Jalife J, eds. Cardiac electrophysiology and arrhythmias. New York: Grune & Stratton, Inc., 1985; 419–33.
4. Wellens HJJ, Farre J, Bär FW. The Wolff-Parkinson-White syndrome. In: Mandel WJ, ed. Cardiac arrhythmias. Their mechanisms, diagnosis and management. Philadelphia, London, New York: J. P. Lippincott Co., 1987; 274–96.
5. Prystowsky EN. Diagnosis and management of the preexcitation syndromes. Curr Probl Cardiol 1988; 13: 227–96.
6. Clinical perspectives in management of Wolff-Parkinson-White syndrome, Part 1: Recognition, diagnosis, and arrhythmias. Part 2: Diagnostic evaluation and treatment strategies. Mod Concepts Cardiovasc Dis 1989; 58: 43–53.
7. Lemery R, Hammill SC, Wood DL, et al. Value of the resting 12 lead electrocardiogram and vectorcardiogram for locating the accessory pathway in patients with the Wolff-Parkinson-White syndrome. Br Heart J 1987; 58: 324–32.
8. Bär FW, Brugada P, Wellens HJJ. Atrial fibrillation and pre-excitation. In: Kulbertus HE, Olsson SB, Schlepper M, eds. Atrial fibrillation. Mölndal, Sweden: Astra Cardiovas cular, 1982; 179–87.
9. Robinson K, Rowland E, Krikler DM. Latent pre-excitation: Exposure of anterograde accessory pathway conduction during atrial fibrillation. Br Heart J 1988; 59: 53–55.
10. Prystowsky EN, Fananapazir L, Packer DL, et al. Wolff-Parkinson-White syndrome and sudden cardiac death. Cardiology 1987; 74 (Suppl. 2): 67–71.
11. Robinson K, Rowland E, Krikler DM. Wolff-Parkinson-White syndrome: Atrial fibrillation as the presenting arrhythmia. Br Heart J 1988; 59: 578–80.
12. Becquart J, et al. Prognosis for Wolff-Parkinson-White syndrome. Arch Mal Coeur 1988; 81: 695–700.
13. Wiedermann CJ, Becker AE, Hopferwieser T, et al. Sudden death in a young competitive athlete with Wolff-Parkinson-White syndrome. Europ Heart J 1987; 8: 651–55.
14. Klein GJ, Yee R, Sharma AD. Longitudinal electrophysiologic assessment of asymptomatic patients with the Wolff-Parkinson-White electrocardiographic pattern. New Engl J Med 1989; 320: 1230–33.
15. Kerr CR, Gallagher JJ, Smith WM, et al. The induction of atrial flutter and fibrillation and the termination of atrial flutter by esophageal pacing. Pace 1983; 6: 60–72.
16. Waldo AL, Akhtar M, Benditt DG, et al. Appropriate electrophysiologic study and treatment of patients with the Wolff-Parkinson-White syndrome. JACC 1988; 11: 1124–29.
17. Wellens HJJ, Brugada P, Penn OC. The management of preexcitation syndromes. JAMA 1987; 257: 2325–33.
18. Wiener I. Syndromes of Lown-Ganong-Levine and enhanced atrioventricular nodal conduction. Am J Cardiol 1983; 52: 637.
19. Ward DE, Camm J. Mechanisms of junctional tachycardias in the Lown-Ganong-Levine syndrome. Am Heart J 1983; 105: 169.

Chapter 8
Escape rhythm, accelerated rhythm, sinus bradycardia, irregular sinus rhythm and multifocal supraventricular rhythm

Escape rhythm[1]

An escape rhythm is three or more consecutive impulses arising from an ectopic pacemaker as a result of an undue delay in normal impulse formation or conduction.

ECG diagnosis

The characteristic features of an escape rhythm are those of ectopy and a rate equal to the inherent rate of the corresponding ectopic pacemaker (Fig. 1.6, page 5).

AV nodal escape rhythm (Figs. 8.1 A and B) is characterized by:

- QRS complexes of supraventricular type. Retrograde P waves may precede the complex, be hidden within it or appear in the ST segment following the complex (Fig. 3.13, page 48)

- The recording of three or more of such PQRS complexes in a row and at a rate in the range of (35)40–60/min.

Ventricular escape rhythm (Fig. 8.1 C) is characterized by:

- QRS complexes of ventricular type (Fig. 3.16, page 50)

- The recording of three or more of such complexes in a row and at a rate in the range of 20–40/min.

Symptoms

Unstable escape rhythms with sudden failure of impulse formation can result in Stokes Adams attacks (Figs. 10.8, page 260/261 and 10.10, page 263) or sudden death. When complicating disease states with limited cardiac reserve, slow escape rhythms can contribute to the development of congestive failure and shock.

Aetiology

Escape rhythms develop in response to block and bradycardia. They maintain the activation of the ventricles and thereby the vital pumping activity of the heart.

Episodes of AV nodal escape rhythm may be induced by high vagal tone, e.g. by vagal manoeuvres. They are not uncommon findings in apparently healthy athletes or children. They are secondary to sinus bradycardia (Fig. 8.1 A), SA block (Figs. 11.5–11.7, page 284 – page 287) or AV block of monofascicular type (Fig. 8.1 B). They may occur as an early sign of digitalis overdosage.

The common cause of a ventricular escape rhythm is third degree AV block (Fig. 8.1 C)(Chapter 10, page 248).

Management

Treatment is indicated only if the rate of the escape rhythm is inadequate to maintain an appropriate pumping activity of the heart or if it becomes unstable with episodes of ventricular arrest (Figs. 10.8 and 10.10, page 263) or attacks of torsade de pointes ventricular tachycardia (Fig. 10.11, page 265).

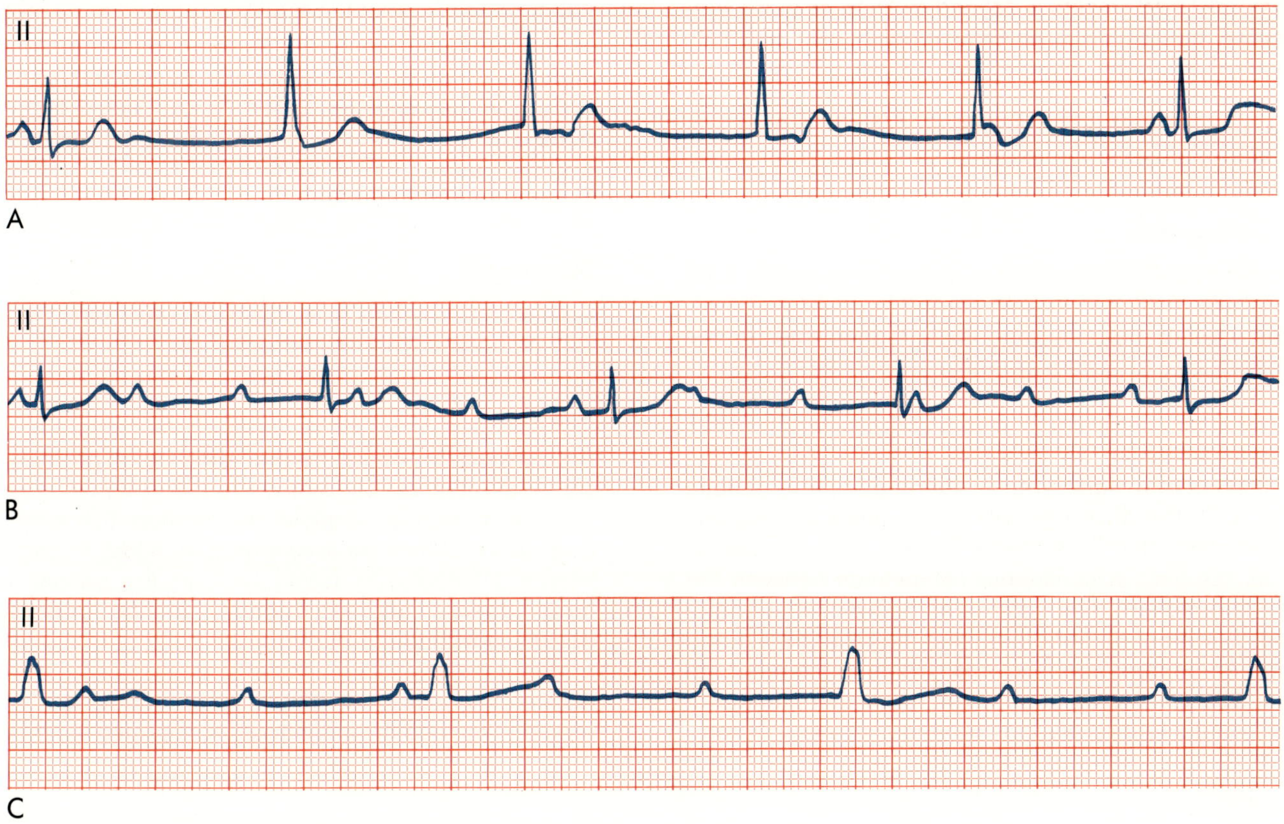

Fig. 8.1
Escape rhythms

A *AV nodal escape rhythm alternating with sinus bradycardia. There are a few sinus P waves (↑), two at the start and two at the end of the ECG; only the first and last are AV conducted. The rate of the sinus rhythm, as judged from the two pairs of sinus P waves, ranges from 40 to 65/min. Complex Nos. 2–5 represent an episode of AV nodal escape rhythm with a rate of 48/min. The AV nodal origin of these complexes is confirmed by the absence of preceding sinus P waves and their normal width (QRS = 0.11 s). Despite their AV nodal origin, the complexes are not quite identical to those of sinus rhythm (Nos. 1 and 6), but differ slightly in QRS axis and amplitude. Retrograde P waves are visible in the ST segment of complexes 3 and 4, but are absent in complexes 2 and 5 due to atrial capture by the sinus node.*

B *AV nodal rhythm in third degree AV block. There are sinus P waves at a rate of 118/min and QRS complexes at a slower and independant rate of 38/min.*

C *Ventricular escape rhythm in third degree AV block. There are sinus P waves at a rate of 72/min and wide, bizarre QRS complexes (QRS = 0.18 s) at an independant rate of 28/min.*

Accelerated rhythm [1–7]

An accelerated rhythm is defined as three or more consecutive impulses from an ectopic pacemaker at a rate above that of the inherent rate of the ectopic pacemaker but less than 100/min i.e. a rate of 60 to 100/min in accelerated AV nodal rhythm and of 40 to 100/min in accelerated ventricular rhythm.

ECG diagnosis

Accelerated AV nodal rhythm is characterized by QRS complexes similar to those recorded in an AV nodal escape rhythm but occurring at a higher rate, in the range of 60–100/min (Fig. 8.3).

Accelerated ventricular rhythm is characterized by QRS complexes similar to those in a ventricular escape rhythm but at a higher rate, in the range of 40–100/min (Fig. 8.2). The discharge rate of the ventricular ectopic pacemaker often fluctuates within the range of the SA node, resulting in continuous competition between the two pacemakers. The ventricular pacemaker is sometimes dominant and at other times the SA node is dominant. At the transition from one rhythm to the other, fusion QRS complexes occur, their width and configuration being intermediate between those of the QRS complexes recorded during ventricular rhythm and those recorded during sinus rhythm. Fusion complexes (FC in Fig. 8.2) are created by dual activation of the ventricular myocardium due to the simultaneous formation of impulses in the ectopic ventricular pacemaker and the arrival, in the ventricles, of an AV conducted sinus impulse. The fusion complexes in Fig. 8.2 are preceded by a sinus P wave at an interval equal to or almost equal to the normal PR interval.

Symptoms

Accelerated rhythms are clinically silent arrhythmias with no haemodynamic consequence.

Aetiology

Accelerated AV nodal rhythm showing a gradual increase in rate from 60 to 80 up to 100–140/min may be seen as a sign of digitalis intoxication (Chapter 12, page 292). Otherwise accelerated AV nodal rhythm is a benign phenomenon found both in the patient with heart disease and occasionally in the apparently healthy individual.

Accelerated ventricular rhythm is by contrast rarely observed in the healthy individual. Accelerated ventricular

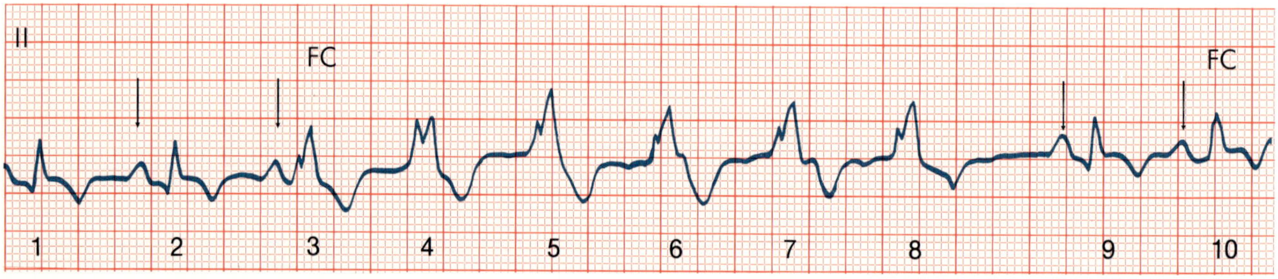

Fig. 8.2
Accelerated ventricular rhythm.
ECG from a 46-year-old man with recent inferior myocardial infarction.
QRS complexes Nos. 4–8 represent accelerated ventricular rhythm with a consecutive bizarre configuration (QRS = 0.16 s) at a rate of 90/min. Complex Nos. 1, 2 and 9 are genuine sinus complexes (PR = 0.19 s, QRS = 0.11 s), whereas complexes Nos. 3 and 10 are fusion complexes (FC) (PR is slightly shorter = 0.17–0.18 s, QRS is intermediate in width and configuration between those of sinus and ventricular origin). There is AV dissociation during the entire period of accelerated ventricular rhythm with sinus P waves.

rhythm frequently occurs during the acute stage of acute myocardial infarction. It is a benign arrhythmia with little or no tendency for acceleration to ventricular tachycardia or fibrillation and without indication for treatment. It has been found to occur especially following thrombolysis and is suggested as a useful marker for successful thrombolysis with reperfusion of the infarcted region.

Prognosis

Prognosis relates to underlying heart disease if present, otherwise the arrhythmia has no independent prognostic significance. Digitalis induced accelerated AV nodal rhythm may precede more serious digitalis induced arrhythmias (Chapter 12, page 293).

Management

Accelerated rhythms are benign arrhythmias which require no active intervention.

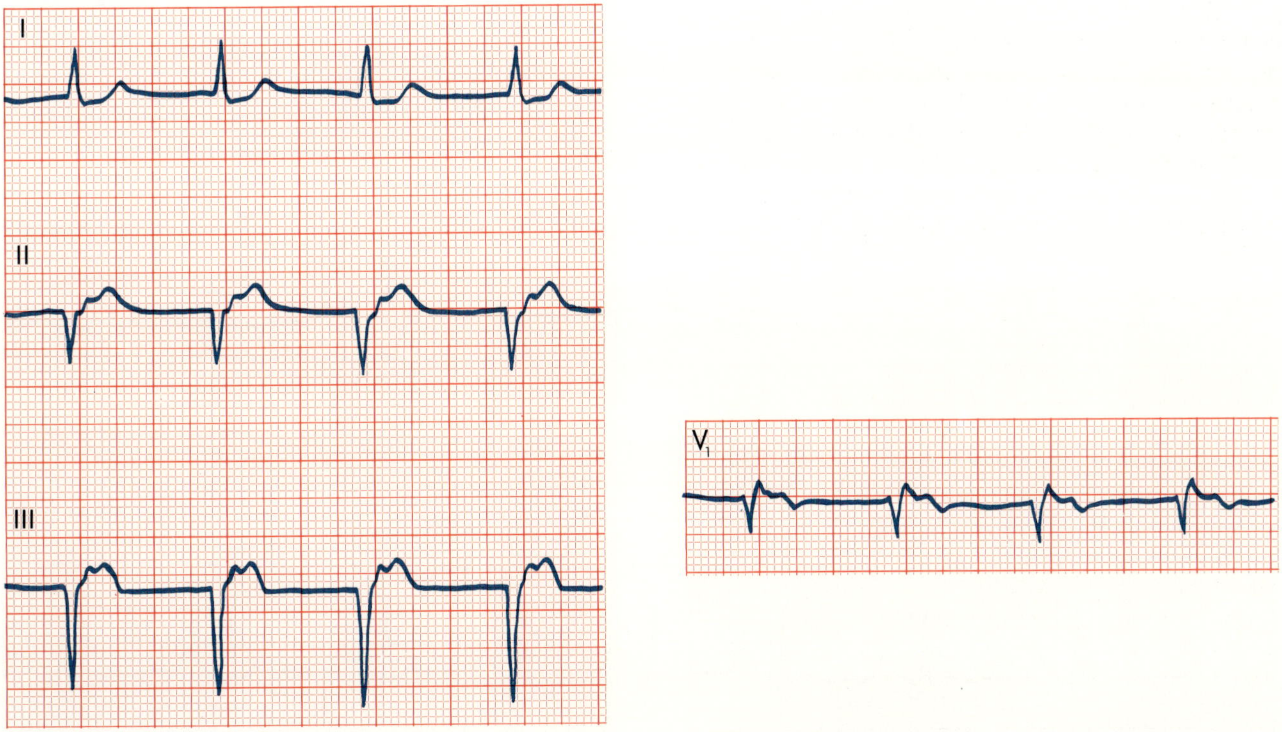

Fig. 8.3
Accelerated AV nodal rhythm.
There are QRS complexes of normal width (QRS = 0.08 s) at a regular rate of 75/min. Retrograde P waves are visible in the ST segment after the QRS complex.

Sinus bradycardia and irregular sinus rhythm [1, 8–10]

ECG diagnosis

Sinus bradycardia is defined as sinus rhythm at a rate below 50/min, usually within the range of 35–50/min (Fig. 8.4).

Irregular sinus rhythm is sinus rhythm characterized by a continuous variation in the PP interval (Fig. 8.5). The variation in cycle length usually is related to respiration, showing an increase during expiration. The term sinus arrhythmia is often used synonomously but this is classified as a "non-preferred term" by the WHO/ISFC task force on definitions of cardiac rhythms.

Sinus bradycardia and irregular sinus rhythm often alternate with each other in the same ECG tracing.

Differential diagnosis

Second degree type I sinoatrial block (SA block) may closely resemble irregular sinus rhythm but the former is characterized by a repetitive pattern over three to four P waves of progressive shortening of the PP interval followed by a long PP interval and then again progressive shortening of the PP interval and so on (Fig. 11.1, page 280).

Symptoms

Symptoms usually are absent but sinus bradycardia with a rate below 35/min may contribute to the development of hypotensive shock in the vasovagal syndrome (see below) and the hypersensitive carotid sinus (Fig. 11.5, page 284).

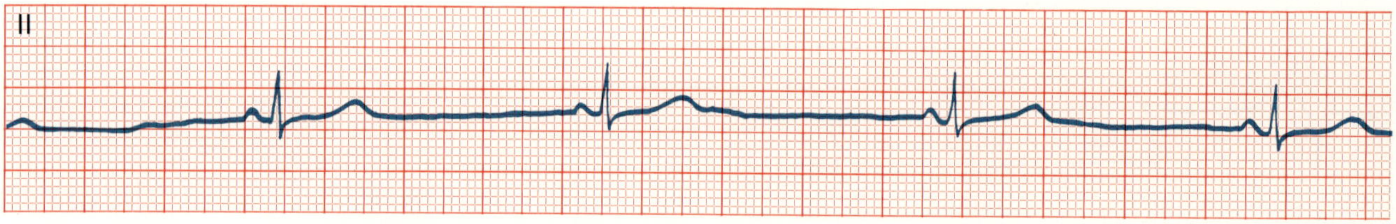

Fig. 8.4
Sinus bracycardia at a rate of 36/min. Bipolar precordial lead

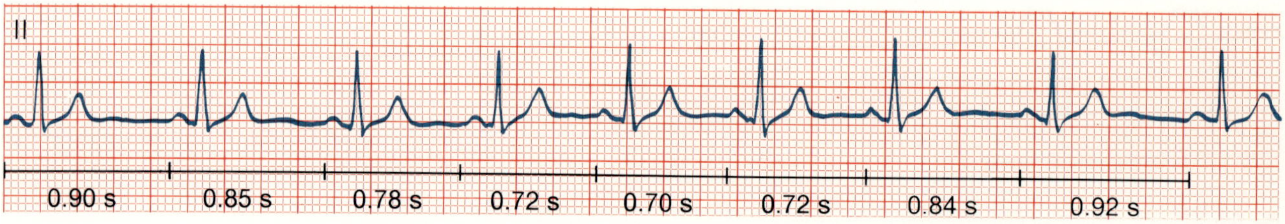

Fig. 8.5
Irregular sinus rhythm with a variation in the PP interval corresponding to a rate variation from 65/min to 86/min.

Aetiology

Sinus bradycardia often reflects high vagal tone and commonly is observed in children and athletes. It is seen during treatment with beta blocking agents. It is a prominent feature of the vasovagal syndrome (episodes of bradycardia and hypotension related e.g. to morphine injection in the early stage of myocardial infarction, arterial puncture and occasionally carotid sinus massage).

Irregular sinus rhythm may alternate with sinus bradycardia in children and athletes and like the sinus bradycardia is related to high vagal tone.

Management

Bradycardia and the hypotension in the vasovagal syndrome can be alleviated by the intravenous injection of atropine or ipratroprium bromide.

Multifocal supraventricular rhythm [1, 9, 10]

In multifocal supraventricular arrhythmia some impulses originate in the SA node whereas others originate from various atrial foci and the AV node. An often used synonym is "wandering pacemaker" but this term has been discouraged by the WHO/ISFC task force on definitions of cardiac rhythm, as it implies a mechanism which remains unsubstantiated.

ECG diagnosis

Multifocal supraventricular rhythm is a slightly irregular rhythm at a rate below 100/min and is characterized by P waves of changing shape and with varying PR intervals (Fig. 8.6).

Aetiology, prognosis and management

Multiform supraventricular rhythm is a frequent finding in normal individuals, particularly children. It is benign and, as a normal variant, requires no treatment.

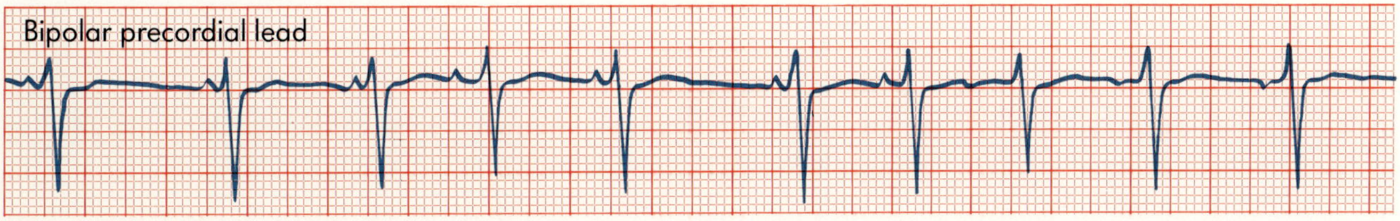

Fig. 8.6
Multifocal suptaventricular rhythm. The rhythm is irregular with a rate variation from 75/min to 100/min with a varying P wave configuration and changing PR interval.

1. WHO/ISFC Task Force. Definition of terms related to cardiac rhythm. Europ J Cardiol 1978; 8: 127–44.
2. Schamroth L. Idioventricular rhythm and tachycardia. Basic concept and diagnosis. In: Sandøe E, Flensted-Jensen E, Olesen KH, eds. Cardiac arrhythmias. Södertälje, Sweden: Astra, 1970; 308–11.
3. Medvedowsky J-L, Donzeau J-P, Nicolai P, et al. Accelerated idioventricular rhythm. In: Puech P, Slama R, eds. The cardiac arrhythmias by the Arrhythmia Working Group of the French Cardiac Society. Paris: Corbière and Roussel, 1979; 218–27.
4. Wellens HJJ. The electrocardiogram in digitalis in toxication. In: Yu PN, Goodwin JF, eds. Progress in cardiology. Philadelphia: Lea & Febiger, 1976; 271–90.
5. Marriott HJL, Conover MH, eds. Advanced concepts in arrhythmias. Digitalis dysrhythmias. St. Louis: The C.V. Mosby Co., 1983; 324–38.
6. Cercek B, Horvat M. Arrhythmias with brief, high-dose intravenous streptokinase infusion in acute myocardial infarction. Europ Heart J 1985; 6: 109–13.
7. Gorgels APM, Vos MA, Letsch IS, et al. Usefulness of the accelerated idioventricular rhythm as a marker for myocardial necrosis and reperfusion during thrombolytic therapy in acute myocardial infarction. Am J Cardiol 1988; 61: 231–35.
8. Bjerregaard P. Mean 24 hour heart rate, minimal heart rate and pauses in healthy subjects 40-79 years of age. Europ Heart J 1983; 4: 44–51.
9. Huston TP, Puffer JC, MacMillan Rodney W. The athletic heart syndrome. New Engl J Med 1985; 313: 24–32.
10. Nizet PM, Borgia JF, Horvath SM. Wandering atrial pace maker. (Prevalence in French hornists.) J Electrocardiol 1976; 9: 51–52.

Chapter 9
Intraventricular block

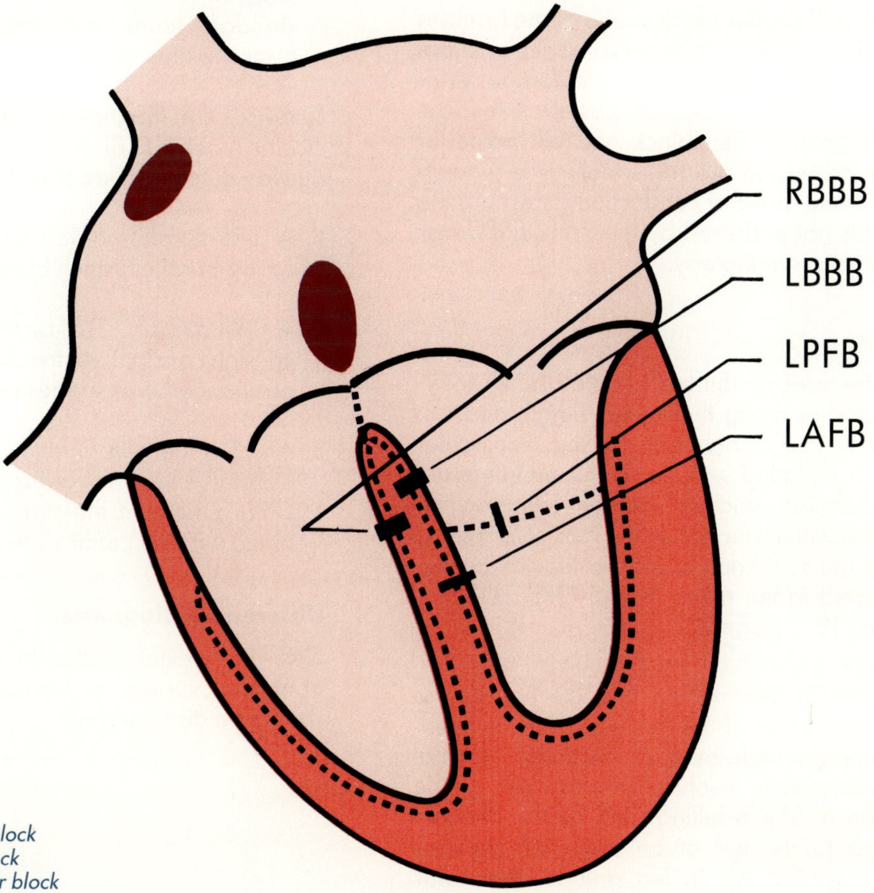

Fig. 9.1
Intraventricular block
RBBB = Right bundle branch block
LBBB = Left bundle branch block
LPFB = Left posterior fascicular block
LAFB = Left anterior fascicular block

Intraventricular block [1]

Blocks in the intraventricular conduction system are classified as (Fig. 9.1):

- Fascicular block (FB) with block in one of the fascicles of the left bundle branch, left anterior FB (LAFB) with block in the anterior fascicle, or left posterior FB (LPFB) with block in the posterior fascicle

- Bundle branch block (BBB) with block in either the right bundle branch (RBBB) or the left (LBBB)

- Incomplete right bundle branch block – a term referring to an ECG appearance which may be due (but not always) to minor conduction delay in the right bundle branch.

Since the upper portion of the intraventricular conduction system forms part of the AV conduction system (Fig. 9.1), intraventricular block may merge with AV block caused by the combined occurrence of a right bundle branch block plus a left bundle branch block or of a right bundle branch block plus block of both left fascicles (Fig. 10.1, page 247).

Fascicular block (FB) [1–7]

Fascicular block (FB) implies block in one of the fascicles of the left bundle branch. *Left anterior fascicular block (LAFB)* is block in the left anterior fascicle, *left posterior fascicular block (LPFB)* in the left posterior fascicle. Hemiblock, left anterior hemiblock and left posterior hemiblock have been (and still are) widely used synonymous terms for these forms of conduction defect but the term hemiblock is not endorsed by the WHO/ISFC task force on arrhythmia terminology.

ECG diagnosis

Since the two fascicles of the left bundle branch interconnect via branches along their entire length and fascicular block is limited to only one fascicle, ventricular activation is accomplished with no or minimal time delay. Thus QRS duration which reflects ventricular activation time remains within normal limits. Fascicular block, however, alters the sequence of left ventricular activation causing a shift in the mean frontal QRS axis (Fig. 1.25–1.28, page 19 – page 22).

The critical factor in determining the direction of the QRS axis is the activation of the free wall of the left ventricle, the dominant muscle mass of the heart. Normal activation simultaneously involves both fascicles of the left bundle branch. The resulting QRS axis is directed downwards and to the left at an angle of approximately +60° (Fig. 9.2 A). In left anterior fascicular block (LAFB) activation occurs solely through the left posterior fascicle with a corresponding shift of the QRS axis upwards and to the left at an angle of −45° or more (Fig. 9.2 B). In left posterior fascicular block (LPFB) activation is solely through the left anterior fascicle with a shift of the frontal QRS axis downwards and to the right at an angle of +110° or more (Fig. 9.2 C).

The diagnostic criteria for *left anterior fascicular block (LAFB)* as an *isolated* conduction lesion are (Fig. 9.2 B):

1 A QRS duration of less than 0.12 s thus excluding a complicating bundle branch block

2 A QRS axis of −45° or more suggesting a diagnosis of LAFB

3 A (q)R pattern in leads I, aVL and an rS pattern in leads II, III and aVF is the typical LAFB-pattern in the standard leads and when combined with (2) confirms the diagnosis.

Likewise, the diagnostic criteria for *left posterior fascicular block (LPFB)* as an *isolated* intraventricular conduction defect include (Fig. 9.2 C):

1 A QRS duration of less than 0.12 s excluding complicating bundle branch block

2 A QRS axis of +110° or more in the absence of clinical signs of right ventricular disease or of a vertically positioned heart suggests a diagnosis of LPFB

3 An rS pattern in leads I and aVL and a qR pattern with tall R waves in leads II, III and aVF is the typical LPFB-pattern in the standard leads and when combined with (2) confirms the diagnosis.

Differential diagnosis

QRS axis deviation due to ventricular hypertrophy or abnormal vertical or horizontal position of the heart should be distinguished.

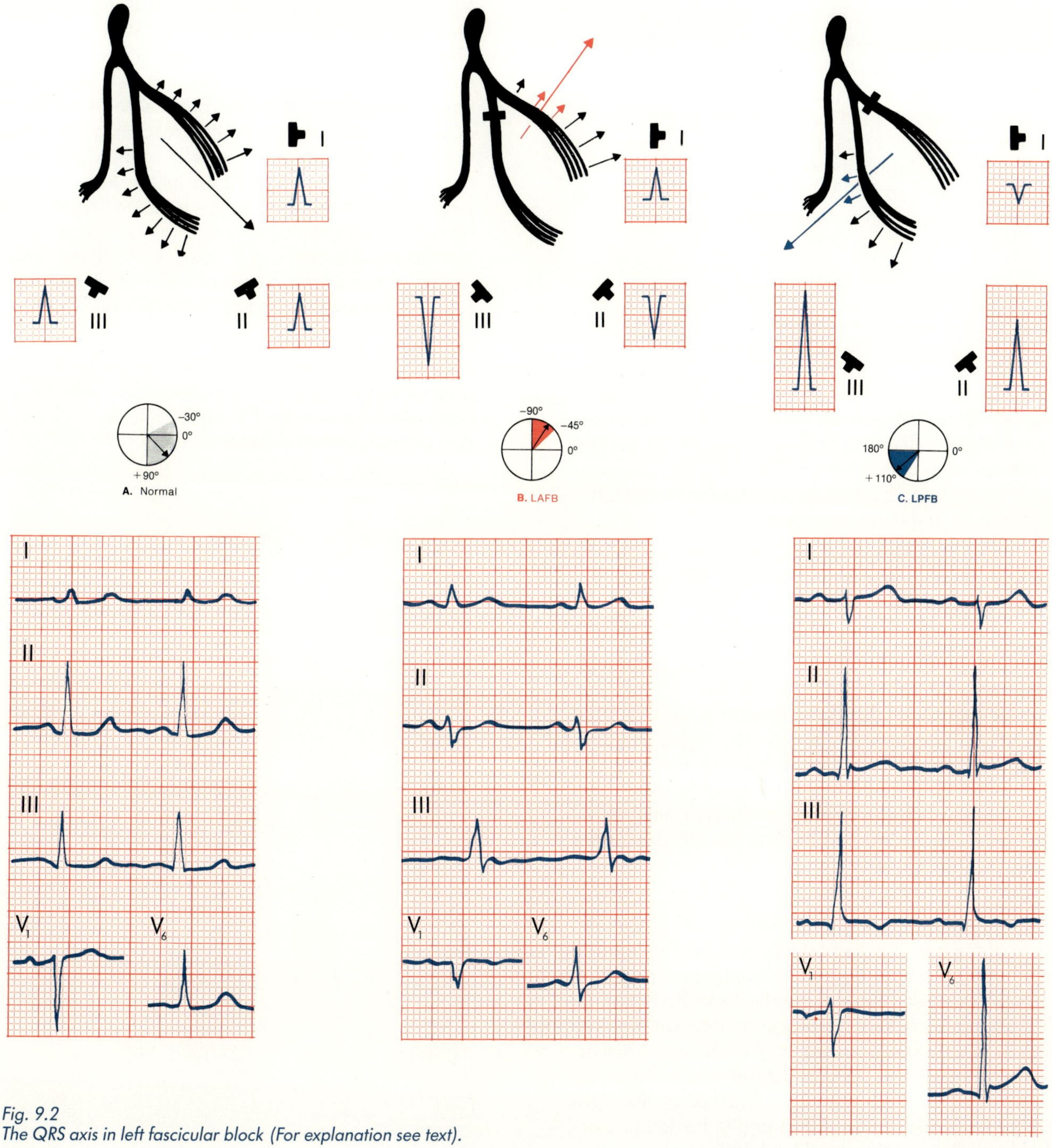

Fig. 9.2
The QRS axis in left fascicular block (For explanation see text).

Aetiology and prognosis

LAFB is a not uncommon finding in the normal population with an incidence increasing from 0.5–2 % below the age of 40 years up to approximately 10 % around the age of 60, and 15–20 % at the age of 70. It is benign and is unassociated with cardiac morbidity or mortality. It does not imply worsening in prognosis when it develops during the course of cardiac disease. LAFB can progress to LBBB. LPFB as an isolated lesion is rare and like LAFB it has no prognostic significance.

Bundle branch block (BBB) [8–12]

Bundle branch block (BBB), right bundle branch block (RBBB) or *left bundle branch block (LBBB),* indicate impulse conduction delay or failure in one of the bundle branches of such a magnitude that the corresponding ventricle is activated by impulse conduction through the bundle branch of the opposite side.

The electrophysiological events in BBB, RBBB (Fig. 9.3 B) or LBBB (Fig. 9.3 C) include:

1 *Normally timed activation of the intraventricular septum from the septal branches of the non-blocked bundle branch.* In RBBB, activation proceeds from the left bundle branch towards the right; in LBBB, from the right bundle branch towards the left. The associated ECG event is a small positive deflection, an r wave, which in RBBB is seen in the right precordial leads (V_{1-2}) and in LBBB in the left precordial leads (V_{5-6}) and in lead I.

2 *Normally timed activation of the free wall of the ventricle of the non-blocked bundle branch.* The impulse reaches the Purkinje fibres with impulse propagation through the non-blocked bundle branch. From the Purkinje fibres activation proceeds through the free wall in a direction opposite to that of septal activation. The result is a sudden downstroke in the initial upstroke of the QRS complex observed in the right precordial leads (V_{1-2}) in RBBB and in the left precordial leads (V_{5-6}) and/or lead I in LBBB.

3 *Late and prolonged free wall activation of the ventricle of the blocked bundle branch.* Activation is initiated by slow impulse propagation from the non-blocked ventricle through the muscle mass of the apical region and septum. Within the free wall, activation proceeds in a direction parallel to that of septal activation and results in the recording of a late, broad, positive wave, R′ in RBBB in the right precordial leads (V_{1-2}) and in LBBB in the left precordial leads (V_{5-6}) and in lead I. The leads facing the heart from the opposite side record a mirror image of R′ in the form of a broad s or S wave. In RBBB the latter is recorded in the left precordial leads (V_{5-6}) and in lead I; in LBBB in the right precordial leads (V_{1-2}).

4 Abnormal ventricular activation is followed by a correspondingly *abnormal repolarization* with ST segment displacement and T wave polarity opposite to that of the terminal deflection of the QRS complex.

Fig. 9.3
The formation of the precordial QRS complex in bundle branch block

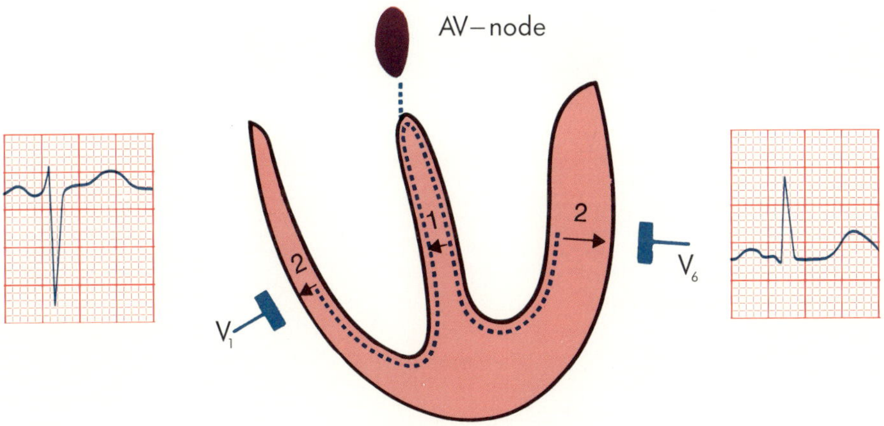

A Normal intraventricular conduction
1 Septal activation from both bundle branches but primarily from the left
2 Free-wall activation occuring simultaneously in the two ventricles

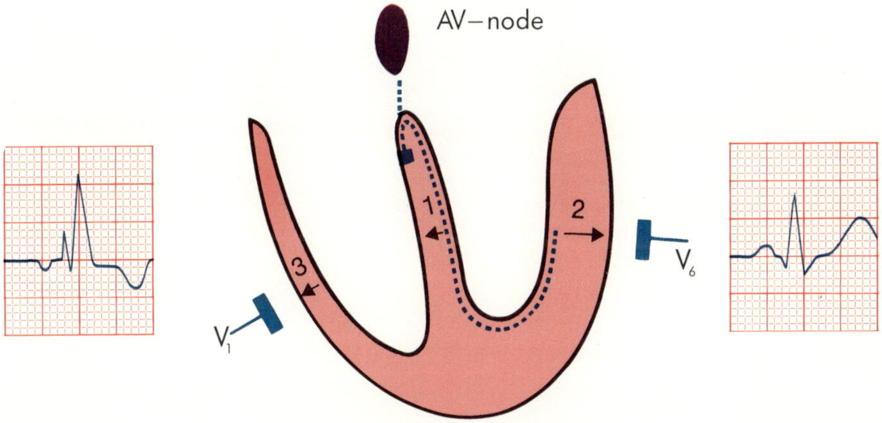

B Right bundle branch block (RBBB)
1 Septal activation from the intact left bundle branch
2 Free-wall activation in the left ventricle by normally timed impulse propagation through the intact left bundle branch
3 Late unopposed free-wall activation in the right ventricle by impulse propagation from the left ventricle

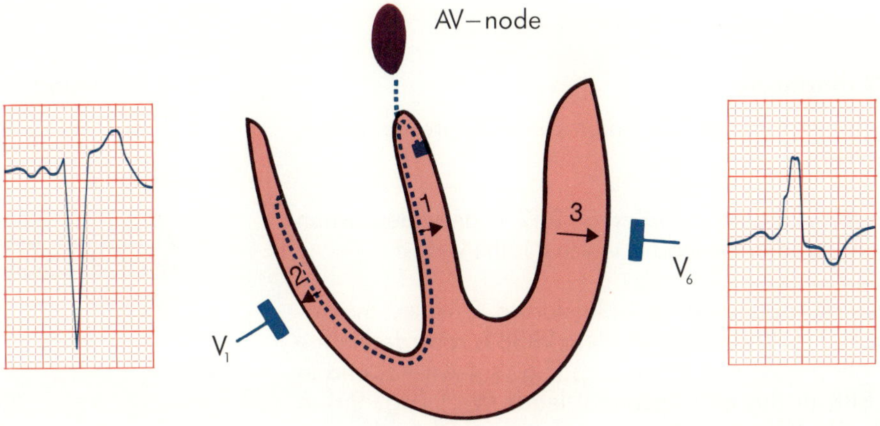

C Left bundle branch block (LBBB)
1 Septal activation from the intact right bundle branch
2 Free-wall activation in the right ventricle by normally timed impulse propagation through the intact right bundle branch
3 Late unopposed free-wall activation in the left ventricle by impulse propagation from the right ventricle

Fig. 9.4
Bundle branch block (BBB) pattern

A An rR′ or wide slurred R recorded in leads V_1–V_2 in right bundle branch block (RBBB) and in leads V_5–V_6 in left bundle branch block (LBBB)

B A late broad s or S recorded in leads V_5–V_6 in right bundle branch block (RBBB) and in leads V_1–V_2 in left bundle branch block (LBBB)

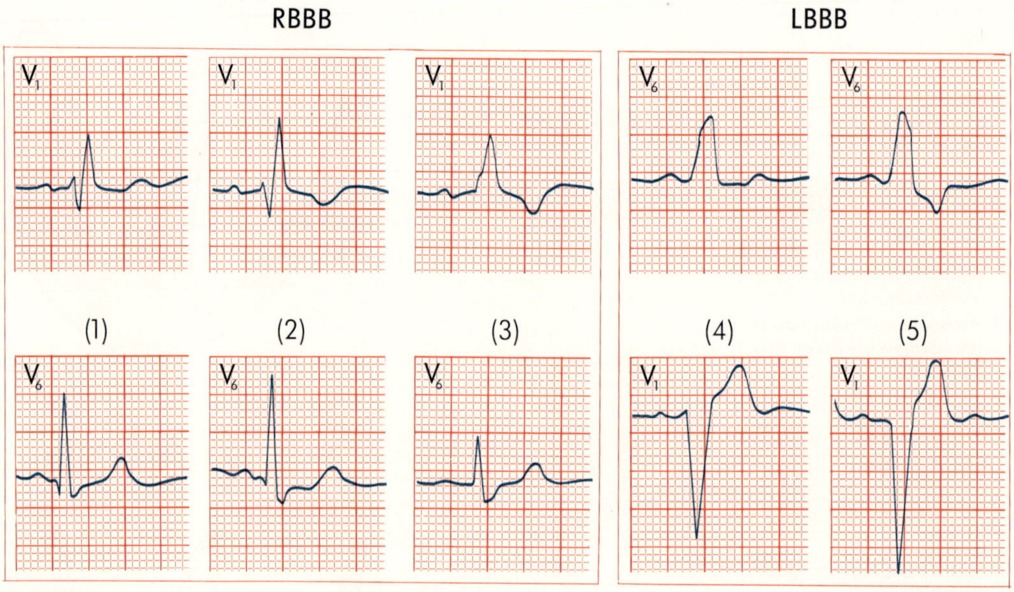

ECG diagnosis

The characteristic ECG features of BBB are as follows (Fig. 9.4):

1 *A broad QRS complex* of 0.12 s or wider, when measured in the lead in which it is the widest

2 An rR′ pattern or a wide slurred R wave, the so-called *BBB pattern,* which in RBBB is recorded in the right precor dial leads (V_{1-2}) (Fig. 9.4 A 1–3) and in LBBB in the left precordial leads (V_{5-6}) (Fig. 9.4 A 4–5) and/or lead I

3 *A late broad s or S,* which in RBBB (Fig. 9.4 B 1–3) is recorded in the left precordial leads (V_{5-6}) and in lead I and in LBBB (Fig. 9.4 B 4–5) in the right precordial leads (V_{1-2})

4 *ST segment displacement and T wave polarity* opposite in direction to the terminal deflection of the QRS complex.

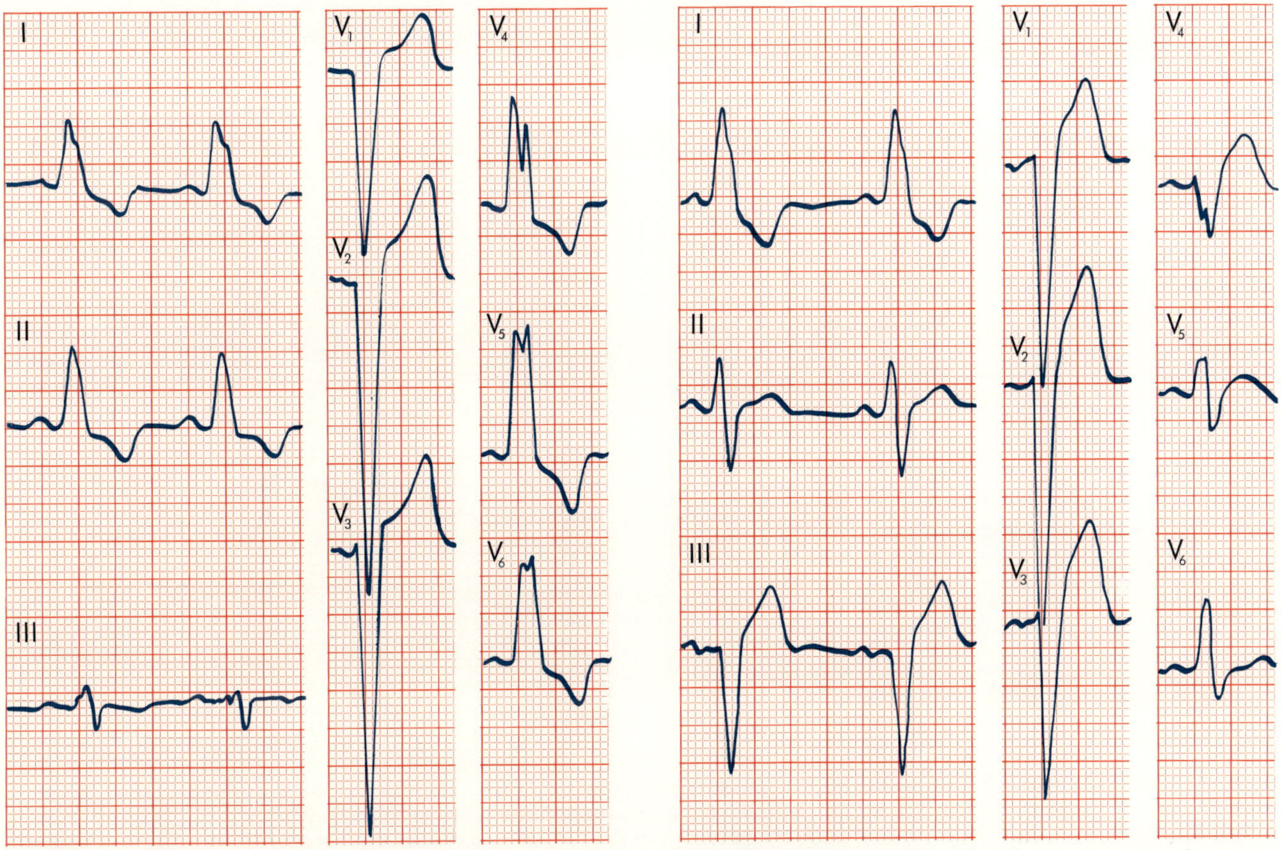

A ECG from a 54-year-old male with aortic stenosis

B ECG from a 62-year-old female with coronary artery disease and stable angina

Fig. 9.5
Left bundle branch block (LBBB) recorded in patients with various types of cardiac disease. The diagnosis of LBBB is based on sinus rhythm with: (1) a wide QRS complex of 0.12 s or wider, (2) broad slurred R waves in leads V_6 and I, and a late boad S wave in leads V_1 and V_2.

For LBBB the characteristic ECG findings (Fig. 9.5) include:

1 *A broad QRS complex* of 0.12 s or more measured in the lead in which it is widest

2 *A wide slurred R wave* in V_5, V_6 and/or lead I

3 *A late broad S wave* in V_1 and/or V_2

4 *ST displacement and T waves* opposite in direction to the terminal deflection of the QRS complex.

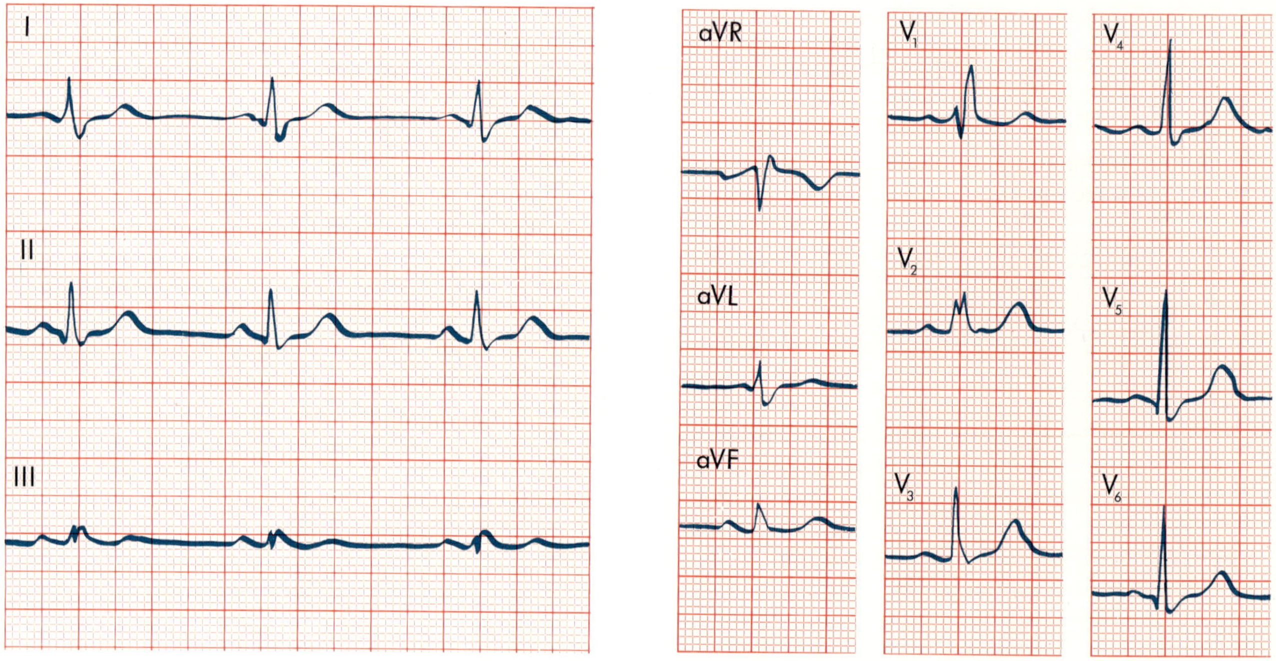

Fig. 9.6
Right bundle branch block (RBBB)

The ECG is from an apparently healthy 78-year-old man.

The diagnosis of RBBB is based on sinus rhythm with: (1) a broad QRS complex of 0.12 s or wider, (2) an rR′ pattern in leads V_{1-2} and (3) late broad s in leads V_{5-6} and I. There is no co-existing left fascicular block since the QRS axis lies within the normal range (+80°) (for estimation of the QRS axis see Figs. 1.26–1.28, p. 20–22). The PQRS rate is regular (56/min), and the PR interval is normal (0.16 s).

For RBBB, the characteristic ECG features (Fig. 9.6) include:

1 *A broad QRS complex* of 0.12 s or more measured in the lead in which the QRS complex is the widest

2 *An rR′ pattern or a wide slurred R wave* in leads V_1 and/or V_2

3 *A late, broad s or S* in leads V_5, V_6 and/or I

4 *ST displacement and T waves* opposite in direction to the terminal deflection of the QRS complex.

Based on the mean frontal QRS axis a distinction can be made between (Fig. 9.7):

– Right bundle branch block as an isolated lesion (RBBB): *A mean QRS axis in the limb leads within the range of* +110° to −45°

– Right bundle branch block with left anterior fascicular block (RBBB + LAFB): A QRS axis in the limb leads of −45° or more; a (q)R in leads I and aVF; and an rs leads II, III and aVF

– Right bundle branch block with left posterior fascicular block (RBBB + LPFB). A QRS axis in the limb leads of +110° or more; an rS pattern in lead I and aVF; and a (q)R pattern with tall R waves in leads II, III and aVF.

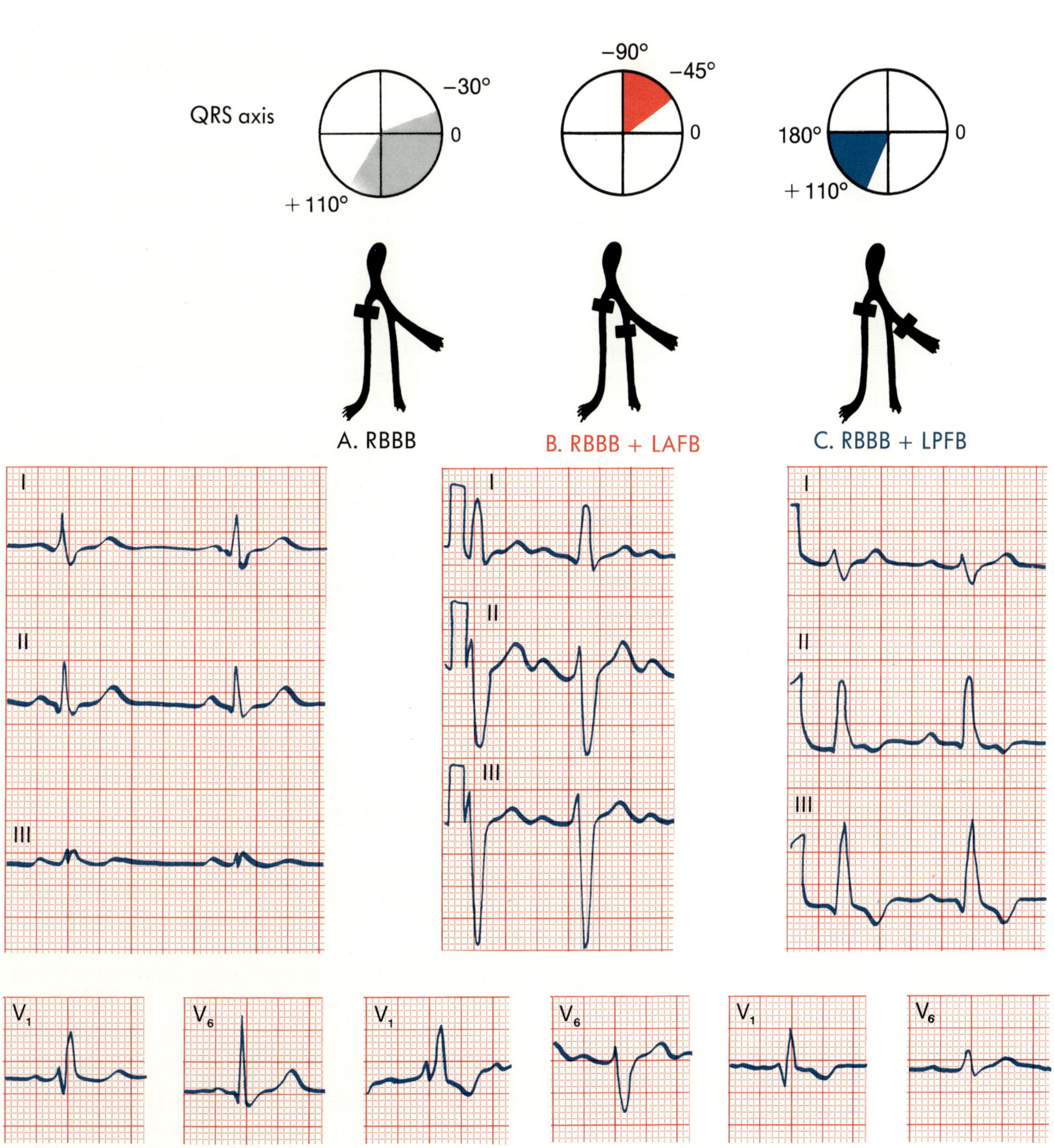

Fig. 9.7
The QRS axis in bundle branch block.
RBBB: right bundle branch block, LAFB: left anterior fascicular block, and LPFB and left posterior fascicular block

Differential diagnosis

A broad QRS complex is recorded in other conditions than bundle branch block, e.g. in:

- *Ventricular pre-excitation of the WPW type.* A WPW pattern type A (Fig. 7.5 A, page 193) may resemble right bundle branch block and WPW pattern type B (Fig. 7.5 B) may resemble left bundle branch block. The diagnosis of pre-excitation is evident from the associated short PR interval.

- *Ventricular arrhythmia.* The diagnosis is suggested by the "ventricular" configuration of the QRS complex; (Fig. 3.16, page 50) by AV dissociation, or occasionally by retrograde atrial activation.

On an ECG of bundle branch block with typical widening of the QRS complex, the major potential for misinterpretation relates to the accompanying QT prolongation, ST segment deviation and T wave inversion. By their "first-glance" impressiveness these secondary block changes may capture the attention of the unexperienced investigator. If the primary and diagnostically more pivital widening of the QRS complex are missed then a straightforward diagnosis of bundle branch block may become long QT syndrome, myocardial ischaemia or ventricular strain.

Symptoms

The altered sequence of ventricular activation in BBB is of no haemodynamic consequence and BBB causes no symptoms of its own.

Aetiology

BBB occurs in a great variety of conditions:

1 BBB is seen in ventricular disease with ventricular *dilatation and/or hypertrophy;* RBBB in right ventricular disease and LBBB in left. Thus, RBBB occurs in chronic cor pulmonale, recurrent pulmonary embolism and congenital heart disease such as atrial septal defect, ventricular septal defect, pulmonary stenosis, Fallot's tetralogy and Eisenmenger's syndrome. RBBB is a frequent although usually transient finding in acute pulmonary embolism (Fig. 14.24, page 341). LBBB frequently is observed in aortic valvular disease, in hypertrophic cardiomyopathy, and arterial hypertension.

2 RBBB and LBBB are common complications in *acute myocardial infarction* where they usually have grave prognostic implications (see next section).

3 LBBB may appear as an early manifestation of severe *coronary artery disease* (two or three vessel disease). RBBB is of minor diagnostic significance in this context as there is a fairly high prevalence of RBBB in the elderly part of the population (see later).

4 RBBB is a common finding in *Stokes-Adams* syndrome with fainting related to paroxysms of AV block (Chapter 10). LBBB is observed occasionally.

5 RBBB and LBBB are recorded in a *great variety of pathological conditions with myocardial involvement*: cardiomyopathy, myocarditis of various types including Chagas' disease (Cruzi trypanosomiasis), cardiac tumours, collagenosis, sarcoidosis, giant cell arteritis, leukaemia and lymphogranulomatosis. Surgery for congenital heart disease with a *right ventriculotomy* may be associated with RBBB or an RBBB-like pattern in the ECG without widening of the QRS complex.

6 *Aberrant ventricular conduction* of supraventricular extrasystoles and tachycardias may result in a pattern of RBBB or rarely LBBB (Fig. 3.11, page 46).

7 *Rate dependent bundle branch block* is a rare condition with aberrant ventricular conduction which oc-

curs in sinus rhythm at critical heart rates within the physiological range.

8 Lastly, RBBB is a not uncommon finding in the *apparently healthy individual.* Due to a very slow but steadily progressive fibrosis of the intraventricular conduction system occurring over the course of a lifetime, the incidence of RBBB increases from less than a quarter of a percent in adolescence to about 1 % at the age of 60 years, and up to 5–6 % in the seventh decade of life. Thus, the mere recording of RBBB in an otherwise healthy individual with no other signs or symptoms of cardiac disease and no history of fainting or dizzy spells can be considered benign and as having no prognostic significance. LBBB, how ever, is rarely recorded in the healthy individual. One to two-year follow-up of such an individual often reveals that LBBB has appeared as an early manifestation of severe coronary artery disease or cardiomyopathy.

Like RBBB, RBBB + LAFB often can be seen in an apparently healthy individual and, like RBBB, its frequency increases with age. Moreover, RBBB + LAFB is observed in a great many of *the same pathological conditions as RBBB,* e.g. in right ventricular disease, coronary artery disease, acute myocardial infarction and Stokes-Adams syndrome. The same applies to RBBB + LPFB but this combination is much more rare.

Clinical significance and prognosis

Recognition of a bundle branch block (BBB) pattern is important from several points of view:

- Whereas RBBB is fairly often recorded in the apparently healthy individual the recording of LBBB is a reliable *indicator of cardiac disease*

- The recording of bundle branch block, usually RBBB but occasionally LBBB is one of the more easily available pieces of *circumstantial evidence* for *a cardiac origin of fainting and dizzy spells* in the patient with Stokes-Adams syndrome (Figs. 10.10, page 263, 10.12, page 266/267, 10.15, page 272/273).

Since RBBB + LAFB blocks two of the three fascicles in the AV conduction pathway, and RBBB only one, it has long been held that RBBB + LAFB reflects an extensive conduction defect, with a more serious prognosis. Prospective studies, however, indicate a similar prognosis of RBBB + LAFB and RBBB as long as the two types of conduction defects occur in the same clinical setting and with the same aetiological background.

The combination of RBBB + LPFB is generally thought to represent a more extensive lesion of the intraventricular conduction system than RBBB + LAFB and to be associated with a more serious prognosis with a high risk of third degree AV block. Clinical experience, however, is scanty.

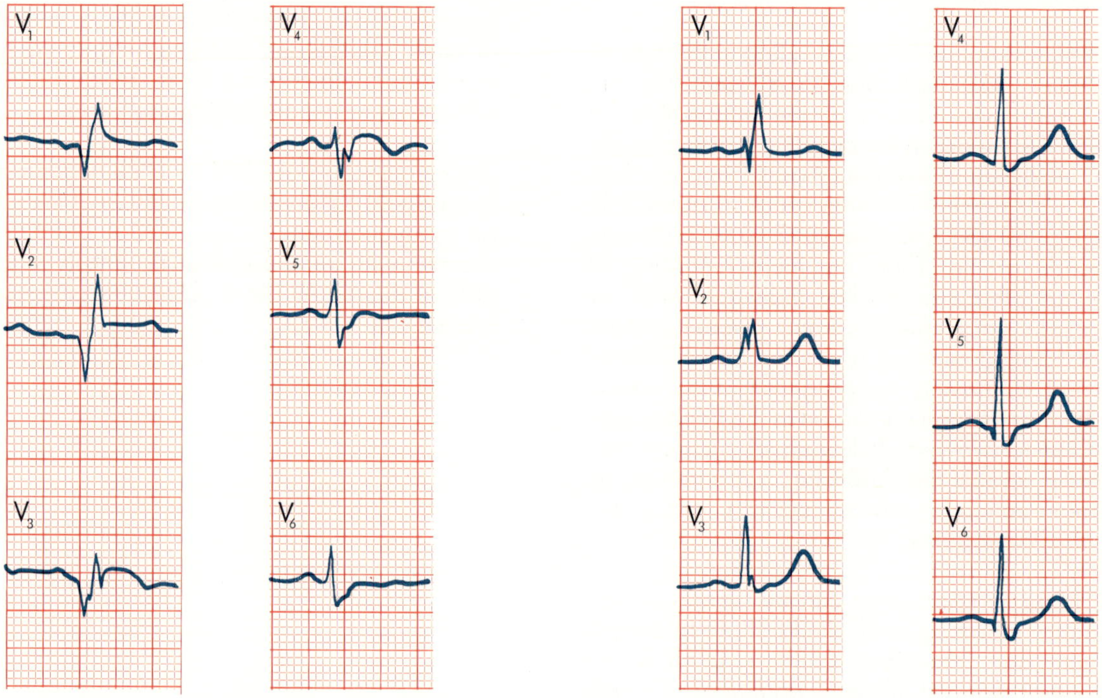

A Right bundle branch block and anteroseptal infarction

B For comparison right bundle branch block without underlying infarction

Fig. 9.8
The pattern of anteroseptal myocardial infarction in the patient with right bundle branch block

Bundle branch block (BBB) in acute myocardial infarction [13–18]

BBB develops in 10–15 % of patients with acute myocardial infarction: RBBB or RBBB + LAFB each in 3–4 %, LBBB in 5 % and RBBB + LPFB in less than 1 %. The underlying lesion is usually either a very large anteroseptal or anterior infarct or more rarely, an anterolateral infarct related to occlusion of the anterior descending branch of the left coronary artery. While far more common in acute anterior infarction, BBB does occur in acute inferior infarction, but most often in patients who have already suffered an anterior infarct.

ECG diagnostic problems

The presence or the development of left bundle branch block (LBBB) makes it impossible to recognize a new myocardial infarction. In *right bundle branch block* (RBBB), septal and left ventricular activation occurs in an almost normally timed sequence (compare Figs. 9.3 A and 9.3 B, page 227). Abnormal Q waves, the cardinal sign of a transmural myocardial infarct (Fig. 14.6, page 316) will thus still be recorded. Since RBBB frequently occurs as a complication of an anteroseptal infarct, Q waves are most often recorded in the right precordial leads where the rR′ pattern of the uncomplicated case of RBBB (Fig. 9.8 B) is modified to a qR′ or QR′ pattern (Figs. 9.8 A, 9.9, page 237 and 9.10, page 238/239). A q or Q wave in the initial part of the QRS complex (i.e. the first 0.04 – 0.06 s) discloses the infarct, while RBBB is exposed by an R′ deflection in the terminal part of the complex.

Prognosis

The occurrence of BBB in acute myocardial infarction (RBBB, LBBB, RBBB + LAFB or RBBB + LPFB) is associated with at least a two-fold increase of in-hospital mortality. The main cause of death is pump failure but sudden arrhythmic death due to AV block or, more often, ventricular fibrillation, also takes its toll.

Within the first days after an infarction, *third degree AV block* develops in about 30 % of the patients with RBBB or RBBB + fascicular block (Fig. 9.9) but in only 15 % of the patients with LBBB.

Late in-hospital ventricular fibrillation, defined as ventricular fibrillation developing in the second to fourth week after the onset of the infarct, occurs in about 30 % of the first-week-survivors who have RBBB and an anteroseptal infarct (Fig. 9.10). These late attacks usually develop after a phase of rapid ventricular tachycardia which deteriorates into fibrillation. This contrasts with the ventricular fibrillation observed in the very early stages of the infarct which follows a single ventricular extrasystole or a short run of ventricular tachycardia. The outcome of late in-hospital ventricular fibrillation is often fatal because it usually develops after the patient has been transferred from the CCU to a general ward and is no longer under ECG monitoring. Most victims of late in-hospital ventricular fibrillation have enlarged hearts. They present with signs of congestive failure, or would do so if they were not treated with diuretics. Patients with BBB who are discharged from hospital, have a poor long-term prognosis, primarily due to progressive heart failure. Furthermore, a substantial number of patients die suddenly. The cause of sudden death is not fully clarified but accumulated evidence favours ventricular fibrillation as the likely mechanism.

For the few patients with BBB who survive an episode of third degree AV block in the early phase of the infarct, the risk of late sudden death due to recurrence of the AV block may be increased, but statistical evaluation of this risk is lacking.

Management

The high incidence of late in-hospital ventricular fibrillation in anteroseptal infarct complicated by BBB has in some centres led to a policy of prolonged ECG monitoring for a couple of weeks for this group of patients.

In the long-term, the patient who through immediate resuscitation survives an attack of "late" ventricular tachycardia/fibrillation in AMI, will face a high risk of recurrence and sudden death. Thus all options for effective long-term antitachycardia prophylaxis should be considered including medication, antitachycardia surgery and the implantation of an automatic implantable cardioverter/defibrillator (AICD implant). Such entails that the patient should be referred to a centre with facilities for electrophysiologic studies.

The indications and contraindications for prophylactic artificial pacing in acute myocardial infarction with BBB are discussed in the section on the management of AV block in acute myocardial infarction (Chapter 10, page 257).

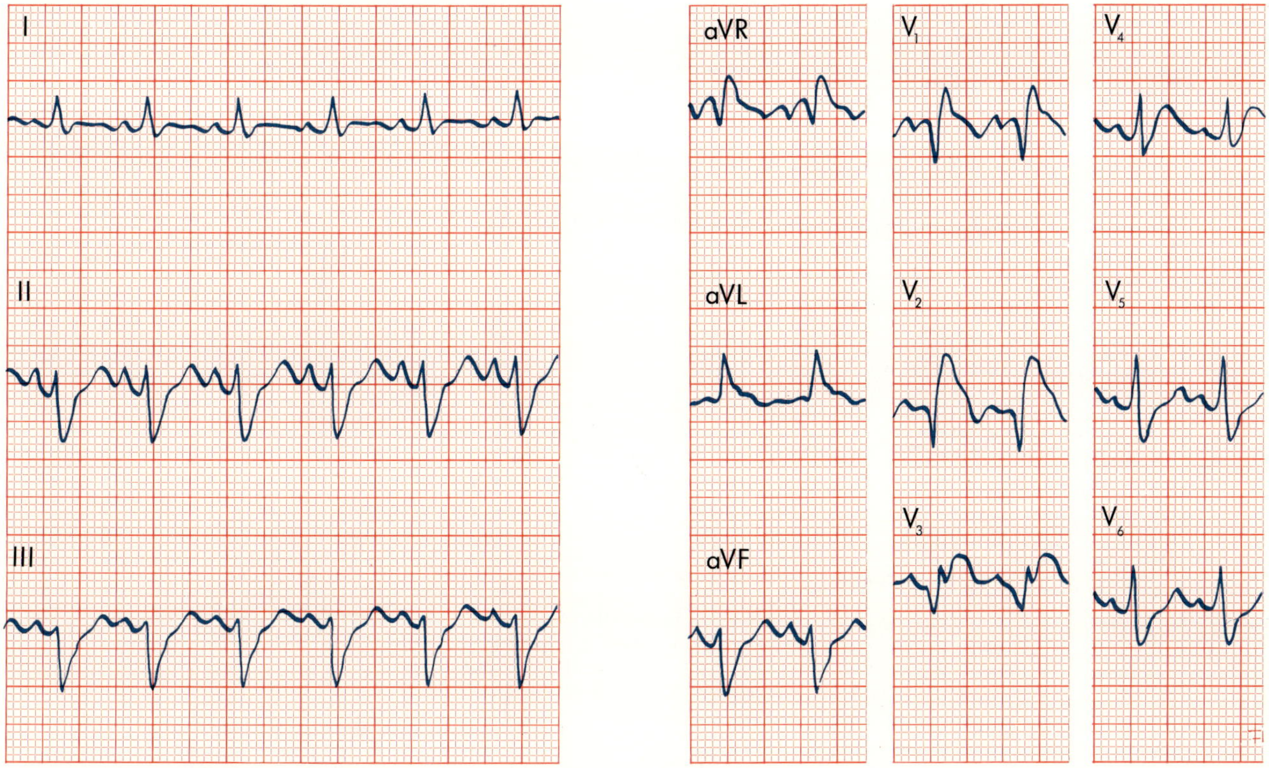

A ECG from the second day after onset of chest pains. There is a right bundle branch block (RBBB) and a left anterior fascicular block (LAFB). The diagnosis of RBBB is based on: (1) a wide QRS (0.16 s), (2) a qR' wave pattern in leads V_1 and V_2, and (3) a late broad s wave in leads V_5 and V_6. The hallmarks of concomitant LAFB include: (1) a QRS axis to the left (−70°) (for the estimation of the QRS axis, see Figs. 1.26–1.28, p. 20–22) and (2) a (q)R wave pattern in leads I and aVL, and an rS wave pattern in leads II, III and aVF. Deep Q waves in leads V_1, V_2 and V_3 suggest an anteroseptal infarction (see Fig. 9.8).

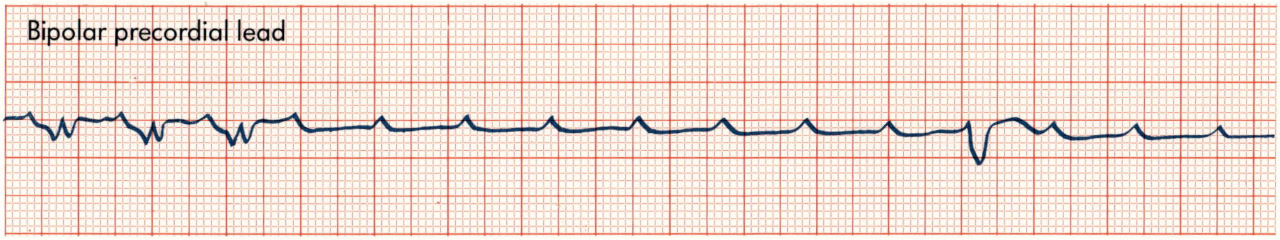

B A sequence from the continuous ECG monitoring recorded shortly afterwards. The first three complexes in the tracing represent sinus rhythm with bundle branch block. Sudden block in the AV conduction associated with ventricular arrest after the third sinus complex. Artifical pacing was initiated and continued for a period of 2 weeks before the pacing electrodes were withdrawn. Continued ECG monitoring for a period of 2 weeks showed neither recurrence of the AV block nor attacks of ventricular tachycardia. Echocardiography and isotope cardiography (MUGA) before discharge confirmed the diagnosis of an extensive myocardial infarction with a severely reduced ejection fraction.

Fig. 9.9
Anteroseptal myocardial infarction and bundle branch block, complication with third degree AV block and ventricular arrest.
ECG recordings from a 65-year-old female with acute myocardial infarction

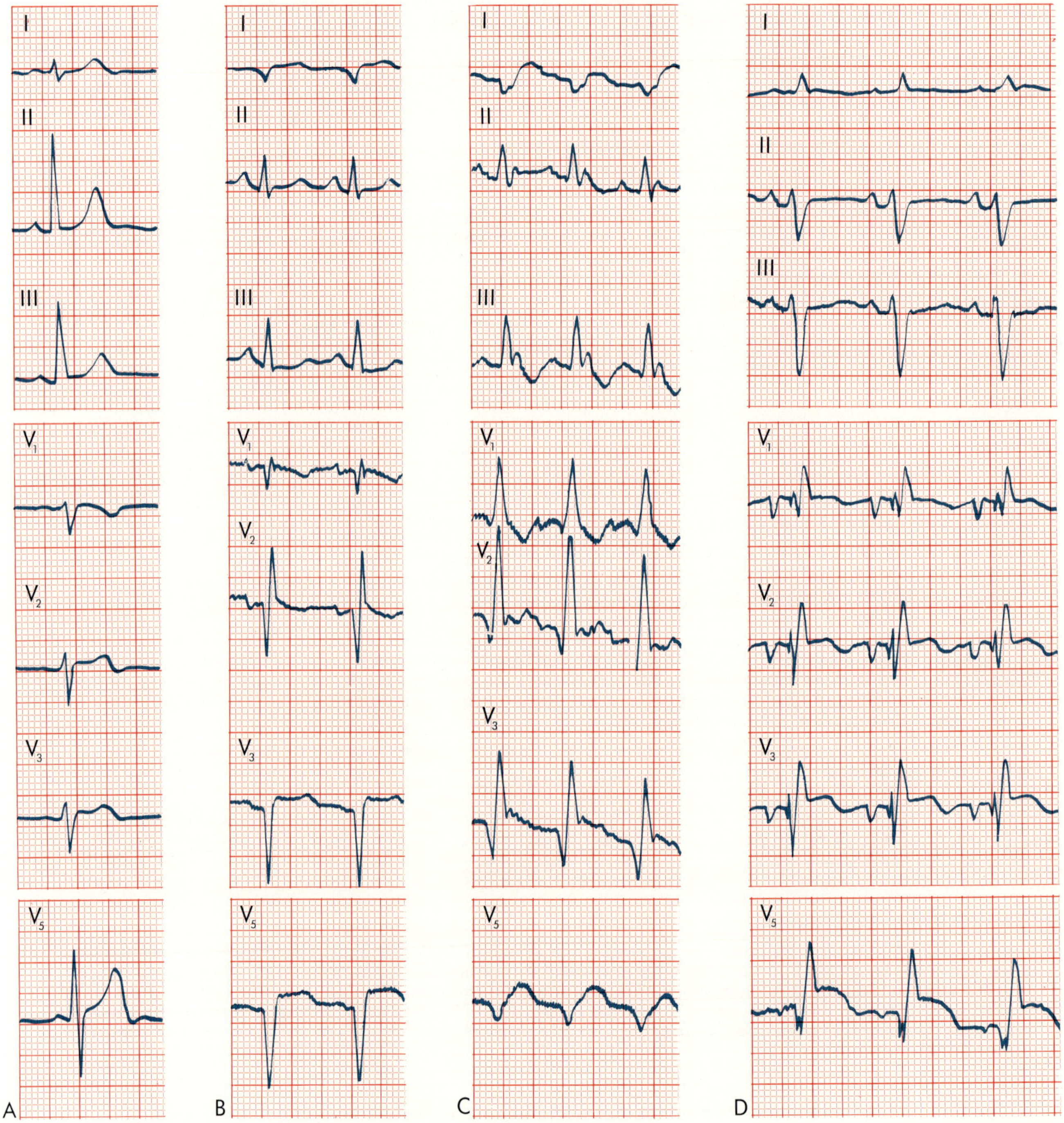

(to be continued next page)

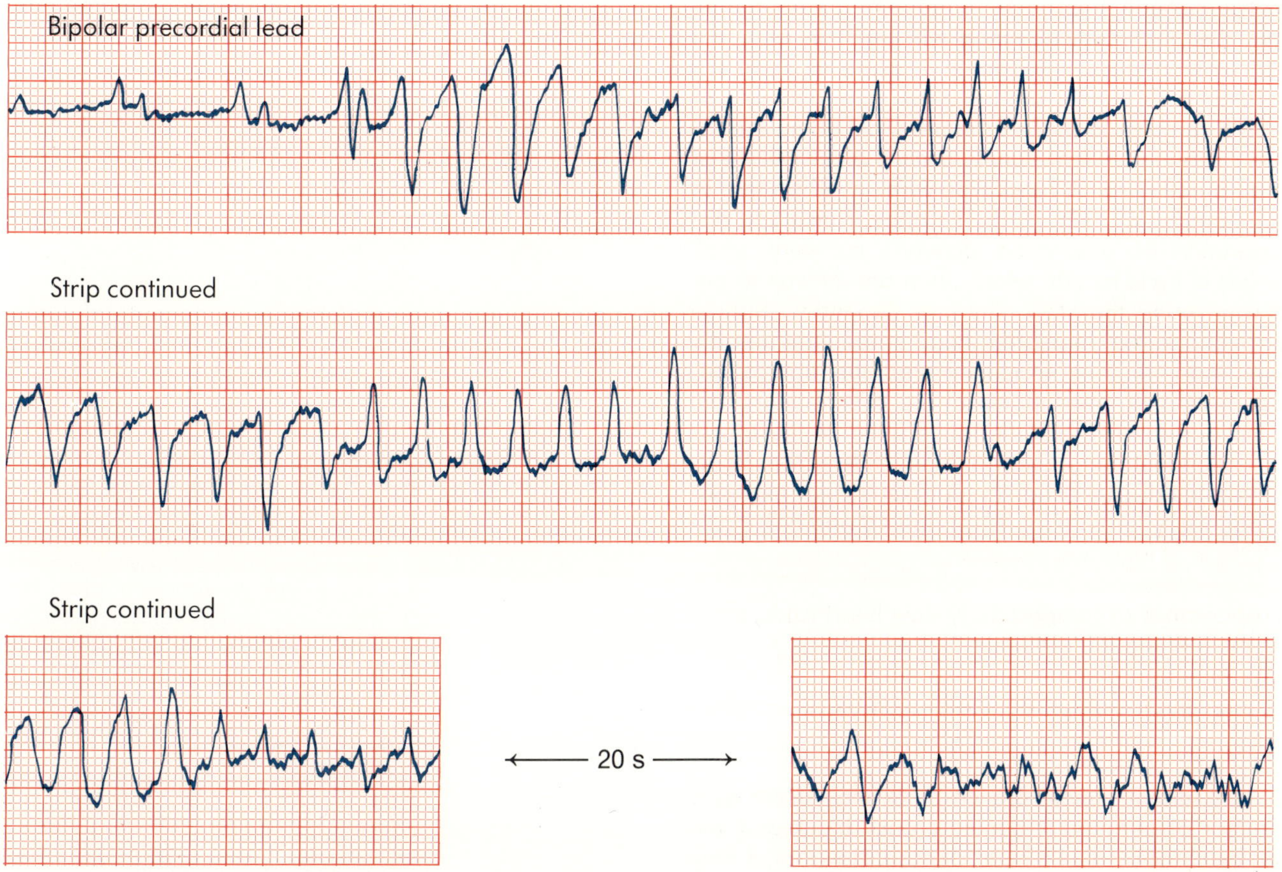

Fig. 9.10
Anteroseptal myocardial infarction, right bundle branch block and late in-hospital ventricular fibrillation.
The ECG-recordings are from a 59-year-old male who during hospital admission for a leg fracture developed an acute myocardial infarction.

A The ECG 1 week before the infarction. Normal PQRST complexes in the precordial leads
B The ECG from the second day after infarction. There is an extensive anterior infarction with Q waves starting in lead V_1 and continuing towards the left to lead V_5 and also present in lead I. A qR′ wave pattern in leads V_1 and V_2 combined with a QRS complex of only 0.11 s supports a diagnosis of incomplete right bundle branch block.
C The ECG on the second day, a few hours later. There is now RBBB with a wide QRS complex (0.13 s) and a qR′ wave pattern starting in lead V_1.
D The ECG on the tenth day with a slightly slower PQRS rate than in C but otherwise unchanged with signs of extensive anterior infarction with RBBB and as well as LAFB.
E A sequence from continuous ECG monitoring recorded very shortly after the ECG shown in D. The first three complexes show sinus rhythm with bundle branch block (P waves not clearly visible due to a low quality, noisy ECG signal). The third sinus beat is followed by a ventricular extrasystole which releases fast ventricular tachycardia with a rate of 200–210/min which after 30 s degenerates into ventricular fibrillation. Sinus rhythm was re-established by an immediately applied DC countershock.

Rate dependent bundle branch block[21]

In a few patients heart rate increase to a certain rate within the physiological range will result in aberrant ventricular conduction (Chapter 3, page 45) and the recording of a bundle branch block with widening of the QRS complex to 0.12 s or more. Most often, the recorded *rate dependent bundle branch block* will be of the left bundle branch block type with an rR′ pattern in leads I and/or V_{5-6} (Fig. 9.11). The appearance and disappearance of aberration depends on very small changes in cycle length, which often are difficult to detect even using the ECG. The rate dependent bundle branch block may persist at heart rates considerably slower than the one which initiated the aberration. Thus, there is an overlapping of the critical heart rate for the appearance and disappearance of the block. Rate dependent bundle branch block differs from aberrant ventricular conduction in supraventricular extrasystole and tachycardia (Fig. 3.11, page 46 and 6.3, page 128/129) in at least two respects:

- Appearance at comparatively slow heart rates, often in the range of 60–140/min

- Predominance of left bundle branch block morphology.

Rate dependent bundle branch block may occur as a precursor of permanent bundle branch block and will often be associated with heart disease. However, it may also be observed on a "routine" exercise ECG as a benign finding without clinical significance in the otherwise healthy individual.

The development of a "rate dependent" bundle branch block during the recording of an exercise ECG (Chapter 14) should not be regarded as an indicator of ischaemia. ST segment depression can be considered supportive of a diagnosis of ischaemic heart disease only if it remains following a decrease in heart rate with disappearance of the block pattern immediately after cessation of exercise. Even then the diagnostic validity of such ST segment displacement has been questioned. A decrease in heart rate to values which may result in the alleviation of the block often can be induced by carotid sinus massage (Fig. 7.1, page 189).

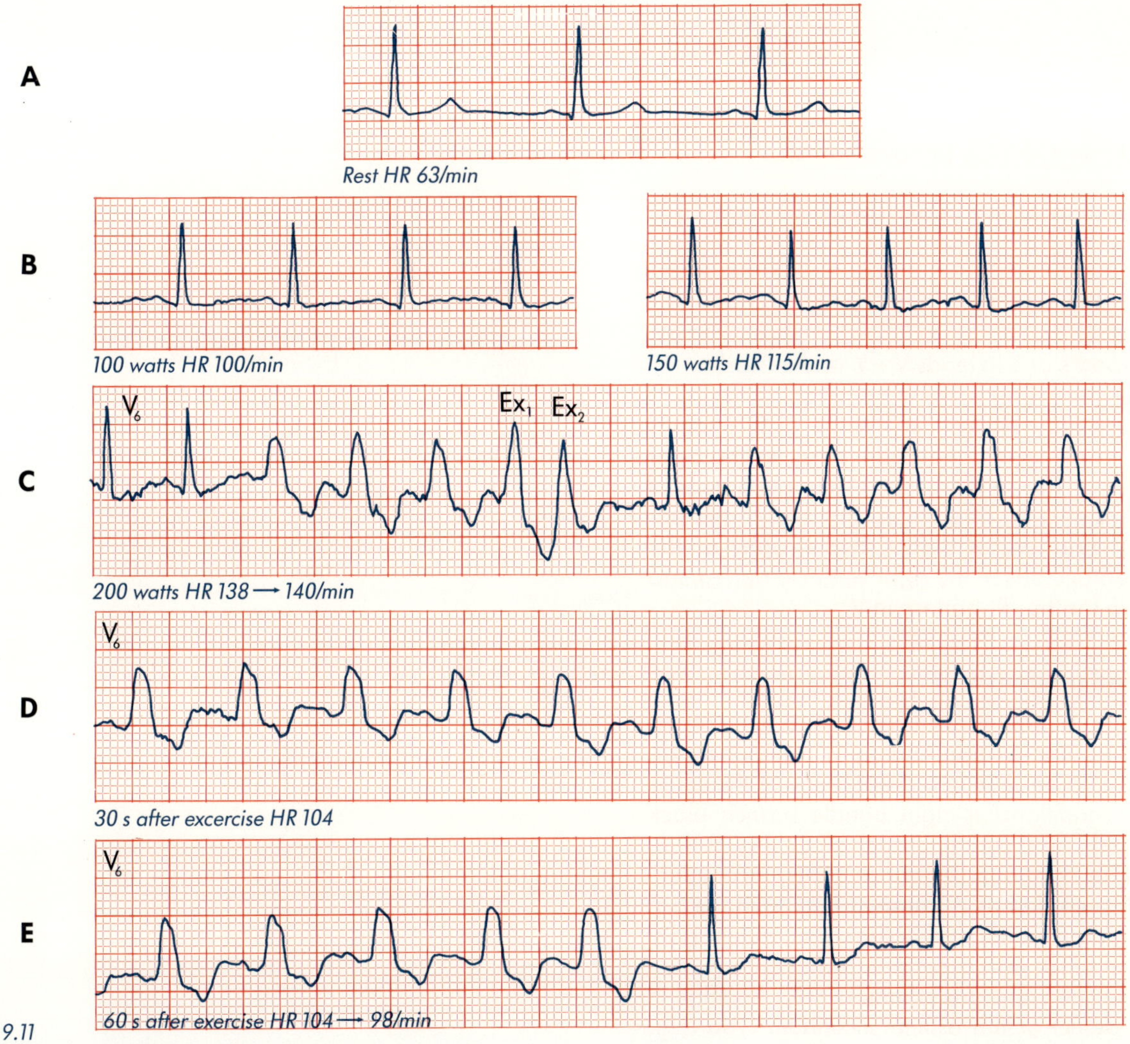

Fig. 9.11
Rate dependent bundle branch block
Routine exercise ECG from a 40-year-old healthy pilot with no signs of heart disease and in particular no signs of ischaemic heart disease (myocardial scintigraphy normal).
ECG recording in lead V_6 during a graded exercise test on a bicycle ergometer. Stepwise increase in workload, 50 watts every 3 min starting at a workload of 100 watt.
A Resting ECG, heart rate (HR) 63/min, QRS 0.10 s and, thus, no bundle branch block (BBB).
B 100 watt/3 min – 150 watt/3 min, HR 100/min – 115/min.
C 200 watt/3 min, HR 138 – 140/min, sudden QRS widening from 0.10 s to 0.16 s with the development of a left BBB pattern. Following three complexes with BBB, two pairs of ventricular extrasystoles (marked $Ex_1 – Ex_2$) which induce a long compensatory pause and result in the disappearance of the BBB pattern for a single complex. However, the following shortening of the RR interval results in the immediate reappearance of the BBB.
D 30 s after discontinuance of exercise. HR 104/min – 98/min, unchanged left BBB pattern.
E 60 s after discontinuance of exercise. HR 104 – 98/min, change from left BBB pattern to normal QRS configuration with reduction in QRS duration from 0.16 s to 0.10 s.

Incomplete right bundle branch block [19, 20]

ECG diagnosis

The term incomplete right bundle branch block (Fig. 9.12) is used to describe the combination of:

1 A QRS duration at the upper range of normal i.e. 0.10–0.11 s.

2 An rR′ pattern in lead V_1.

3 Often a broad s or S in leads V_5–V_6 and in lead I.

The term block may be justified as the ECG findings might relate to a minor conduction delay in the right bundle branch. The underlying electrophysiological mechanism is, however, often more obscure. In the patient with an atrial septal defect, hypertrophy of the crista supraventricularis in the right ventricle appears to be responsible for the rR′ pattern in V_1.

Aetiology and prognosis

Incomplete right bundle branch block often is recorded as an incidental and benign finding in a healthy individual. It can also be seen in a great many of the same pathological conditions as right bundle branch block and can precede right bundle branch block (Fig. 9.10 B, page 239). Like right bundle branch block, incomplete block often is recorded as a transient finding in the patient with acute pulmonary embolism. Incomplete right bundle branch block with a normal frontal QRS axis or a QRS axis to the right are common ECG findings in atrial septal defect of the ostium secundum type (Fig. 9.12). Incomplete right bundle branch block associated with left anterior fascicular block and a QRS axis to the left are the usual findings in atrial septal defect of the ostium primum type and in common atrioventricular canal.

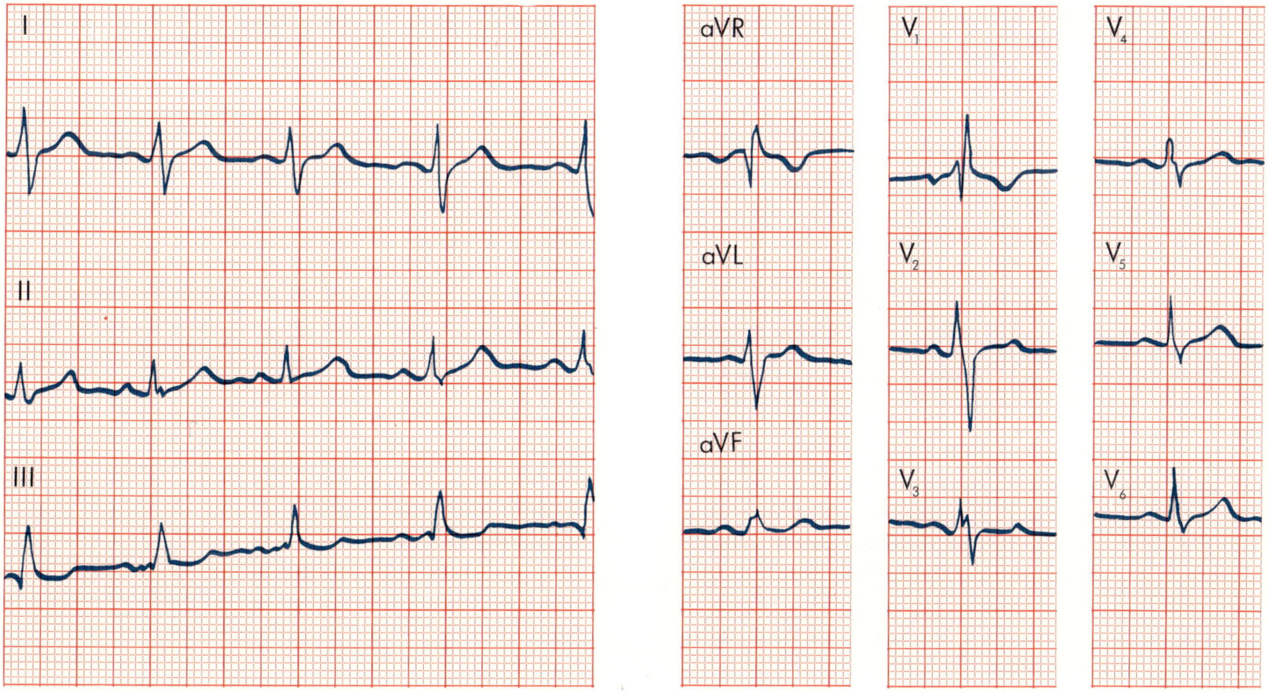

Fig. 9.12
Incomplete right bundle branch block

The ECG is from a 17-year-old female with an atrial septal defect of secundum type associated with an arteriovenous shunt and normal pressures in the right ventricle and pulmonary artery. The diagnosis is based on sinus rhythm with: (1) a narrow QRS complex (0.10 s), (2) an rR′ wave pattern in lead V_1 and (3) late broad s or S wave in leads V_5, V_6 and I. The QRS axis is to the right (+ 95°).

References Chapter 9

1. WHO/ISFC Task Force. ed. Definition of terms related to cardiac rhythm. Europ J Cardiol 1978; 8: 127–44.
2. Rosenbaum MD, Elizari MV, Lazzari JO. The hemiblocks. Tampa tracings. Florida: Oldsmar, 1970.
3. Kulbertus HJE, Demoulin JC. Pathological basis of concept of left hemiblock. In: Wellens HJJ, Lie KL, Janse MF, eds. The conduction system of the heart. Philadelphia: Lea & Febiger, 1976; 287–95.
4. Kulbertus HE. The hemiblocks. Ten years experience. Ingelheim am Rhein: Boehringer Ingelheim Postgraduate Medical Services, 1978.
5. Demoulin J-C. The conduction system of the heart. Ingelheim am Rhein: Boehringer Ingelheim, 1988.
6. Davies MJ, Anderson RH, Becker AE. The conduction system of the heart. London, Boston: Butterworths, 1983.
7. Spodick DH. Left axis deviation and left anterior fascicular block. Am J Cardiol 1988; 61: 869–70.
8. Rowlands DJ. Left and right bundle branch block, left anterior and left posterior hemiblock. Europ Heart J 1984; 5 (Suppl. A): 99–105.
9. Kreger BE, Anderson KM, Kannel WB. Prevalence of intraventricular block in the general population: The Framingham Study. Am Heart J 1989; 117: 903–10.
10. Freedman RA, Alderman EL, Sheffield LT, et al. Bundle branch block in patients with chronic coronary artery disease: Angiographic correlates and prognostic significance. JACC 1987; 10: 73–80.
11. Flowers NC. Left bundle branch block: A continuously evolving concept. In: Surawicz B, Fisch C, eds. Seminar on the changing role of electrocardiography in clinical practice – IV. JACC 1987; 9: 684–97.
12. Ross DL. Approach to the patient with bundle branch block. In: Wellens HJJ, Kulbertus HE, eds. What's new in electrocardiography. The Hague, Boston, London: Martinus Nijhoff Publishers, 1981; 111–30.
13. Roos JC, Dunning AJ. Bundle branch block in acute myocardial infarction. Europ J Cardiol 1978; 6: 403–24.
14. Becker AE, Lie KI, Anderson RH. Bundle-branch block in the setting of acute anteroseptal myocardial infarction. Clinicopathological correlation. Br Heart J 1978; 40: 773–82.
15. Lie KI, Manger Cats V, Durrer D. CCU findings useful for identification of sudden death candidates in the post hospital phase of myocardial infarction. In: Kulbertus HE, Wellens HJJ, eds. Sudden death. The Hague, Boston, London: Martinus Nijhoff Publishers, 1980; 232–36.
16. Watson RDS, Glover DR, Page AJF, et al. The Birmingham Trial of permanent pacing in patients with intraventricular conduction disorders after acute myocardial infarction. Am Heart J 1984; 108: 496–501.
17. Pagoni F, Finzi A, Valentini R, et al. Long-term prognostic significance and electrophysiological evolution of intraventricular conduction disturbances complicating acute myocardial infarction. Pace 1986; 9: 91–100.
18. Twidale N, Tonkin AL, Tonkin AM. Programmed stimulation after anterior myocardial infarction complicated by bundle branch block – Late ventricular tachyarrhythmias and out come. Pace 1988; 11: 1024–31.
19. Moore EN, Boineau JP, Patterson DF, Incomplete right bundle-branch block: An electrocardiographic enigma and possible misnomer. Circulation 1971; 44: 678–87.
20. Liao YL, Emidy LA, Dyer A et al. Characteristics and prognosis of incomplete right bundle branch block: An epidemiologic study. J. Am. Coll. Cardiol. 1986; 7: 492–9.
21. Fisch D, Zipes DP, McHenry PL. Rate dependent aberrancy. Circulation 1973; 48: 714–24.

Chapter 10
Atrioventricular (AV) block

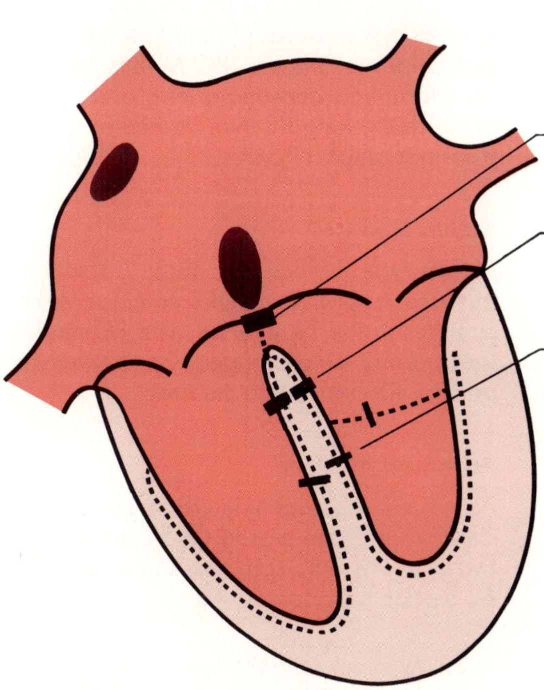

Fig. 10.1
Sites of AV block in the AV conduction pathway

Atrioventricular (AV) block [1–3]

Atrioventricular (AV) block is a delay or a failure of impulse conduction from the atria to the ventricles. The sequential mono-, bi- and trifascicular composition of the AV conduction pathway forms a basis for classification of the AV blocks (Fig. 10.1):

- *Monofascicular AV block* in which conduction is interrupted in the AV node or in the bundle of His

- *Bifascicular AV block* in which conduction is interrupted in both bundle branches (RBBB + LBBB, often called bilateral BBB)

- *Trifascicular AV block* in which conduction is interrupted in the right bundle branch and both the anterior and posterior fascicles of the left bundle branch (RBBB + LAFB + LPFB).

A simplified classification of AV blocks related exclusively to their site above or below the bifurcation of the bundle of His is preferred by the authors. The classification differentiates:

- *Proximal AV block* located proximal to the bifurcation of the bundle of His, and

- *Distal AV block* located distal to this point.

With reference to the definitions for mono-, bi- and trifascicular block (Fig. 10.1) proximal AV block is synonymous with monofascicular AV block, while distal AV block includes both, bi- and trifascicular AV block.

ECG diagnosis

Depending upon the severity of the AV conduction disturbance AV blocks are classified as of first, second and third degree.

First degree AV block

First degree AV block (Fig. 10.2, 1 A and 1 B, Figs. 10.3 and 10.4, page 250) is characterized by a prolonged PR interval of 0.23 s or longer but with each P wave followed by a QRS complex. A PR interval of 0.23–0.25 s is so frequent as to be almost a physiological variant in the elderly. A PR interval of 0.26–0.30 s is common in cardiac disease. A PR interval of up to 0.50–0.60 s may be observed (Fig. 10.3). When associated with a high basic heart rate, PR interval prolongation can lead to the superimposition of the P wave on the preceding T wave with the result that the P wave is hidden by the T wave (Fig. 10.3).

Second degree AV block

Second degree AV block (Fig. 10.2, 2 A and 2 B) is the intermittent failure of AV conduction of a P wave with a "missed" QRS complex. The pattern often is repetitive, e.g. with AV conduction of two out of three P waves (Fig. 10.7 B, page 259) or three out of four P waves resulting in an AV conduction ratio of 3:2, 4:3 etc. (the denominator in the ratio is the number of P waves recorded, the numerator the ones that elicit a QRS complex). Second degree AV block is subdivided into Mobitz type I block (Wenckebach block), Mobitz type II block and advanced AV block.

Mobitz type I

Mobitz type I block (Figs. 10.2, 2 A and 10.7 B), also called Wenckebach block is characterized by a progressive lengthening of the PR interval over successive P-QRS complexes, usually three (Fig. 10.7 B) or, occasionally four (Fig. 10.2, 2 A), until a QRS complex is missed. The subsequent pause enables the AV node to recover. Thus, the PR interval of the following P-QRS complex shortens to its original length and a new block cycle starts. While the PR interval progressively lengthens over the block cycle, the increment of the lengthening decreases progressively. In the typical case this particular electrophysiological feature of Mobitz type I block leads to a progressive *shortening* of the RR interval in the course of the block cycle. Thus, in a block cycle of three P waves (3:2 Mobitz type I block) there is an alternation between a long and a short RR interval in which the long RR interval relates to the failure of AV transmission of a P wave.

Mobitz type II

Mobitz type II block (Fig. 10.2, 2 B) is characterized by an occasional missed QRS complex without preceding changes in the PR interval. The PR interval may be either normal or prolonged, but remains constant from one P-QRS complex to the next.

Advanced AV block

Advanced AV block (Fig. 10.5, page 251) is characterized by alternate missed QRS complexes, or the loss of two or more QRS complexes in a row. Thus, advanced AV block encompasses:

- 2:1 AV block with AV conduction of one out of two P waves such that every second QRS complex is missed (Fig. 10.5 A)
- 3:1 AV block with AV conduction of one out of three P waves such that two out of three QRS complexes are missed (Fig. 10.5 B)
- 4:1 AV block with AV conduction of one out of four P waves such that three out of four QRS complexes are missed (Fig. 10.5 C).

Third degree AV block (complete AV block)

Third degree AV block (Fig. 10.2, 3 A and 3 B) is characterized by complete interruption of AV impulse conduction. The SA node usually continues to activate the atria at an unchanged rate, whereas ventricular activation is taken over by a slow firing ectopic pacemaker which in proximal AV block is located in the AV node, in distal AV block in the bundle branches or Purkinje fibers. Instability of the ectopic pacemaker activity can result in episodes of ventricular arrest, or sometimes in torsade de pointes ventricular tachycardia.

(continued page 252)

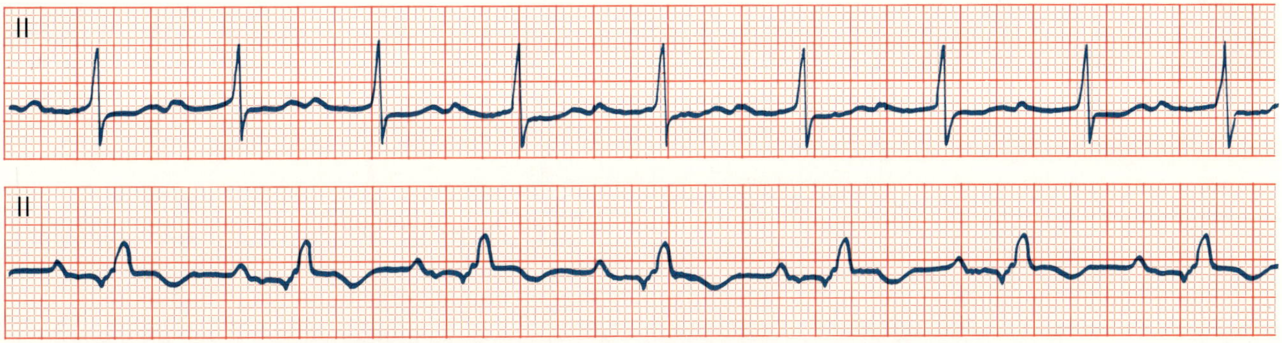

1 *First degree AV block associated with (A) normal intraventricular conduction and (B) bundle branch block*

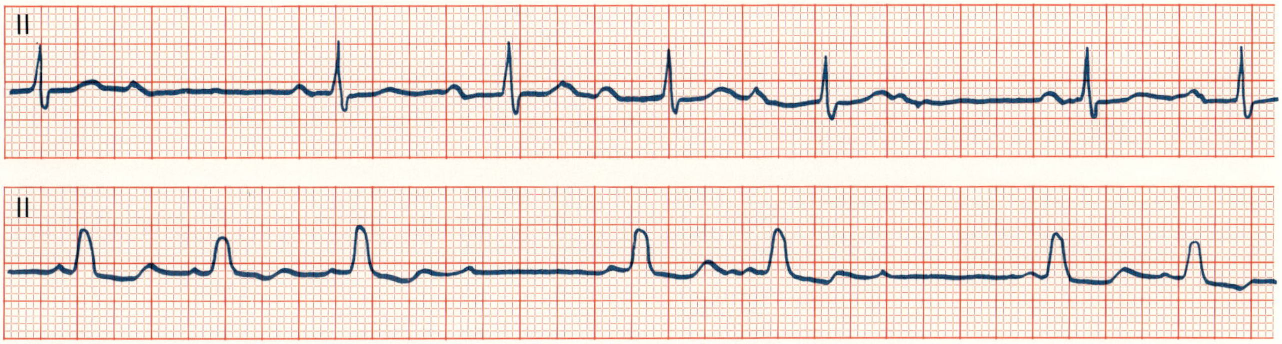

2 *Second degree AV block (A) Mobitz type I (5:4 conduction) associated with normal intraventricular conduction and (B) Mobitz type II with bundle branch block*

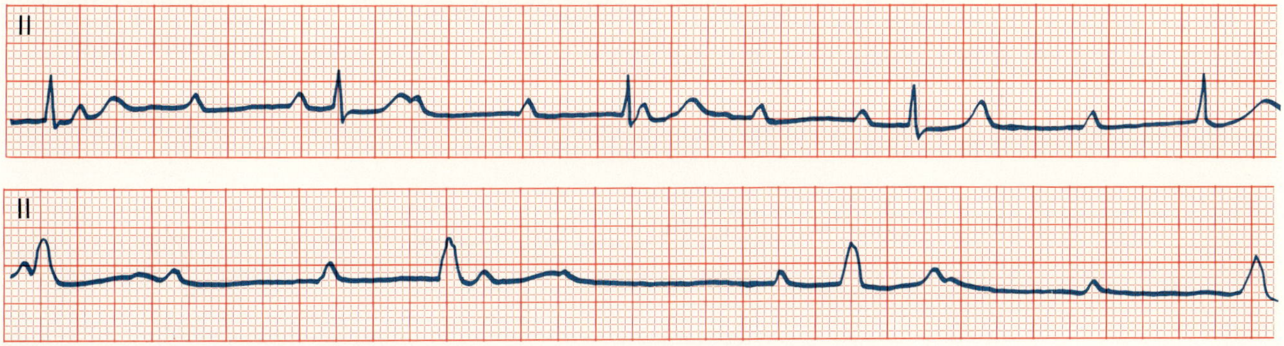

3 *Third degree AV block with (A) AV nodal escape rhythm and (B) ventricular escape rhythm*

Fig. 10.2
AV block of first (1), second (2) and third (3) degree

Fig. 10.3
First degree AV block caused by digitalis intoxication.
ECG from a 77-year-old female who had received 250 micrograms of digoxin daily for 1 year

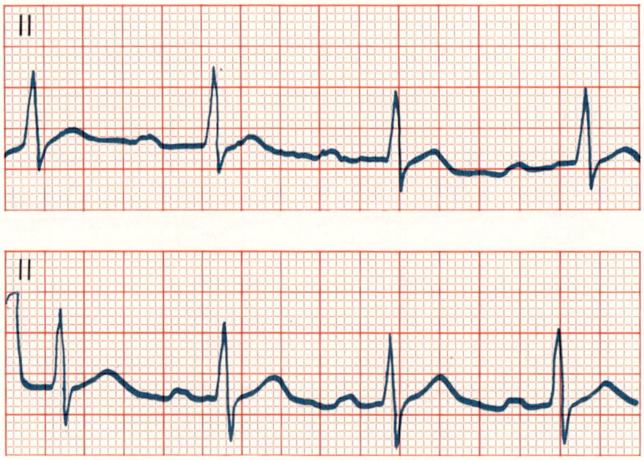

A ECG at admission. First degree AV block with prolonged PR interval (= 0.36 s)

B ECG 3 days after cessation of digoxin therapy. PR interval normal (=0.22 s)

Fig. 10.4
First degree AV block, concealment of the P wave by the preceding T wave.
ECG recording from a graded exercise test on a bicycle ergometer. The PR interval in all three tracings is prolonged to 0.48 s

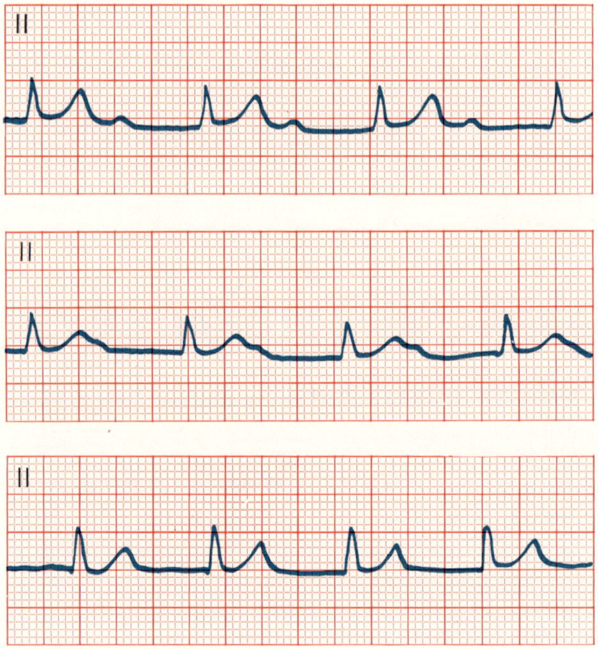

A Heart rate 64/min: The P wave is seen distinctly shortly after the preceding T wave

B Heart rate 70/min: The P wave merges with the T wave

C Heart rate 81/min: The P wave is now concealed by the preceding T wave

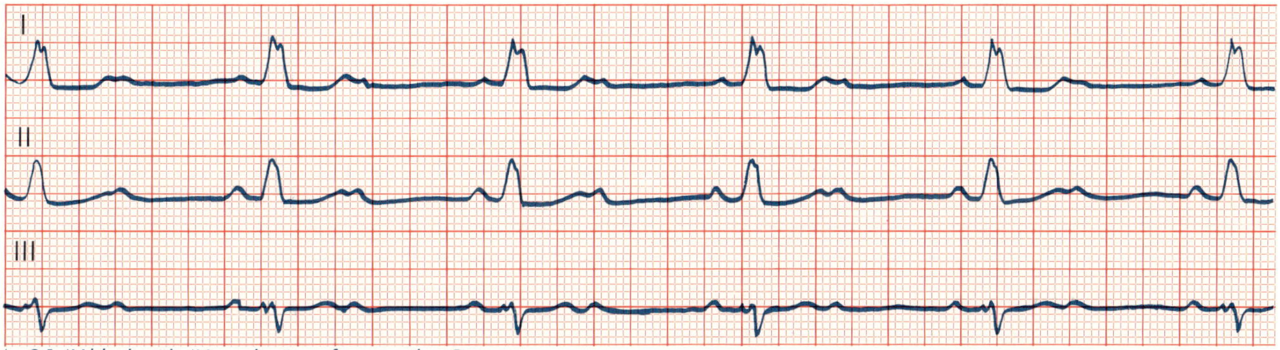

A 2:1 AV block with AV conduction of every other P wave

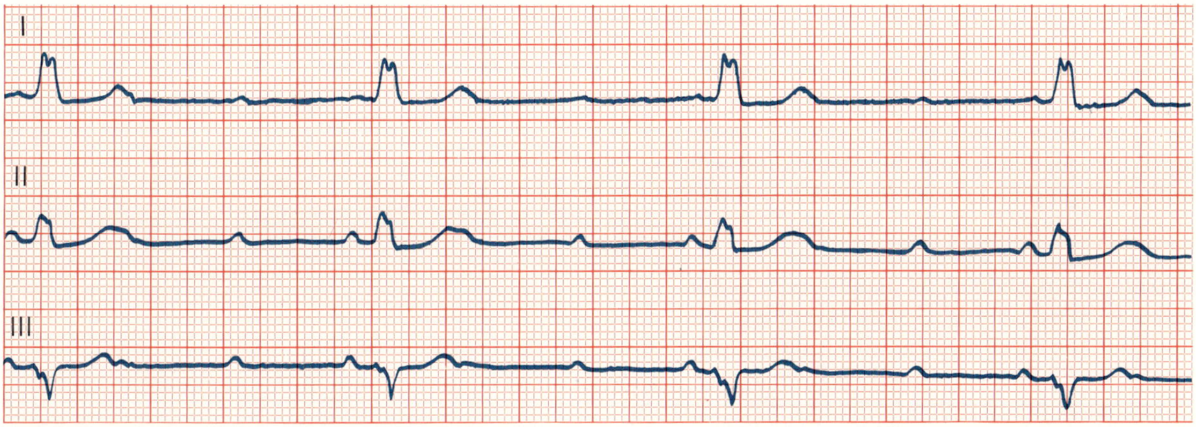

B 3:1 AV block with AV conduction of every third P wave

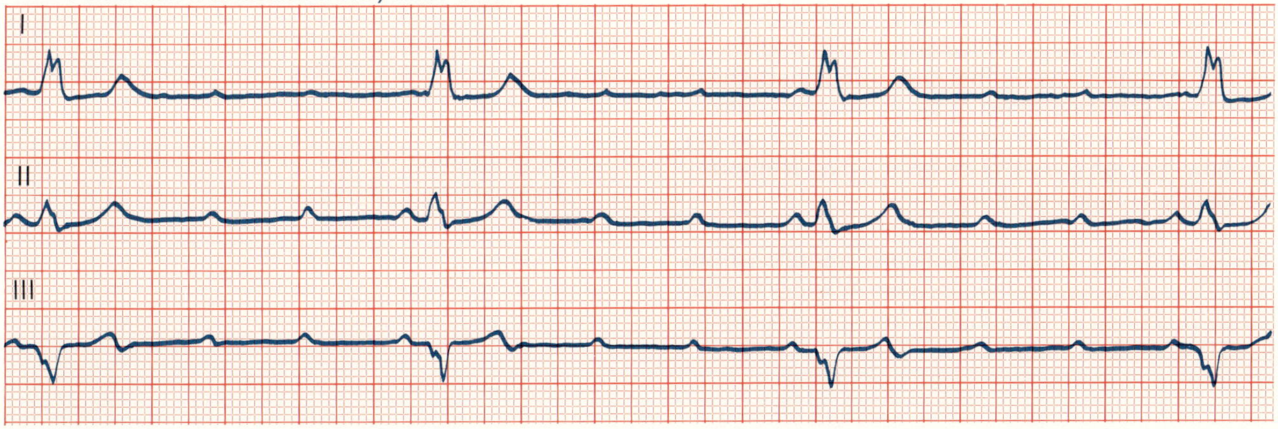

C 4:1 AV block with AV conduction of every fourth P wave

Fig. 10.5

Advanced AV block

The AV blocks in all tracings are most likely of distal location, since the AV conducted P waves are followed by wide QRS complexes with a bundle branch block pattern. In the actual case there was a left bundle branch block pattern with a wide QRS = 0.16 s and a rR' wave pattern in lead I.

The ECG criteria for third degree AV block are:

1 *Evidence of atrial activity* usually in the form of sinus P waves (Fig. 10.2, 3 A and 3 B, page 249), more rarely atrial tachycardia, AV nodal tachycardia, atrial fibrillation (Fig. 10.6, page 254/255) or atrial flutter.

2 An *AV nodal escape rhythm* (Fig. 10.2, 3 A) or *ventricular escape rhythm* (Fig. 10.2, 3 B), sometimes alternating with short or sometimes long-lasting attacks of ventricular arrest (Fig. 10.10 A, page 263) or torsade de pointes ventricular tachycardia (Fig. 6.33, page 164)

3 *AV dissociation* with independent atrial and ventricular activity. In the case of SA node activation of the atria, AV dissociation is revealed by sinus P waves occurring at a regular rate and thus associated with a constantly changing PR interval (Fig. 10.2, 3 A and B).

Despite complete interruption of AV impulse conduction in third degree AV block, the ECG may reveal interdependence between the atrial and the ventricular activity manifest by a short PP interval when two P waves surround a QRS complex and a somewhat longer PP interval when there is no intervening QRS complex (Fig. 10.14, page 271). This phenomenon, *ventriculo-phasic sinus arrhythmia,* is seen particularly in third degree AV block of congenital type. The underlying mechanism may be the mechanical effect of the ventricular contraction on the SA node structures which by increasing blood flow through the AV node artery, may temporarily accelerate SA node discharge.

In the patient with *atrial fibrillation* a transition from normal AV conduction to third degree AV block is indicated by a change in QRS rhythm from perpetually irregular to completely regular (Fig. 10.6).

ECG diagnosis of site of AV block [4–7]

The site of the AV block can be fairly accurately defined by recording a His bundle electrogram (Fig. 3.21, page 55) during an electrophysiological study. A reasonable estimate on the site of a block to differentiate between proximal and distal AV blocks is possible from a simple analysis of the ECG. The primary clue in assessing the site of an AV block is the width of the QRS complex:

1 *A narrow QRS complex* of less than 0.12 s implies an intact intraventricular conduction system and strongly suggests a proximal AV block.

2 *A wide QRS complex* of 0.12 s or wider implies impairment of the intraventricular conduction system and suggests a distal AV block.

Based on the ECG features of the AV block itself, a general rule is that second degree Mobitz type I block is related to a proximal site and Mobitz type II block or advanced block to a distal site of the AV block.

Considering both types of AV block and the width and pattern of the QRS complex three groups of ECG changes should be recognized:

1 Those which favour a *proximal site of AV block:*

- First degree AV block without bundle branch block (Fig. 10.2 1 A)
- Second degree AV block without bundle branch block (Fig. 10.2 2 A)
- Third degree AV block with an AV nodal escape rhythm (Fig. 10.2 3 A)

2 Those which favour a *distal site of AV block:*

- Second degree AV block Mobitz type II which usually will be associated with bundle branch block (Fig. 10.2, 2 B)
- Third degree AV block with a ventricular escape rhythm (Fig. 10.2, 3 B)
- Alternation between right and left bundle branch block (RBBB and LBBB) (Figs. 10.8, page 260, 10.12, page 266 and 10.15, page 272) or between right bundle branch complicated by left anterior fascicular block and left posterior fascicular block (RBBB + LAFB and RBBB + LPFB).

3 The concurrent recording of first degree AV block (prolonged PR) and bundle branch block (QRS ≥0.12 s), is compatible *with either a proximal and or a distal site* of the block (Fig. 10.16, page 274). Supplementary investigation by His bundle electrography (Fig. 3.21, page 55) is required to locate the site of the AV block in patients with these ECG features.

Symptoms

The bradycardia itself usually is not noticed by the patient but the effect of hypotension or low cardiac output can cause significant clinical symptoms.

Haemodynamic consequences. In third degree AV block of *proximal type* the resting rate of the AV nodal escape rhythm lies in the range of (35–)40–60/min (Figs. 10.1, 3 A, page 247 and 10.8). With exercise the decrease in vagal tone and the increase in adrenergic activity often will significantly increase the heart rate to 70–120/min. Thus, the functional capacity of the patient with third degree AV block of the proximal type often is normal or at worst is only slightly restricted. In third degree AV block of the *distal type* the escape rhythm is of ventricular origin with a resting rate of (25–)30–50/min and the rate increases slightly if at all in response to exercise. Depending on the balance between the severity of bradycardia and the associated pathology of the myocardium or coronary arteries, symptoms vary from shortness of breath or angina on exercise to congestive failure or shock at rest.

Neurological symptoms. Particularly in the elderly, episodes of severe bradycardia can cause confusion, dizziness or mental tiredness. Fainting or severe dizzy spells, however, are the major symptoms and are caused by episodes of ventricular arrest or attacks of torsade de pointes ventricular tachycardia (see section later in the chapter on Stokes-Adams syndrome, page 262).

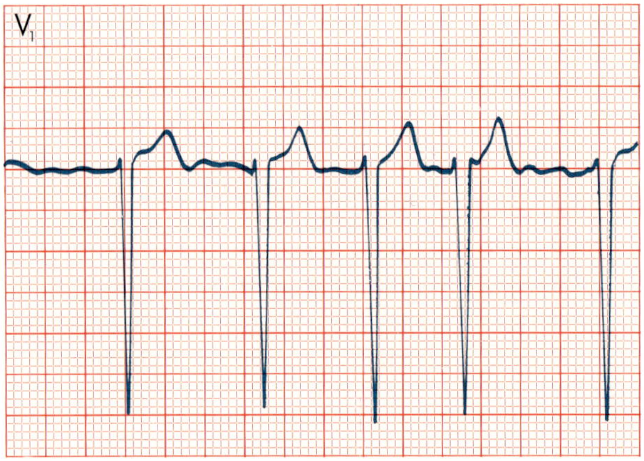

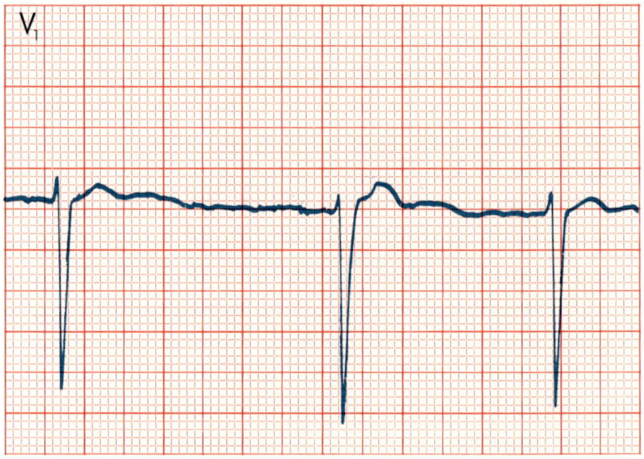

A1

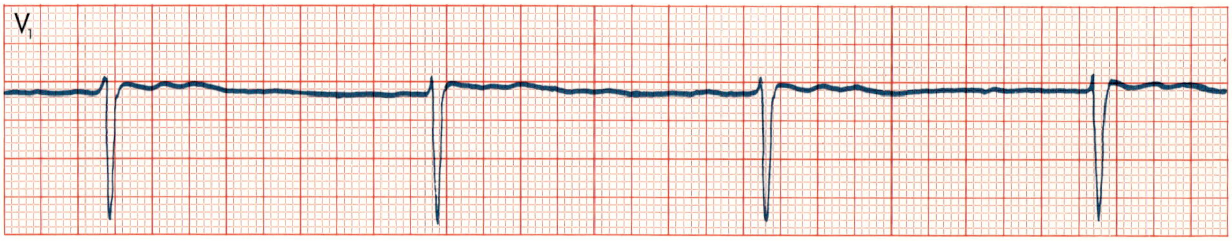

A2

Fig. 10.6
Development of third degree AV block in atrial fibrillation

A1 and B1. Uncomplicated atrial fibrillation characterized by (1) absence of P waves and (2) a base line with fibrillatory waves (fast irregular oscillations) and (3) narrow QRS complexes in a totally irregular rhythm.
A2 and B2. Atrial fibrillation complicated by third degree AV block. Atrial fibrillation is present with (1) absence of P waves and (2) fibrillatory wavelets on the base line, but (3) the QRS rhythm has become regular, which can only be explained by the development of third degree AV block. The QRS complexes recorded in A2 most likely represent an AV nodal escape rhythm as they are narrow and identical to those recorded in uncomplicated atrial fibrillation (A1). The QRS complexes in B2 most likely represent a ventricular escape rhythm as the complexes are wide and different from those recorded before the development of the AV block (B1).
A1 and A2 are ECG tracings recorded during digitalization of a 60-year-old female with congestive heart failure. Digoxin dosage is unknown. Serum digoxin at the time of the recording shown in A2 was 6 nanogram/ml. The third degree AV block disappeared 2 days after digoxin was discontinued.
B1 and B2 are tracings from a 68-year-old male, the first before the start of digoxin treatment and the other after 1 month of treatment with 500 microgram digoxin daily. Digoxin was discontinued, but the patient continued to have recurrent episodes of third degree AV block. The block was intermittently complicated by attacks of torsade de pointes ventricular tachycardia (B3) which were first suppressed after the implantation of an artificial pacemaker (B4).

Bipolar precordial lead

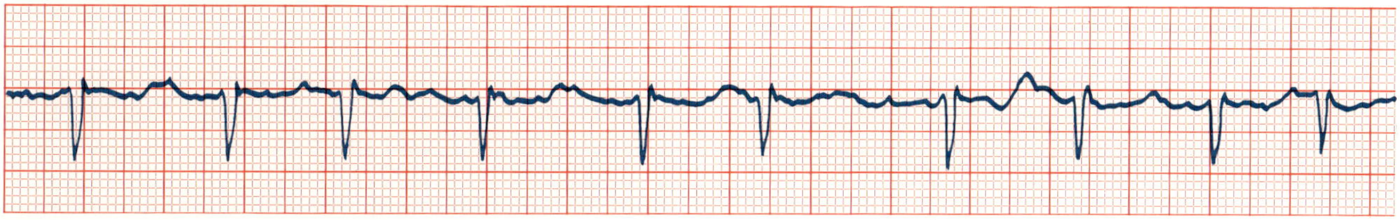

B1

Bipolar precordial lead

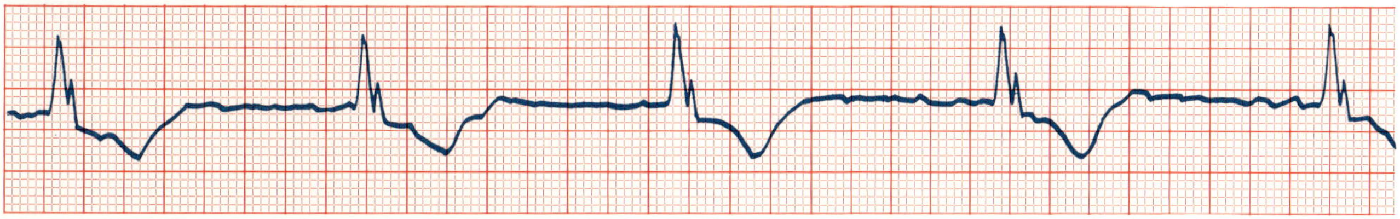

B2

Bipolar precordial lead

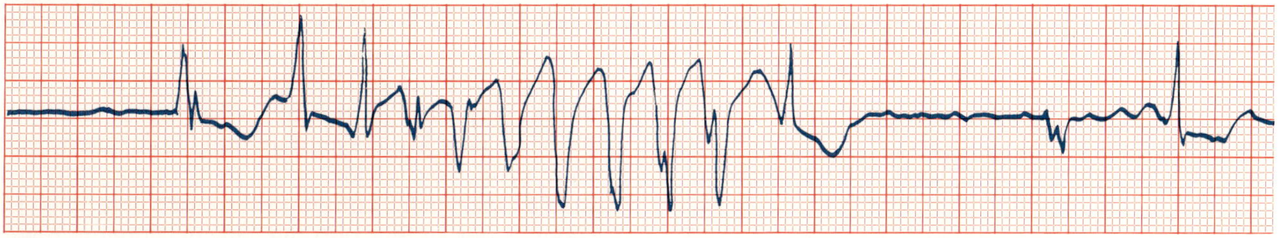

B3

Bipolar precordial lead

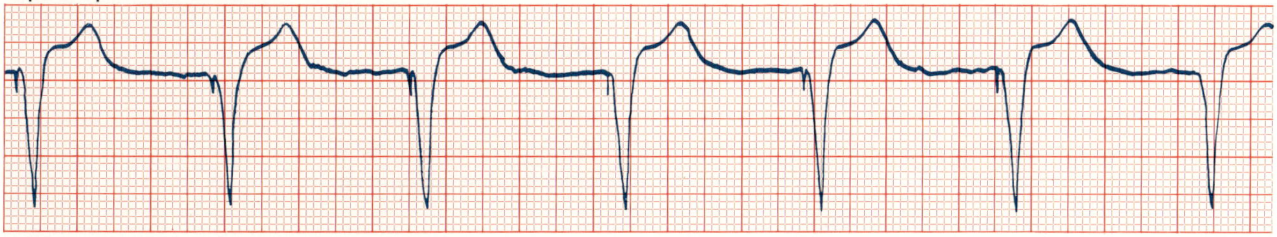

B4

Fig. 10.6
(continued)

Table 10.1

Aetiological factors in AV block

A. Acute AV block	
Cardiac disease:	Myocardial infarction [2, 14, 16] Prinzmetal's variant angina [23]
	Bacterial endocarditis particularly with affection of the aortic valves and abscess formation in the summit of the ventricular septum [24]
	Myocarditis (rheumatic, viral, bacterial) [2]
Drug overdosage/ intoxication:	Digitalis (Chapter 12, p. 293)
	Antiarrhythmic drugs (Chapter 4, p. 76)
	Tricyclic antidepressants [25, 26]
	Phenothiazines [25]
Electrolyte derangements:	Hyperkalaemia (Chapter 13, p. 298)
B. Recurrent or chronic AV block	
Cardiac disease:	Lenègre's and Lev's disease with idiopathic fibrosis of the conduction system or cardiac skeleton [2, 27, 28]
	Coronary artery disease [2]
	Cardiomyopathy [2]
	Aortic stenosis and particularly aortic insufficiency following spondylitis [29]
	Surgical heart block [2]
	Congenital AV block [2, 22]
	Cruzi trypanosomiasis [2]
Connective tissue disorders:	Sarcoidosis, scleroderma, amyloidosis, systemic lupus [2]
Hormonal disorders:	Myxoedema [2]
Abnormal vagal reflexes:	Exercise, cough and swallowing induced syncope [30–35]

Aetiology of AV block [8–16, 22–35]

PR interval prolongation is a not infrequent finding in apparently healthy individuals, particularly the elderly. It often occurs as a benign and fully reversible phenomenon in relation to infectious disease, both viral and bacterial. PR prolongation and second degree AV block type I (and SA block) are frequent findings in the well trained athlete. A survey of the many pathological conditions associated with second and third degree AV block are presented in Table 10.1. AV block related to digitalis treatment (Figs. 10.3, page 250 and 10.6 A, page 254) and to antiarrhythmic drug therapy are discussed in Chapters 4 (page 71) and 12 (page 293). The following sections of the present chapter deal with AV block in acute myocardial infarction, Stokes-Adams syndrome, congenital AV block and the development of AV block in the apparently healthy individual.

Prognosis

A useful rule of thumb is that proximal AV block is associated with few if any symptoms and has a good prognosis. Distal AV block has a far more serious outlook. Exceptions to this rule are, however, not uncommon. Proximal AV block can be associated with Stokes-Adams attacks (Fig. 10.13, page 269), while patients with distal AV block may live a symptom-free life for many years. Thus, proper evaluation of the significance of AV block should take into consideration not only the ECG changes per se, but also the clinical situation in which the block is observed including history, complaints and symptoms of the patient and the aetiology of the block.

Management

Management is discussed in the next sections on AV block in acute myocardial infarction, Stokes-Adams syndrome, congenital AV block and AV block in the apparently healthy individual.

AV block in acute myocardial infarction [14–16]

First and second degree AV block have been reported in 12–15 % of patients with acute myocardial infarction, while the incidence of third degree AV block has been reported to vary between 2 % and 10 %. AV block usually develops within the first hours or days after the infarction. Third degree AV block is two or three times as common in inferior infarction as in anteroseptal and anterior infarction. AV block following inferior and anterior infarction differ in many aspects and will therefore be discussed separately.

In *acute inferior myocardial infarction* AV block is usually of the proximal type with a narrow QRS complex: AV block of first degree, AV block of Mobitz type I or occasionally third degree AV block with an AV nodal escape rhythm (Fig. 10.7, page 259). The frequent occurrence of AV block of the proximal type in inferior infarction may relate to the common source of blood supply of the AV node and the inferior wall of the ventricles. The AV block usually is fully reversible, lasting for only a few hours or days, rarely as long as a week. The bradycardia associated with third degree AV block usually is moderate with few haemodynamic consequences, but it may aggravate shock or congestive failure in the patient with a severely injured myocardium. Complications of prolonged ventricular arrest or torsade de pointes ventricular tachycardia are rare, but do occur. The prognosis is good with no significant difference between survival rates for inferior infarct patients with or without complicating third degree AV block.

In *acute anteroseptal or anterior myocardial infaction* complication with AV block occurs more rarely and is usually seen only with very large infarcts. The AV block is usually of the distal type with bundle branch block, Mobitz type II AV block, or third degree AV block with a ventricular escape rhythm. The prognosis is poor, approaching an 80–90 % mortality, particularly with the development of third degree AV block. The primary cause of death is pump failure but some patients die suddenly of ventricular arrest or fibrillation. The progression from bundle branch block to third degree AV block can occur gradually (Fig. 10.8, page 260/261) but often is very sudden (Fig. 9.9, page 237). The initial attack of third degree AV block may be lethal due to complicating ventricular arrest, torsade de pointes ventricular tachycardia or fibrillation. Paced or unpaced, a substantial number of patients die from pump failure. For the patients who survive the initial transient complication to leave hospital with third degree AV block of distal type, the risk of dying within the first month or year is high. A substantial number of patients with bundle branch block die from pump failure; some die suddenly. The cause of late sudden death may be paroxysms of AV block, ventricular tachycardia or fibrillation. Exceptionally distal AV block may be associated with death when complicating an acute inferior infarction. This outcome is more common in patients with previous anteroseptal, anterior or anterolateral infarction.

Management

In *AV block of proximal type complicating inferior infarction* treatment usually can be restricted to the withdrawal of digitalis and other antiarrhythmic drugs. Bradycardia leading to shock, congestive failure or bursts of ventricular ectopic activity should be treated by intravenous injection of atropine or ipratropium bromide. An isoprenaline infusion, temporary transthoracic pacing or transvenous pacing (Figs. 4.14, page 90, 4.15, page 90) may be needed in the rare situation in which intravenous atropine is ineffective.

In the early stage of an *anteroseptal or anterior* infarct the mere development of left or right bundle branch block or right bundle branch block complicated by left fascicular block does not warrant inserting transvenous pacing electrode (Fig. 4.15). Prophylactic transvenous pacing might be considered for the patient who develops:

1 Alternating bundle branch block (Fig. 10.8, page 260/261) with alternation between RBBB and LBBB or between RBBB + LAFB and RBBB + LPFB

2 Second degree AV block, Mobitz type II or advanced AV block

3 Third degree AV block with a ventricular escape rhythm.

Despite transvenous pacing, a substantial number of patients die of pump failure. Furthermore, pacing in acute myocardial infarction is not without hazards. Insertion of the pacing electrode into the right ventricle can provoke ventricular fibrillation by mechanical irritation of the unstable ischaemic myocardium. Pacing in the vulnerable period of the ventricular myocardium is a potential hazard because loss of viable myocardium may decrease the amplitude of the intracavity electrogram with the risk of pacemaker undersensing. The fibrillatory threshold of the ischaemic myocardium is low and the risk of inducing ventricular fibrillation by pacing in the vulnerable period of the ventricles is high (Fig. 10.9, page 261).

In the rare patient who in the second or third week after an infarct still has a second or third degree AV block, the indication for pacemaker implantation is clear. Whether survivors of a transient distal AV block should undergo pacemaker implantation before discharge from hospital remains a matter of controversy. Many believe it to be indicated for the patient with persistent right bundle branch block and left anterior (or posterior) fascicular block. It is possible, though not proven, that such an intervention might decrease the risk of sudden death.

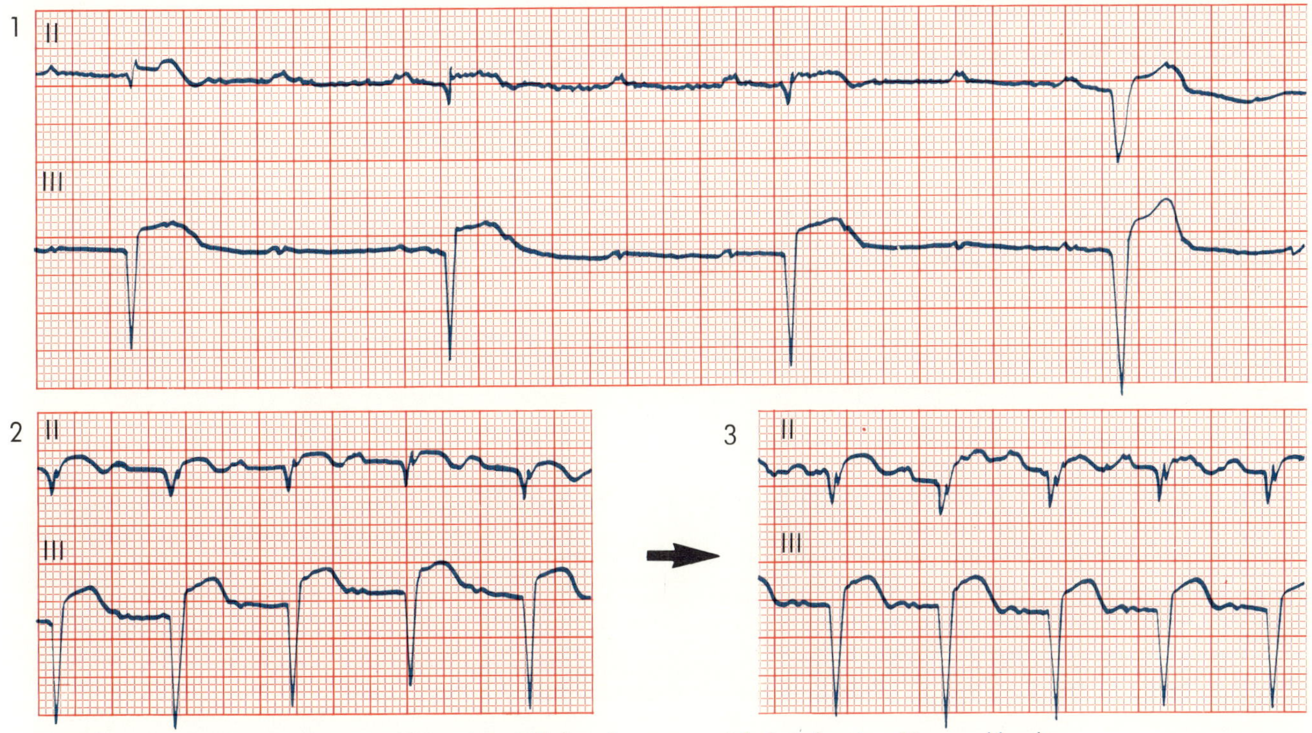

A ECG tracings from the first (1), second (2) and third (3) day after an acute inferior infarct in a 68-year-old male

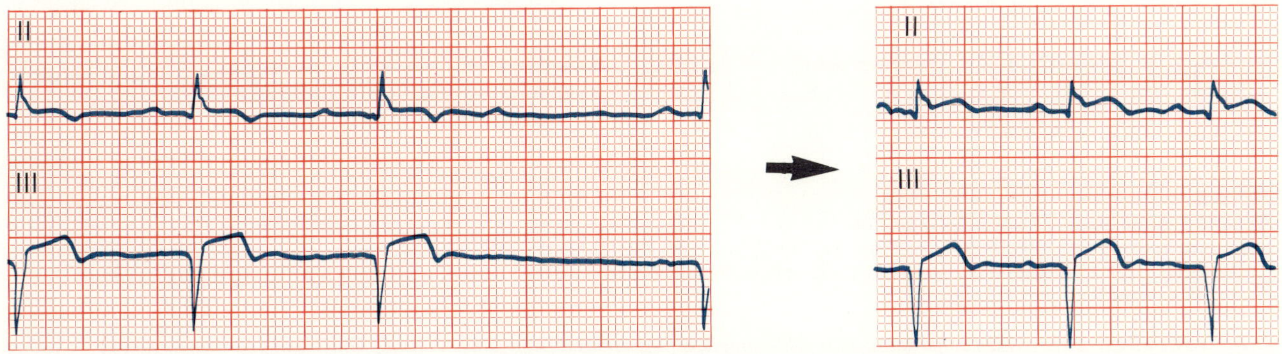

B ECG tracings from the second and seventh day after an acute inferior infarct in a 50-year-old female

Fig. 10.7
AV block in acute inferior myocardial infarction.
The diagnosis of acute inferior myocardial infarction (Chapter 14) is based on the recording of abnormal Q waves and ST segment elevation in leads II, III and aVF.
The recorded AV blocks are all of proximal location: third degree AV block with AV nodal escape rhythm (A1), second degree AV block Mobitz type I (4:3 conduction) (B) and first degree AV block (A2).

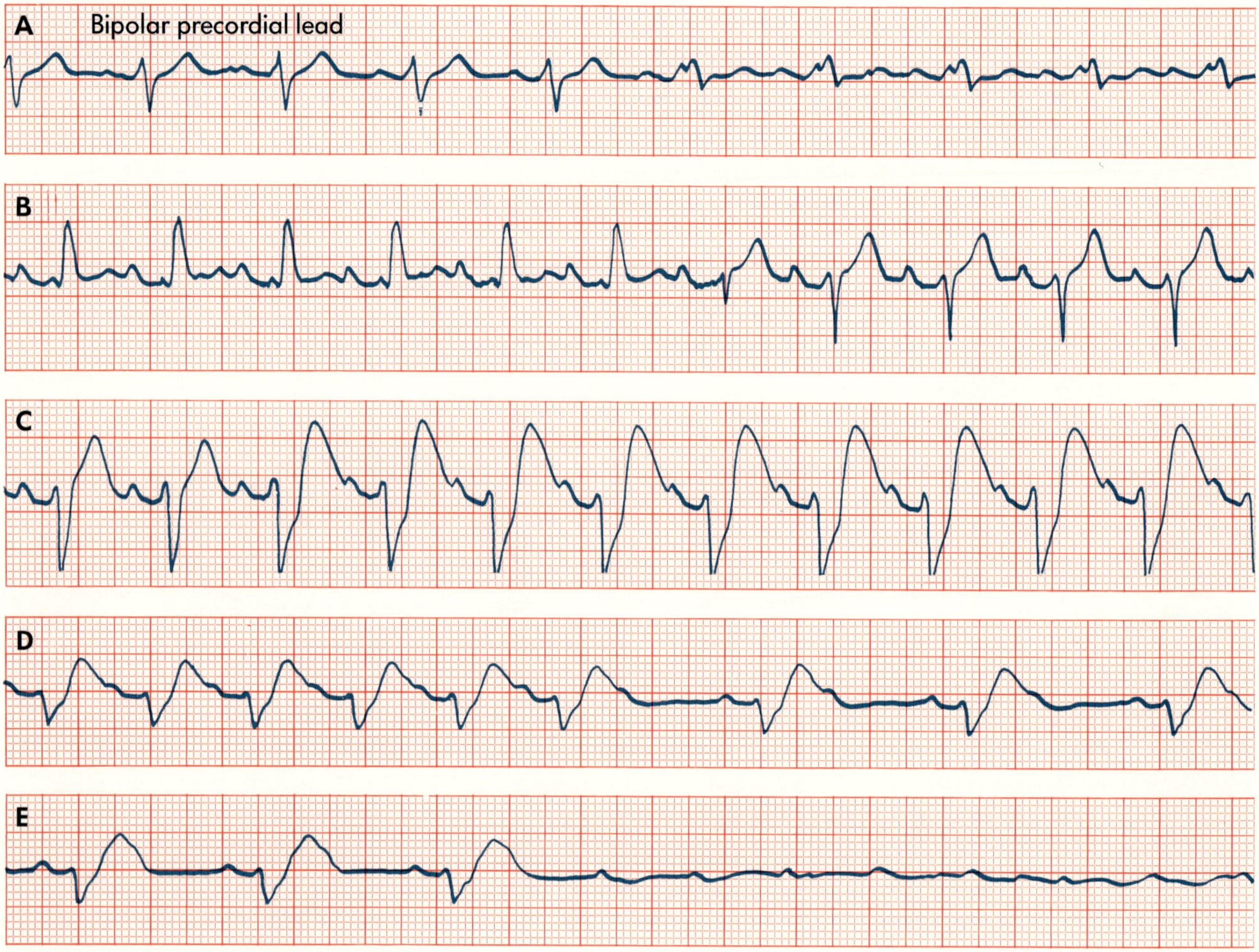

Fig. 10.8
AV block in acute anterior myocardial infarction.
Sequences from the first 24-hour ECG monitoring in the CCU of a 60-year-old male with an acute anterior myocardial infarction Infarct diagnosis and site localization of the subsequently developed bundle branch blocks of various types have been assessed by repeated 12-lead ECG recordings (not shown).

A A transition from narrow QRS complexes to wide QRS complexes represents a change from normal intraventricular conduction to right bundle branch block.
B The amplification of the ECG amplifier was changed with a subsequent change in QRS amplitude. The first six wide QRS complexes signify the continued presence of right bundle branch block; the transition to narrow QRS complexes indicates the disappearance of the bundle branch block associated with development of left anterior fascicular block.
C Gradual progression from left anterior fascicular block with narrow QRS complexes to left bundle branch block with wide QRS complexes.
D Continued left bundle branch block first associated with 1:1 AV conduction of the P waves, later complicated by 2:1 AV block.
E Continued 2:1 AV block with left bundle branch block followed by the sudden development of third degree AV block with ventricular arrest.

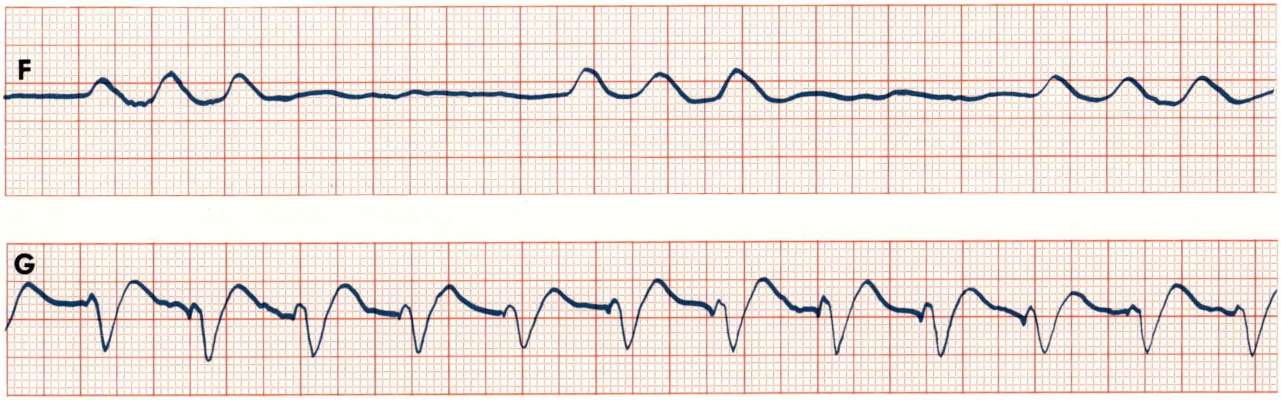

Fig. 10.8
(continued)

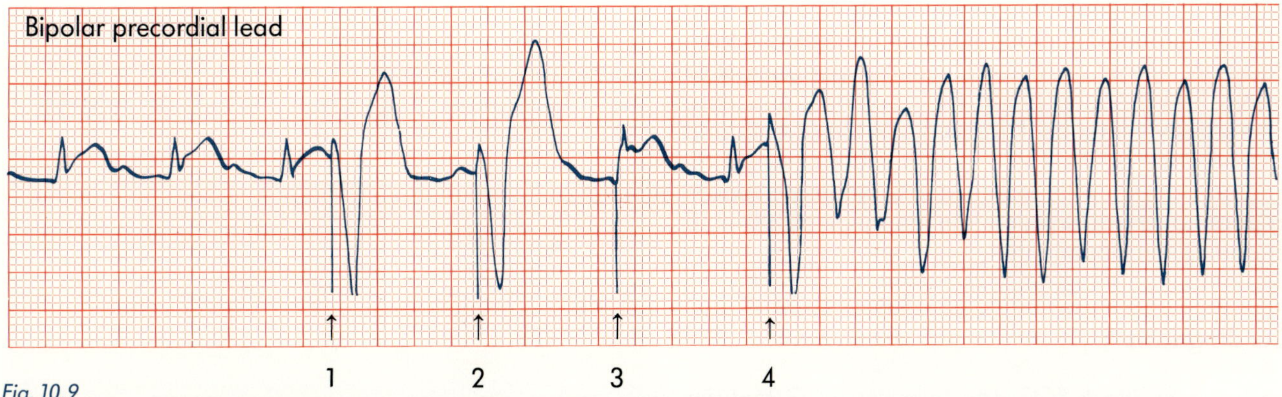

Fig. 10.9
Pacing induced ventricular flutter/fibrillation in acute myocardial infarction.
50-year-old male with acute inferior myocardial infarction. Third degree AV block developed shortly after admission. Artificial pacing through a transvenously inserted pacing electrode was started soon afterwards due to complication with bradycardia and hypotension. The figure presents a sequence from the ECG monitoring a few hours later. Sinus rhythm has recurred but there is still a first degree AV block (PR interval 0.28 s). Pacemaker undersensing of the third sinus complex in the ECG strip is followed by a brief period of fixed rate pacing including four pacemaker spikes (marked 1–4). The fourth spike falls on the ascending part or summit of the T wave of the preceding complex i.e. within the vulnerable period of the ventricles. It triggers an attack of ventricular flutter with subsequent transition to ventricular fibrillation (not shown). Sinus rhythm was immediately restored by DC countershock.

Stokes-Adams syndrome [17–21]

A Stokes-Adams attack is the common term for a faint or near faint caused by a transient cardiac arrest with spontaneous recovery (Chapter 3, page 62). Some patients suffer recurrent Stokes-Adams attacks occurring at varying time intervals over periods of weeks, months or years. The underlying cause of repeated Stokes-Adams attacks are:

1 In about 50–60 % of patients *paroxysmal or chronic AV block* with ventricular arrest (Fig. 10.10) or, more rarely, torsade de pointes ventricular tachycardia (Figs. 6.33, page 164 and 10.11, page 265).

2 In approximately 30–40 % of patients, sinoatrial block with ventricular arrest often alternating with paroxysms of supraventricular tachycardia, the "sick sinus syndrome" (Fig. 11.7, page 287).

3 In a few percent of patients the attacks are unrelated to heart block but are caused by paroxysms of fast tachycardia or fibrillation, either ventricular (Figs. 6.35, page 168, 6.38, page 174, 6.41, page 178, 6.44, page 183 and 14.22, page 336) or supraventricular (Figs. 6.18, page 144, 7.11, page 199, 7.13, page 202 and 7.14, page 204).

The term Stokes-Adams syndrome usually is reserved for the major group of patients in whom the Stokes-Adams attacks are related to AV block, whether paroxysmal or chronic. Stokes-Adams syndrome is primarily a disease of the elderly with a peak frequency in the seventh and eighth decade of life. The annual number of newly diagnosed patients with Stokes-Adams syndrome requiring pacemaker implantation is in the range of 100–150 per one million inhabitants.

ECG diagnosis

The between-attack-ECG. The following ECG features may be detected:

1 In half the patients there is chronic third degree AV block, most often with ventricular escape rhythm, (Figs. 10.10 A and 10.2, 3 B, page 249) or advanced AV block (Fig. 10.5, page 251) or a Mobitz type II block associated with a BBB pattern (Fig. 10.2, 2 B).

2 The other patients with Stokes-Adams syndrome are in sinus rhythm between attacks but:

A A majority have a widened QRS complex signifying bundle branch block (Fig. 10.12, page 266), usually a right bundle branch block with or without left anterior fascicular block.

B Rarely the ECG is without any sign of AV or intraventricular conduction disturbance (Fig. 10.13, page 269).

ECG during a Stokes-Adams attack. An ECG recorded during a faint or near faint will show:

– In about 90 % of patients, episodes of ventricular arrest lasting for 5–10 s or longer (Fig. 10.10).

– In the remaining 10 %, attacks of torsade de pointes ventricular tachycardia (Figs. 6.33, page 164 and 10.11).

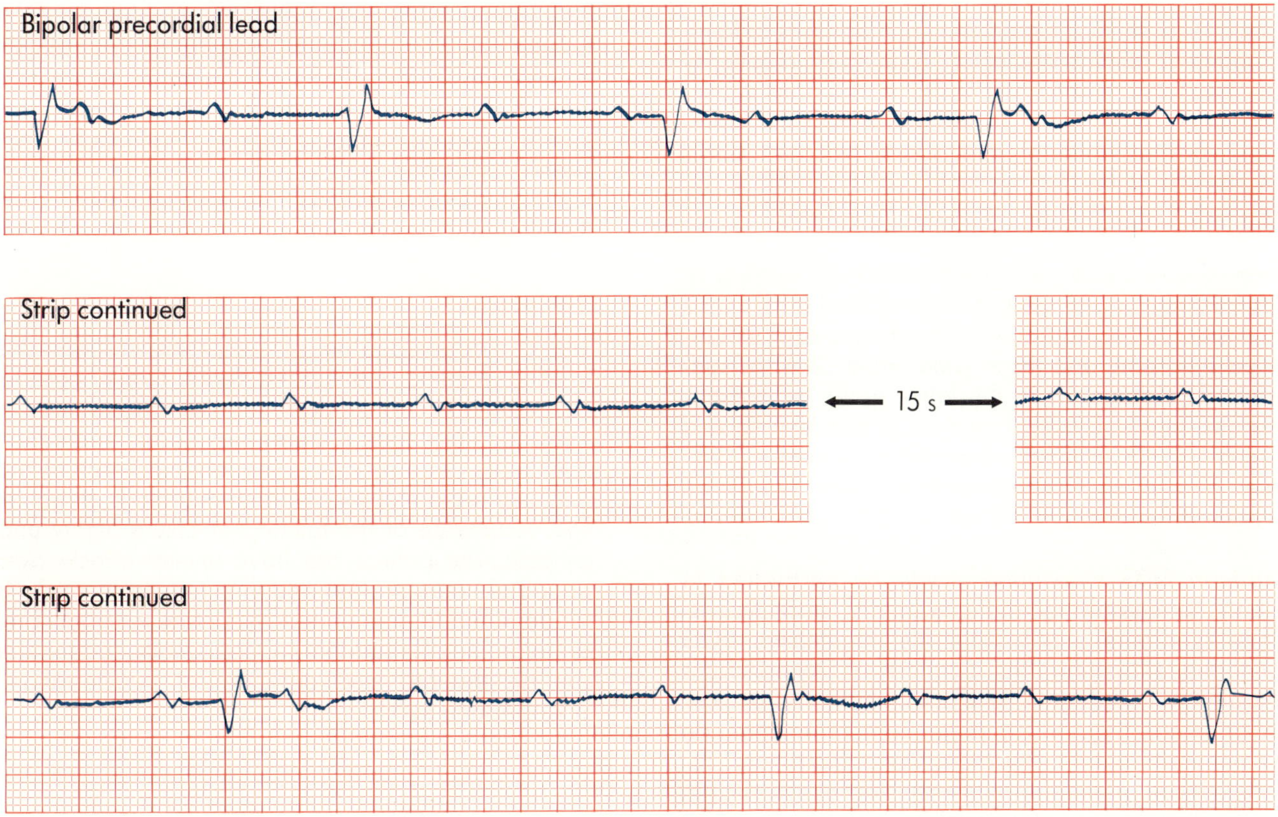

A *Third degree AV block with ventricular rhythm at a rate of 34/min (upper strip), sudden loss of ventricular activation for a period of 20 s (middle strip) and spontaneous recurrence of ventricular escape rhythm at a slowly accelerating rate of 25 to 35/min (lower strip). From a 83-year-old male with repeated fainting spells during the previous 2 months.*

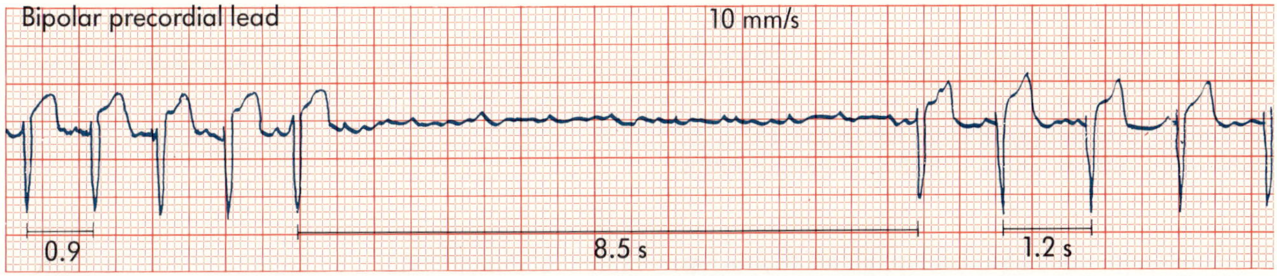

B *Sinus rhythm and bundle branch block with a sudden attack of third degree AV block complicated by ventricular arrest for a period of 8 s followed by spontaneous recurrence of sinus rhythm. ECG monitoring from a 70-year-old male with repeated attacks of fainting or near fainting 1 year prior to admission (Paper speed 10 mm/s).*

Fig. 10.10
Stokes-Adams syndrome with fainting due to episodes of ventricular arrest (ECG monitoring by telemetry)

Differential diagnosis

In the clinical setting, the differential diagnoses of fainting and near fainting are legion, ranging from epilepsy and transitory cerebral ischaemia to hypoglycaemia, orthostatic hypotension, hypersensitive carotid sinus, cough, postmicturitional and vagal syncope, aortic stenosis and other arrhyhmias (sinoatrial block or, rarely to paroxysmal tachycardia or fibrillation).

When recorded in a patient with attacks of fainting or near fainting, any of the ECG events listed in (1) might be considered corraborative of the diagnosis of Stokes-Adams syndrome and those listed under (2 A) as suggestive. The diagnosis in the latter group of patients (and also those of 2 B), should be further investigated by long-term ECG monitoring. When diagnostic difficulties remain an electrophysiologic study should be considered.

Long-term ECG monitoring should be performed in hospital, preferably by radio telemetry, since Stokes-Adams syndrome is potentially life threatening. ECG monitoring will confirm the diagnosis of Stokes-Adams syndrome if third degree AV block complicated by ventricular arrest (Fig. 10.10, page 263) or torsade de pointes ventricular tachycardia (Fig. 10.11) are recorded. It can provide strong circumstantial evidence in favour of the diagnosis by revealing:

1 Third degree AV block with an escape rhythm usually of ventricular origin (Fig. 10.2, 3 B, page 249)

2 Second degree AV block of Mobitz type II (Fig. 10.2, 2 B)

3 Alternating bundle branch block with a shift between RBBB and LBBB or between RBBB + LAFB and RBBB + LPFB.

ECG monitoring can also be useful in disproving Stokes-Adams syndrome by the recording of a normal and undisturbed cardiac rhythm up to and during an episode of near fainting, fainting or whatever other symptoms the patient may experience.

His bundle electrography (Fig. 3.21, page 55) has been used widely in the evaluation of patients with suspected Stokes-Adams syndrome. The diagnostic and prognostic implications of a prolonged HV interval in the His bundle electrogram which suggests a distal block remains a matter for debate. A reasonable diagnostic approach is to first use long-term ECG monitoring and to turn to electrophysiologic studies (His bundle electrography, sinus node recovery time, testing for substrates for re-entry tachycardias) in the (rare) situation in which the diagnosis remains in doubt.

Symptoms

The characteristic triad of symptoms includes: Near fainting, fainting and sudden death. Loss of consciousness usually occurs suddenly without any cardiac symptoms. Clonic or tonic seizures may occur. Trauma is frequent. Besides a sudden onset, a typical feature of the faint is a rapid recovery without neurological sequelae. The occurrence of the fainting attacks is highly unpredictable. The patient can have several attacks over a period of hours or days and then remain symptom free for days, weeks or even months before the attacks recur or before he dies suddenly. Occasionally, sudden death can be the first and only clinical manifestation of Stokes-Adams syndrome.

Aetiology

A survey of the various aetiological factors for AV block and thus Stokes-Adams syndrome is presented in Table 10.1. The most common cause is widespread fibrosis in the intraventricular conduction system, *Lenegre's disease*. A slow accumulation of fibrotic tissue occurs normally with advancing age. Although the incidence of fascicular block and bundle branch block (LAFB, RBBB and RBBB + LAFB) increases significantly with age, the rate of progression of fibrosis is so slow that an AV conduction defect rarely develops before death. In the patient with Lenegre's disease the fibrotic process accelerates for reasons unknown, with loss of conduction tissue and pacemaker cells. This results in intraventricular block and distal AV block with complicating episodes of ventricular arrest or torsade de pointes ventricular tachycardia.

Fibrosis and calcification causing AV block and fainting are also seen with degenerative change in the skeleton of the heart, particularly in the central fibrous body and the pars membranacea of the ventricular septum (*Lev's disease*). There is often an overlap between Lenegre's and Lev's diseases, but the former predominantly affects the distal part of the bundle branches while the latter affects the more proximal part of the conducting system near the central fibrous body. Calcification of diseased aortic valves, as in aortic stenosis, can extend into the central fibrous body or into the intraventricular septum and cause AV block.

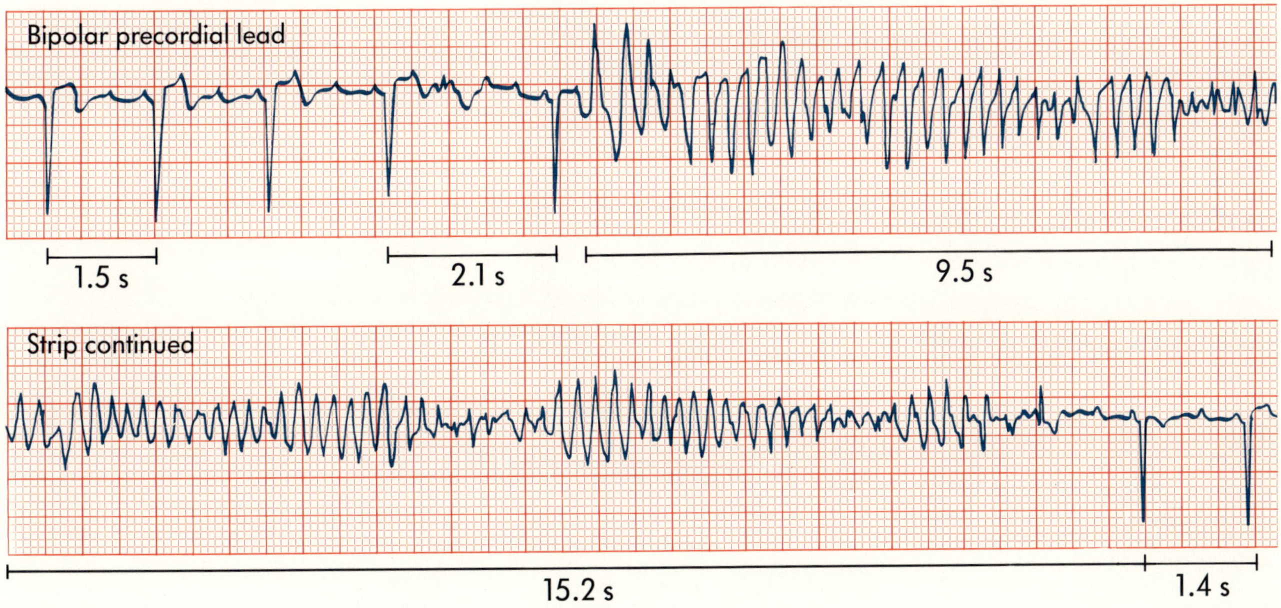

Fig. 10.11
Stokes-Adams syndrome with fainting due to attacks of torsade de pointes ventricular tachycardia.
The ECG is from a 59-year-old female with a slow pulse and one fainting spell in the year prior to admission. Sequences from continuous telemetric ECG monitoring. Note that the paper speed is 10 mm/s. The first part of the tracing shows a 3:1 AV block with transition to a 5:1 AV block followed by torsade de pointes ventricular tachycardia. The tachycardia associated with fainting continued for a period of 23 s before sinus rhythm with 3:1 AV block recurred.

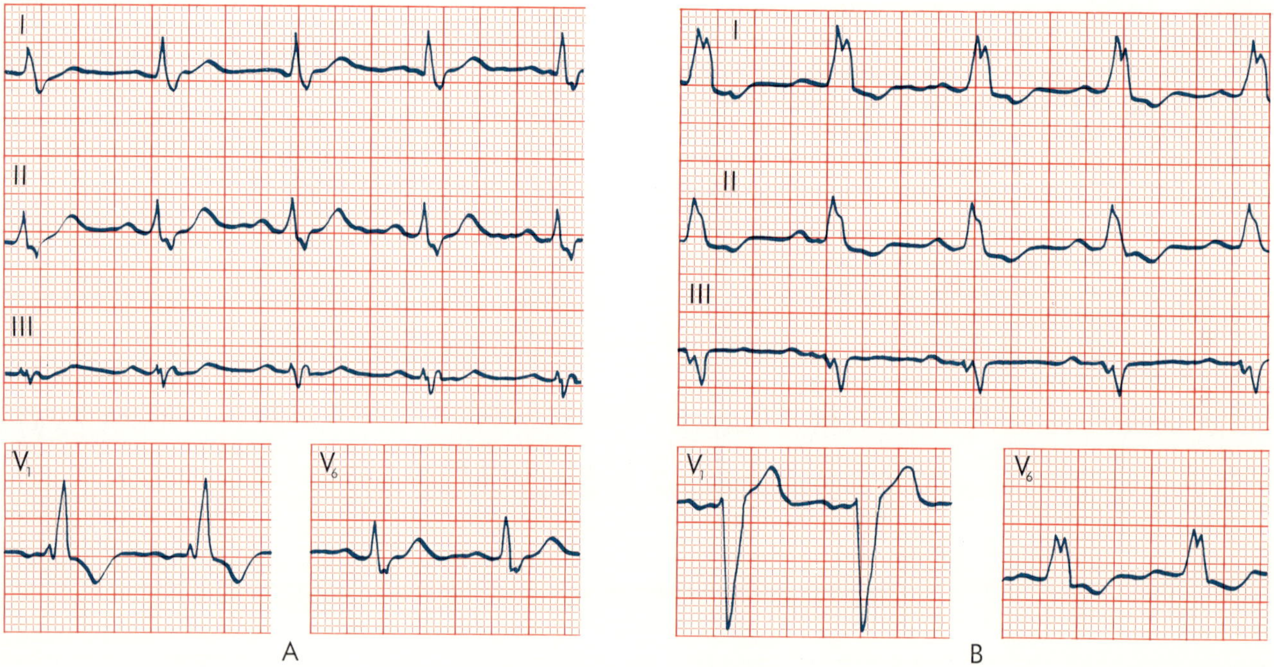

Fig. 10.12
Alternating bundle branch block in Stokes-Adams syndrome.

A *ECG at the first admission of a 77-year-old female who, shortly before admission, had experienced a brief attack of unconsciousness. The ECG showed right bundle branch block (a QRS of 0.16 an rR′ pattern in V_1 and late broad s in V_6 and I). There were no symptoms during the following 2 weeks of hospital admission. Continued ECG monitoring consistently showed sinus rhythm with 1:1 AV conduction and right bundle branch block. It was considered that the fainting was not of cardiac origin and the patient was discharged without any treatment.*

B *ECG 1 year later when the patient was readmitted due to recurrent fainting spells during the 2 months prior to admission. The ECG now shows sinus rhythm with left bundle branch block (wide QRS=0.16 s, an rR′ like pattern in V_6 and I, and a late broad S in V_1 and V_2).*

C *2:1, 3:1 and 4:1 AV blocks were observed during the following days (see ECG's presented in Fig. 10.5, which are from this patient) and finally as shown in this tracing, an episode of third degree AV block with ventricular escape rhythm. An artifical pacemaker was implanted. At a follow-up 2 years after pacemaker implantation the patient had experienced no further fainting attacks.*

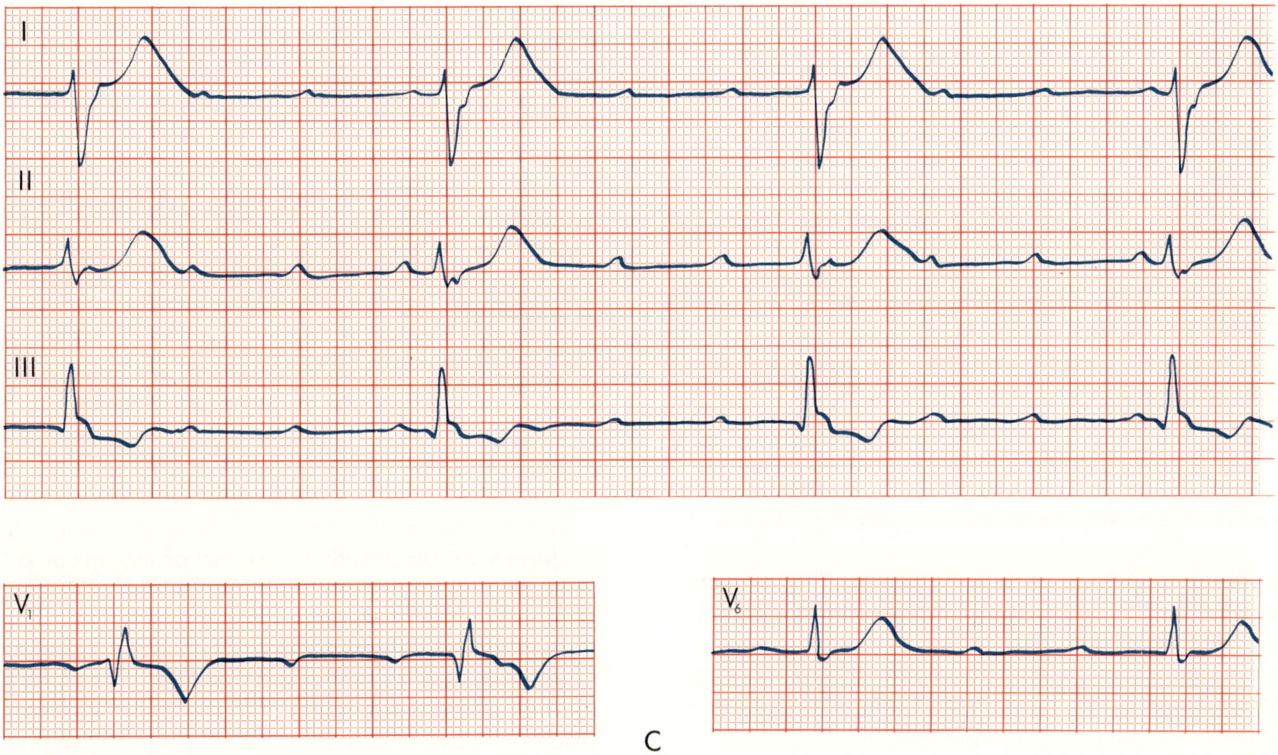

C

Fig. 10.12
(continued)

The reported incidence of coronary artery disease in Stokes-Adams syndrome varies between 30–50 %. As the mean age of the patient population is high, however, coronary artery disease may be more a coincidental phenomenon than a causal disease. Hence, while the nature of the fibrotic changes of Lenegre's and Lev's diseases is debated, there is universal agreement that they are *not* due to coronary artery disease.

Prognosis

Untreated long-term prognosis is poor with a mortality of around 50 % within the first years after the initial attack.

Lenegre's disease, however, usually is confined to the conduction system of the heart and interferes little if at all with pumping. Thus, with an artificial pacemaker, the prognosis is good with a survival rate that approaches that for the normal population.

Management

In an emergency with ventricular arrest and before transthoracic pacing can be arranged (Fig. 4.14, page 90), or a pacing cathether (Fig. 4.15, page 90) can be inserted treatment with intravenous adrenaline can be followed by an intravenous infusion of isoprenaline. Atropine might be effective in block of proximal type.

Long-term oral treatment with isoprenaline or orciprenaline for the prevention of Stokes-Adams attacks is very unreliable and should be considered only in patients for whom pacemaker implantation is inappropriate or impossible. The one and only effective treatment is that of pacemaker implantation.

Pacemaker implantation

The physician's dilemma is primarily diagnostic. He should not misdiagnose the condition nor postpone pacemaker implantation lest the correct diagnosis of Stokes-Adams syndrome be revealed by the sudden death of the patient. Nor should he implant a pacemaker on scanty evidence as this latter approach will lead to many unneccessary pacemaker implantations with attendant risks of morbidity, mortality and psychological problems. Once the diagnosis of Stokes-Adams syndrome has been established, treatment of the otherwise healthy patient should be by pacemaker implantation.

Ventricular pacing by implantation of a ventricular inhibited pacemaker (VVI pacemaker, Fig. 4.20, page 96) has been and still is the most commonly used treatment for Stokes-Adams' syndrome. It is a comparatively inexpensive device and is easy to implant. With the increased reliability and technical sophistication of the dual chamber pacemaker (DDD pacemaker, Fig. 4.26, page 100), however, many centres have adopted this type of pacemaker as a routine in all patients with Stokes-Adams' syndrome. This type of pacemaker preserves the physiological heart rate response and protects against AV asynchrony and thus against the pacemaker syndrome (page 289). Dual chamber pacemaker implantation seems the ideal treatment not only for chronic third degree AV block but also for AV block of the paroxysmal type since:

- a fair number of the patients with paroxysmal AV block who undergo implantation of a VVI pacemaker suffer from the pacemaker syndrome related to episodes of AV asynchrony induced by the transitory ventricular pacing during their shortlasting but not infrequent attacks of AV block, and

- a majority of these patients develop chronic third degree AV block within a period of months or a few years.

Before the implantation of a DDD pacemaker, sinus node response to exercise should be tested by the recording of an exercise ECG. The implantation of a rate responsive pacemaker (VVI-R, page 99) should be considered in patients with AV block and an inadequate sinus node response to exercise or AV block combined with atrial fibrillation or flutter.

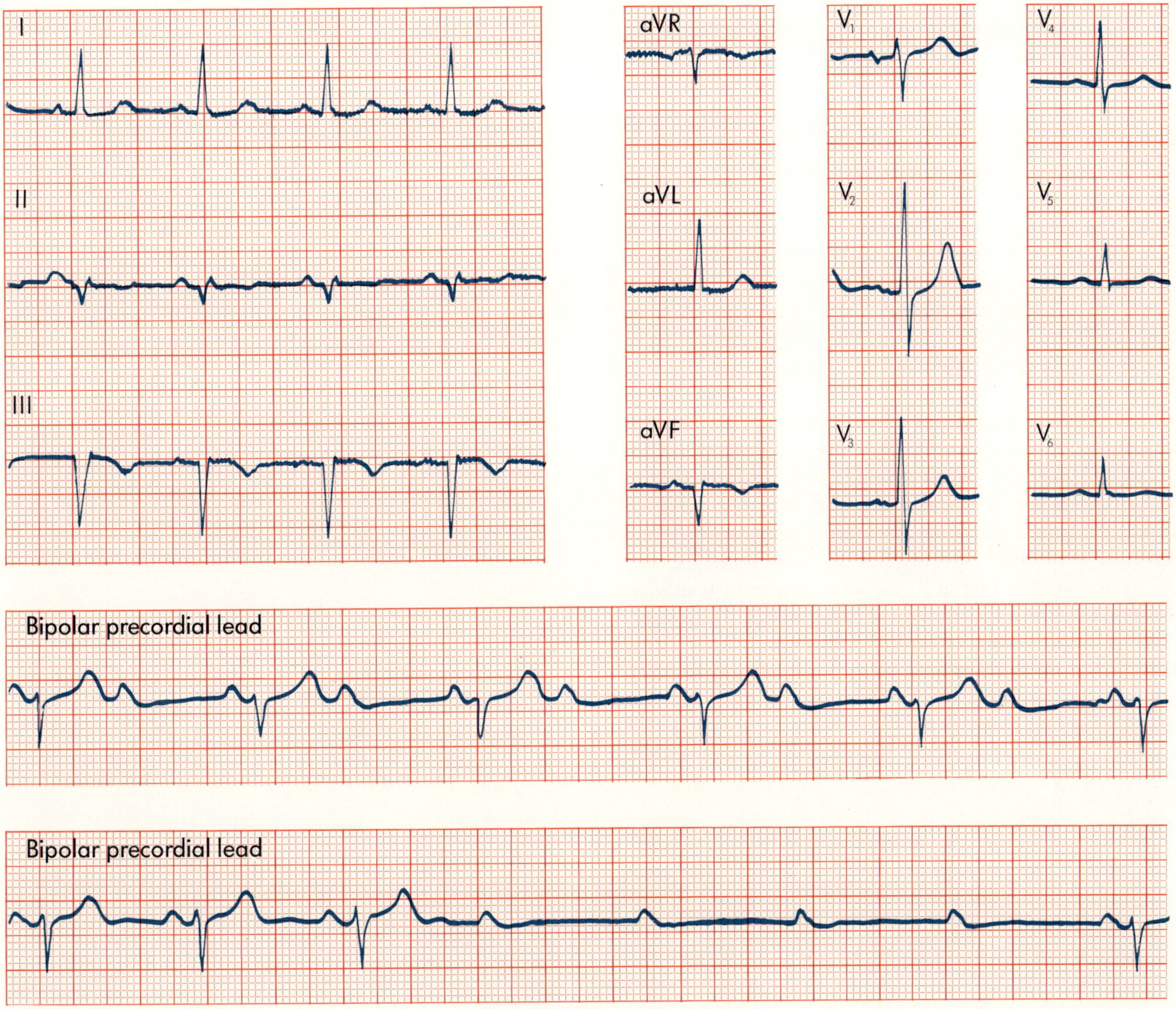

Fig. 10.13
Stokes-Adams syndrome in a patient with apparently normal AV and intraventricular conduction (ECG recording without AV or bundle branch block between attacks).
The ECG is from a 68-year-old male who had been admitted to another hospital 4 years earlier with an uncomplicated inferior myocardial infarct. He was readmitted due to repeated fainting spells during the previous 2 months. There were no complaints of angina or signs of recurrence of the myocardial infarct.
The ECG shows signs of an old inferior myocardial infarction with Q waves and negative T waves in leads II, III and aVF. There is sinus rhythm, all P waves are AV conducted, the PR interval is normal (0.16 s) and the QRS complex is narrow (0.09 s). However, continuous telemetric ECG monitoring for a period of 1 week revealed repeated episodes of third degree AV block with prolonged ventricular arrest that caused occasional fainting.

Congenital AV block [22]

Third degree AV block may occur as a congenital lesion when the block is usually of proximal type with an AV nodal escape rhythm. The resting rate is 50–90/min in the infant and (35–)40–60/min in the child and young adult (Fig. 10.14). Submaximal and maximal exercise usually increase the rate to 90–120/min.

In the first weeks of life, congenital third degree AV block may be associated with Stokes-Adams attacks or life threatening bradycardia. In the newborn this means a heart rate of below 50/min. After the age of one month children with AV block usually are symptom free and continue to grow and develop normally.

The prognosis depends primarily on any associated congenital heart disease which is present in about one third of the children. Most patients without underlying heart disease live a normal life and possibly have a normal life span. The long-term prognosis has not yet been fully evaluated and regular ECG surveillance, including an exercise test at 2 to 3 year intervals, is advisable. Pacemaker implantation is indicated in the event of Stokes-Adams attacks and should be seriously considered if the ventricular rate slows progressively or fails to increase on exercise.

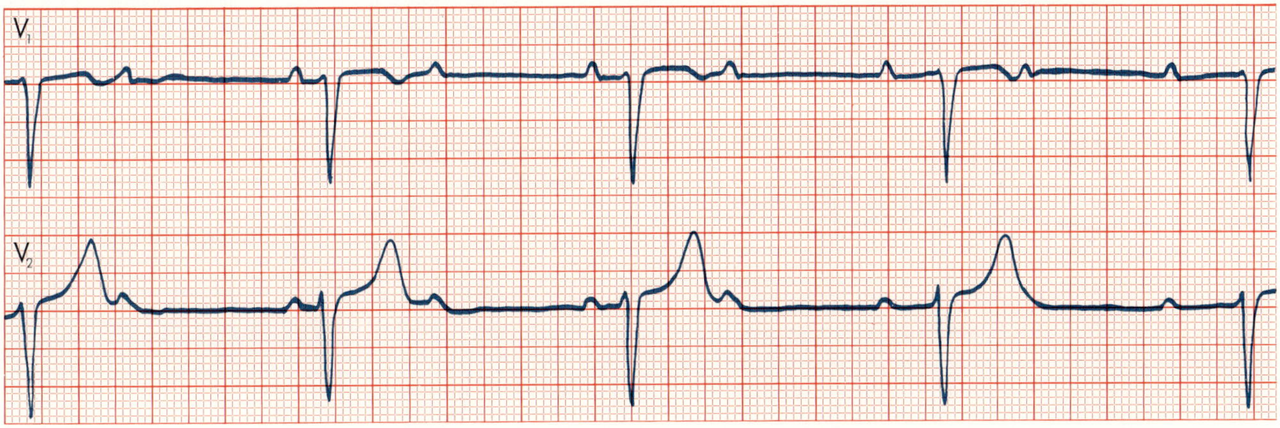

Fig. 10.14
Third degree AV block with AV nodal escape rhythm and ventriculophasic irregularity of sinus rhythm.
ECG from a 18-year-old man with congenital third degree AV block. Sinus P waves in an irregular rhythm at a rate of 73/min and narrow QRS complexes (0.11 s) at a regular but slower rate of 36/min. The irregularity of the sinus P waves seems to be related to ventricular rhythm as the PP segments are shorter (0.76 s) when two P waves surround a QRS complex and somewhat longer (0.81–0.88 s) when there is no intervening QRS complex.

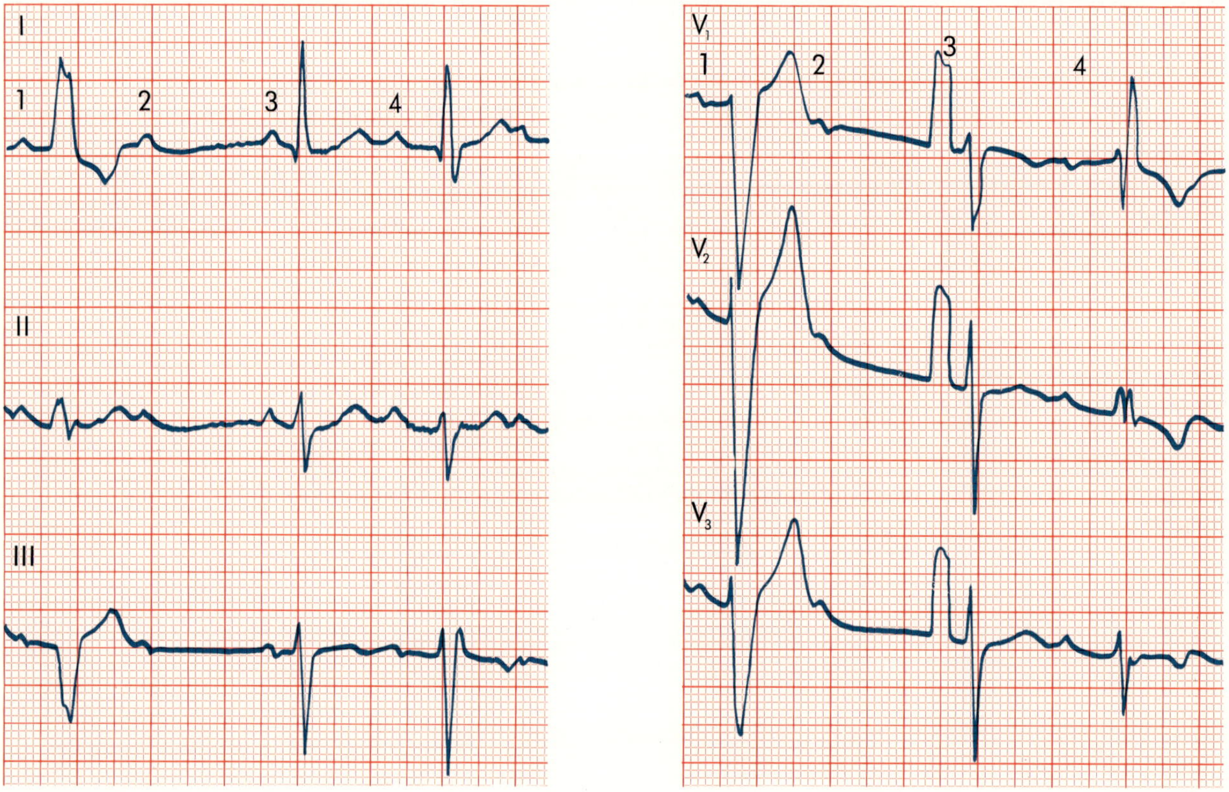

Fig. 10.15
Alternating bundle branch block and Mobitz type II AV block in an asymptomatic individual.
ECG from a 76-year-old male with no history of fainting, cardiac complaints or signs of cardiac disease. With reference to the numbering of the P waves in the ECG recording, the following conduction defects can be noted:

1 Normal AV conduction, left bundle branch block (LBBB)
2 Second degree AV block Mobitz type II
3 Normal AV conduction, left anterior fascicular block (LAFB)
4 First degree AV block, right bundle branch block and left anterior fascicular block (RBBB + LAFB)

It was concluded that the AV block was of distal type since it was Mobitz type II and because there was alternation between LBBB and RBBB + LAFB.
Although the patient was without symptoms, a pacemaker was implanted to reduce the risk of Stokes-Adams attacks and sudden death.

AV block in the asymptomatic individual [11–13, 32–35]

The physician sometimes is faced with the problem of an atrioventricular conduction defect in an apparently healthy symptom free individual (Fig. 10.15). The recording of such a conduction abnormality should initiate a search for underlying heart disease. Attention should be paid to block precipitating factors such as electrolyte derangement (e.g. hyperkalaemia) or treatment with digitalis, antiarrhythmic drugs or tricyclic antidepressants. The risk of sudden death related to AV block is small in the great majority of cases, but is greater in:

1 Third degree AV block with an escape rhythm of ventricular origin (Figs. 10.2, 3 B, page 249)

2 Mobitz block type II or advanced AV block combined with wide QRS complexes of more than 0.12 s (RBBB or LBBB)(Figs. 10.2, 2 B and 10.5, page 251)

3 Alternating bundle branch block with a shift between RBBB and LBBB (Fig. 10.15) or between RBBB + LAFB and RBBB + LPFB

4 Bundle branch block associated with progressive lengthening of the PR interval (Fig. 10.16, page 274) and found to be related to HV prolongation at His bundle electrography.

Many feel that in these groups of patients, especially groups (1) to (3), the circumstantial evidence of an increased risk of sudden death is sufficient to justify prophylactic implantation of a pacemaker, particularly if the patient is otherwise well. This strategy is accepted and practicized by the authors of this book.

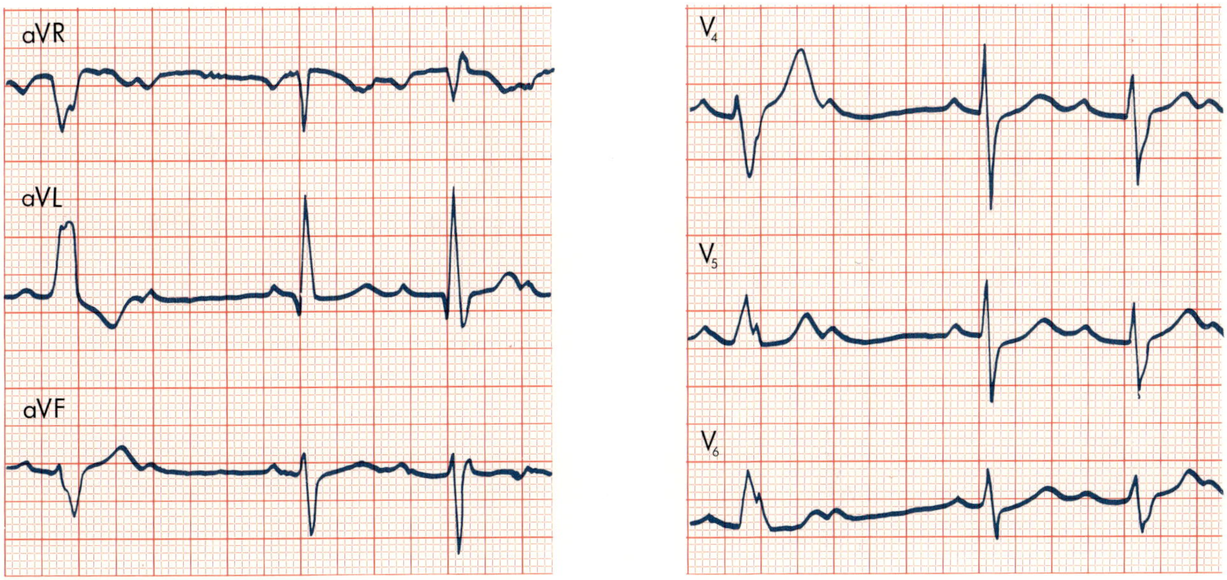

Fig. 10.15 (continued)

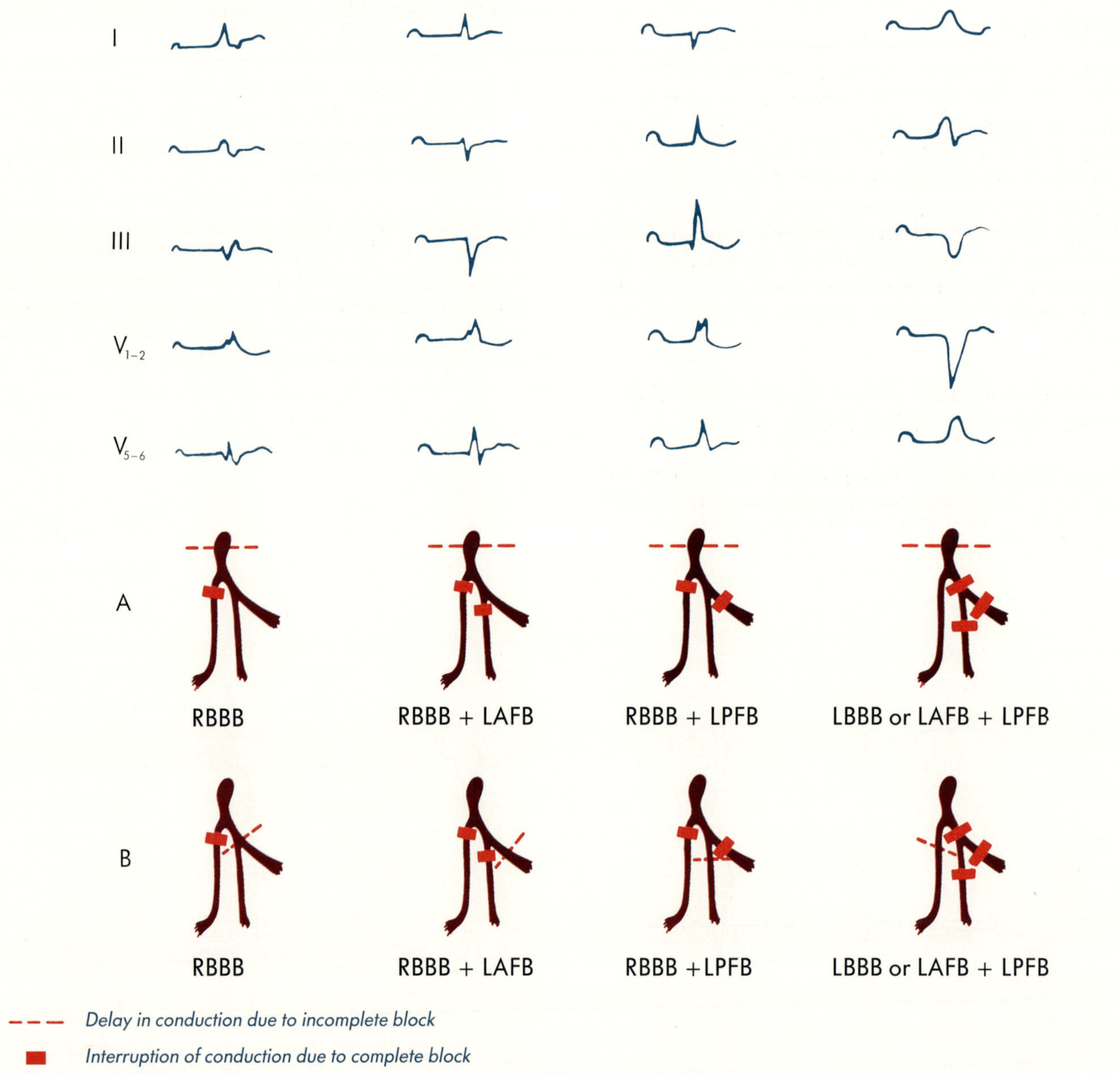

Fig. 10.16
Alternative sites of the first degree AV block in the patient in whom the ECG shows both first degree AV block (prolongation of the PR interval) and bundle block (widening of the QRS complex and BBB pattern) and maybe fascicular block (QRS axis deviation to the left or the right).

A Two-level lesion with proximal first degree AV block
B One-level lesion with distal first degree AV block

1. WHO ISFC Task Force, Definition of terms related to cardiac rhythm. Europ J Cardiol 1978; 8: 127–44.
2. Davies MJ, Anderson RH, Becker AE. The conduction system of the heart. London, Boston: Butterworths, 1983.
3. Demoulin J-C. The conduction system of the heart. Ingelheim am Rhein: Boehringer Ingelheim, 1986.
4. Puech P, Grolleau R. Localization of atrioventricular block. In: Puech P, Slama R, eds. The cardiac arrhythmias by the Arryhthmia Working Group of the French Cardiac Society. Paris: Corbière and Roussel, 1979; 139–50.
5. Slama R, Motte G, Grolleau R. Paroxysmal atrioventricular block. Indications for electrophysiological investigation and permanent pacing in patients in sinus rhythm. In: Puech P, Slama R, eds. The cardiac arrhythmias by the Arrhythmia Working Group of the French Cardiac Society. Paris: Corbière and Roussel, 1979; 151–63.
6. Puech P, Wainwright RJ. Clinical electrophysiology of atrioventricular block. In: Zipes DP, ed. Cardiol Clin 1983; 1: 209–24.
7. Fujimura O, Yee R, Klein GJ, et al. The diagnostic sensitivity of electrophysiologic testing in patients with syncope caused by transient bradycardia. New Engl J Med 1989; 321: 1703–07.
8. Bexton RS, Camm AJ. First degree atrioventricular block. Europ Heart J 1984; 5 (Suppl. A): 107–09.
9. Bexton RS, Camm AJ. Second degree atrioventricular block. Europ Heart J 1984; 5 (Suppl. A): 111–14.
10. Bjerregaard P. Mean 24 hour heart rate, minimal heart rate and pauses in healthy subjects at 40–79 years of age. Europ Heart J 1983; 4: 44–51.
11. Ingerslev J, Bjerregaard P. Prevalence and prognostic significance of cardiac arrhythmias detected by ambulatory electrocardiography in subjects 85 years of age. Europ Heart J 1986; 7: 570–75.
12. Huston TP, Puffer JC, MacMillan Rodney W. The athletic heart syndrome. New Engl J Med 1985; 313: 124–32.
13. Viitasalo MT, Kala R, Eisalo A. Ambulatory electrocardiographic findings in young athletes between 14 and 16 years of age. Europ Heart J 1984; 5: 2–6.
14. Roos JC, Dunning AJ. Bundle branch block in acute myocardial infarction. Europ J Cardiol 1978; 6: 403–24.
15. Haft JL. Clinical implications of atrioventricular and intraventricular conduction abnormalities. II. Acute myocardial infarction. Cardiovasc Clin 1977; 8: 65–77.
16. Tans AC, Lie KL, Durrer D. Clinical setting and prognostic significance of high degree atrioventricular block in acute inferior myocardial infarction. A study of 144 patients. Am Heart J 1980; 99: 4–8.
17. Johansson BW. Adams-Stokes syndrome. A review and follow-up study of forty-two cases. Am J Cardiol 1961; 8: 76–93.
18. Friedberg CK, Donoso E. Stein WG. Non-surgical aquired heart block. Ann NY Acad Sci 1964; 111: 835–47.
19. Edhag O, Swahn A. Prognosis of patients with complete heart block or arrhythmic syncope who were not treated with artifical pacemakers. A long-term follow-up study of 101 patients. Acta med scand 1976; 200: 457–63.
20. Jensen G, Sigurd B, Meibom J, et al. Adams-Stokes syndrome caused by paroxysmal third-degree atrioventricular block. Br heart J 1973; 35: 516–20.
21. Perelman M, Rowland E, Krikler DM. Torsade de pointes. A review. Int Med 1983; 11: 126–31.
22. Camm AJ, Bexton RS. Congenital complete heart block. Europ Heart J 1984; 5 (Suppl. A): 115–17.
23. Vilhelmsen R, Mortensen SA, Sandøe E. Diagnostic fallacies and drug management in Prinzmetal's variant angina. In: Mason DT, Collins JJ, eds. Myocardial revascularization. Medical and surgical advances in coronary disease. New York: Yorke Medical Books, 1981: 122–37.
24. Roberts NK, Somerville J. Pathological significance of electrocardiographic changes in aortic valve endocarditis. Br Heart J 1969; 31: 395–96.
25. Fowler NO, McCall D, Chou T-C, et al. Electrocardiographic changes and cardiac arrhythmias in patients receiving psychotropic drugs. Am J Cardiol 1976; 37: 223–30.
26. Hultén B-Å, Heath A. Clinical aspects of tricyclic antidepressant poisoning. Acta med scand 1983; 213: 275–78.
27. Lev M, Bharati S. Atrioventricular and intraventricular conduction disease. Arch Intern Med 1975; 135: 405–10.
28. Lenègre J. Bilateral bundle branch block. Cardiologia 1966; 48: 134–47.
29. Jensen G, Sigurd B. Atrioventricular block in aortic in sufficiency. Mechanism, ECG features and clinical consequences. Acta med scand 1972; 192: 391–94.
30. Wenger TL, Dohrmann ML, Strauss HC, et al. Hypersensitive carotid sinus syndrome manifested as cough syncope. Pace 1980; 3: 332–39.
31. Tomlinson IW, Fox KM. Carcinoma of the oesophagus with swallow syncope. Br Med J 1975; 2: 315–16.
32. Rasmussen V, Haunsø S, Skagen K. Cerebral attacks due to excessive vagal tone in heavily trained persons. A clinical and electrophysiologic study. Acta med scand 1978; 204: 401–05.
33. DiNardo-Ekery D, Abedin Z. High degree atrioventricular block in a marathoner with 5-year follow-up. Am Heart J 1987; 113: 835–37.
34. Northcote RJ, Rankin AC, Scullion R, et al. Is severe bradycardia in veteran athletes an indication for a permanent pacemaker? Br Med J 1989; 298: 231–32.
35. Bharati S, Dreifus LS, Chopskie E, et al. Conduction system in a trained jogger with sudden death. Chest 1988; 93: 348–51.

Chapter 11
Sinoatrial (SA) block and sinus arrest

Sinoatrial (SA) block and sinus arrest [1]

Sinoatrial (SA) block conceptually induces a ring of block around the normal pacemaker of the heart, the SA node. The block inhibits or halts impulse conduction from the SA node to the surrounding atrial myocardium. Like AV blocks, SA blocks are classified into blocks of first, second and third degree with a subclassification of the second degree block into types I and II. Within this spectrum of SA blocks, SA block of the first degree produces no ECG changes and SA block of second degree type I produces only minor changes in the form of a somewhat irregular sinus rhythm. Over a sequence of three or more P waves, the PP interval becomes slightly shorter, is then followed by a fairly long pause, then the PP interval shortens again and so on (Fig. 11.1, page 280). As neither of these types of SA blocks are of clinical significance the following section will focus on the clinically and ECG diagnostically more important forms of SA block: SA block of second degree type II, advanced SA block and SA block of third degree.

Sinus arrest is the failure of impulse formation in the SA node. Sinus arrest can be paroxysmal or persistent.

ECG diagnosis

Second degree SA block (type II)

Second degree SA block type II is characterized by an intermittent interruption in sinoatrial conduction recorded in the ECG by a missed PQRS complex. The PP interval which includes the missed PQRS complex is twice the length of the normal PP interval (Fig. 11.2). *Advanced* (second degree) SA block (Figs. 11.3 and 11.4, page 283) is characterized by alternate missed PQRS complexes (2:1 SA block) or of two or more successive PQRS complexes. Differentiating sinus bradycardia can be difficult unless the recording shows either the onset of the block when the rate suddenly halves or its termination when the rate suddenly doubles (Fig. 11.3). In advanced SA block the long pauses are multiples of the usual PP (or RR) interval (Figs. 11.3 and 11.4).

Third degree SA block and sinus arrest

The characteristic ECG finding in both third degree SA block and sinus arrest is an isoelectric line (without P waves) which continues until an escape rhythm, usually an AV nodal escape rhythm, supervenes or sinus rhythm is restored (Figs. 11.4–11.7, page 283 – page 287). While pauses due to SA block are multiples of the normal PP interval (Fig. 11.4) no such relationship is seen in sinus arrest. Third degree SA block is otherwise impossible to differentiate from sinus arrest.

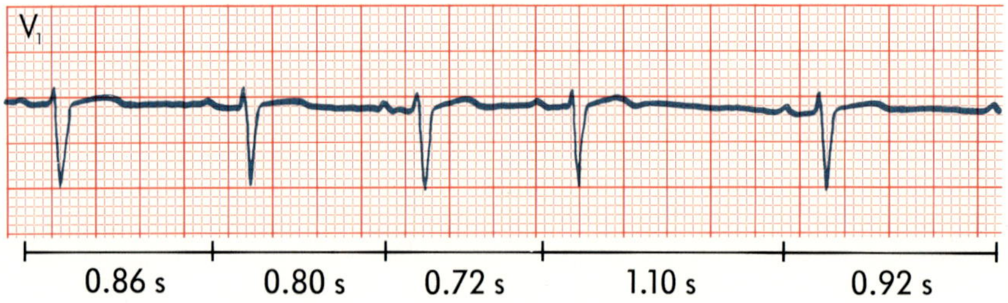

A Block cycle of four SA node impulses with a long pause followed by progressively shorter PP/RR intervals over two cycles and another long pause (4:3 conduction).

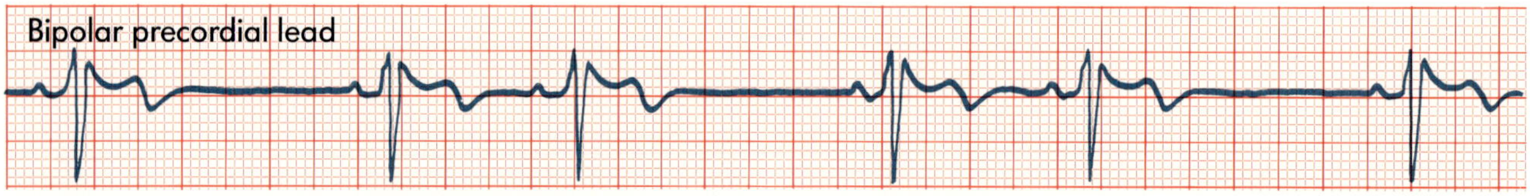

B Block cycle of three SA node impulses alternating between long and short PP/RR intervals (3:2 conduction). The differential diagnosis of atrial extrasystole with bigemy cannot be excluded, but the identical shape and height of the P waves favour the diagnosis of SA block type I. There is a widening and splitting of the QRS complex.

Fig. 11.1
Second degree SA block type I (Wenckebach block)

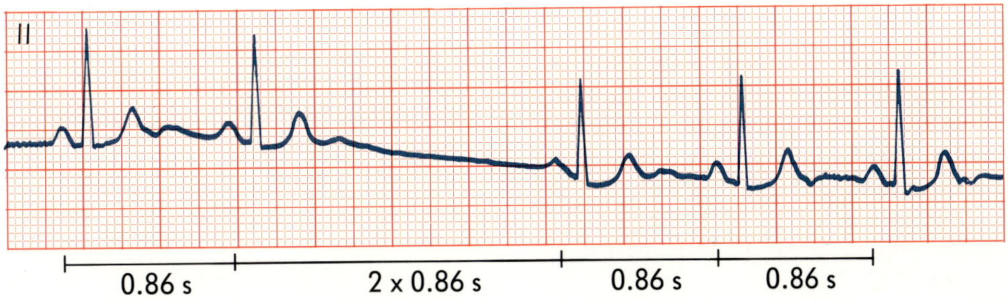

Fig. 11.2
Second degree SA block type II with dropout of a PQRS complex

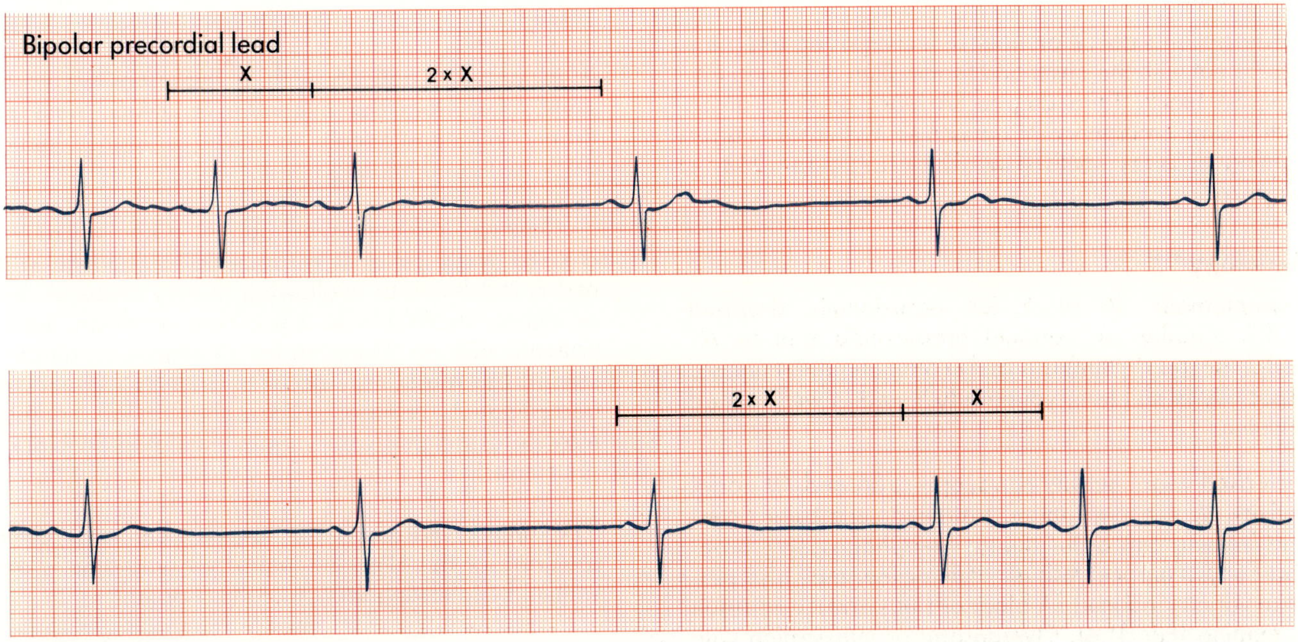

Fig. 11.3
Onset and termination of 2:1 SA block
The sinus rate is halved at the onset of the 2:1 SA block and doubled when it stops. The strips are not continuous. (Reduced size)

Differential diagnosis

The long (non-compensatory) pause after a blocked supraventricular extrasystole (Fig. 5.11 B, page 114) may be mistaken for second degree SA block or transitory sinus arrest. Due to its short coupling interval, the P wave (the only ECG manifestation of the extrasystole) will be superimposed on the T wave where its presence might be revealed only by a slight indentation in the contour of the T waves. Alternatively the P waves may be completely obscured by the T wave in which case they can be visualized by an oesophageal ECG. The differential diagnosis between 2:1 SA block (Fig. 11.3, page 281) and sinus bradycardia (Fig. 8.4, page 218) has been mentioned already (see ECG diagnosis).

SA block second degree type I (Fig. 11.1, page 280) resembles irregular sinus rhythm (Fig. 8.5, page 218) but is characterized by a repetitive pattern of progressive shortening of the PP interval with an occasional intervening long pause between P waves.

Symptoms

A few patients notice an uneasy feeling of an irregular heart beat with the onset and termination of second degree SA block. Third degree SA block or sinus arrest with a slow emergence of an escape rhythm can cause fainting or dizzy spells (Figs. 11.4–11.7, page 283 – page 287).

Aetiology [2–18]

Asymptomatic SA block (an occasionally dropped PQRS complex or transient bradycardia due to AV nodal escape rhythm) is a fairly common phenomenon, especially in children, young adults and in well trained athletes.

Increased vagal activity can suppress SA and AV nodal activity. By this mechanism, sustained ventricular arrest and fainting can occur during oesophagoscopy, bronchoscopy, pleurocentesis etc. Pain or fear may also provoke vagally induced SA block or sinus arrest and result in fainting (Fig. 11.6). Overdosage or intoxication with digitalis, verapamil or diltiazem, beta blocking agents, amiodarone or rarely other antiarrhythmic drugs can provoke SA block of second and third degree or sinus arrest.

Long-term antipsychotic treatment with lithium salts may cause sustained SA block and fainting.

Sinus bradycardia often alternating with AV nodal escape rhythm and sometimes with episodes of third degree SA block or sinus arrest are common arrhythmias during the first minutes and hours of an acute inferior infarction. Other causes of SA block and sinus arrest include myocarditis, cardiomyopathy and Prinzmetal's variant angina.

Hypersensitive carotid sinus. Gentle pressure on the one side of the neck in the region of the carotid sinus (Fig. 4.1, page 70) will in some individuals, particularly the elderly, induce an exaggerated vagal response resulting in:

– episodes of ventricular arrest due to SA block and sinus arrest (Fig. 11.5) or sometimes due to AV block, and/or

– hypotension due to vagally induced vasodepression unrelated to a slowing of the heart rate.

A minority of patients with a hypersensitive carotid sinus suffer from the *hypertensive carotid sinus syndrome* with spontaneous episodes of vagally induced dizzy spells and fainting.

Swallowing induced syncope. A pathologically increased vagal reflex is responsible for fainting which occurs in relation to swallowing. It may cause SA block or sometimes AV block. It is a rare condition, seen in patients with an oesophageal diverticulum, tumor or spasm, but rarely may occur in patients without overt oesophageal disease. Glossopharyngeal neuralgia may be associated with vagally mediated SA block or sinus arrest.

Sick sinus syndrome. The aetiological and clinical spectrum of this clincially important syndrome is dealt with in the following section of the chapter.

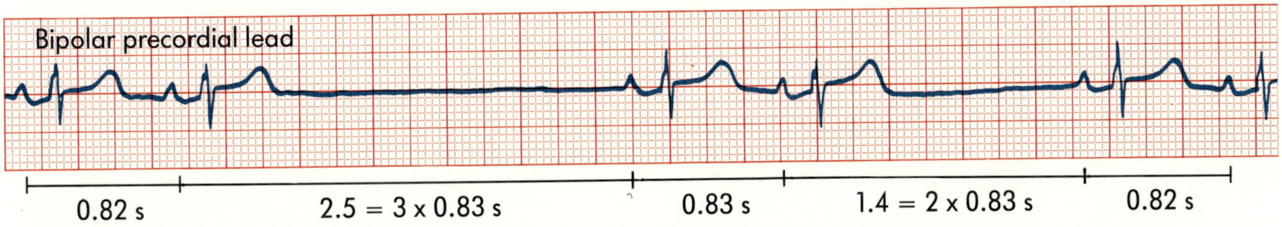

A 3:1 and 2:1 SA block

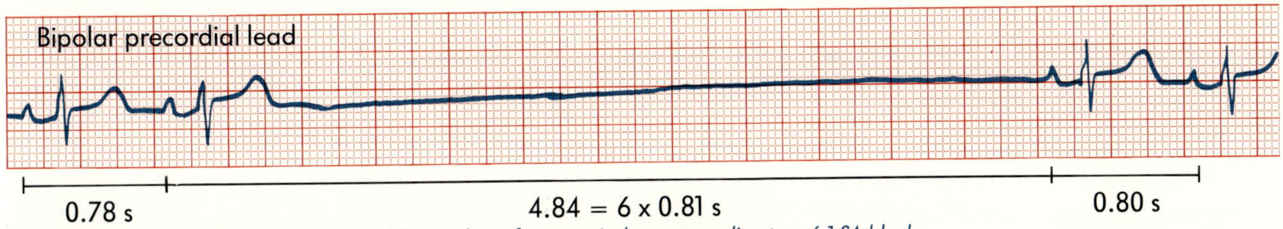

B A period of arrest without P waves or QRS complexes for a period corresponding to a 6:1 SA block

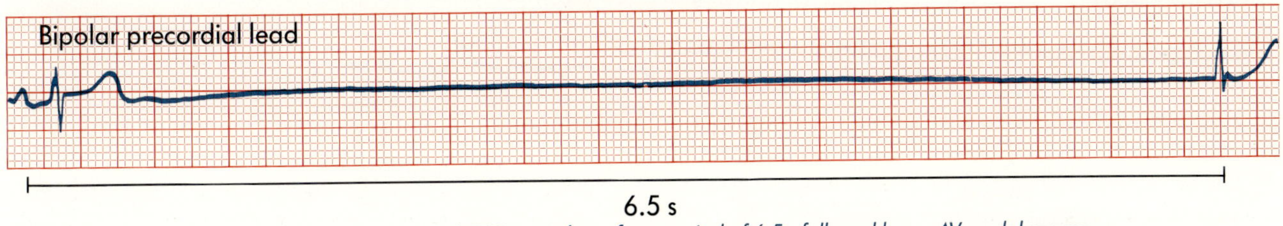

C Third degree SA block with missing P waves and QRS complexes for a period of 6.5 s followed by an AV nodal escape

Fig. 11.4
Advanced SA block and third degree SA block

ECG from a 73-year-old female with episodes of dizziness and fainting during the previous month. During 2 weeks of telemetric ECG monitoring there were repeated episodes like the one shown above associated with dizziness and occasional fainting. The symptoms disappeared with the implantation of a pacemaker.

Prognosis

Third degree SA block or sinus arrest as an isolated lesion (not accompanied by other conduction defects) rarely if ever causes death. The many subsidiary pacemaker centres in the conduction system, however, may be slow to respond with a risk of several seconds of ventricular arrest. Nonetheless they will, in time, take over the pacing of the heart and avert death.

Management

In an emergency, third degree SA block or sinus arrest will often respond to intravenous atropine or ipratropium bromide, or if these drugs fail, to an isoprenaline infusion. The possibility of drug intoxication should always be kept in mind. Treatment with drugs like beta blocking agents, verapamil, digitalis and various other antiarrhythmic drugs may predispose to block/bradycardia.

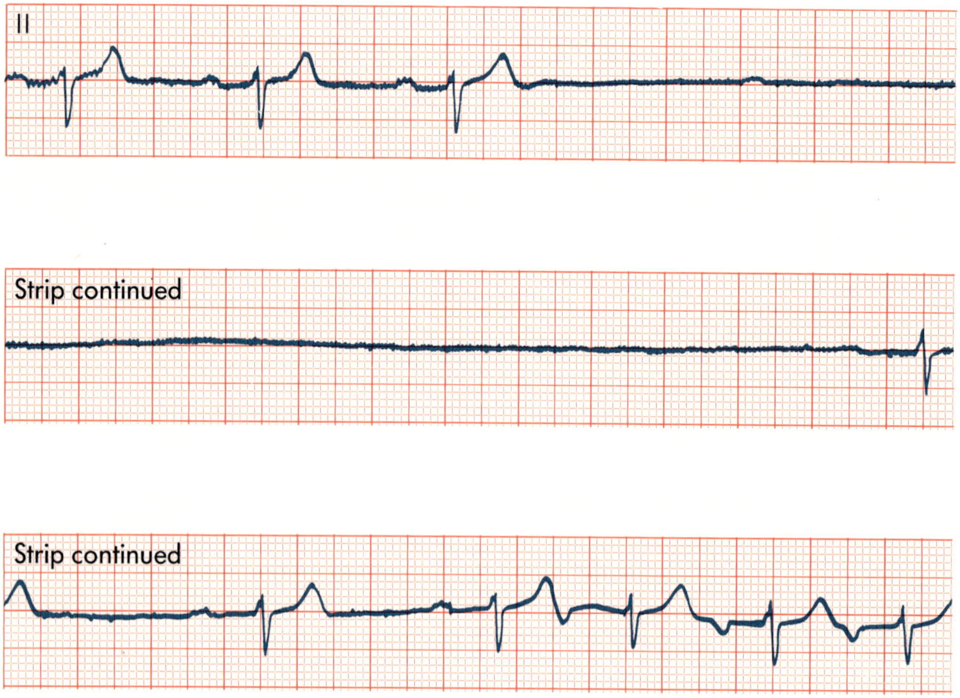

Fig. 11.5
Hypersensitive carotid sinus.

ECG recording during right carotid sinus massage (Fig. 4.1, p. 70). At the onset of the tracing, three sinus complexes at a rate of 56/min followed by third degree SA or sinus arrest with missing P waves and QRS complexes for a period of 8 s, sinus bradycardia at a rate of 42/min and later by AV nodal rhythm at a rate of 80/min.
The ECG is from a 73-year-old male with complaints of dizziness and black-outs related to turning his head quickly. The bradycardic reaction to carotid sinus massage could be suppressed by the i.v. injection of atropine.

In patients with symptoms due to *hypersensitive carotid sinus syndrome* (and other conditions with pathologically increased vagal reflexes) oral treatment with atropine or ipratropium bromide can be tried to prevent attacks of SA block and fainting. Such treatment, however, often proves impractible because effective dose causes intolerable side effects such as dryness of the mouth, blurred vision or urinary retention. The reported symptomatic relief achieved by the implantation of ventricular pacemakers (VVI) for some reason or another has been disappointing. Relatively good symptomatic relief has been achieved using atrial pacemakers (AAI) for patients with episodes of SA block or sinus arrest and dual chamber pacemakers (DDD) for patients with AV block or combined SA and AV block. Since pacemaker implantation does not counteract the vasodepressor effect of increased vagal tone, pacemaker therapy will be unsuccessful in patients in whom vagally induced vasodepression contributes significantly to their symptoms.

In the *sick sinus syndrome*, pacemaker implantation often is required to alleviate dizzy spells and fainting (see next section).

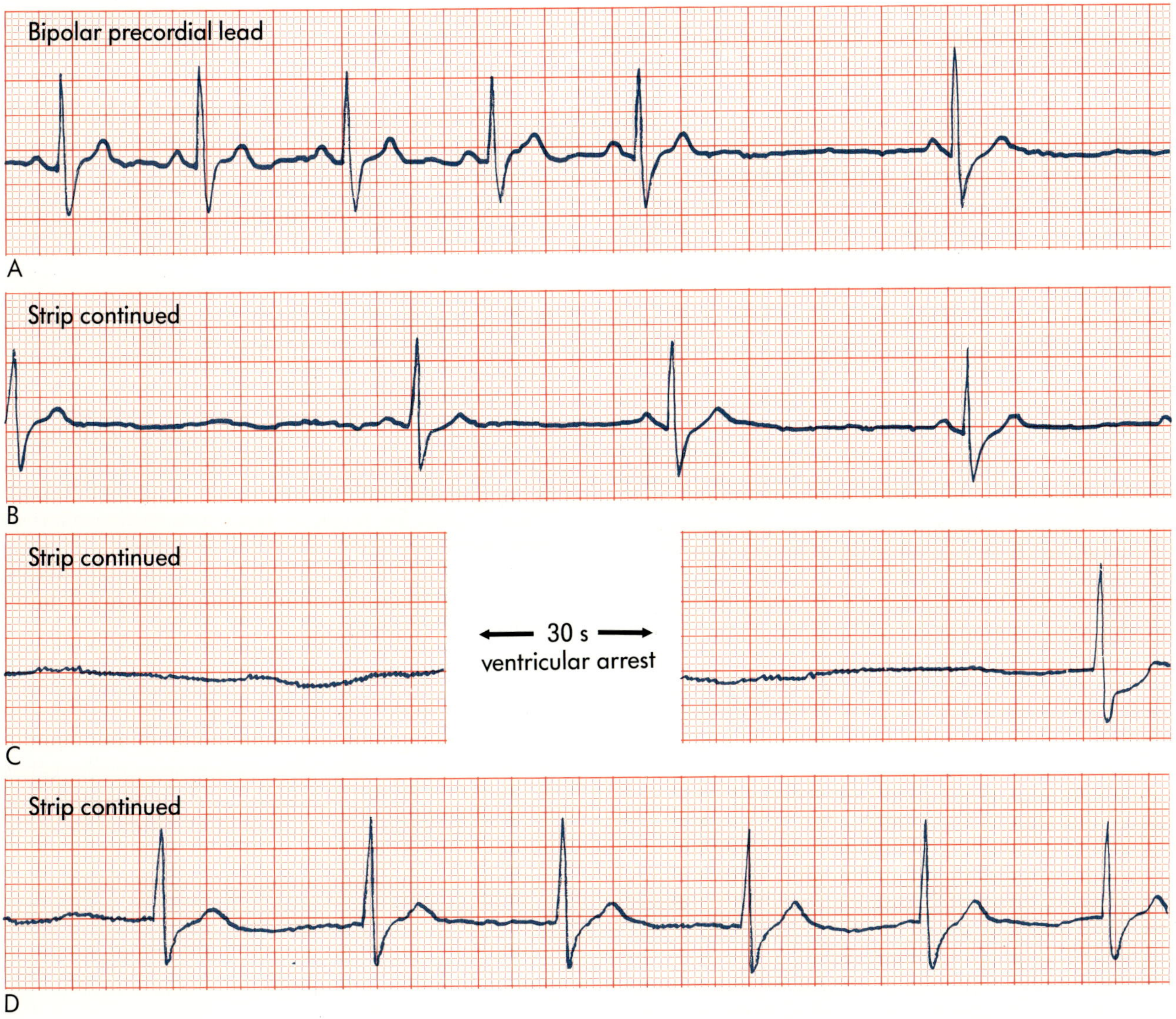

Fig. 11.6
Fear/anxiety induced SA block causing fainting
ECG monitoring during a fainting attack in a 35-year-old healthy male. After the fourth child he had been persuaded by his wife to undergo vasectomy but he remained reluctant toward and apprehensive for the operative procedure. Lying on the operation table – and while the nurse was loading the syringe for the local anaesthesia – he suddenly passed out. He soon recovered and after application of the local anaesthesia the vasectomy was performed without further complications.
A Sinus rhythm of a rate of 65–70/min with a sudden change to a 2:1 SA conduction
B Sinus bradycardia, irregular sinus rhythm and/or SA block
C Sinus arrest for 35 seconds
D AV nodal escape rhythm (rate 55/min)

Sick sinus syndrome [19, 20]

The term sick sinus syndrome is used to describe a chronic condition with episodic or persistent supraventricular arrhythmias *combined with* recurrent faints or near faints due to SA block or sinus arrest.

The sick sinus syndrome can develop at any age but is most frequent in the sixth and seventh decades of life, a decade earlier than the Stokes-Adams syndrome. The annual rate of new cases of sick sinus syndrome requiring pacemaker implantation, is around 100 per million; a figure of the same order of magnitude as that for Stokes-Adams syndrome.

ECG diagnosis

Some patients suffer only from supraventricular bradycardia (Fig. 11.5, page 284): sinus bradycardia, AV nodal escape rhythm, SA block of second degree, atrial extrasystole with prolonged postextrasystolic pauses or occasionally atrial fibrillation or flutter with slow ventricular rate. More than half of the patients, however, have the so-called tachycardia/bradycardia syndrome characterized by alternation between (Fig. 11.7):

- Attacks of tachycardia, most often atrial fibrillation or flutter (with fast ventricular rate) or, occasionally, AV nodal or atrial tachycardia, and
- Episodes of supraventricular bradycardia of the forementioned types.

Both groups of patients have intermittent attacks of SA block or sinus arrest with sustained ventricular arrest lasting long enough (5 s or more) to cause fainting or near fainting (Figs. 11.4, page 283, 11.5 and 11.7). In the tachycardia/bradycardia syndrome the episodes of ventricular arrest follow the attacks of tachycardia (Fig. 11.7). Sinus rhythm can exist for long periods of time, weeks or months.

Concomitant bundle branch block is seen in 15–20 % of the patients and AV block in additional 10 %.

Differential diagnosis [21, 22]

The diagnosis of sick sinus syndrome should always be considered when recurrent attacks of fainting or dizzy spells develop after the age of 50–60 years especially in association with complaints of palpitation or a history of prior episodes of tachycardia. As in Stokes-Adams syndrome the clinical differential diagnoses are many (see Stokes-Adams syndrome, differential diagnosis, page 264).

As the between-attack ECG in patients with the sick sinus syndrome is non-diagnostic or at best only suggestive of the diagnosis, the primary diagnostic tool is long-term ECG monitoring.

This may be performed by telemetry in the hospitalized patient, or, since the suspected arrhythmia usually is not life threatening, by ambulatory ECG monitoring with a small portable tape recorder (Holter monitoring). Positive evidence of "sick sinus" induced fainting or dizzy spells is provided by the simultaneous ECG recording of an episode of ventricular arrest (> 4 seconds) related to third degree SA block or sinus arrest often alternating with paroxysms of tachycardia (Fig. 11.7). Definite evidence against a cardiac origin of the fainting would be the finding of undisturbed cardiac activity on the ECG at the time of symptoms.

An electrophysiologic study which reveals a prolonged SA node recovery time following rapid atrial pacing is strongly suggestive of a diagnosis of sick sinus syndrome. The recording of a normal sinus node recovery, however, does not preclude the diagnosis as in about half the patients with recurrent fainting due to SA block or sinus arrest the test is normal.

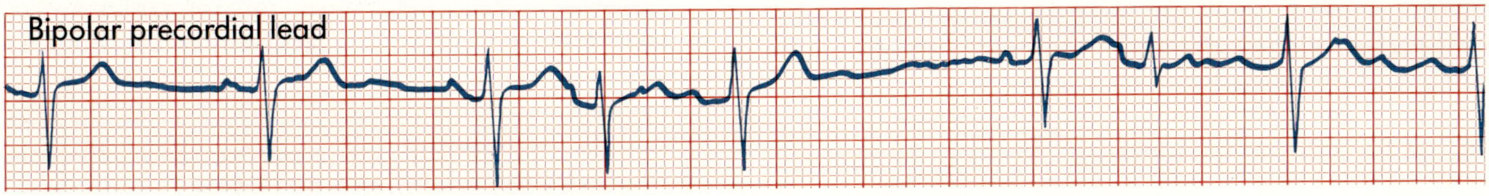

A Alternation between sinus bracycardia and atrial flutter

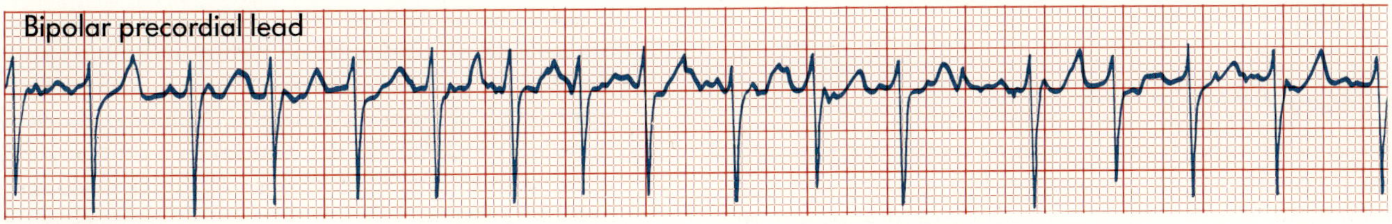

B Atrial flutter

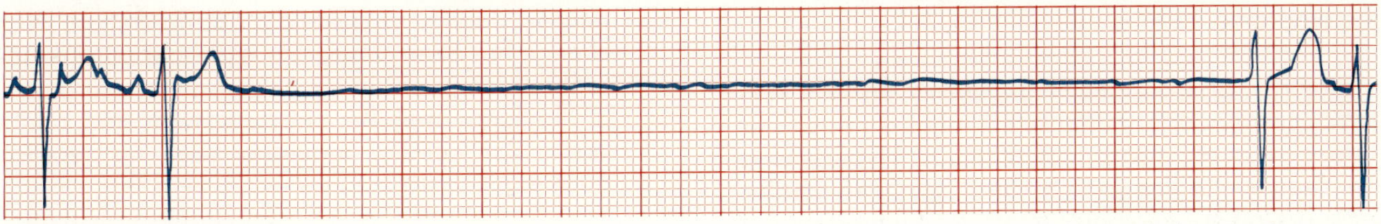

C The end of an episode of atrial flutter followed by SA block or sinus arrest with no signs of atrial activity for a period of 5.5 s ending with an AV nodal escape

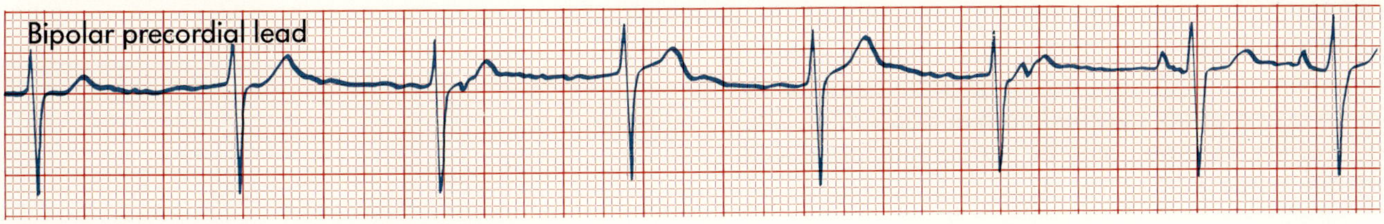

D AV nodal rhythm followed by two sinus complexes

Fig. 11.7
Sequences from continuous telemetric ECG monitoring in the sick sinus syndrome
ECG from a 78-year-old male with a 20-year history of attacks of palpitations sometimes associated with dizzy spells or fainting. The attacks of tachycardia had become more frequent and troublesome in recent years. Treatment with digoxin and later beta blockade was associated with an increased tendency for fainting. Implantation of an artificial pacemaker supplemented by continued antiarrhythmic treatment finally led to satisfactory management of the block as well as of the tachycardia.

Symptoms

Fainting and dizzy spells are the principal symptoms of the "bradycardia syndrome". Alternate palpitations, fainting and dizzy spells are characteristic of the tachycardia/bradycardia syndrome. Congestive failure or angina can be induced by sustained attacks of tachycardia.

Cerebrovascular accidents due to arterial embolism can occur in the tachycardia/bradycardia syndrome (see prognosis).

Aetiology [22–25]

Most clinical reports of sick sinus syndrome patients have detailed a high percentage (40–70 %) *without* concomitant heart disease. Pathological studies on a limited number of autopsied cases have revealed severe fibrosis of the SA node and parts of the atrium and sometimes the AV node as the histological background of the syndrome.

The majority of the remaining patients present with chronic coronary artery disease e.g. angina pectoris or a history of an old myocardial infarction. Hypertensive heart disease, cardiomyopathy and rheumatic cardiac disease are other aetiologic factors in an important but smaller group of patients.

Prognosis [26–32]

Survival in patients with sick sinus syndrome but without concomitant heart disease does not differ significantly from an age and sex matched normal population. The quality of life, however, may be severely impaired and morbidity increased due to:

- Recurrence of the attacks of fainting or dizzy spells over years at unpredictable time intervals. While the underlying arrhythmias do not endanger life, intermittent syncope makes patients feel insecure and fearful. Eventually unexpected fainting can be complicated by trauma or the blackouts can cause traffic accidents.

- Systemic embolism which occurs in patients with tachycardia/bradycardia syndromes, primarily those with known organic heart disease and/or an enlarged hearts. The annual rate of cerebrovascular accidents in tachycardia/bradycardia syndromes is in the range of 5–10 %.

Over time the clinical and electrocardiographic profile of the sick sinus syndrome may change:

- From fainting due to paroxysms of SA block or sinus arrest to fainting secondary to paroxysms of AV block; i.e. a change from sick sinus syndrome to Stokes-Adams syndrome or a mixture of the two syndromes. In patients with no AV block at the initial diagnosis of sick sinus syndrome (including those with bundle branch block) the annual rate of newly developed second and third degree AV block does not exceed 1–2 %.

- In the tachycardia/bradycardia syndromes paroxysms of atrial fibrillation may give way to phases of relative stability in chronic atrial fibrillation. Such a change has been claimed to represent possible spontaneous remission. In fact, conversion to chronic atrial fibrillation may be associated with slow unstable ventricular activity, requiring back up ventricular pacing.

Management [28–36]

While there is no absolute indication for pacemaker implantation in the patient who has only a few attacks of fainting with months or maybe years in between, pacing is the treatment of choice to improve the quality of life for the patient who has frequent recurrent attacks.

The optimal pacing mode has been a matter of debate. When feasible atrial pacing is preferable to ventricular pacing as there is a five to ten fold higher conversion rate from paroxysmal to chronic atrial fibrillation with ventricular pacing (30 % over a period of some years, compared to 2–4 % only in atrial pacing). Suspected but not confirmed is a higher incidence of thromboembolic complications in the ventricular paced patients (significantly increased in one series, not in others). Moreover, whereas atrial pacing ensures AV synchrony, ventricular pacing is apt to produce AV asynchrony with associated side effects in the form of the pacemaker syndrome (a feeling of uneasiness, weakness and distressing pulsations in the neck or chest related to simultaneous atrial and ventricular activations, Chapter 4, page 99).

In the patient with AV and/or intraventricular conduction defects the minor risk of cardiac arrest due to AV block can be avoided by the implantation of a dual chamber pacemaker. To avoid pacemaker mediated AV transmission of fast atrial tachycardias, the pacemaker should be programmed for DDI pacing. In the DDI mode (Table 4.3, page 91) the pacemaker provides both atrial and ventricular pacing when required, but the AV logistics of the pulse generator will be "locked", so that atrial sensing will not trigger subsequent ventricular pacing as would be the case with DDD pacing.

For the patient with a depressed sinus node response to exercise and stress, the optimal pacemaker would be one of the rate responsive type (AAI-R or DDI-R).

Most patients with tachycardia/bradycardia syndromes require supplementary antiarrhythmic treatment for their attacks of supraventricular tachycardia. Prior to pacemaker implantation such antiarrhythmic treatment could well have precipitated fainting but after pacing, antiarrhythmic drugs can be administered without concern for further depression of SA node function.

Long-term anticoagulation treatment should be considered for patients with tachycardia/bradycardia syndrome when there is associated organic heart disease and/or an enlarged heart.

References Chapter 11

1. WHO/ISFC Task Force. ed. Definition of terms related to cardiac rhythm. Europ J Cardiol 1978; 8: 127–44.
2. Bjerregaard P. Mean 24 hour heart rate, minimal heart rate and pauses in healthy subjects at 40-79 years of age. Europ Heart J 1983; 4: 44–51.
3. Ingerslev J, Bjerregaard P. Prevalence and prognostic significance of cardiac arrhythmias detected by ambulatory electrocardiography in subjects 85 years of age. Europ Heart J 1986; 7: 570–75.
4. Scott O, Williams GJ, Fiddler GI. Results of 24 hour ambulatory monitoring of electrogram in 131 healthy boys aged 10 to 13 years. Br Heart J 1980; 40: 304–08.
5. Brodsky M, Wu D, Denes P, et al. Arrhythmias documented by 24 hour continuous electrocardiographic monitoring in 50 male medical students without apparent heart disease. Am J Cardiol 1977; 39: 390–95.
6. Guilleminault C, Pool P, Motta J, et al. Sinus arrest during REM sleep in young adults. New Engl J Med 1984; 311: 1006–10.
7. Huston TP, Puffer JC, MacMillan Rodney W. The athletic heart syndrome. New Engl J Med 1985; 313: 24–32.
8. Viitasalo MT, Kala R, Eisalo A. Ambulatory electrocardiographic findings in young athletes between 14 and 16 years of age. Europ Heart J 1984; 5: 2–6.
9. Shaw DB, Southall DP. Sinus node arrest and sino-atrial block. Europ Heart J 1984; 5 (Suppl. A): 83–87.
10. Rasmussen V, Haunsø S, Skagen K. Cerebral attacks due to excessive vagal tone in heavily trained persons. A clinical and electrophysiologic study. Acta med scand 1978; 204: 401–05.
11. Wik B, Hillestad L. Deglutition syncope. Br Med J 1975; 2: 747.
12. Tomlinson JW, Fox KM. Carcinoma of the oesophagus with "swallow syncope". Br Med J 1975; 2: 315–16.
13. Jacobsen RR, Ross Russell RW. Glossopharyngeal neuralgia with cardiac arrhythmia. A rare but treatable cause of syncope. Br Med J 1979; 1: 379–80.
14. Montalescot G, Levy Y, Hatt PY. Serious sinus node dysfunction caused by therapeutic doses of lithium. Int J Cardiol 1984; 5: 94–96.
15. Adgey AAJ, Geddes JS, Mulholland HC, et al. Incidence, significance, and management of early bradyarrhythmia complicating acute myocardial infarction. Lancet 1968; 2: 1097–1101.
16. Hatte L, Bathen J, Rokseth R. Sinoatrial disease in acute myocardial infarction. Long-term prognosis. Br Heart J 1976; 38: 410–14.
17. Morley CA, Sutton R. Carotid sinus syncope. Int J Cardiol 1984; 6: 287–93.
18. Strasberg B, Sagie A, Erdman S, et al. Carotid sinus hypersensitivity and the carotid sinus syndrome. Prog Cardiovasc Dis 1989; 31: 379–91.
19. Ferrer MI. The sick sinus syndrome. Circulation 1973; 47: 635–41.
20. Sigurd B, Jensen G, Meibom J, et al. Adams-Stokes syndrome caused by sinoatrial block. Br Heart J 1973; 35: 1002–08.
21. Reiffel JA. Electrophysiologic evaluation of sinus node function. Cardiol Clin 1986; 4: 401–16.
22. Fujimura O, Yee R, Klein GJ, et al. The diagnostic sensitivity of electrophysiologic testing in patients with syncope caused by transient bradycardia. New Engl J Med 1989; 321: 1703–07.
23. Demoulin J-C, Kulbertus HE. Histopathological correlates of sinoatrial disease. Br Heart J 1978; 40: 1384–89.
24. Davies MJ, Anderson RH, Becker AE. The conduction system of the heart. London, Boston: Butterworths, 1983.
25. Demoulin J-C. The conduction system of the heart. Ingelheim am Rhein: Boehringer Ingelheim, 1988.
26. Shaw DB, Holman RR, Gowers JI. Survival in sinoatrial disorder (sick-sinus syndrome). Br Med J 1980; 280: 139–41.
27. Rasmussen K. Chronic sinus node disease: Natural course and indications for pacing. Europ Heart J 1981; 2: 455–59.
28. Breivik K, Ohm O-J, Segadal L. Sick sinus syndrome treated with permanent pacemaker in 109 patients. Acta med scand 1979; 206: 153–59.
29. Simonsen E, Nielsen JS, Nielsen BL. Sinus node dysfunction in 128 patients: A retrospective study with follow-up. Acta med scand 1980; 208: 343–48.
30. Simonsen E. Sinus node dysfunction. A prospective clinical study with special reference to the diagnostic value of ambulatory electrocardiography, electrophysiologic study and exercise testing. Odense: CAVI, 1987.
31. Sutton R, Kenny R-A. The natural history of sick sinus syndrome. Pace 1986; 9: 1110-14.
32. The natural history of sick sinus syndrome and automatic disturbances of heart rate control: Sick sinus syndrome, carotid sinus syndrome and malignant vasovagal syndrome. New Trends Arrhythmias 1989; V: 125–29.
33. Rosenqvist M, Obel IWP. Atrial pacing and the risk for AV block: Is there a time for change in attitude? Pace 1989; 12: 97.
34. Rosenqvist M, Brandt J, Schüller H. Long-term pacing in sinus node disease: Effects of stimulation mode on cardiovascular morbidity and mortality. Am Heart J 1988; 116: 16.
35. Hatano K, Kato R, Hayashi H, et al. Usefulness of rate responsive atrial pacing in patients with sick sinus syndrome. Pace 1989; 12: 16.
36. Markewitz A, Schad N, Hemmer W, et al. What is the most appropriate stimulation mode in patients with sinus node dysfunction? Pace 1986; 9: 1115–20.

Chapter 12
Digitalis and the ECG

"Digitalis effects" on the ECG[1,2]

In many but not all patients receiving a digitalis preparation in therapeutic doses, the ECG will show characteristic changes referred to as "digitalis effects" (Fig. 12.1). The changes usually are most prominent in leads with tall R waves and include:

1 Flattening or inversion of the T wave

2 Downward sloping ST segment depression. The depression often has a characteristic sagging with its concavity upwards

3 Slight shortening of the QT interval

4 Modest PR prolongation up to 0.24 s.

"Digitalis effects" are associated with digitalis therapy but provide no clue as to whether the given digitalis dose is toxic, adequate or too low. Digitalis effects, however, introduce diagnostic problems in respect of the ST segment and T wave as in ventricular hypertrophy, myocardial infarction and ischaemia (Fig. 14.36, page 358).

Digitalis intoxication[1,3–5]

With increasing severity of digitalis intoxication a wide spectrum of arrhythmias may occur including benign sinus bradycardia, ventricular extrasystoles, SA block or AV block of first degree or Mobitz type one second de-

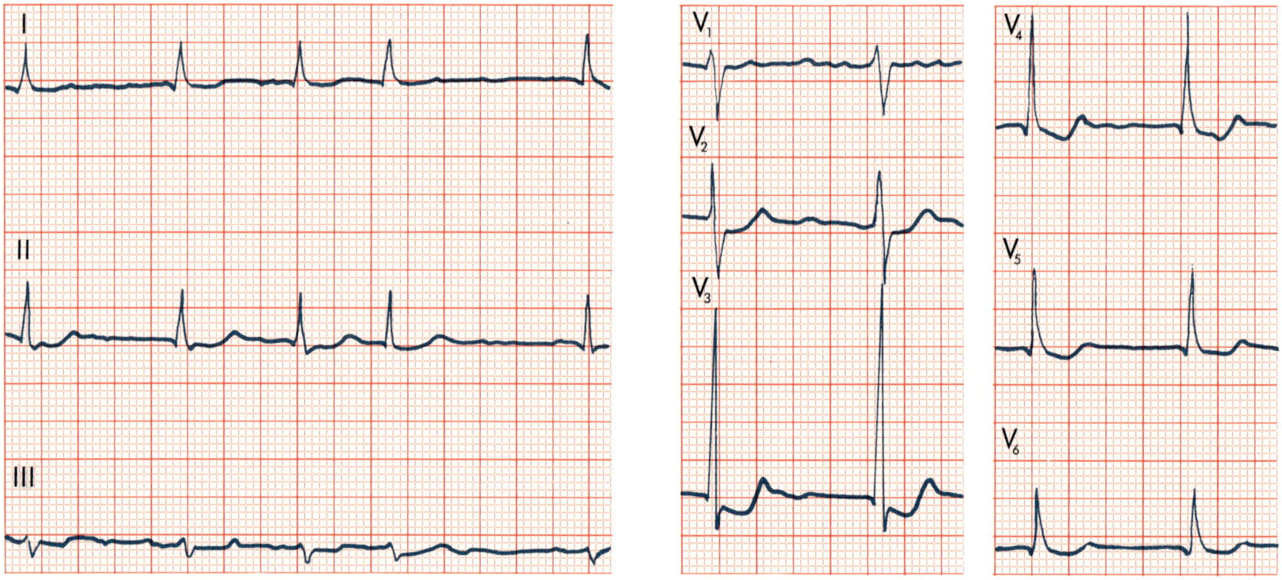

Fig. 12.1
Digitalis treated atrial fibrillation
The irregular QRS rate is 75–80/min and there is no ventricular ectopic activity so the atrial fibrillation is "well regulated" by the digitalis treatment. A "digitalis effect" (Cohn effect) in the form of a concave ST segment depression is apparent in several leads.

gree, and life threatening ventricular tachycardia and fibrillation. The arrhythmias may be preceded or accompanied by non-cardiac side effects in the form of nausea, vomiting, diarrhoea, blurred vision or, rarely, disturbed colour vision (green or yellow halos around lights). Often, however, arrhythmias are the sole manifestation of digitalis intoxication. The therapeutic action of digitalis probably is related to an indirect electrophysiological effect on the cardiac cell mediated via the autonomic nervous system but the arrhythmias are a direct effect of the drug on the cardiac cell.

Low serum potassium, low serum magnesium and high serum calcium increase sensitivity to digitalis. Myxoedema is associated with high sensitivity to digitalis and thyrotoxicosis with a lowered sensitivity. Patients with chronic pulmonary disease and cor pulmonale are particularly prone to develop digitalis induced arrhythmias.

Combination treatment with quinidine reduces the renal excretion of digoxin by approximately 50 % and combined treatment with amiodarone and verapamil by 30 and 10–15 % respectively. Thus, to avoid digoxin intoxication the daily digoxin intake has to be halved in the quinidine treated patient and reduced somewhat in the patient who receives amiodarone or verapamil.

Digitalis induced arrhythmias[6–8]

The spectrum of digitalis induced arrhythmias changes with the severity of the digitalis intoxication:

A *Arrhythmias observed with slight digitalis overdosage*

- Sinus bradycardia or in patients with atrial flutter or fibrillation a slow ventricular rate of 40–60/min

- First degree AV block with a PR of 0.25–0.40 s (Fig. 10.3, page 250)

- Ventricular extrasystoles and often periodic or persistent bigeminy or trigeminy

- Second degree SA block

- Second degree AV block of Mobitz type I (Wenckebach's block).

Management. The drug should be withheld for a few days. Serum potassium, serum creatinine and possibly serum digoxin should be checked. Hypokalaemia should be corrected by the administration of a potassium salt and/or a potassium sparing diuretic and if digoxin is to be restarted, its dosage should be adjusted.

B *Arhythmias observed with significant digitalis overdosage*

- Multifocal ventricular extrasystoles and ventricular extrasystoles in pairs or salvos

- AV nodal escape rhythm or accelerated AV nodal rhythm

- Paroxysmal atrial tachycardia with block.

Management. Hospitalization with continuous ECG monitoring in the CCU and the above measures should be considered.

C *Arrhythmias associated with severe intoxication*

- Non-paroxysmal AV nodal tachycardia at a rate of 100–200/min
- Paroxysmal third degree SA block or sinus arrest complicated by ventricular arrest and syncope
- Third degree AV block with AV nodal escape rhythm (Fig. 10.6 A, page 254) sometimes alternating with ventricular arrest and associated with syncope
- Ventricular tachycardia especially bifocal tachycardia (AV nodal and ventricular or atrial and ventricular) or bidirectional tachycardia (Fig. 6.37, page 172)
- Recurrent attacks of rapid ventricular tachycardia and/or ventricular fibrillation.

Management. The risk of cardiac arrest is high and the patient should be hospitalized without delay for continuous ECG monitoring in a CCU. Guidelines for the treatment of the various types of arrhythmias are given in the section on management of serious digoxin intoxication at the end of the chapter.

Differential diagnosis of digitalis induced arrhythmias [4–9]

A common and unsolved question is whether new arrhythmias developing during digitalis treatment are caused by the drug or are merely coincidental arrhythmogenic events for which more digitalis might be indicated. Assessment of the following variables will assist in resolving that problem, e.g.:

A *The degree of digitalis accumulation in the organism.* The digitalis balance can be estimated by comparing the daily digitalis dosage with the assumed daily excretion assessed from the weight, age and renal function of the patient.

B *The serum digoxin level.* Arrythmogenic complications occur most often with serum digoxin concentrations above 2.5 nanomol/l (2.0 nanog/l) or for digitoxin above 30 nanog/l. A serum digoxin less than 1.0 nanomol (0.8 nanog/l) or a serum digitoxin less than 12 nanog/l all but excludes digitalis intoxication, while a serum digoxin of less than 2.5 nanomol/l (2.0 nanog/l) or a serum digitoxin of less than 25 nanog/l makes it less likely.

C *Serum electrolytes.* A low serum potassium and/or low serum magnesium and/or increased serum calcium increases the sensitivity to digitalis and predisposes to digitalis intoxication.

Suicidal ingestion of large amounts of digitalis e.g. 5–20 mg of digoxin often releases potassium from muscle increasing the serum potassium to levels of 6–8 millimol/l. The prognosis is bad for patients with a digitalis induced hyperkalaemia when levels are above 6.5 millimol/l.

D *The type of arrhythmia.* Although digitalis can induce almost any arrhythmia, some are rarely if ever induced by digitalis intoxication. These include parasystole, second degree AV block of Mobitz type II, atrial flutter and bundle branch block. Infrequently atrial fibrillation may be induced by digitalis.

E *Non-cardiac symptoms of digitalis intoxication.* Symptoms such as nausea, vomiting, diarrhoea, blurred vision or disturbed colour vision (green or yellow halos around lights) favour a diagnosis of digitalis intoxication.

F *Time correlation between digitalis withdrawal and arrhythmia improvement.*

Management of acute serious digoxin intoxication [1, 3–5, 10–15]

In patients who have consumed large quantities of digitalis by mistake or in attempted suicide the stomach should be emptied of all remaining tablets as fast as possible. Oral cholestyramine binds digitalis glycoside and hinders its absorption from the intestine. Cholestyramine is indicated in all cases of *digitoxin* intoxication because it inhibits the enterohepatic cycle of digitoxin (digitoxin is eliminated via the bile but reabsorbed again by the small intestine).

Obviously, all digitalis medication should be stopped. When there is hypokalaemia, potassium salts should be administered. Perhaps, even the normokalaemic patient's serum potassium concentration should be brought to the upper end of normal. In AV block, potassium should be given only when the serum potassium is low because a high serum potassium and perhaps rapid increase in serum potassium can inhibit atrio-ventricular conduction and thus worsen an atrio-ventricular block.

Ventricular tachycardia and ventricular fibrillation are treated with lignocaine, diphenylhydantoin or beta blocking agents. At present there is inadequate data to determine which is best. Good results have also been reported with intravenous magnesium sulfate, even in patients with normal serum magnesium levels. Quinidine and amiodarone should not be used as they interact with digoxin at the renal level.

As there is a risk of precipitating new and dangerous arrhythmias, DC cardioversion should be used only in attacks of life threatening tachycardia and should employ the lowest possible power setting, e.g. starting at 10 J. For symptomatic AV and SA block atropine should be given intravenously. If ineffective, temporary pacing is required.

Life threatening cardiac arrhythmias caused by severe *digoxin* intoxication can be successfully suppressed within 30–60 min by the intravenous administration of digoxin specific antibody fragments (FAB). It is an expensive treatment but as severe digoxin intoxication has a bad prognosis, it should be started as soon as possible in the patient:

- Who has taken 10 mg or more of digoxin or who by mistake has been given an i.v. injection of 5 mg or more.
- With digoxin induced rise in serum potassium to 6.0 millimol/l or more.
- With recurrent attacks of ventricular tachycardia or fibrillation refractory to lignocaine.

References Chapter 12

1. Smith TW. Digitalis. Mechanisms of action and clinical use. In: Epstein FH, ed. Mechanism of disease. New Engl J Med 1988; 77: 358–76.
2. Saner HE, Lange HW, Pierach CA, et al. Relation between serum digoxin concentration and the electrocardiogram. Clin Cardiol 1988; 11: 752–56.
3. Marcus FI, Opie LH, Sonnenblick EH. Digitalis, sympathometics and inotropic-dilators. In: Opie LH. Drugs for the heart. Orlando, New York, London: Grune & Stratton, Inc., 1987; 91–110.
4. Smith TW, Antman EM, Friedman PL, et al. Digitalis glycosides: Mechanisms and manifestations of toxicity. Prog Cardiovasc Dis 1984; 27: 21–56.
5. Storstein L. Digitoxin intoxication. Am Heart J 1977; 93: 434–43.
6. Wellens HJJ. The electrocardiogram in digitalis in toxication. In: Yu PN, Goodwin JF, eds. Progress in cardiology. Philadelphia: Lea & Febiger, 1976; 271–90.
7. Marriott HJL. Conover MH. Advanced concepts in arrhythmias. Digitalis dysrhythmias. St. Louis: The C.V. Mosby Co., 1983; 324–38.
8. Fisch C, Knoebel SB. Digitalis cardiotoxicity. JACC 1985; 5: 91–98.
9. Surawicz B. Factors affecting tolerance to digitalis. JACC 1985; 5: 69–81.
10. Smith TW, Butler VP Jr, Haber E, et al. Treatment of life-threatening digitalis intoxication with digoxin-specific Fab fragments. Experience in 26 cases. New Engl J Med 1982; 307: 1357.
11. Lignian H, Vincent JL, Hallemans R. Treatment of severe digitoxin intoxication by digoxin-specific Fab antibody fragments. Acta Cardiol 1984; 39: 301–05.
12. Citrin D, Stevenson IH, O'Malley K. Massive digoxin over dose. Observations on hyperkalaemia and plasma digoxin levels. Scott Med J 1972; 17: 275.
13. Bismuth C, Motté G, Fréjaville JP, et al. L'hyperkaliémie dans l'intoxication digitalique massive. Valeur pronostique et implications thérapeutiques. Arch Mal Coeur 1973; 66: 1537–41.
14. Wenger TL, Butler VP, Haber E, et al. Treatment of 63 severely digitalis-toxic patients with digoxin-specific antibody fragments. JACC 1985; 5: 118–23.
15. Proudfoot AT. A star treatment for digoxin overdose? Br Med J 1986; 293: 642–43.

Chapter 13
Electrolytes and the ECG

Electrolyte disturbances and the ECG[1]

Electrolyte disturbances, particularly of potassium and to a lesser degree of magnesium and calcium, may cause changes in the ECG and contribute to the development of cardiac arrhythmias. The effects produced by the electrolyte abnormalities depend on:

- The relative concentrations of the individual ions one to another
- The ratio between the concentration of the ions at the cellular level and the extracellular level (the former usually is unknown, the latter is equivalent to the serum concentration of the ion), and
- The functional status of the heart and concurrent drug treatment e.g. with digitalis.

The resulting ECG changes and arrhythmias are non-specific and cannot be differentiated from those caused e.g. by myocardial infarction or ischaemia or drugs.

For these and other reasons, an ECG recording is *no* substitute for the measurement of the serum concentration of potassium or magnesium or calcium. In fact, knowledge of the serum electrolyte concentrations are often mandatory to interpret ECG changes and to best manage the associated arrhythmias.

Hyperkalaemia[1–4]

A high ionic serum concentration of potassium, *hyperkalaemia*, can produce ECG changes. These become increasingly more severe as the level of the potassium rises (Fig. 13.1), though the correlation between the serum level of potassium and the induced ECG changes are neither precise nor consistent. The following changes are associated with an elevated serum potassium (Fig. 13.1):

1 The earliest change is the development of tall, peaked T waves in the precordial leads (Fig. 13.2, page 301).

2 A reduction in P wave amplitude with its subsequent disappearance (Fig. 13.2). The ECG may suggest an accelerated AV nodal rhythm but evidence from animal models indicates that the SA node remains the pacemaker of the heart with the SA node impulse conveyed to the AV node via strands of still functioning atrial fibres in an otherwise paralyzed non-contractile atrial myocardium.

3 A reduction in R wave height, a widening of the QRS complex, ST segment depression or elevation and/or a PR prolongation.

4 Progressive widening of the QRS complex and the appearance of ventricular extrasystole.

5 Cardiac arrest threatens when the serum potassium con centration exceeds 7–8 mmol/l. An ECG recording during the cardiac arrest shows a flutter-like picture with very wide QRST complexes at a fast regular rate (a sinusoidal wave form). The flutter may degenerate to ventricular fibrillation or alternate with episodes of AV block and ventricular arrest.

Hyperkalaemia causing cardiac arrest occurs as a complication of uraemia or is induced by long-term therapy with potassium sparing diuretics (spironolactone or amiloride) and/or a daily potassium salt supplement in the elderly hypertensive or cardiac patient with reduced renal function. Life threatening hyperkalaemia can also develop as an acute complication of diabetic keto-acidosis, severe burns, multiple trauma and drowning.

Management

Serious arrhythmias due to hyperkalaemia are rapidly suppressed by a bolus injection of calcium salt. The calcium ion antagonizes the cardiotoxic effect of hyperkalaemia but does not reverse the hyperkalaemia itself. The next step is to reduce the plasma level of potassium rapidly by the injection of a glucose and insulin solution and by alkalinization. Alkalinization with sodium bicarbonate is most effective in the presence of acidosis but is also effective in hyperkalaemia without associated acidosis. With such alkalinization the serum-potassium level can be reduced by 1–2 mmol/l within 15–30 min. The situation is stabilized by continued infu-

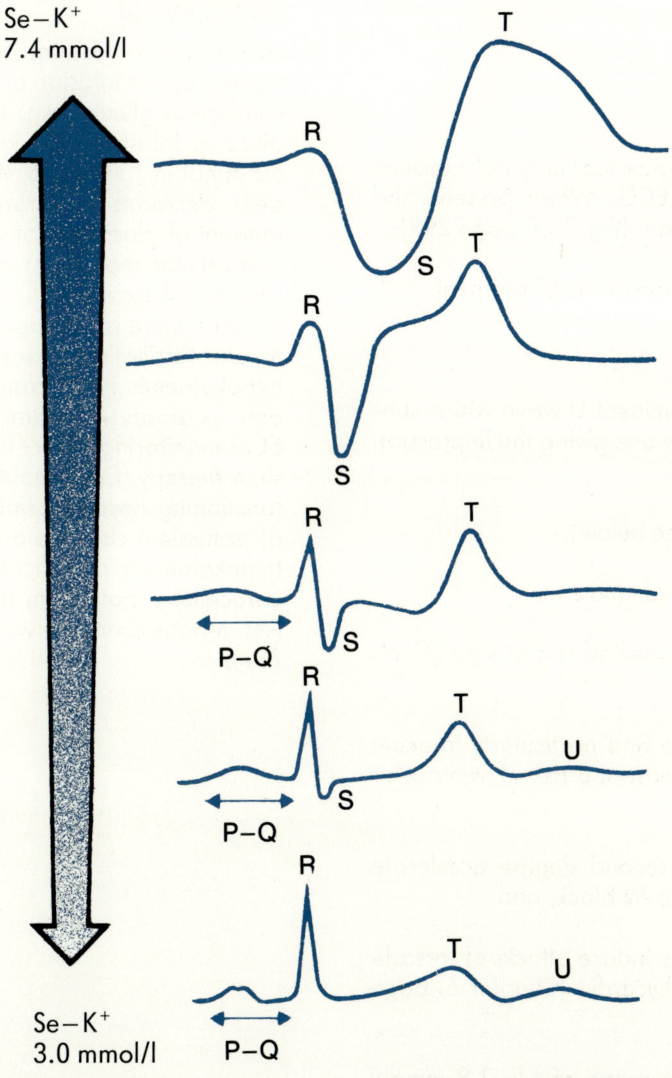

Fig. 13.1
ECG changes in potassium disturbances
See text for explanation

sion of 10 % glucose and by an enema with a cation exchange resin e.g. sodium sulfonate. If available haemodialysis will effect a significant reduction of the serum potassium within 15 min, and peritoneal dialysis within 2 h.

Hypokalaemia [1, 5–8]

Low serum potassium, hypokalaemia, may not produce significant changes on the ECG. When present, the most common ECG changes are (Fig. 13.1, page 299):

- A steeply concave depression of the ST segment
- Flattening of the T wave
- The development of a prominent U wave which subsequently fuses with the T wave giving the impression of QT prolongation, and
- Ventricular arrhythmias (see below).

Moderate and severe hypokalaemia can:

- In digitalis treatment increase the risk of side effects (Chapter 12, page 292)
- In coronary artery disease and particularly in acute myocardial infarction increase the risk of ventricular tachycardia or fibrillation
- In AV block of first and second degree accelerate progression to third degree AV block, and
- In AV block of third degree induce attacks of torsade de pointes ventricular tachycardia (Chapter 6, page 163).

Severe hypokalaemia (in the range of 1.5–1.8 mmol/l or lower) can trigger attacks of torsade de pointes ventricular tachycardia even in an individual with a healthy heart, but this is a very rare clinical event.

Hypokalaemia is a common complication of both short-term and long-term diuretic therapy. Vomiting, diarrhoea and insulin treatment of diabetic coma may lead to severe hypokalaemia. Familiar hypokalaemic periodic paralysis may be associated with attacks of torsade de pointes ventricular tachycardia.

Management

Low serum potassium causing serious arrhythmias is treated by the infusion of a strong solution of potassium chloride in glucose e.g. 100 mmol KCl in 1 litre of 5 % glucose. Infusion of weaker KCl glucose solutions e.g. 50 mmol in 1 litre of 5 % glucose can result in a transient *decrease* in serum potassium since the large amount of glucose relative to potassium, may cause an intracellular movement of potassium. The infusion rate should not exceed 0.5–1 mmol per min, and even at this rate there is a danger of transient AV block or ventricular fibrillation as seen in hyperkalaemia, since the hypokalaemic heart can be extremely sensitive to sudden increases in serum potassium. Thus, continuous ECG monitoring is necessary during intensive i.v. potassium therapy. Care should be taken that the i.v. drip is functioning normally since extravascular extravasation of potassium chloride produces necrosis of the skin. In hypokalaemia complicated by hypomagnesaemia the intracellular potassium deficit cannot be corrected unless magnesium is given to reactivate membrane ATPase.

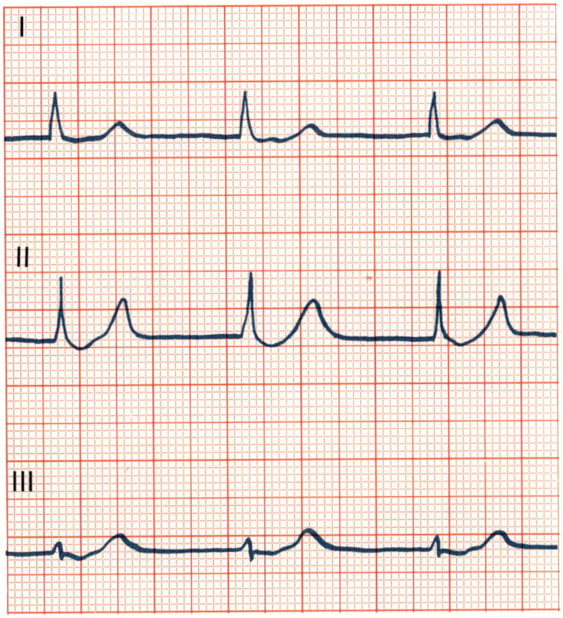

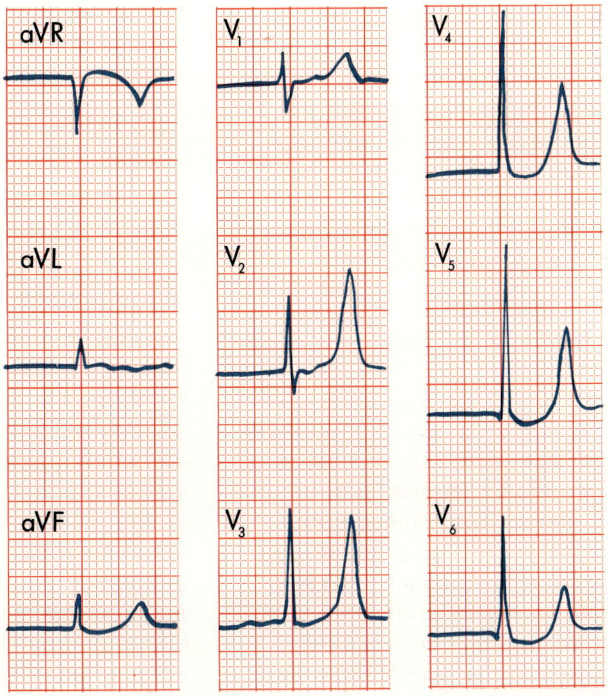

Fig. 13.2
An ECG from a patient with severe hyperkalaemia. The QRS complex is not widened and is without a preceding P wave; regular rate of 58/min. The T wave is steep and spiked. The ECG from a 60-year-old woman admitted to hospital in diabetic keto- acidosis with a serum potassium level of 8.4 mmol/l and pH 7.10.

Hypernatraemia and hyponatraemia [1]

Changes in the serum concentration of sodium are not associated with ECG changes or cardiac arrhythmias.

Hypomagnesaemia [1, 9]

The ECG changes of hypomagnesaemia are similar to those of hypokalaemia. Hypomagnesaemia often develops concurrently with hypokalaemia, and its clinical significance relates primarily to an intensification of the arrhythmogenic effect of the hypokalaemia.

Hypomagnesaemia may be associated with hypokalaemia during long-term diuretic treatment. It is a frequent finding in chronic severe enteropathies and occurs in chronic alcoholism. Severe hypomagnesaemia may develop during prolonged parenteral nutrition with magnesium free solutions.

Management [10–12]

Hypomagnesaemia complicated by serious arrhythmias is treated by an i.v. infusion of 10–20 ml of a 20 % magnesium sulfate solution over a 10-minute period. Infusion of a similar amount of magnesium sulfate has also been recommended for the treatment of ventricular tachycardia and fibrillation in patients with normal serum magnesium. Recent reports indicate that this may be effective against drug-induced torsade de pointes ventricular tachycardia (Chapter 6, page 163).

Hypercalcaemia [1]

In hypercalcaemia with a significantly increased level of *ionized* calcium in the serum, the ST segment is shortened or absent and the QT interval is shortened correspondingly. The U wave is either normal or augmented. AV block has been observed in a few patients with hypercalcaemia when related to hyperparathyroidism. The incidence of ventricular extrasystoles does not seem to be increased. Sudden death in the hypercalcaemic crises of hyperparathyroidism are thought to be due to attacks of ventricular fibrillation, but this has not been proven by ECG monitoring. There is a synergistic action between calcium and digitalis. Digitalis and/or hypokalaemia induced arrhythmias may be worsened catastrophically by the i.v. injection of a calcium salt given as an emergency to increase cardiac contractility.

Hypocalcaemia [1, 13]

Hypocalcaemia with a significantly decreased level of *ionized* calcium in the serum is characterized by a prolongation of the ST segment with associated prolongation of the QT interval. There are usually no T or U wave abnormalities, and the condition is rarely associated with a propensity to torsade de pointes ventricular tachycardia.

Acidosis [14]

Acidosis is not in itself arrhythmogenic but it may precipitate arrhythmias by accentuating preexisting hyperkalaemia. Acute and severe acidosis occurs in sustained cardiac arrest or shock. It lowers the contractility of the myocardium, diminishes the oxygen carrying capacity of the blood and contributes to the persistance of ventricular fibrillation. For these reasons, treatment of acidosis is a significant element in the management of sustained cardiac arrest and shock.

Management

The mainstay of the control of the acid-base balance in the cardiac arrest patient is to ensure adequate alveolar ventilation by artificial respiration. Hyperventilation corrects respiratory acidosis by removing carbon dioxide, which is freely diffusible across cellular and organic membranes including the blood-liquid barrier. Buffering of the acidosis by intravenous infusion of a concentrated hydrobicarbonate solution has been widely used to combat the acidosis of cardiac arrest, but few data are available, indicating that this or other types of buffering therapy improve outcome. Evidence to the contrary includes laboratory and clinical data indicating that bicarbonate has the following adverse effects:

- It does not improve the ability to defibrillate or improve survival in experimental animals.

- It shifts the oxyhaemoglobin saturation curve, inhibiting the release of oxygen.

- It induces hyperosmolarity and hypernatraemia.

- It produces paradoxical acidosis due to the production of carbon dioxide, which is freely diffusible into myocardial and cerebral cells and which may depress function, especially in ischaemic myocardium, and

- It induces adverse effects due to extracellular alkalosis.

In the patient with cardiac arrest and preexisting acidosis bicarbonate may be of benefit. When bicarbonate is given, no more than 0.5–1 mmol per kg body weight should be given as the initial dose. Ideally, the pH, plasma standard bicarbonate and base deficit should be measured as rapidly as possible, and the result used to calculate the bicarbonate dose.

References Chapter 13

1. Surawicz B, Braun HA, Crum WB, et al. Quantitative analysis of the electrocardiographic pattern of hypopotassemia. Circulation 1957; 16: 750–3.
2. Ettinger PO, Hega J, Oldewurtel A. Hyperkalemia, cardiac conduction and the electrocardiogram: A review. Am Heart J 1974; 88: 360–1.
3. Ettinger PO, Regan TJ, Oldewurtel HA, et al. Ventricular conduction delay and asystole during systemic hyperkalemia. Am J Cardinol 1974; 33: 876–8
4. Chakko SC, Frutchey J, Gheorghiade M. Life-threatening hyperkalemia in severe heart failure. Veterans Administration Center, Salem, Va. Am Heart J 1989; 117: 1083–1.
5. Helfant RH. Hypokalemia and arrhythmias. Am J Med 1986; 80 (Suppl. 4A): 13–2.
6. Nordrehaug JE, von der Lippe G. Hypokalaemia and ventricular fibrillation in acute myocardial infarction. Br Heart J 1983; 50: 525–9.
7. Nordehaug JE, von der Lippe G. Serum potassium concentrations are inversely related to ventricular, but not to atrial, arrhythmias in acute myocardial infarction. Europ Heart J 1986; 7: 204–9.
8. Blomström-Lundqvist C, Caidahl K, Olsson SB, et al. Electrocardiographic findings and frequency of arrhythmias in Bartter's syndrome. Br Heart J 1989; 61: 274–9.
9. Surawicz B. Is hypomagnesemia or magnesium deficiency arrhythmogenic? JACC 1989; 14: 1093–6.
10. DiCarlo LA, Morady F, de Buitleir M, et al. Effects of magnesium sulfate on cardiac conduction and refractoriness in humans. JACC 1986; 7: 1356–2.
11. Rasmussen HS, Suensson M, McNair P, Nørregard P, Balsløv S. Magnesium infusion reduces the incidence of arrhythmias in acute myocardial infarction. A double-blind, placebo-controlled study. Clin Cardiol 1987; 10: 351–6.
12. Abraham AS, Rosenmann D, Kramer M, et al. Magnesium in the prevention of lethal arrhythmias in acute myocardial infarction. Arch Intern Med 1987; 147: 753–5.
13. Akiyama T, Batchelder J, Worsman J, et al. Hypocalcemic torsades de pointes. Electrocardiology 1989; 22: 89–2.
14. Jaffe AS. New and old paradoxes. Acidosis and cardiopulmonary resuscitation. Circulation 1989; 80: 1079–3.

Chapter 14
ECG interpretation in sinus rhythm and supraventricular arrhythmia

Diagnostic limitations of the ECG in ventricular pre-excitation, bundle branch block and ventricular arrhythmia

A normal sequence of the activation of the various parts of the ventricular myocardium is an important element for the reliable interpretation of the ECG for signs of ventricular hypertrophy, myocardial infarction and ischaemia. In ventricular arrhythmias, ventricular pre-excitation and bundle branch block the spread of activation through the ventricular myocardium is abnormal. Under these circumstances ECG interpretation is limited to recognizing the arrhythmia/conduction anomaly. No reliable conclusion can be reached as to the nature of the underlying lesion of the ventricular myocardium. An exception is right bundle branch block in which it is possible to identify the abnormal Q waves of transmural myocardial infarction (Fig. 9.8, page 234).

This chapter focuses on the diagnostic potential of the ECG during sinus rhythm or supraventricular arrhythmia and without ventricular pre-excitation or bundle branch block (i.e. with a PR interval of more than 0.12 s and a QRS complex of less than 0.12 s). The first section on atrial enlargement refers solely to the ECG recording in sinus rhythm.

Atrial enlargement [1–4]

Atrial enlargement is reflected by changes in the form, height and/or width of the sinus P wave. The changes usually are most distinct in lead II and lead V_1. Sometimes the term atrial hypertrophy is used synonymously with atrial enlargement. Since there is no significant correlation between P wave changes and atrial weight this terminology is inappropriate for an ECG diagnosis.

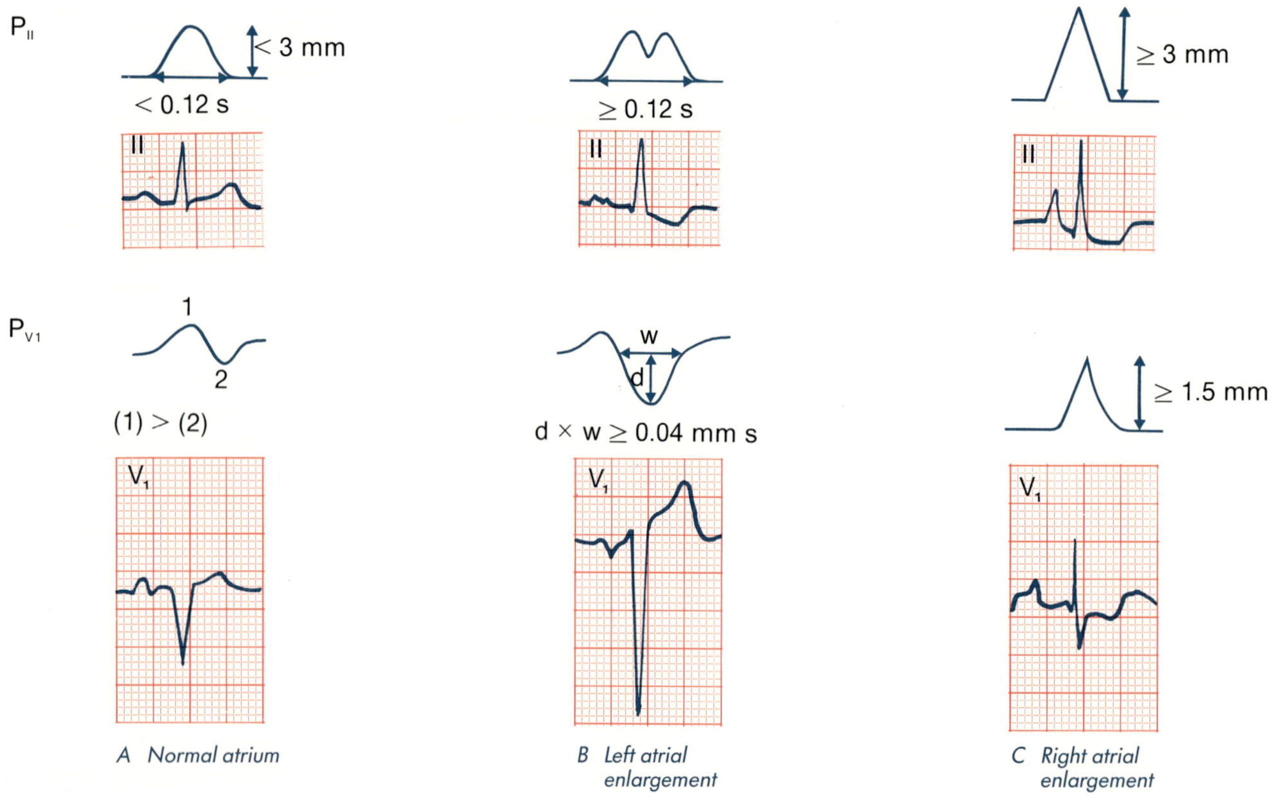

Fig. 14.1
Atrial enlargement. Principal P wave changes.

The normal sinus P wave

For reference, a normal P wave has these features (Fig. 14.1 A):

– In lead II the P wave is less than 2 mm in height and less than 0.12 s in width, and

– In lead V_1 the P wave often is biphasic with an initial positive and a subsequent negative component. The latter does not exceed that of the preceding positive component. Alternatively the P wave is only a small positive deflection.

Left atrial enlargement

Left atrial enlargement (Fig. 14.1 B) is manifest by a broad notched P wave in lead II of 0.12 s or more in width, so-called P mitrale. In lead V_1 left atrial enlargement may be reflected by a P wave with a dominant negative component which in depth (d) is more than or equal to 1 mm or in width (w) is more than or equal to 0.04 s – or which in net area = (d x w) exceeds 0.04 mm.

ECG evidence of left atrial enlargement is seen in mitral stenosis and in many conditions which impose a load

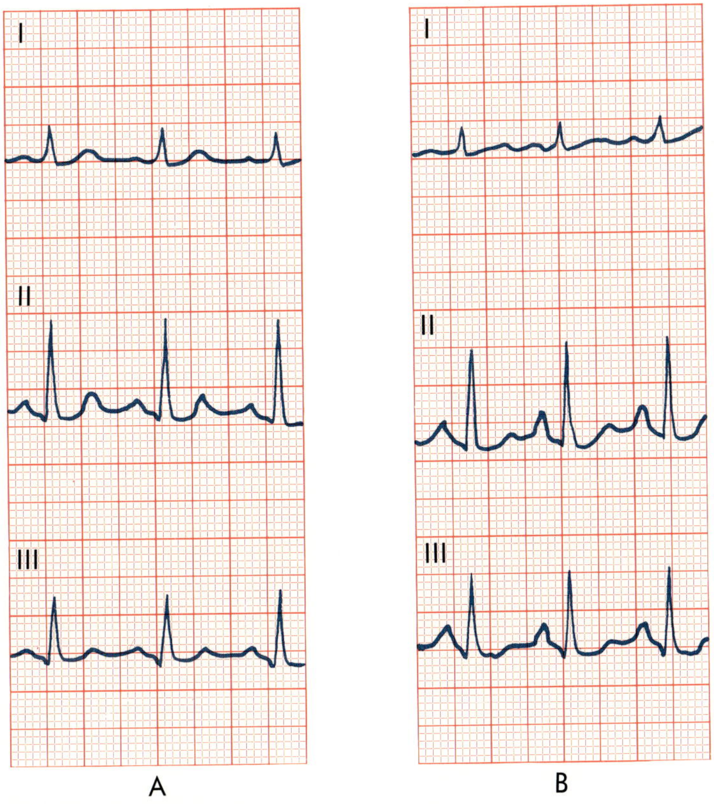

Fig. 14.2
Atrial enlargement. Acute development of P pulmonale in asthma bronchiale. 20-year-old girl with attacks of asthma bronchiale for several years. The ECG in between attacks (A) shows a normal P wave (blunt P wave = 2 mm in lead II) while an ECG recording during a sustained severe attack (B) shows a P pulmonale (pointed P wave = 3.5 mm in lead II). Regression to a normal P wave after the attack (not shown).

on the left ventricle, leading to dilatation of the left atrium (see section on left ventricular hypertrophy).

Right atrial enlargement

Right atrial enlargement (Fig. 14.1 C) may be manifest by a tall, slender peaked P wave larger than or equal to 3 mm in lead II, so-called P pulmonale. Similarly tall P waves are often seen in leads III and aVF. The typical finding in lead V_1 is a P wave with an initial tall, slender positive component larger than or equal to 1.5 mm.

ECG evidence of right atrial enlargement is seen in many conditions which impose a load on the right ventricle, leading to dilatation of the right atrium (see section on right ventricular hypertrophy). Acute, transitory and fully reversible development of P pulmonale may occur in an acute attack of bronchial asthma and acute pulmonary embolism (Fig. 14.2).

Ventricular hypertrophy[1–4]

Several features suggest hypertrophy (thickening) of the wall of the left or right ventricles. They may be summarized as follows:

- *Hypertrophy patterns* (Fig. 14.3 B–C) with abnormally tall R waves in the left precordial leads (V_{5-6}) in left ventricular hypertrophy and in the right precordial leads (V_1 and/or V_2) in right ventricular hypertrophy. Tall S waves are often recorded in the contralateral leads.
- *Strain patterns* (Fig. 14.3 B–C) with ST segment depression and/or T wave inversion in the left precordial leads (V_{5-6}) and/or lead I in left ventricular hypertrophy and in the right precordial leads (V_{1-3}) in right ventricular hypertrophy.
- *QRS axis deviation* (Fig. 1.28, page 22) particularly of right axis deviation in right ventricular hypertrophy.
- *Atrial enlargement* (Fig. 14.1 B–C, page 308) with the recording of a P mitrale in left ventricular hypertrophy, and a P pulmonale in right ventricular hypertrophy.

These criteria vary in the sensitivity and specificity. In general, the greater the number of criteria fulfilled, the more likely the diagnosis of ventricular hypertrophy.

The normal QRST complex

The features of the normal QRST are:

- In the precordial leads (Fig. 14.3 A) an rS pattern in lead V_1 and a qR(s) pattern in leads V_{5-6} with V_{5-6} of less than 27 mm and a sum of R in V_5 or V_6 plus S in V_1 of less than 35 mm; the ST segment is isoelectric and the T wave is positive in leads V_{5-6}.
- In the limb leads a mean QRS axis (Fig. 1.28) in the range −30° to 90°; the ST segment is isoelectric and the T wave positive in lead I.

Left ventricular hypertrophy

Left ventricular hypertrophy (thickening of the wall of the left ventricle) may produce the following ECG features:

- *Left ventricular hypertrophy pattern* (Fig. 14.3 B and 14.4 A, page 313) with an abnormally tall R wave in lead V_{5-6} and often an abnormally deep S wave in lead V_{1-2} with the R in V_5 or V_6 larger than or equal to 27 mm and/or a sum of R in V_5 or V_6 plus the S in V_1 larger than or equal to 35 mm.
- *Left ventricular strain pattern* (Figs. 14.3 B and 14.4 A) with ST depression equal to or exceeding 1 mm and/or a negative T wave in leads V_{5-6} or lead I. Strain and hypertrophy patterns are often recorded simultaneously but can be observed separately as isolated ECG manifestations of left ventricular hypertrophy.
- *Left axis deviation* (Fig. 1.28) is an inconsistent finding but is seen if the underlying left ventricular disease is complicated by left anterior fascicular block (Fig. 9.2, page 225).
- *P mitrale in lead II and/or a P in V_1 with a prominent negative component* (Fig. 14.1 B). Enlargement of the left atrium frequently is associated with left ventricular disease. Correspondingly, ECG evidence of left atrial enlargement is a common indirect marker of left ventricular hypertrophy.

The ECG patterns of left ventricular hypertrophy and/or strain occur in many conditions which impose a load on the left ventricle e.g. systemic hypertension, aortic valvular disease and mitral incompetence. They are common in hypertrophic cardiomyopathy (Fig. 14.29, page 347) and occur also in dilated cardiomyopathy (Fig. 14.28, page 346) and in coronary artery disease.

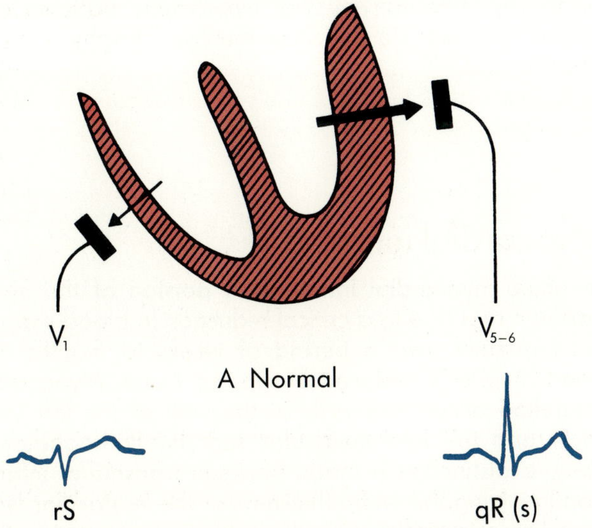

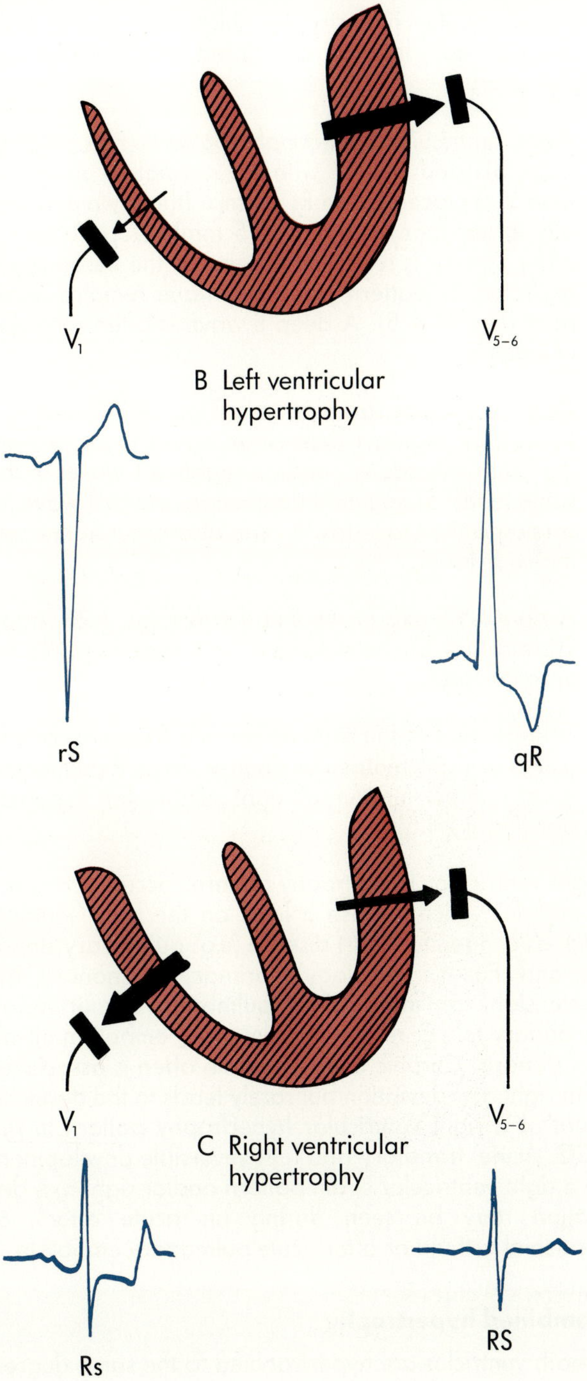

Fig. 14.3
Vectorial background of the hypertrophy patterns.
The spread of the activation wave through the free wall of the right and left ventricle can be conceived as a single vector, the free wall vector (see Fig. 1.30, p. 25). The direction and magnitude of this vector reflects the relative thickness of the free wall of the two chambers of the heart and is mirrored by the configuration of the QRS complex in the precordial leads.

A In the normal heart the free wall vector is directed away from lead V_1 and towards leads V_{5-6}. The result is the recording of an rS pattern in lead V_1 and a qR(s) pattern in lead (see also Fig. 1.30).

B In left ventricular hypertrophy, like in the normal heart, the free wall vector is directed away from lead V_1 and towards leads V_5 or V_6. However, it is of larger magnitude. The result is the recording of an abnormally tall R wave in leads V_5 or V_6 and/or an abnormally deep S wave in lead V_1 ($Rv_{5-6} \geq 27$ mm and/or$Rv_{5-6} + Sv_1 > 35$ mm).

C In right ventricular hypertrophy the free wall vector is directed towards V_1 and more or less away from leads V_{5-6}. The result is the recording of an Rs pattern in lead V_1 and often an RS pattern in leads V_{5-6}.

Right ventricular hypertrophy

Right ventricular hypertrophy, thickening of the right ventricular wall, may be associated with the following ECG features:

- *Right ventricular hypertrophy pattern* (Figs. 14.3 C, page 311 and 14.4 B) with the normal rS pattern in lead V_1 replaced by an Rs pattern (the R wave is usually larger than or equal to 5 mm). Occasionally a qR(s) pattern is recorded instead of the theoretically expected Rs pattern but the R wave remains dominant (Fig. 14.4 B). A deep S wave is often recorded in leads V_{5-6}.
- *Right ventricular strain pattern* (Figs. 14.3 C and 14.4 B) with ST segment depression equal to or exceeding 1 mm in leads V_{1-3} and/or negative T waves in the same leads. ST segment depression and/or T wave inversion limited to leads V_{1-2} can also occur in the normal individual.
- *A right QRS axis in the limb leads* (Figs. 1.28, page 22 and 14.4 B) characterized by a negative QRS net area in lead I.
- Enlargement of the right atrium is a frequent complication of right ventricular disease. Thus, P pulmonale is an indirect marker of right ventricular hypertrophy (Fig. 14.4 B).

Right ventricular hypertrophy patterns occur with many conditions which impose a load on the right ventricle such as congenital heart disease (e.g. pulmonary stenosis and Fallot's tetralogy), primary pulmonary hypertension, or more often pulmonary hypertension secondary to e.g. recurrent pulmonary embolism or mitral stenosis. Chronic cor pulmonale often is associated with right axis deviation but rarely leads to the development of a right ventricular hypertrophy pattern in the ECG. Acute, transitory and fully reversible development of a right ventricular strain pattern and/or right axis deviation may be seen during an acute attack of bronchial asthma or after acute pulmonary embolism.

Combined hypertrophy

If both ventricles are hypertrophied to the same degree their electrical fields will balance each other resulting in an ECG with no diagnostic evidence of ventricular hypertrophy. Alternatively the hypertrophy patterns will reflect the ventricle in which the hypertrophy is most pronounced.

Myocardial infarction [1, 2, 5–9]

In acute myocardial infarction a portion of the myocardium dies due to a critical reduction in blood supply. Subsequently over a period of weeks to months the dead muscle is replaced by fibrous tissue. Myocardial infarction occurs primarily in the wall of the left ventricle and the interventricular septum. Pathoanatomically, a distinction is made between transmural infarction involving the entire thickness of the ventricular wall and subendocardial infarction which is restricted to the inner half to two thirds of the wall.

The pathophysiological mechanism underlying the principal ECG changes of transmural myocardial infarction can be illustrated by an animal model in which acute transmural infarction has been induced by a temporary ligation of a major branch of one of the coronary arteries (Fig. 14.5, page 315).

The upper drawing (A) in Fig. 14.5 shows two unipolar electrodes placed directly on the epicardial surface of the ventricular wall of the exposed animal heart. One electrode is placed over the dead muscle in the center of the infarction and the other electrode on the injured, but still viable muscle in the periphery of the infarction.

Different patterns are recorded by the two electrodes:

1 The electrode located centrally over the infarction "looks" through the electrically inert "window" formed by the dead muscle into the ventricular cavity. It "sees" the activation of the viable muscle of the opposite wall moving away from it. The result is the recording of a monophasic negative complex, a *QS complex* i.e. the typical recording of an electrode facing a dead or fibrotic portion of the ventricular wall.

Fig. 14.4
Ventricular hypertrophy

ECG recording from a 35-year-old female with previous recurrent pulmonary embolism (A) and a 60-year-old male with severe aortic stenosis (B)

A Left ventricular hypertrophy

- *left ventricular hypertrophy pattern (R in V_6 + S in V_1 = 46 mm); and*
- *left ventricular strain pattern (1–2 mm ST segment depression and negative T wave in leads V_{5-6} and I–III)*

The QRS axis is normal (+70°) and there is no P mitrale (P_{II} less than 0.13 s wide and positive P in V_1)

B Right ventricular hypertrophy

- *Right axis deviation (QRS axis = 100°);*
- *Right ventricular hypertrophy pattern (qR pattern in lead V_1 and RS pattern in lead V_6)*
- *Right ventricular strain pattern (ST segment depression of 1–3 mm in leads V_{2-4}) – P pulmonale (pointed P wave = 3 mm in lead II)*

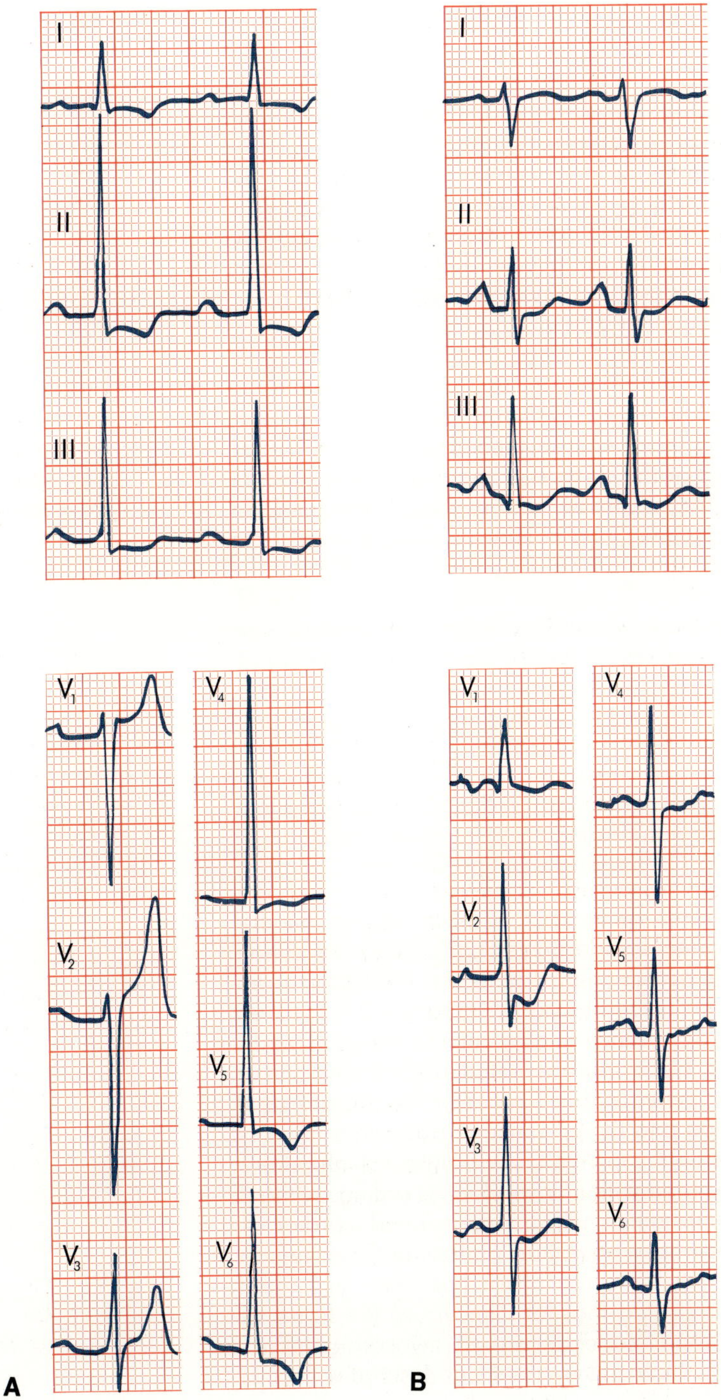

2 The peripheral electrode records a more or less normal QRS complex followed by ST segment elevation (2_1) reflecting cell injury in the border zone of the infarction. Over a period of days the ST segment elevation gradually subsides concurrently with the development of a deeply negative ("inverted"), symmetric T wave (2_2). The gradual reduction and final disappearance of the ST segment elevation reflects that the injured cells which originally produced the pattern either die or recover. The inverted T waves are probably due to abnormal repolarization in the (not fully) recovered cells.

The lower drawing (B) of Fig. 14.5 depicts the same experimental situation but with the ECG recording from an electrode placed at a distance from the ventricular wall, perhaps at the surface of the chest in the precordial region. This electrode "views" the infarcted area in its entirety resulting in a composite ECG pattern. The pattern comprises a broad deep Q wave and a small r wave followed by ST segment elevation ($1-2_1$). The ST segment elevation gradually subsides simultaneous with the development of a deeply negative, symmetric T wave. The final pattern is a broad deep Q wave and a small r wave followed by an isoelectric ST segment and a deeply negative, symmetric T wave ($1-2_2$).

Similar experimental studies on the ECG consequences of subendocardial infarction show loss in amplitude of the R wave and ST/T changes but no Q waves.

From hypotheses generated by such animal experiments it became standard medical practice to divide myocardial infarctions into two types: "transmural infarctions" and "subendocardial infarctions" based on the presence or absence of abnormal Q waves in the 12 lead surface ECG. Autopsy studies, however, have shown major inconsistensies between the mural extent of an infarction and the presence or absence of abnormal Q waves on the in vivo ECG. Transmural infarctions may be associated with in vivo ECG recordings without Q wave abnormalities while some subendocardial infarctions at autopsy have had abnormal Q waves on their ECGs. For these reasons it has been suggested and widely accepted that for clinical use the terms of "transmural" and "subendocardial" myocardial infarction should be replaced by the ECG descriptive terms, *Q-wave* and *non-Q-wave* myocardial infarction.

Despite the inconsistent correlation of the mural extent of the infarction, the classification of the infarctions into *Q-wave* and *non-Q-wave* types is of major clinical interest since it has been found that:

- There is a significantly higher incidence of coronary artery thrombosis in Q-wave infarction than in non-Q-wave infarction (80–90 % versus 20–30 %).

- There is a significantly higher short term mortality in Q-wave infarction than in the non-Q-wave infarction (20 % versus 10 %).

- Long-term (1–2 years) survival is about the same for the two types of infarction, but in some series (not all) a significantly higher reinfarction rate and higher incidence of postinfarction angina in the non-Q-wave infarction has been noted.

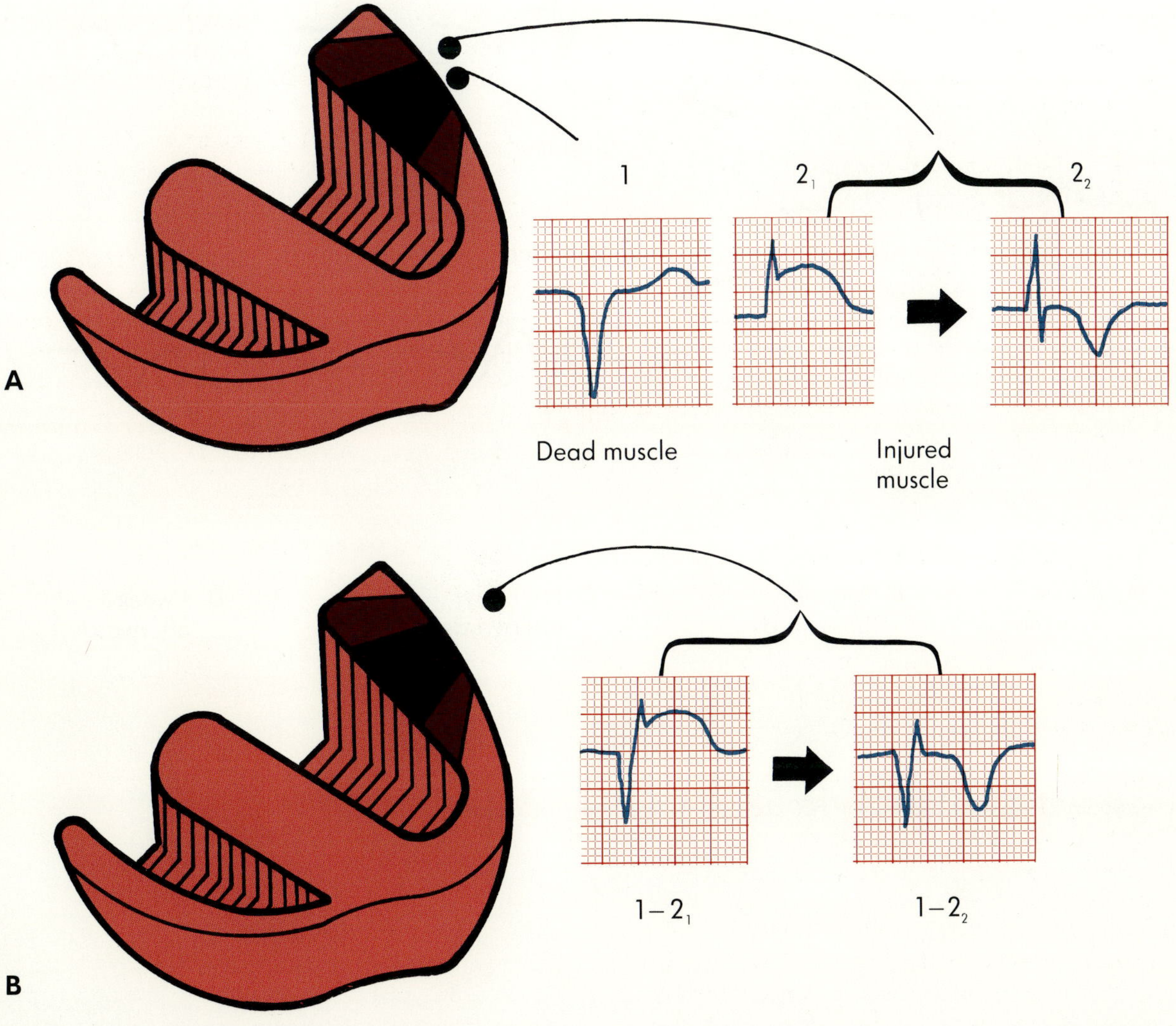

Fig. 14.5
Transmural myocardial infarction. ECG recordings from the exposed heart of an animal model. The schematic drawing shows the situation a few hours after the induction of a myocardial infarction by the temporary ligation of a major branch of one of the coronary arteries. For explanation see text.

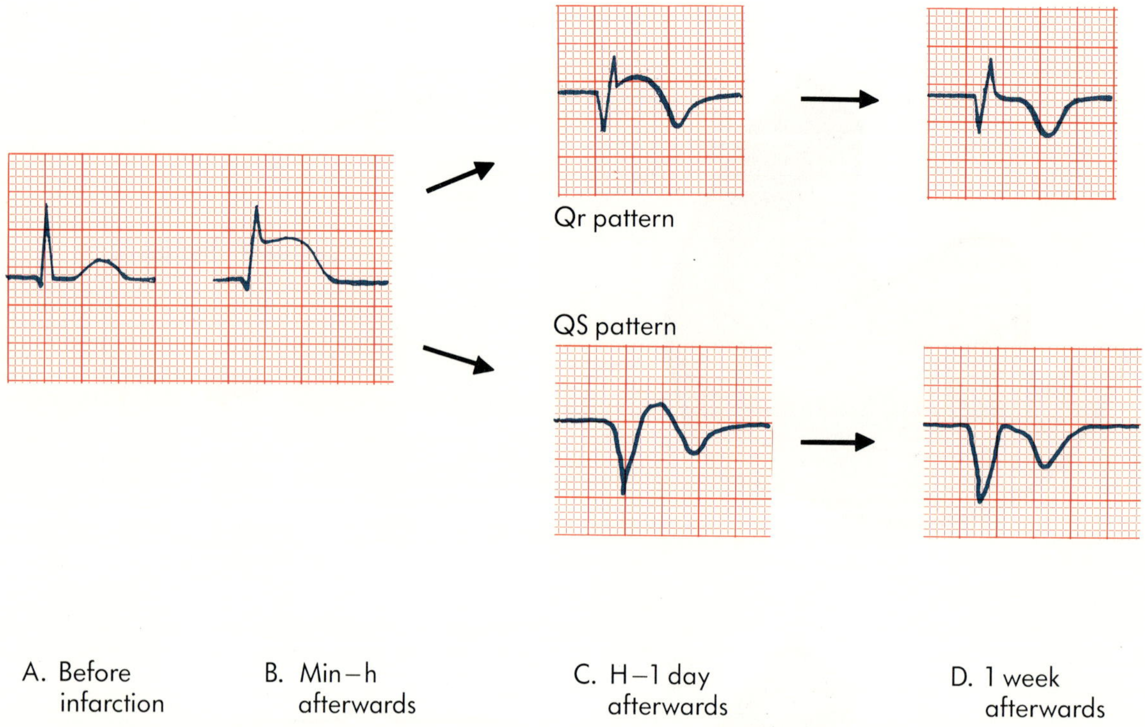

Fig. 14.6
Q-wave myocardial infarction. Sequence of ECG changes in a lead facing the infarction

The Q-wave infarction [1, 2, 5–7]

The sequence of ECG changes

The sequence of typical ECG changes in a lead facing an acute Q-wave infarction are (Fig. 14.6):

A *Before infarction:* A QRS complex dominated by a prominent R wave and followed by a positive T wave.

B *Within minutes or hours:* The swift onset of often substantial ST segment elevation.

C *Within hours or days:* R wave reduction and the appearance of a broad and/or deep Q wave with a change to a Qr pattern or sometimes to a QS complex. The T wave begins to invert.

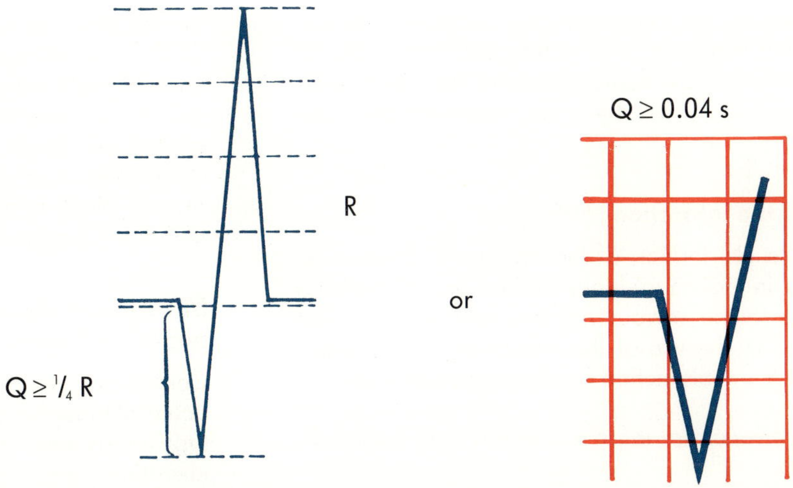

Fig. 14.7
Transmural myocardial infarction. The abnormal Q waves. The abnormality criteria shown apply for all leads with the exception of leads aVR, aVL, V_{1-2} and lead III.

D *Within days, a week or more:* A return of the ST segment to the baseline and the development of a deep, symmetrical negative T wave.

E *Months afterwards:* Persistence of the abnormal Q wave and reduced R wave or QS complex. The deep, symmetrical, negative T wave may remain unchanged, may flatten to become isoelectric or may occasionally become positive.

The abnormal Q wave[1,2,5]

An abnormal Q wave or QS complex is the ECG manifestation of myocardial necrosis or fibrosis and is the fundamental element for the ECG diagnosis of infarction. The criteria for Q wave abnormality are (Fig. 14.7):

- A Q wave exceeding 0.04 s in width, and/or
- A Q wave exceeding 25 % in depth of the following R wave provided the R wave itself is larger than 5 mm.

These criteria for Q wave abnormality apply to all leads with the exception of lead aVR in which a broad and deep Q wave is the usual finding and leads V_{1-2}, III and aVF in which a broad or deep Q wave is an occasional finding in the normal individual.

Myocardial infarction is the most common but not the only cause of abnormal Q waves. Other conditions which can be associated with abnormal Q waves or QS complexes are: pulmonary embolism, cardiomyopathy, chest deformities, muscular dystrophy and cardiac tumours.

Reciprocal changes

Leads opposite to the infarction (Fig. 1.23, page 17) show reciprocal changes compared to those recorded by a lead facing the infarction (Fig. 14.8). The abnormal Q wave is replaced by an abnormal R wave, the ST segment elevation by depression and the deep symmetrical negative T wave by a tall, symmetrically positive T wave.

Location of the infarction [1, 2, 5, 6]

Based on the distribution of the abnormal Q wave or QS complex in individual leads and on the relationship of the leads to the various portions of the ventricular wall (Fig. 1.23), the site of the infarction can be localized (Fig. 14.9). A distinction can be made between:

1 *Anterior myocardial infarction* which may be subdivided into:

   - *Anteroseptal infarction* with abnormal Q waves in leads V_{1-3}
   - *Anterolateral infarction* with abnormal Q waves in leads V_{5-6}, I and aVL
   - *High lateral infarction* with abnormal Q waves in lead aVL, and
   - *Extensive anterior infarction* with abnormal Q waves in leads V_{1-6}, I and aVL (Fig. 14.10, page 320).

2 *Inferior myocardial infarction* with abnormal Q waves in leads III, aVF and often in lead II (Fig. 14.11).

3 *True posterior infarction* with an abnormal R wave in leads V_{1-2} or occasionally V_{2-3} (Fig. 14.9).

Extensive ECG changes representing simultaneous infarction of the anterior and inferior wall can be seen. True posterior infarction is most often seen in combination with an inferior infarction in the form of an inferior-posterior infarction (Fig. 14.12, page 322). Autopsy series indicate a relatively poor correlation between Q wave localization on the 12-lead ECG with the pathoanatomical location and extent of the infarction.

Complication with bundle branch block [9]

Bundle branch block is a frequent complication of acute myocardial infarction. The occurrence of left bundle branch block all but precludes further assessment of the ECG for evidence of myocardial infarction. The presence of right bundle branch block on the other hand still permits identification of abnormal Q waves representing cell death or fibrosis (Fig. 9.8, page 234). The diagnostic and prognostic implications of bundle branch block in myocardial infarction are discussed at length in Chapter 9, page 234.

ST segment elevation and the deep symmetrical negative T wave

Corrobative evidence supporting a diagnosis of an acute myocardial infarction are serial ECGs showing a typical sequence of changes beginning with ST segment elevation subsiding over days concurrently with the development of an abnormal Q wave, R wave reduction and the appearance of deep symmetrical negative T waves. In the acute clinical situation the presence or absence of ST segment elevation helps assess the age of a Q wave infarction. Persistence of the ST segment elevation, however, is seen particularly in extensive transmural infarction involving a major part of the anterior wall. A proportion of such patients with persistent ST elevation have a ventricular aneurysm, i.e. an outward non-contracting bulge on the anterior wall of the left ventricle developed as a complication of the infarction.

ST segment elevation is the common finding in acute pericarditis, a disease which causes sudden chest pain which may be indistinguishable from the pain of acute myocardial infarction. Differential diagnostic features of the ST segment elevation in the two conditions are discussed later.

T wave inversion is a non-specific finding which is associated with a variety of pathological conditions (Fig. 14.36, page 358).

continued page 323

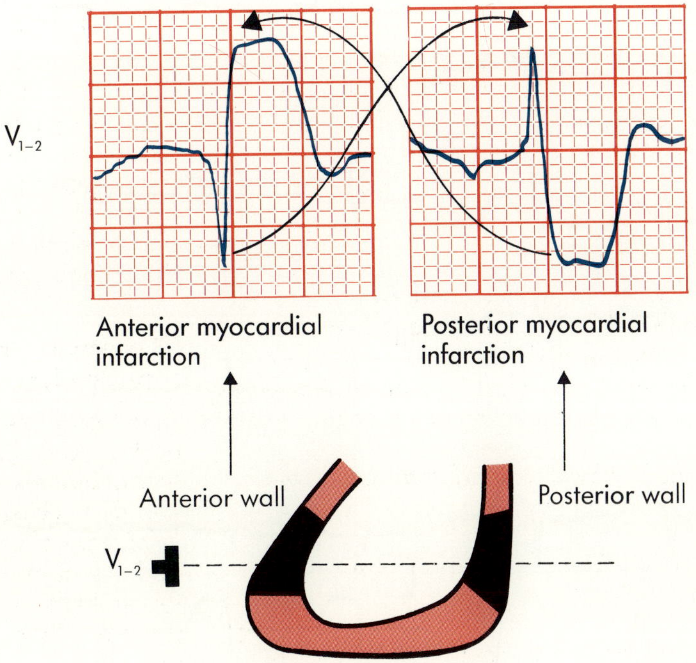

Fig. 14.8
Acute Q-wave myocardial infarction. Changes in lead V_{1-2}, typical infarction changes in an anteroseptal infarction and reciprocal changes in a true posterior infarction.

Fig. 14.9
Q-wave myocardial infarction. Topographical classification and Q wave location in the 12 lead ECG (or in posterior infarction location of the abnormal R wave).

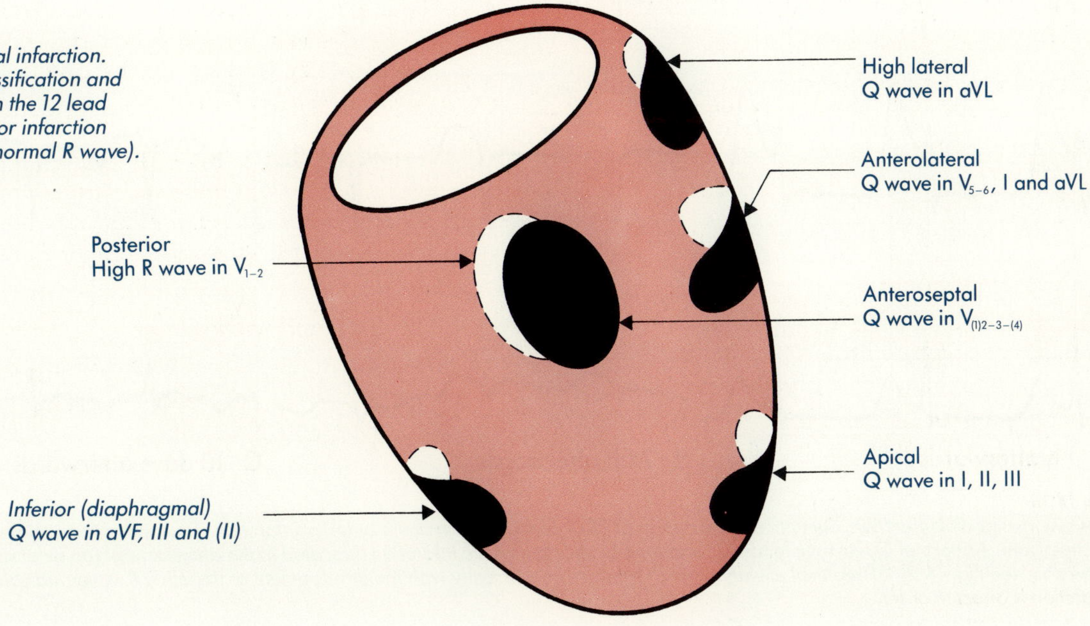

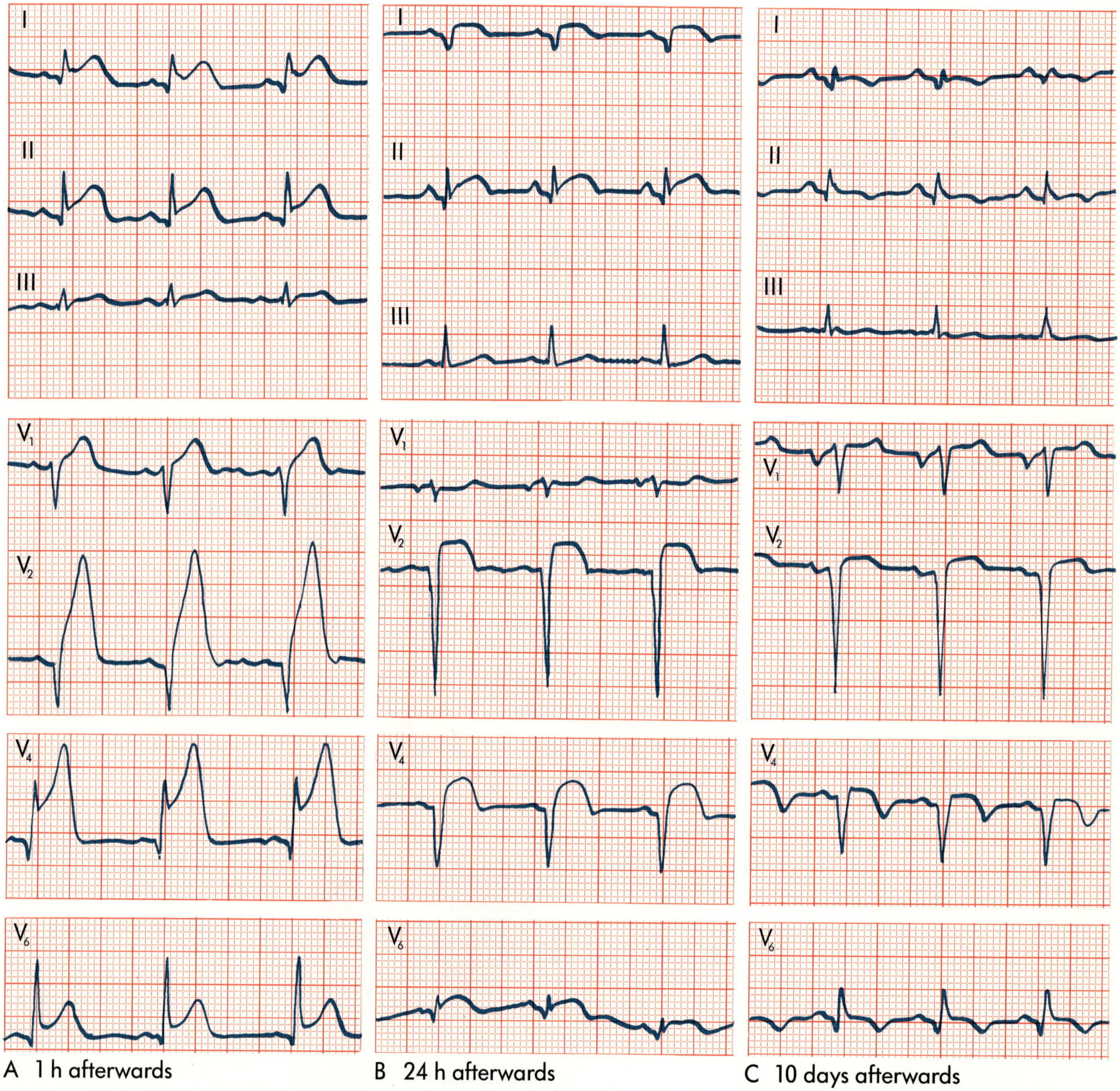

Fig. 14.10
Q wave myocardial infarction. Sequence and location of ECG changes in an acute anterior infarction. Time indications relate to the onset of chest pain. Abnormal Q waves in leads V_{1-6} and lead I indicate that the infarction is located in the anterior wall (an extensive anterior infarction, see Fig. 14.9). ST segment elevation which subsides concurrently with the development of negative T waves indicates that the infarction is of acute onset.

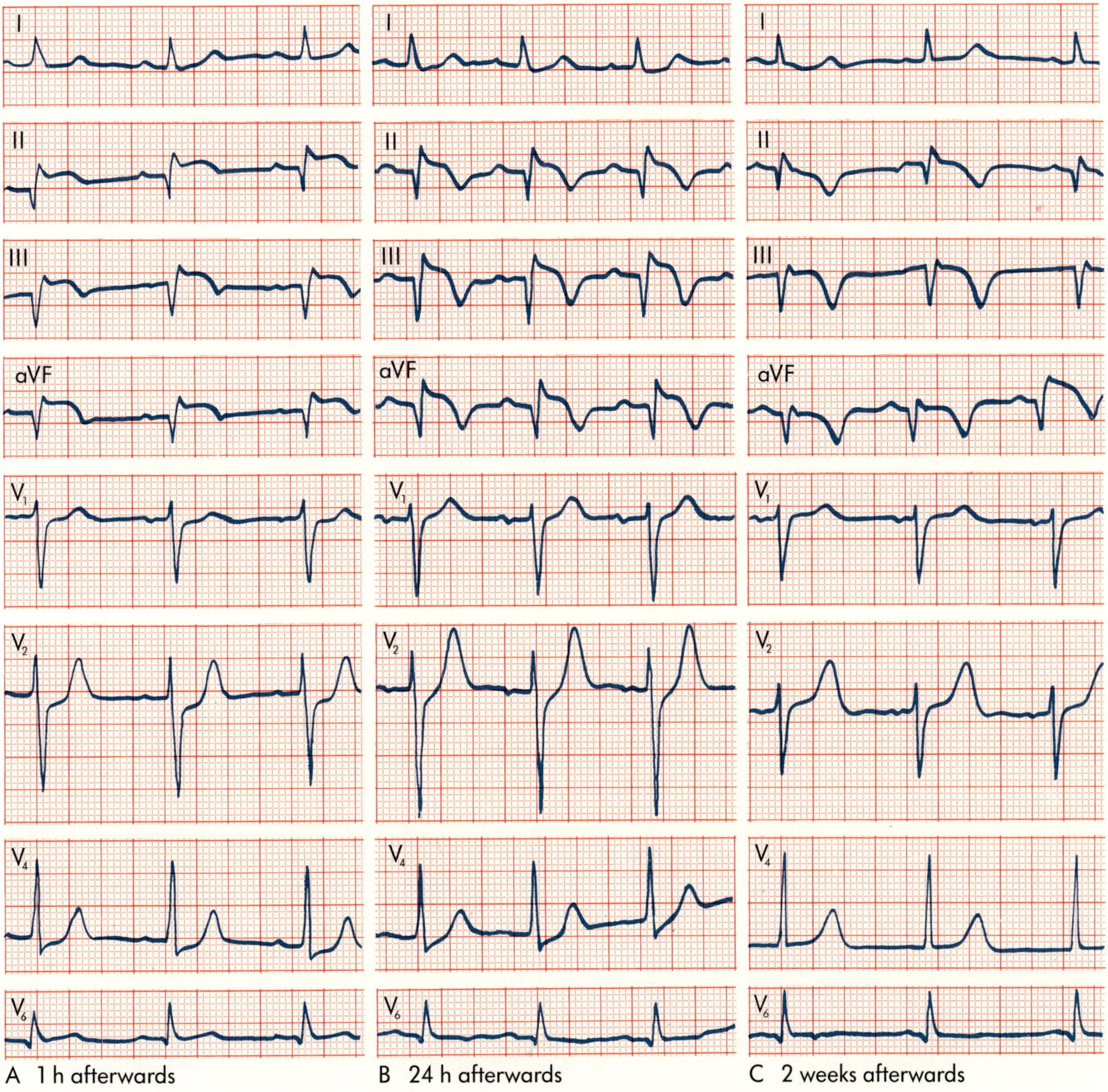

Fig. 14.11
Q-wave myocardial infarction. Sequence and location of ECG changes in an acute inferior infarction. Time indications relate to the onset of chest pain. Abnormal Q waves in leads aVF, II and III indicate that the infarction is located in the inferior wall (an inferior infarction see Fig. 14.9). ST segment elevation which subsides concurrently with the development of negative T waves indicates that the infarction is of acute onset.

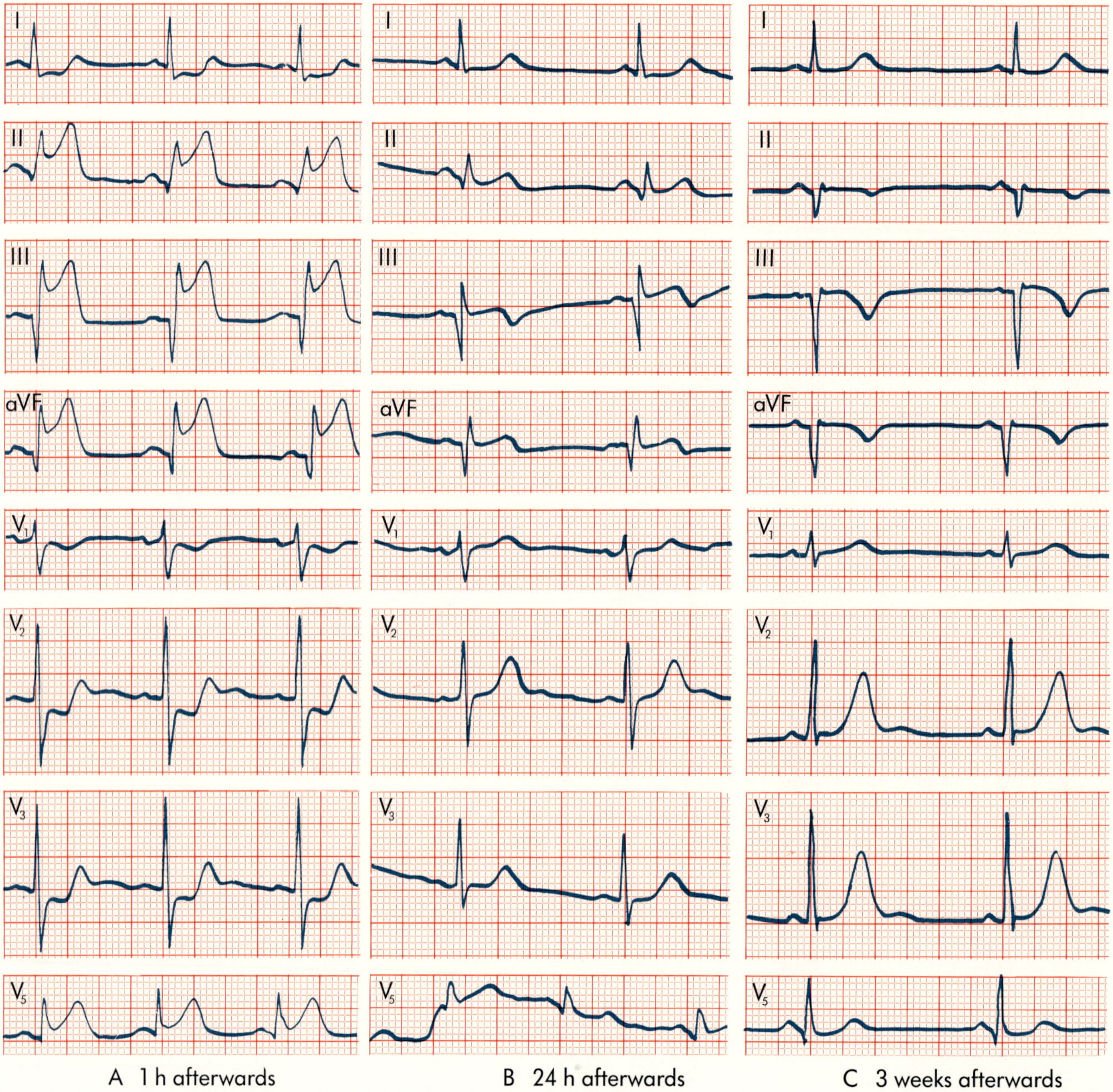

Fig. 14.12
Q-wave myocardial infarction. Sequence and location of ECG changes in an acute posterior–inferior infarction. Time indications relate to the onset of chest pain. The recording of a reciprocal infarction pattern in the form of a tall R wave and ST segment depression which subsequently subsides concurrently with the development of a tall peaked positive T wave suggests a diagnosis of an acute true posterior infarction (see Fig. 14.8). The combined occurrence of a typical infarction pattern (Q wave, ST segment elevation which subsides with sebsequent development of deep symmetrical negative T waves) in leads aVF, II and III indicates a simultaneous involvement of the inferior wall.

Non-Q-wave infarction[7–9]

Non-Q-wave infarction can be associated with a variety of ECG changes (Fig. 14.13):

- ST segment depression, and/or
- Deep symmetrical negative T waves, and/or
- R wave reduction, but by definition *not* the development of abnormal Q waves.

ECG changes usually are reflected in multiple leads because of the tendency of non-Q-wave infarction to encircle the left ventricular cavity. The changes can appear suddenly or may develop gradually over several days. The changes may either subside over the course of some days or within a week (Fig. 14.14, page 324), or they may persist (Fig. 14.15, page 325). ST segment depression and/or T wave changes disappearing shortly after an attack of anginal pain are most likely to be due to transient myocardial ischaemia rather than cell necrosis. Serum enzymes are crucial in the differential diagnosis of infarction and unstable angina. Pericarditis and myocarditis can occasionally present differential diagnostic problems.

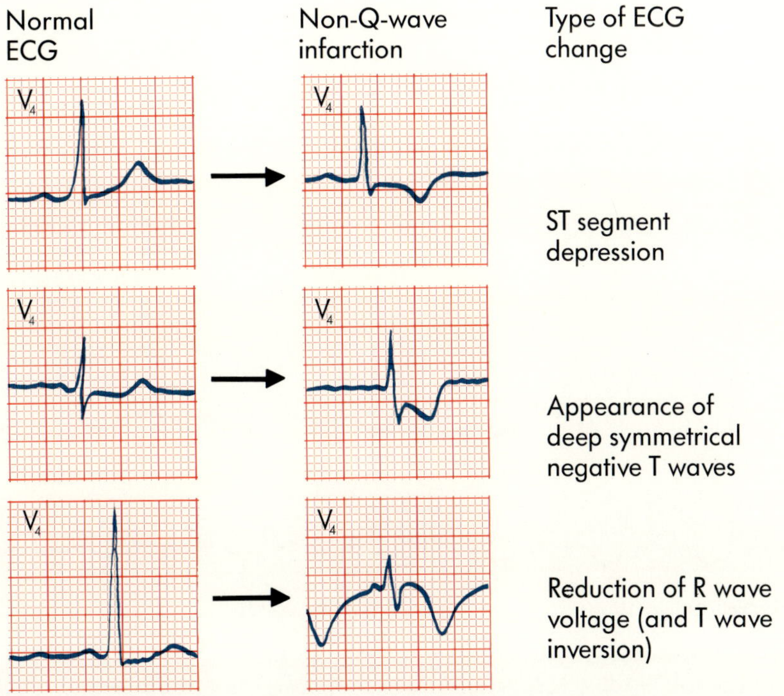

Fig. 14.13
Non-Q-wave infarction. Principal ECG changes

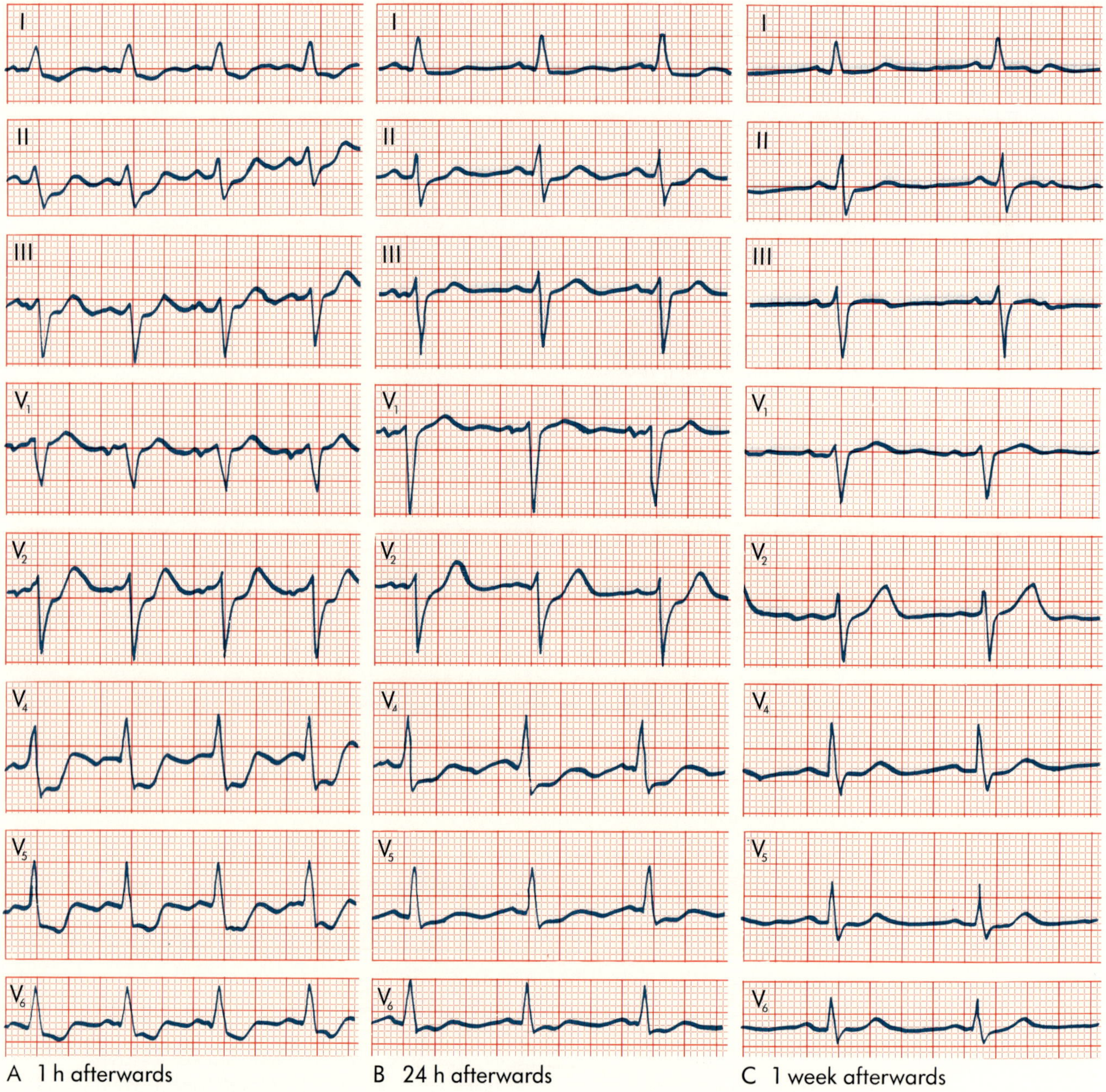

Fig. 14.14
Non-Q-wave infarction. Transitory ECG changes. The ECG recording 1 hour after onset of chest pain shows ST segment depression in multiple leads (V_{2-6}, II and III). The ST segment depression is still present but less impressive at the next recording 24 h later, while there is no significant ST depression in the recording 1 week later.

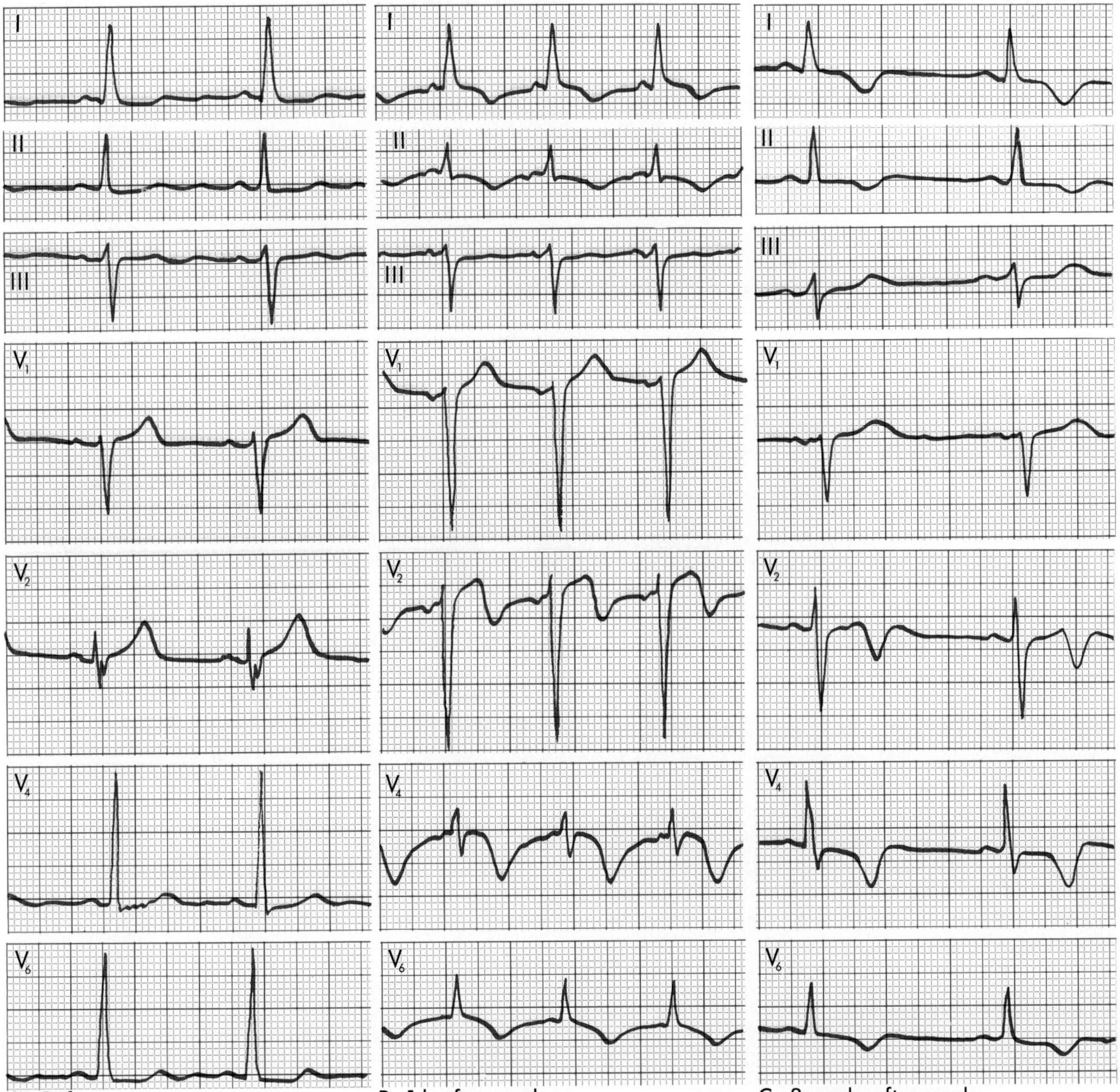

A Before B 1 h afterwards C 3 weeks afterwards

Fig. 14.15
Non-Q-wave infarction. Persistence of ECG changes. There is a reduction in R wave height and the development of deep symmetrical T waves in the ECG recorded shortly after the onset of pain. An ECG recording obtained 3 weeks later shows persistence of the R wave and T wave changes.

Myocardial ischaemia [9–20]

Myocardial ischaemia is a consequence of a lack of oxygen in a portion of the ventricular myocardium and occurs secondary to a temporary and reversible imbalance between oxygen demand and regional blood flow.

Myocardial ischaemia usually is associated with changes in the ST segment. The changes are reversible and come and go with the ischaemia. ECG recording from a lead facing the ischaemic region of the heart may show (Fig. 14.16):

A ST segment depression in subendocardial ischaemia. Subendocardial ischaemia is confined to the inner half to two thirds of the ventricular wall. It is the common form of ischaemia which occurs in effort angina.

B ST segment elevation in the patient with transmural ischaemia. Transmural ischaemia affects the ventricular wall in its entire thickness. Transmural ischaemia is the common finding in Prinzmetal's variant angina. Occasionally, it occurs in unstable angina. It occurs but is rare in effort angina.

Recording of ischaemia by a lead directed away from the ischaemic region will reveal "reciprocal" ECG changes with ST segment elevation in subendocardial ischaemia and ST depression in transmural ischaemia. Angina in the form of *effort angina (stable angina)*, *unstable angina* or *Prinzmetal's variant angina* (vasospastic angina) may accompany the ischaemia. Sometimes ischaemia is *not* associated with chest pain, so-called *silent myocardial* ischaemia.

Effort angina (stable angina) [10, 17]

Effort angina generally occurs with significant coronary artery stenosis (50–90 % occlusion) of often two or three major vessels but occasionally of only one major vessel. The patient is free from symptoms at rest but physical exercise and/or emotional stress induce chest pain. This is because the rise in heart rate, blood pressure and myocardial contractility associated with effort and stress increase the myocardial oxygen demand. The result is myocardial ischaemia since the coronary artery stenoses prevent the required increase in coronary artery blood flow. Myocardial ischaemia generally is of subendocardial type and is associated with ST segment depression usually in multiple leads (Figs. 14.16 A, 14.17 A–B and 14.18, page 328). The ECG recording at rest may be abnormal and show evidence of coronary artery disease e.g. abnormal Q waves related to prior myocardial infarction or ST segment or T wave changes or bundle branch block. Often, however, the ECG at rest is normal but the exercise electrocardiogram will confirm the diagnosis of effort induced myocardial ischaemia.

Exercise electrocardiography [11]

Indications

Exercise electrocardiography traditionally is performed for the diagnosis of coronary artery disease and for the assessment of exercise capacity. Several studies indicate that exercise electrocardiography is useful for identifying patients at high risk for cardiac death among survivors of acute myocardial infarction (i.e. potential candidates for coronary arteriography and subsequent bypass surgery). The relative prognostic significance of ST depression compared to other variables e.g. duration of exercise and ventricular arrhythmias is still unresolved.

continued page 330

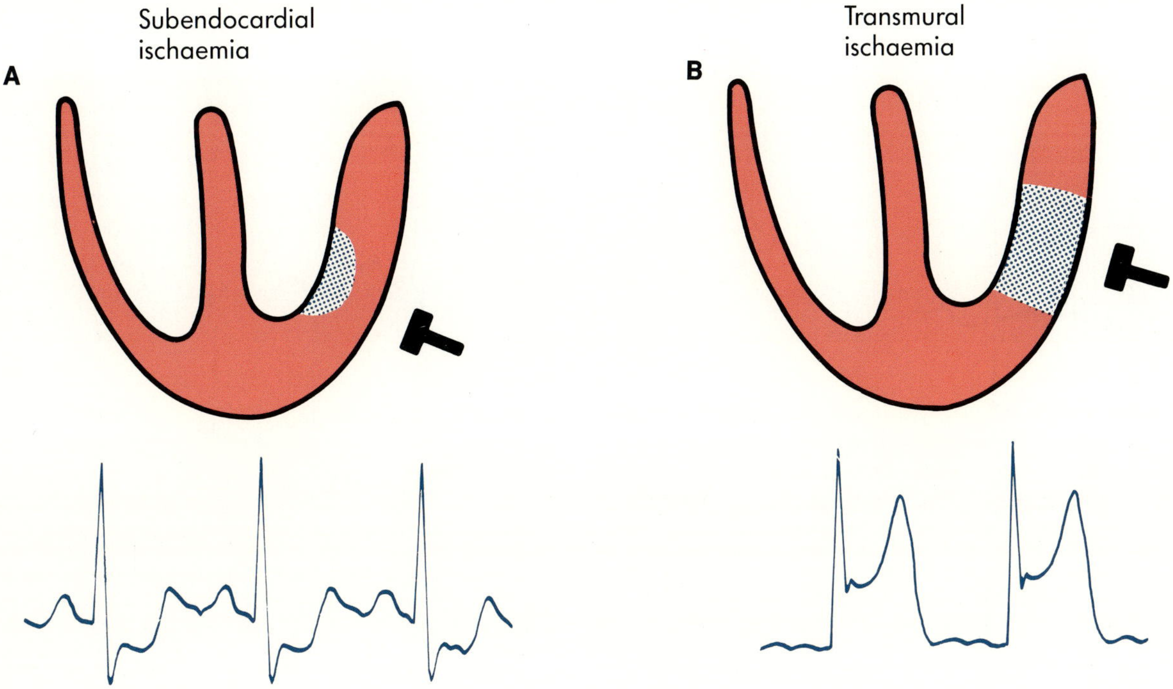

Fig. 14.16
Principal ECG changes in subendocardial (A) and transmural myocardial ischaemia (B)

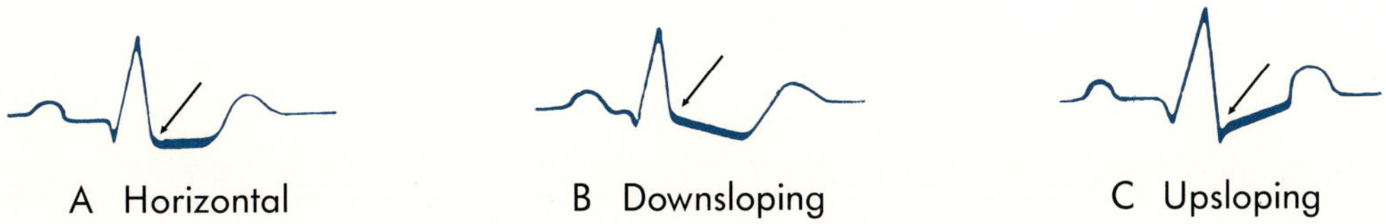

Fig. 14.17
Various types of ST segment depression in subendocardial ischaemi. ST segment depression of the upsloping type is a non-specific finding of minor diagnostic significance. Arrow indicates J point (junction between terminal portion of the QRS complex and the ST segment).

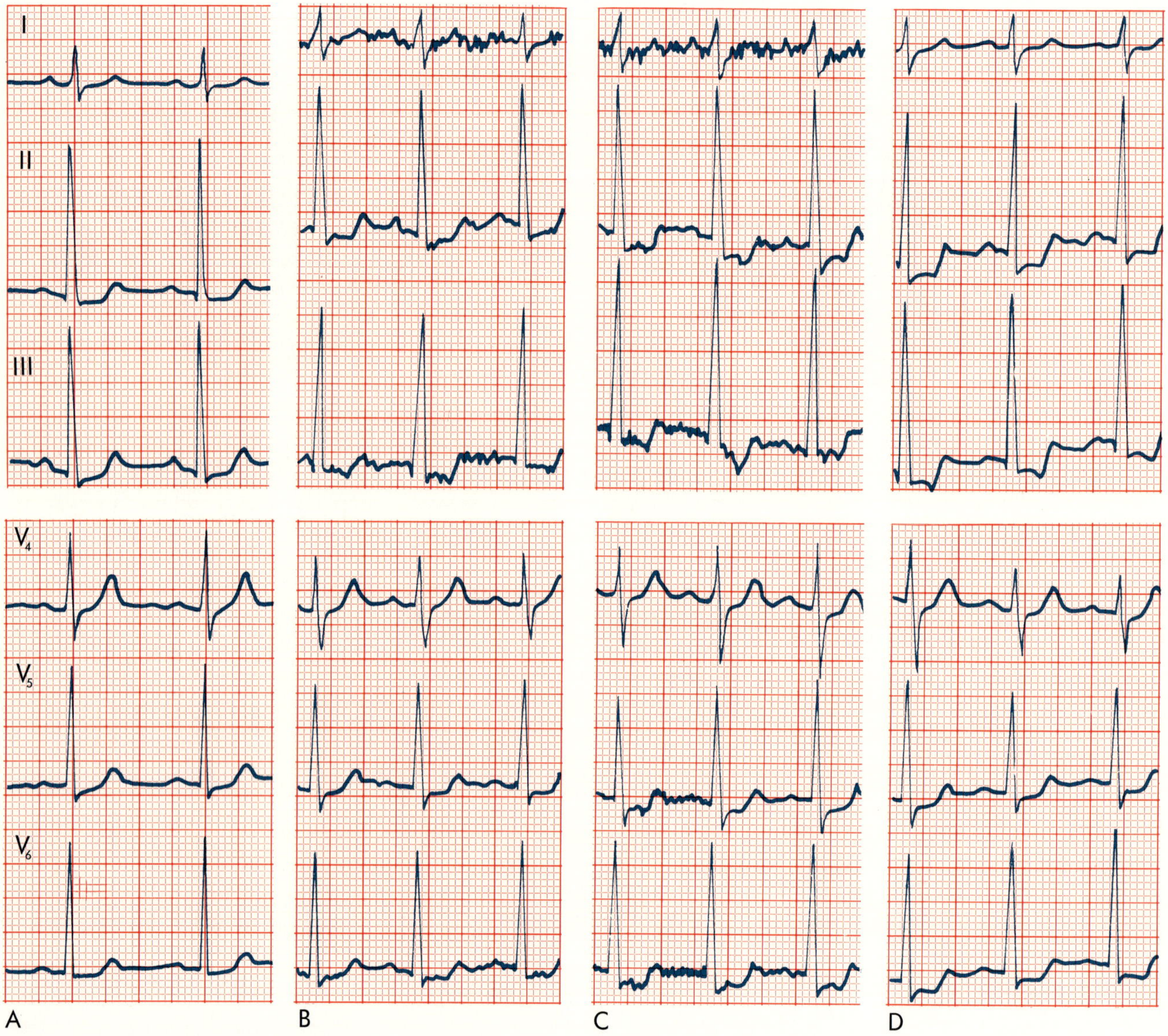

Fig. 14.18
Positive response to exercise electrocardiography in coronary artery disease. 60-year-old male with effort angina pectoris. Subsequent coronary arteriography shows two vessel disease with significant stenosis in the right coronary artery and in the anterior descending branch of the left coronary artery.

A Before exercise test. The patient is without pain, and the ECG is normal
B 50 watts (3 min). Horizontal ST segment depression in many leads
C 75 watts (3 min). Exercise ECG recorded after 6 min of exercise on a bicycle ergometer coinciding with the onset of anginal pain. There is a 1–2 mm horizontal/downsloping ST segment depression in leads I, II, III and V_{5-6}
D After cessation of work. The ST depression continued for approximately 8 min

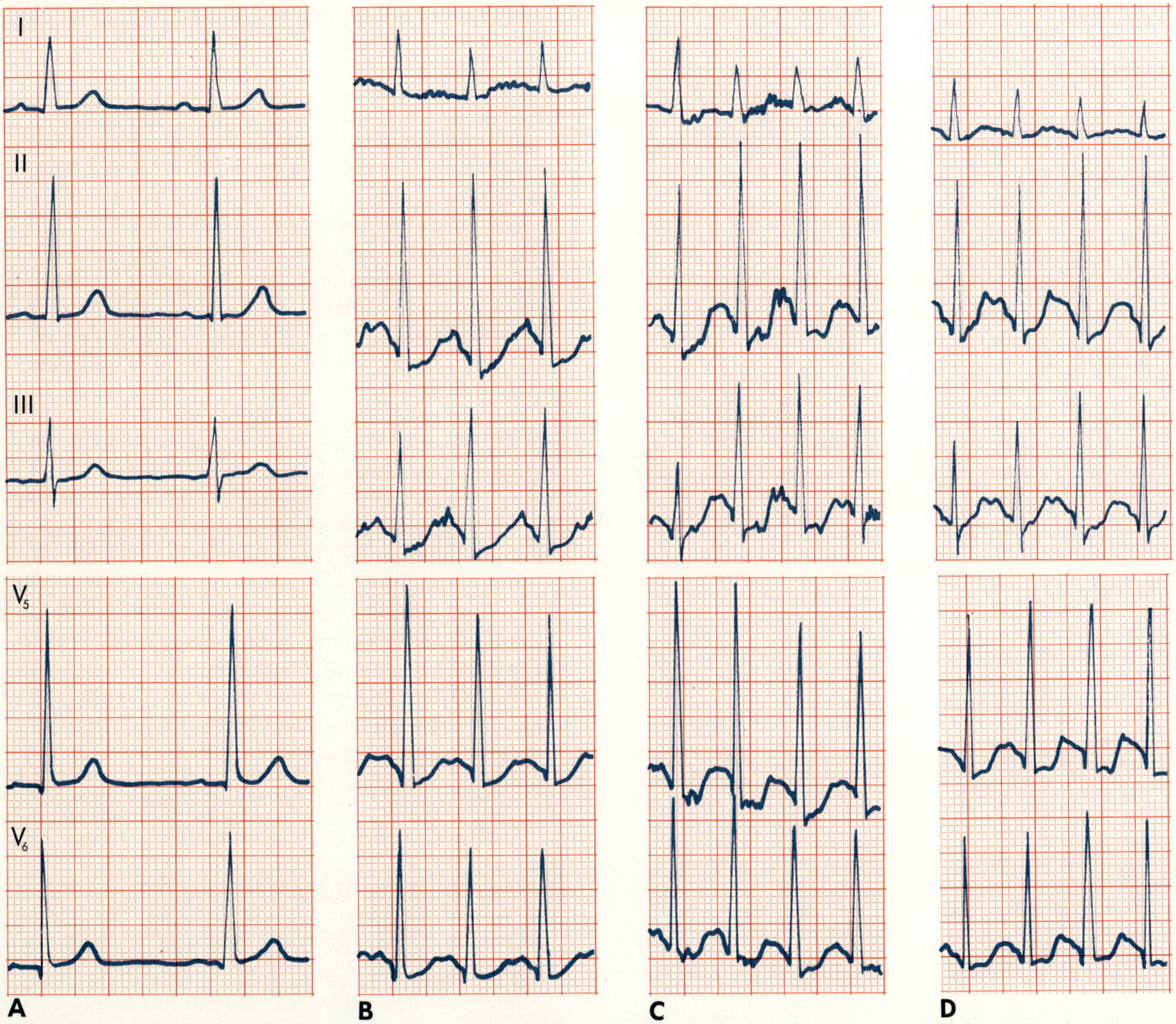

Fig. 14.19
Positive response to exercise electrocardiography in a healthy male. ECG recording from a routine health investigation of 42-year-old airline pilot. He had no cardio-pulmonary complaints. The clinical investigation, chest x-ray, echocardiography and isotope ventriculography combined with exercise testing showed normal conditions. His pilot's licence was suspended following an abnormal response to exercise electrocardiography, but was reinstated unconditionally after a subsequent coronary arteriography and ventriculography showed normal conditions.

A Before exercise test. ECG is normal
B 100 watts (3 min). Upsloping ST segment depression in many leads
C 150 watts (3 min). Horizontal ST segment depression in many leads exceeding 2 mm
D After cessation of work. Unchanged horizontal depression in many leads. The ST segment depression continued for approximately 5 min. The patient felt no chest pain at any time

Exercise electrocardiography can be useful in the diagnosis of effort induced tachycardia or fibrillation. The target patient is the individual with a history of effort induced syncope or dizziness (Figs. 6.41, page 178/179 and 14.22, page 336/337). Exercise electrocardiography is used to provoke the underlying arrhythmia, and may subsequently be repeated to test the efficacy of an antiarrhythmic drug treatment.

Safety

The mortality risk for patients tested by an exercise ECG for coronary artery disease is in the region of 0.5–1 per 10,000 tests with an additional morbidity rate of 2 per 10,000 tests. Mortality is mostly due to cardiac arrest and morbidity due to attacks of angina or cardiac arrhythmias, and occasionally to acute myocardial infarction. Sound clinical judgement should prevail in the selection of patients for the test. The exercise test should *not* be performed in the event of:

- Acute myocardial infarction and during the first week afterwards
- Unstable angina i.e. accelerating angina with more frequent or sustained attacks of angina or episodes of rest angina (see next section)
- Congestive heart failure
- Uncontrolled atrial fibrillation and flutter
- Significant aortic stenosis
- Uncontrolled arterial hypertension (WHO stages III and IV).

Constant supervision including continuous ECG monitoring is mandatory. A doctor should be nearby so as to be able to render assistance within seconds. A defibrillator should be available for immediate use. Emergency drugs including nitroglycerine and atropine must be available as must equipment for i.v. infusion. A resuscitation air bag and oxygen should be available. The staff should be skilled in cardiopulmonary resuscitation. Exercise testing for the purpose of provoking potentially life threatening arrhythmias should be undertaken only in a hospital department where staff are especially skilled in the diagnosis and management of arrhythmias.

Principle

Exercise electrocardiography is best performed as a symptom limited test with gradual increasing workload on a bicycle ergometer or a treadmill. Primary endpoints for patients terminating the test are progressive anginal pain, shortness of breath, fatigue or occasionally dizziness or leg pain. The test should be stopped if the ECG shows complex ventricular arrhythmias, or the patient shows signs of imminent circulatory collapse (pallor, cyanosis, clammy skin, falling blood pressure, respiratory rales).

The ECG is best recorded in 12 leads with a slight modification of standard electrode placement to avoid motion artefacts (arm electrodes placed on the shoulders, leg electrodes on the abdomen just above the right and left anterior superior iliac spine).

The blood pressure response should be monitored by repeated measurements (cuff method). Depending on the functional state of the patient, the initial workload on the bicycle ergomometer might be 25–50 watt with stepwise increase every second minute up to maximum exercise capacity. ECG and blood pressure are recorded:

- At rest before the onset of exercise
- At the end of each 2-minute period of workload, and
- In the post exercise period, immediately after stopping exercise and at 2 to 4-minute intervals until the heart rate has returned to the pre-test level.

The normal response to exercise

The normal ECG response to exercise includes:

- An increased P wave amplitude
- Shortening of the PR interval
- Reduction in height of R waves

- Depression of the onset of the ST segment, *the J point* (J stands for junction between the end of QRS complex and the ST segment) followed by an upsloping ST interval as it merges into the T wave

- Flattening of the T wave.

The heart rate response to exercise decreases with advancing age. Expressed in an easy to remember formula, heart rate at maximum exercise capacity for the normal individual of more than 20 years of age will be at least:

0.85 x (220 – age in years) beats/min.

To ensure that an exercise ECG is truly negative, the patient should be encouraged to work until this age related target heart rate has been achieved. Caution is necessary when the patient has dramatic symptoms (fainting, collapse etc.)

The ischaemic ST segment response to exercise

The typical ECG response to exercise induced subendocardial ischaemia is horizontal ST segment depression (Fig. 14.17 A, page 327) or downsloping depression (Fig. 14.17 B). Upsloping ST segment depression (Fig. 14.17 C) is a normal finding and is of no diagnostic significance.

The magnitude of the ST segment depression is measured by the vertical distance from the isoelectric level of the PR and/or TP segments to the level of the ST segment 80 ms after the J point (junction between QRS complex and ST segment). The commonly applied standard to diagnose abnormal ST segment depression is 1 mm. When multiple leads show ST segment depression (a not uncommon finding) (Fig. 14.18, page 328), the maximum depression should be noted. The most significant ST segment depressions are usually recorded in leads V_{5-6}.

The rate of *false negative responses* to exercise electrocardiography (no ST segment depression despite the presence of significant coronary artery disease) is in the region of 10–20 % if the patient reaches his age related target heart.

If exercise is stopped at a lower heart rate due to nonspecific symptoms e.g. fatigue, shortness of breath or leg pain, the risk of a false negative response is increased. Concurrent administration of a beta adrenergic blocking agent or a calcium channel blocking agent may significantly lower the exercise induced increase in heart rate and blood pressure and may result in a false negative response.

Several conditions can cause a *false positive* ST segment depression with exercise when there is no myocardial ischaemia e.g.:

- Pre-excitation with WPW pattern on the resting ECG

- Left bundle branch block

- Right bundle branch block (while ST segment depression in V_{1-2} is a non-specific finding, ST segment depression in V_{5-6} seems a useful marker of ischaemia)

- Rate dependant bundle branch block (Fig. 9.12, page 243)

- Deep broad Q waves in precordial leads related to an old anterior wall Q-wave infarction (Q waves in limb leads following an inferior wall infarction are of no importance)

- Conditions like valvular disease, systemic hypertension and pulmonary hypertension. Associated ventricular hypertrophy may not be apparent on the resting ECG but reveal itself by ST depression on the exercise ECG and be misinterpreted as subendocardial ischaemia.

Even when all precautions are taken, the false positive rate can be high, as it varies with the prevalence of ischaemic heart disease in the population investigated. The number of false positive responses is low and the specificity of the test is correspondingly high if the prevalence of coronary artery disease is high in the investigated population i.e. if the test is reserved for investigation of patients with angina-like pain. The number of false positive responses increases and the specificity of the test decreases with a decline in the prevalence of coronary artery disease in the investigated population. For screening asymptomatic individuals, uncritical use of the test will result in more false positive than true positive diagnoses. Thus, the odds in favour of a false positive ischaemic ST segment response versus a true one are in the order of 4:1 when the exercise test is performed in an unselected population of forty to sixty-year-old males and may be as high as 10:1 in females and/or younger individuals. Thus, the test may do more to create iatrogenic disease pattern than to detect preclinical coronary artery disease. Practical problems have already been created by the use of the test in the routine health screening of airline pilots (Fig. 14.19, page 329).

Additional ischaemic responses to exercise

ST segment elevation (more than 1 mm) during exercise is most often seen in the patient with a history of a previous myocardial infarction and who has a major dykinetic or akinetic region in the left ventricle. Without previous myocardial infarction, ST segment elevation is rare but it occurs in Prinzmetal's variant angina due to coronary artery spasm. The development of *negative U waves* (e.g. in leads II and V_{5-6}) is an insensitive but specific indicator of coronary artery disease. It is seen particularly in the patient with stenosis of the proximal portion of the left anterior descending coronary artery.

Exercise induced *T wave changes* are frequent but they are non-specific and are of little or no diagnostic importance.

At exercise testing *in the second or third week of recovery from an acute myocardial infarction*, the primary prognostic discriminators between high and low risk patients are:

- A low maximal heart rate and a low rise in systolic blood pressure. A sinister prognostic sign is an actual fall in blood pressure.

- The induction of frequent or repetitive ventricular extrasystole.

In this context, ST segment depression in itself does not add any independent prognostic information.

Unstable angina [12, 13]

Unstable angina is a clinical syndrome characterized by:

- Angina pectoris of new onset brought on by minimal exertion, or
- More severe, prolonged or frequent attacks of angina super-imposed on a prior stable effort angina, or *most often*
- Sustained attacks of angina pectoris at rest.

The attacks of angina usually are associated with reversible ECG changes. These include ST segment depression, or very often ST segment elevation and/or T wave changes, and the development of negative T waves or their change from negative to positive. The condition may progress to myocardial infarction or it may be complicated by cardiac arrest and sudden death. More often the symptoms subside and the situation stabilizes.

The differential diagnosis between unstable angina and subendocardial infarction depends on the regression of the ECG changes after the cessation of pain and the profile of the serum enzymes. Persistence of the ECG changes and/or a significant rise in the serum enzymes indicate that the condition has become complicated by infarction. The differential diagnosis between unstable angina with episodes of ST elevation and Prinzmetal's variant angina of recent onset (see next section) can be made only by observing the patient over a period of time e.g. in the Coronary Care Unit.

Prinzmetal's variant angina (vasospastic angina) [14–16]

Prinzmetal's variant angina or vasospastic angina is caused by spasm in one of the larger coronary arteries resulting in a sudden and total closure of the vessel. This is a rare form of angina seen primarily in younger patients. It is associated with a wide variety of arteriosclerotic lesions ranging from normal coronary arteries to coronary arteries with severe arteriosclerotic lesions. Attacks occur characteristically either late at night or early in the morning when parasympathetic tone is high and sympathetic tone although low is rising. The sudden, total closure of the larger coronary vessels leads to acute transmural ischaemia often associated with very marked ST segment elevation in leads III and aVF if the spasm is located in the right coronary artery (Figs. 14.20 A, page 334 and 14.21, page 335), or in the precordial leads if the spasm occurs in the larger branches of the left coronary artery (Fig. 14.20 B).

The attack often is complicated by arrhythmias e.g. AV block, SA block or ventricular tachycardia, the latter often of torsade de pointes type (Fig. 14.21). The diagnosis of Prinzmetal's variant angina frequently is delayed or overlooked because the attacks of pain and the arrhythmias may be so brief that an ECG cannot be obtained before the attack is over. Occasionally, ST segment depression rather than ST segment elevation is recorded during ECG monitoring in the Coronary Care Unit. ST segment depression occasionally is caused by positive-negative inversion of the monitoring leads compared to the standard limb or precordial lead it was supposed to represent (Fig. 14.21) or ST depression may reflect reciprocal recording of transmural myocardial ischaemia by a lead opposite to the ischaemic region.

A number of studies have corroborated by coronary arteriography that vasospastic angina may sometimes be accompanied by ST segment depression or by an alternation between ST segment depression and ST segment elevation. Spasm responsible for ST segment depression and for subendocardial ischaemia usually is subtotal or localized to smaller branches of the coronary arteries.

continued page 336

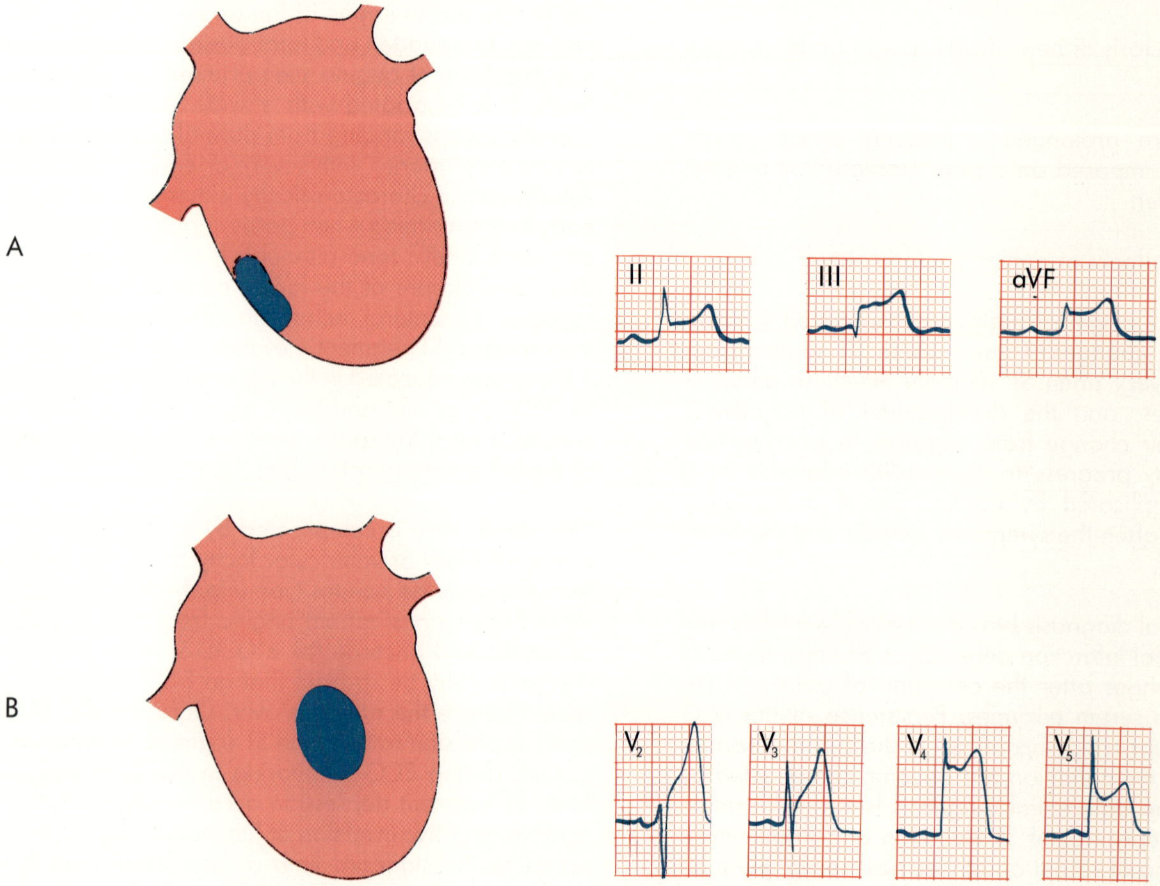

Fig. 14.20
Prinzmetal's variant angina (spasm angina). Location of the ST segment elevation in inferior (A) and anterior (B) wall ischaemia

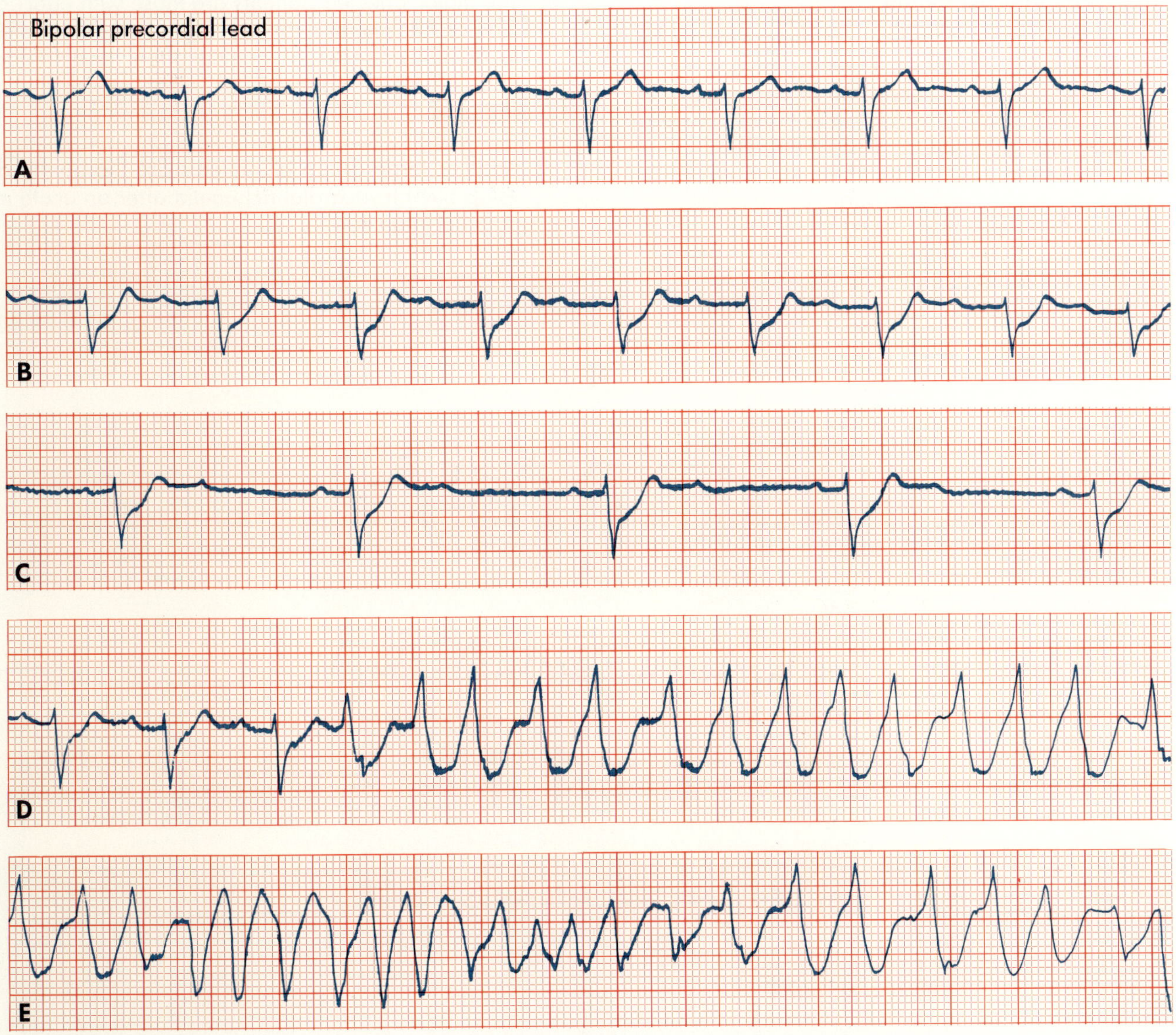

Fig. 14.21
Prinzmetal's variant angina (spasm angina). Complicated by arrhythmias. Strips from the ECG monitoring of the patient whose ECG is shown in Fig. 14.20 A. Strip (A) has been recorded between attacks, strips (B–E) during recurrent episodes of pain. The recordings are from a bipolar chest lead resembling lead aVF (see Chapter 3, Fig. 3.19, p. 54), but the polarity of the lead is reversed so that the transmural ischaemia is reflected by the recording of an ST segment depression instead of an ST elevation.

A No pain. Sinus rhythm, normal PR interval, no ST segment deviation
B Pain. First degree AV block (PR 0.36 s), ST segment depression
C Pain. Second degree AV block (2:1 block), ST segment depression
D Pain. Sinus rhythm with ST segment depression followed by ventricular tachycardia
E Pain. Torsade de pointes ventricular tachycardia

Silent myocardial ischaemia[17–20]

Angina is the common, well-known clinical manifestation of myocardial ischaemia. However, myocardial ischaemia indicated by ST depression or occasionally by ST segment elevation can occur without pain, so-called *silent myocardial ischaemia.*

1 The major affected patients are those with effort angina or Prinzmetal's variant angina, who in addition to painful episodes of angina often have frequent and sustained episodes of silent myocardial ischaemia.

2 Another large group of patients are those who develop silent myocardial ischaemia after an acute myocardial infarction.

REST

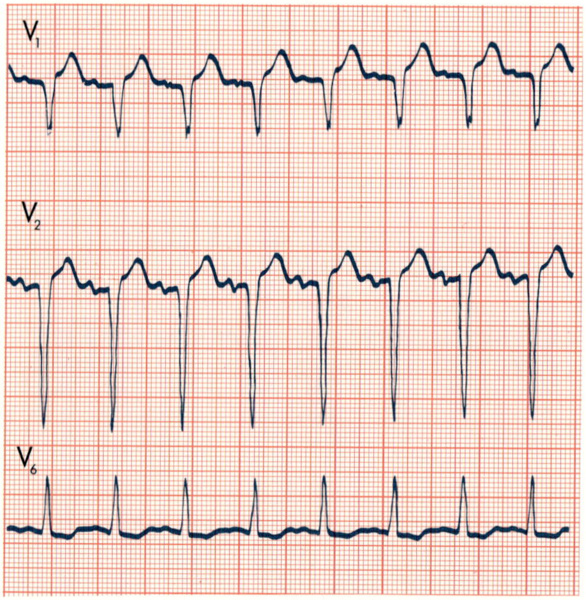

25 mm/s

Fig. 14.22
Exercise induced silent myocardial ischaemia which precipitates attacks of ventricular tachycardia and fibrillation. ECG from a 49-year-old man admitted in ventricular fibrillation. Two attacks of fainting in the week prior to admission, the one in relation to physical strain. No cardiac complaints, no previous angina or myocardial infarction. Exercise on a bicycle ergometer induced horizontal ST segment depression of 3–4 mm in leads I and V_{4-6} at a heart rate of 120/min. No angina but in two of a total of three exercise tests transition from myocardial ischaemia signalled by ST segment depression to multiform ventricular tachycardia which in the last test degenerated into ventricular fibrillation (sinus rhythm was restored by immediate DC conversion). Coronary arteriography showed a 75% stenosis on LAD and a 50% stenosis of the circumflex branch. After coronary bypass surgery the patient did not exhibit either exercise induced myocardial ischaemia or attacks of ventricular tachycardia, fibrillation or fainting (follow-up 2 years).

3 A smaller group of patients are those who have no signs of ischaemic heart disease and have had neither angina, nor acute myocardial infarction. The ECG signs of silent myocardial ischaemia may have been detected by chance (routine health check-ups including exercise ECG or ambulatory ECG monitoring). Because of the high likelihood of false positive, non-ischaemic ST segment deviation in such a symptom free population, a diagnosis of ischaemic heart disease would need confirmation by additional tests, primarily radionucleide scintigraphy. Only if confirmed should invasive investigation by coronary arteriography be considered.

4 min EXERCISE

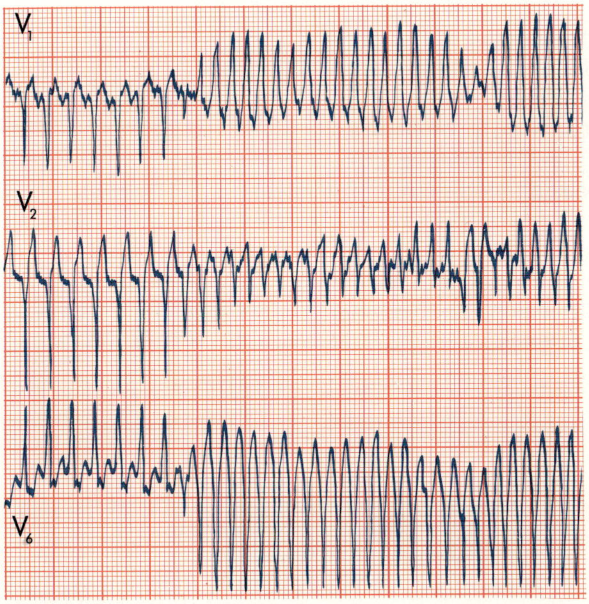

10 mm/s

Fig. 14.22 (continued)

The diagnostic tools for the recognition of silent myocardial include exercise ECG and 24-hour ambulatory ECG monitoring.

These tests can distinguish silent ischaemia with two modes of onset:

- Silent ischaemia induced by an increase in heart rate and blood pressure and thus by an *increased oxygen demand*, is revealed by the exercise ECG, whereas

- Silent ischaemia not preceded by an increase in heart rate or in blood pressure and thus unrelated to an *increase in myocardial oxygen supply* is a frequent finding in ambulatory ECG monitoring.

Apart from the (rare) patient with Prinzmetal's variant angina, ECG monitoring will add few new diagnoses of ischaemic heart disease to those already detected by the exercise ECG, whereas the converse is often true. Thus, from a diagnostic point of view an exercise ECG alone will often suffice when seeking non-painful ischaemic heart disease.

Silent myocardial ischaemia can cause attacks of paroxysmal ventricular tachycardia which may respond to revascularization (Fig. 14.22, page 336/337) or, in "silent" Prinzmetal variant angina to calcium antagonist therapy.

Transitory T wave and/or ST segment changes after an attack of tachycardia [21–23]

T wave inversion (or peaking) and, sometimes, ST segment depression or elevation, may be seen in sinus rhythm immediately after an attack of tachycardia (Fig. 14.23). The changes usually subside gradually within 1 or 2 days to a week, but sometimes may persist for several weeks. The pathophysiological background for these changes is obscure. They seem unrelated to ischaemia, are often recorded in young individuals and are of no prognostic importance.

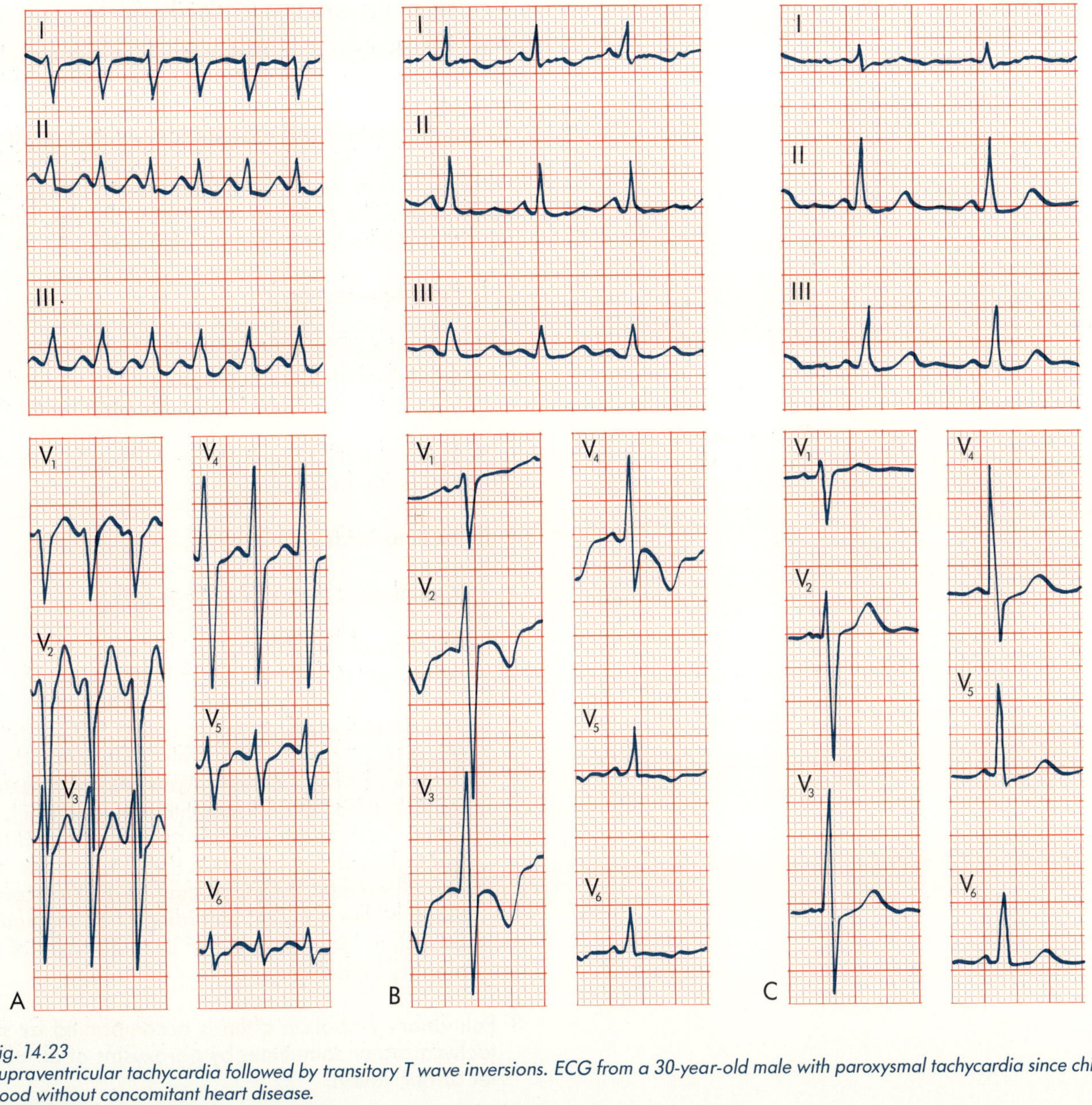

Fig. 14.23
Supraventricular tachycardia followed by transitory T wave inversions. ECG from a 30-year-old male with paroxysmal tachycardia since childhood without concomitant heart disease.

A Supraventricular tachycardia: QRS complexes with a different axis and slightly wider than in sinus rhythm but still < 0.12 s wide. Slight ST segment depression in several leads. QRS rate 200/min. Tachycardia is regular, so atrial fibrillation can be excluded. Further classification is impossible since atrial activity is not visible, but from a statistical point of view the likely diagnosis is AV nodal tachycardia.
B Sinus rhythm, ECG recording 24 hours after an attack of tachycardia: Symmetrical, deeply negative T waves in leads V_{2-4}, slightly negative T waves in I, II, V_{5-6}
C Sinus rhythm, ECG recording 4 days after the attack: The T waves now have become normally positive in all leads

Acute pulmonary embolism [24]

The ECG changes recorded in acute pulmonary embolism vary with the size of the embolus and the strain it imposes on the right ventricle. However, even massive pulmonary embolism may occur without significant ECG changes. The ECG features are usually transient in nature and may be missed if the ECG recording is postponed for some hours or for a day or two. Findings typical of pulmonary embolism include (Fig. 14.24):

1 In the precordial leads:

- A right ventricular strain pattern with a negative T wave and/or ST segment depression in leads V_{1-3} (Fig. 14.24 A–B and Fig. 14.25, page 342), or
- Right bundle branch block, incomplete or complete (Fig. 14.24 C).

2 In the limb leads:

- P pulmonale (Fig. 14.24 D), and/or
- Rotation of the QRS axis to the right with the development of a deep S wave in lead I, and/or
- The development of the so-called $S_I Q_{III} T_{III}$ pattern (Figs. 14.24 E and 14.25). This comprises a deep S wave in lead I, a deep Q wave and an inverted T wave in lead III (and sometimes in lead aVF). The pattern can be very similar to that observed in inferior myocardial infarction (Fig. 14.11, page 321). The differential diagnosis may be further complicated by the transient recording of ST segment elevation in leads III and aVF in some cases of pulmonary embolism.

3 Pulmonary embolism often is accompanied by sinus tachycardia or sometimes by paroxysms of atrial flutter or fibrillation.

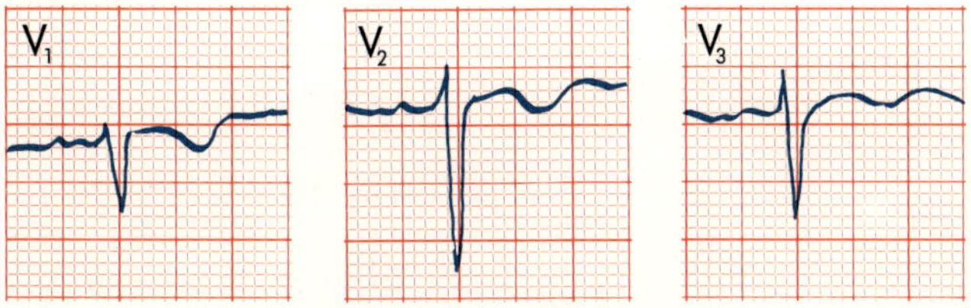

A Negative T in V_{1-3}

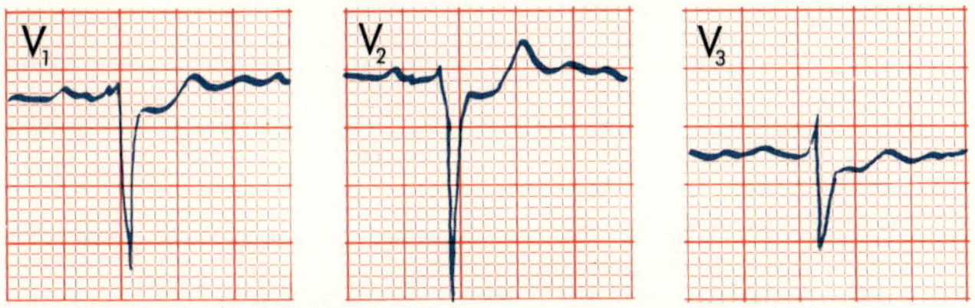

B ST depression in V_{1-3}

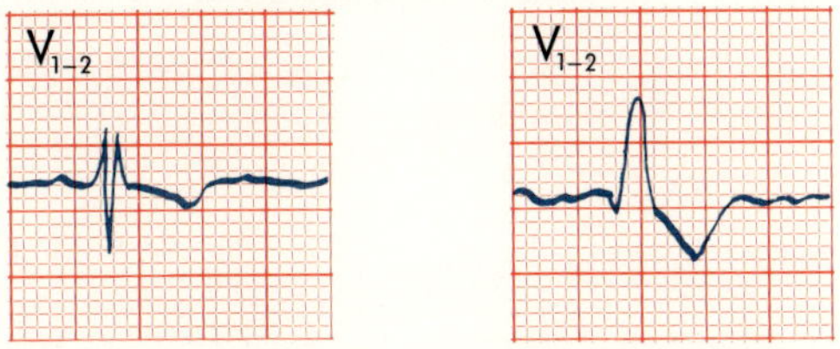

C Incomplete or complete right bundle branch block

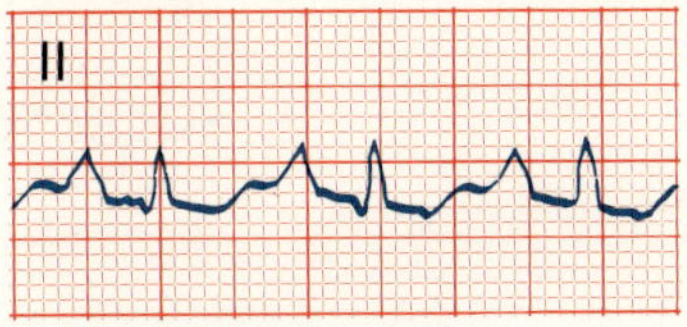

D P–pulmonale

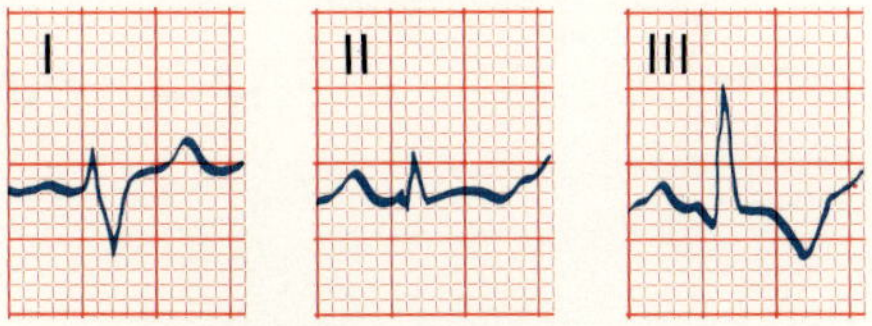

E Right axis deviation, $S_I Q_{III} T_{III}$ pattern

Fig. 14.24
Pulmonary embolism. The spectrum of ECG changes

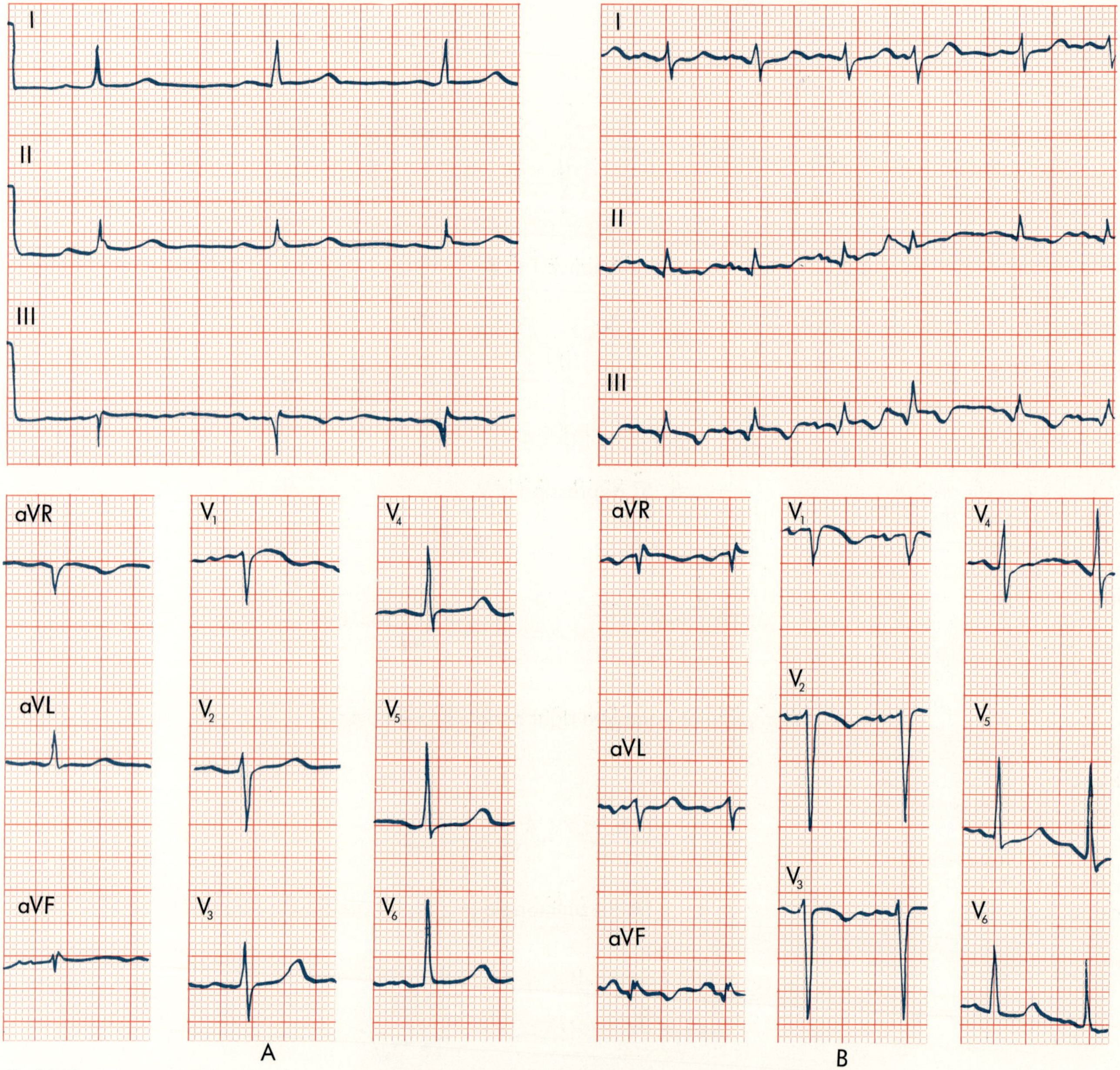

Fig. 14.25
Pulmonary embolism. ECG changes in a 40-year-old woman 1 week after alloplastic operation on the right hip.

A ECG before operation.
B ECG 1 week after operation. Prior to the ECG recording complaints of chest pain and shortness of breath and development of a preshock state with low blood pressure and clamminess of extremities. There is a change from positive to negative T waves in leads V_{1-3}, an axis shift to the right (from 0° to 120°) and the development of an S_IQ_{III} pattern followed by a negative T wave.

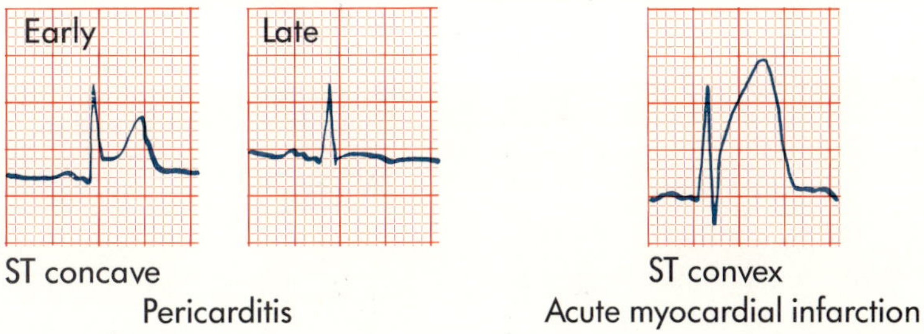

Fig. 14.26
Pericarditis. Early and late ECG changes. For comparison to the right, the ST elevation in an acute transmural infarction

Pericarditis[25–28]

The typical ECG finding in *acute pericarditis* is ST segment elevation (Figs. 14.26 and 14.27 A, page 344) which is present in varying degree in practically all leads of the ECG with the exception of leads III, aVF and V_1 which may show ST segment depression. ST segment elevation in acute myocardial infarction usually is restricted to a few leads and has a convex curvature (Figs. 14.10–14.12, page 320 – page 322 and 14.26). ST elevation of acute pericarditis is recorded in most leads and has an upward concave curvature (Figs. 14.26 and 14.27). Following the initial elevation the ST segment gradually returns towards the isoelectric line, simultaneous with the development of negative T waves (Fig. 14.27 B). Sometimes, negative T waves in multiple leads are the dominant ECG feature even at the very beginning of the pericarditis.

Exudative pericarditis with the accumulation of pericardial fluid often is followed by a reduction in QRS amplitude to produce a "low voltage" pattern in the limb leads (a QRS amplitude of less than 5 mm).

Chronic constrictive pericarditis with fibrotic thickening of the pericardium usually is associated with widespread T wave inversion and sometimes a "low voltage" pattern.

Low voltage of the QRS complex in the limb leads is not limited to exudative or chronic pericarditis but occurs in other pathological conditions including myxoedema, cardiomyopathy, severe coronary artery disease, – and in normal individuals.

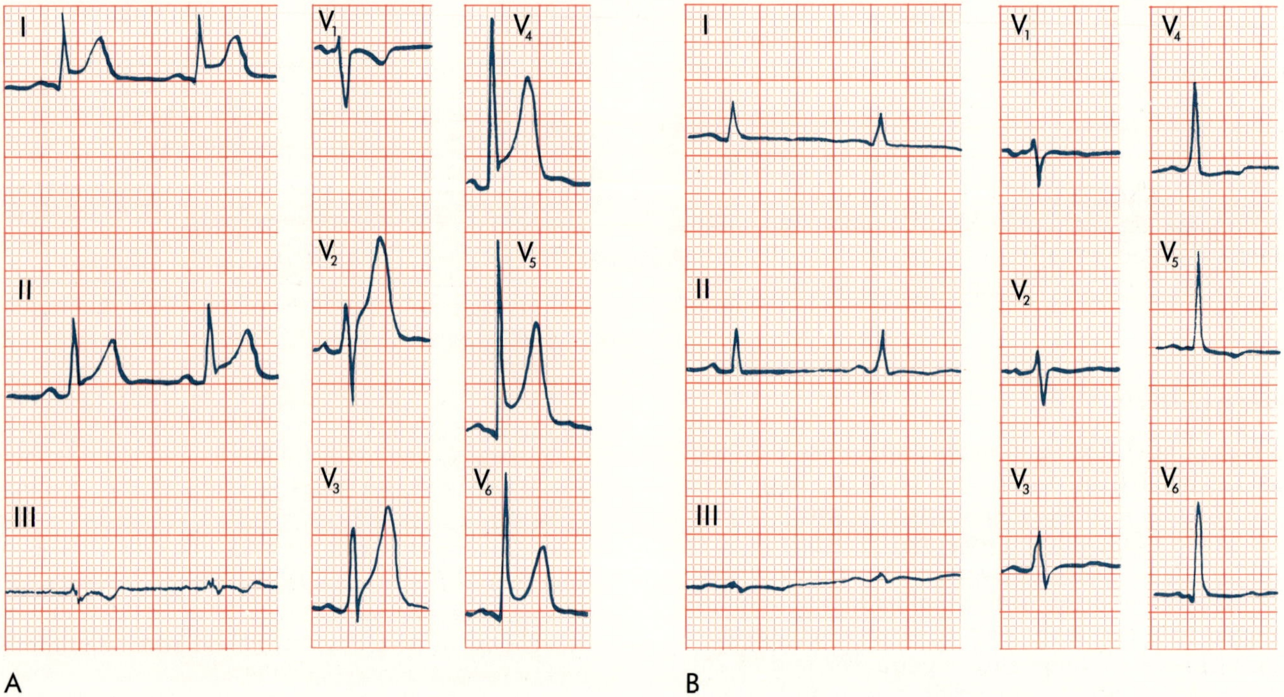

Fig. 14.27
Pericarditis. ECG recording from a 20-year-old male with possible viral pericarditis. The patient was admitted after several days of low grade fever and severe chest pain. At the time of admission, a pericardial friction rub could be heard over the precordium. Radiographic examination revealed a slightly enlarged heart image. Echocardiography demonstrated slight pericardial exsudate. Symptoms and exsudate disappeared over the course of a few weeks. There was no enzyme (LDH) elevation.

A ECG at the time of admission. ST elevation in several leads suggest pericarditis. No abnormal Q waves

B ECG at the time of discharge. T waves range from isoelectric to negative in most leads

Myocarditis [29, 30]

In *rheumatic myocarditis* as presenting in acute rheumatic fever the most common ECG changes are first degree AV block, ST segment depression and T wave inversion.

Many *viral diseases* e.g. mumps, infectious mononucleosis, hepatitis and Coxsackie virus infection are associated with transient ECG changes usually ST depression and/or T wave inversion or occasionally AV block.

Cardiomyopathy [31–33]

Dilated cardiomyopathy. A wide variety of non-specific ECG changes may be seen in dilated (congestive) cardiomyopathy. Left ventricular hypertrophy and/or strain patterns (Fig. 14.28, page 346), bundle branch block (principally left bundle branch block) and low voltage are common findings. Cardiac arrhythmias such as ventricular extrasystoles, atrial fibrillation, ventricular tachycardia and ventricular fibrillation are common complications and may occur early in the disease as debut symptoms. AV block and SA block can occur but are less common.

Hypertrophic cardiomyopathy. The ECG invariably is abnormal usually showing left ventricular hypertrophy and strain pattern (Fig. 14.29, page 347), left bundle branch block (Fig. 14.30 A, page 348), or occasionally a WPW-like pattern (Fig. 14.30 B, page 349). Abnormal Q waves ("pseudo-infarction" pattern) frequently are observed in the limb leads or in the precordial leads (Fig. 14.29). Ventricular arrhythmias are common complications: ventricular extrasystoles, paroxysmal ventricular tachycardia and fibrillation.

Restrictive cardiomyopathy. Patients with Löeffler's endocarditis/endomyocardial fibrosis may show low voltage, features of left atrial enlargement and supraventricular arrhythmias.

continued page 350

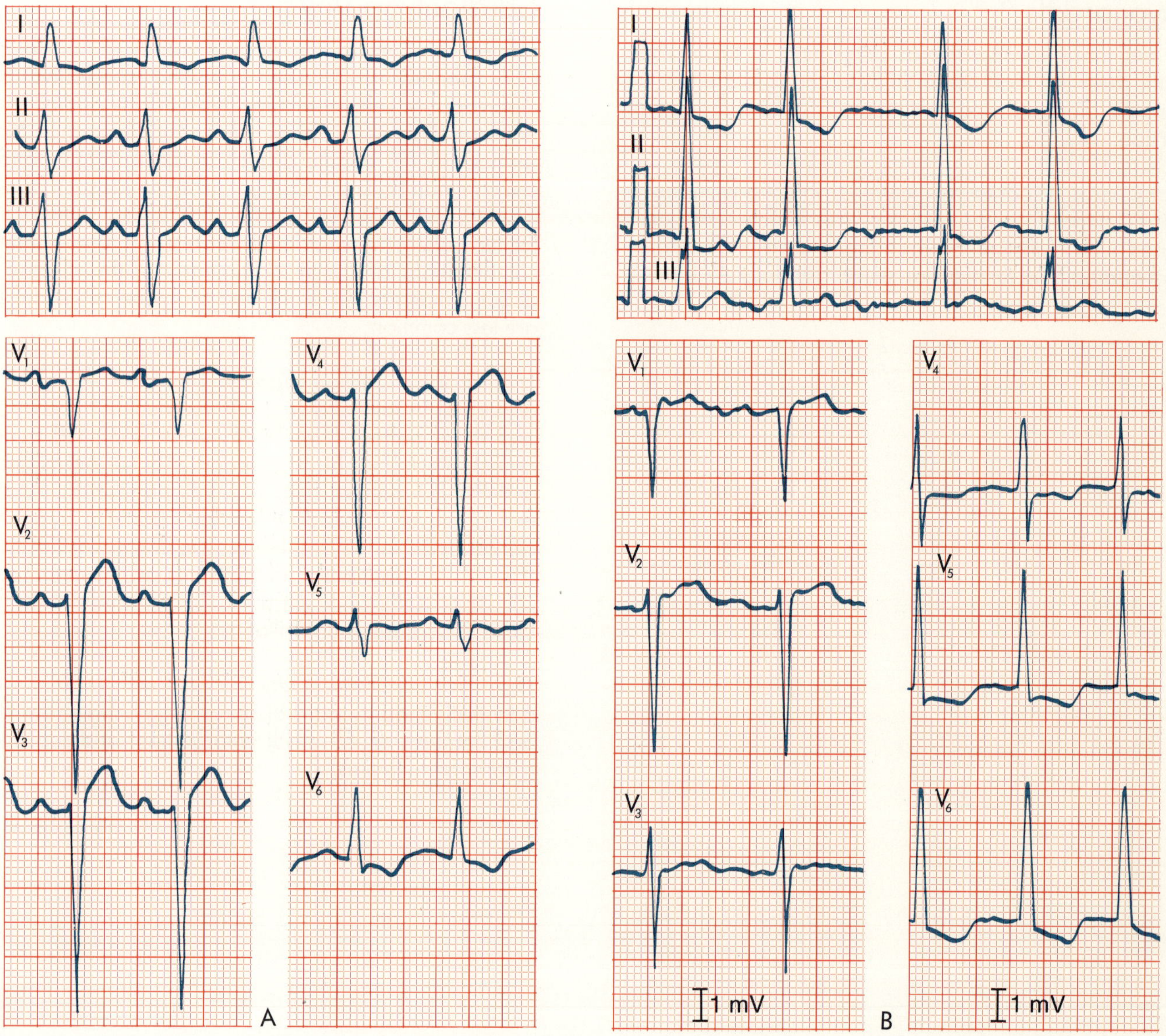

Fig. 14.28
Dilated cardiomyopathy. Two young males, a 32-year-old chronic alcoholic and a formerly healthy 16-year-old boy with no family history of heart disease. Both patients had suffered from shortness of breath on exertion increasing in intensity over a period of 1–2 years and were admitted in congestive failure (combined left and right venticular failure). X-ray of the chest showed a greatly enlarged heart and echocardiography revealed dilated ventricular cavities with a decreased shortening fraction.

A Left ventricular strain with (borderline) ST segment depression and negative T waves in leads V_{5-6} and I

B Atrial fibrillation, left ventricular hypertrophy with abnormally tall R waves in leads V_{5-6} and left ventricular strain with ST segment depression and T wave negativity in leads V_{5-6} and I

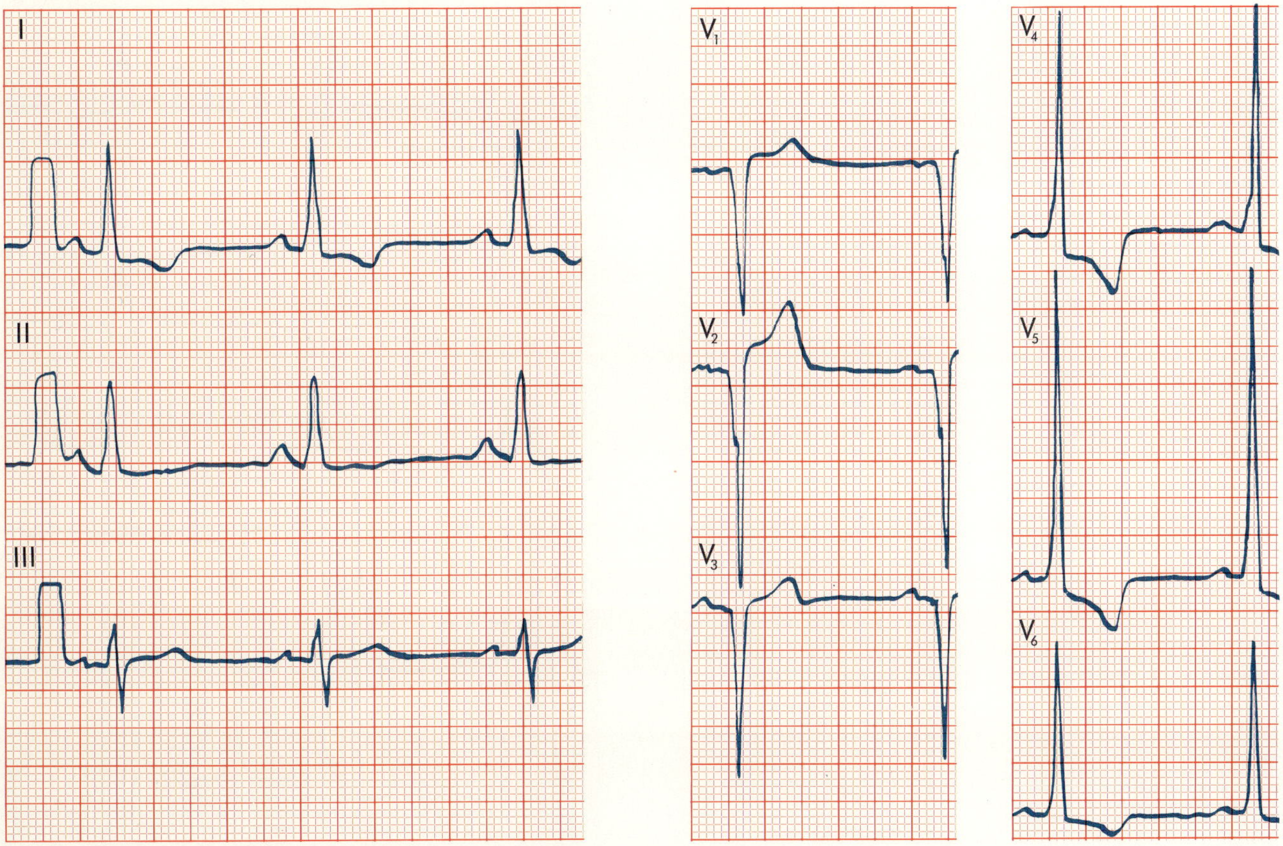

Fig. 14.29
Hypertrophic cardiomyopathy (non-obstructive) . 18-year-old youth. His father died suddenly at the age of 25. For 1 year, the young man had had shortness of breath and angina at exercise. Echocardiography showed diffuse hypertrophy of the left ventricle. ECG shows sinus rhythm, left ventricular hypertrophy and strain patterns.

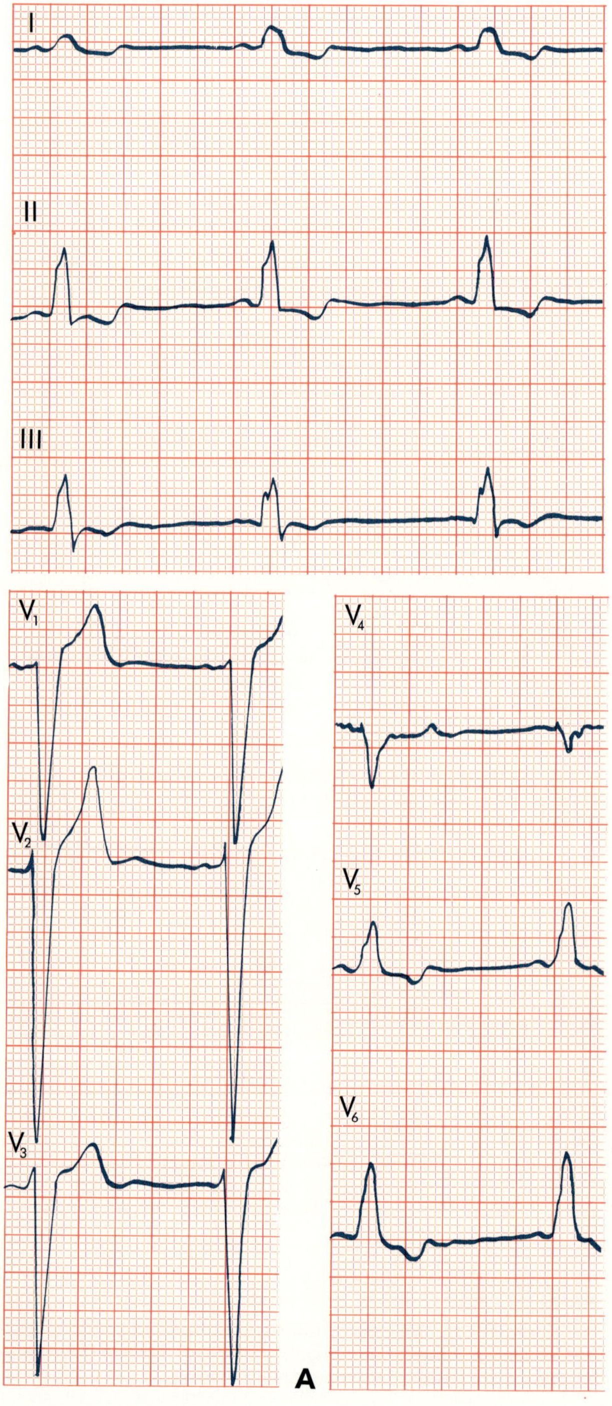

Fig. 14.30
Hypertrophic obstructive cardiomyopathy . Two teenage brothers. Both died before their 18th birthday, one suddenly (A) and the other during an admission for bacterial endocarditis (B). Echocardiography showed asymmetrical left ventricular hypertrophy with massive hypertrophy of the ventricular septum. The ECG shows sinus rhythm and in (A) left bundle branch block, and in (B) a WPW pattern with a very short PR.

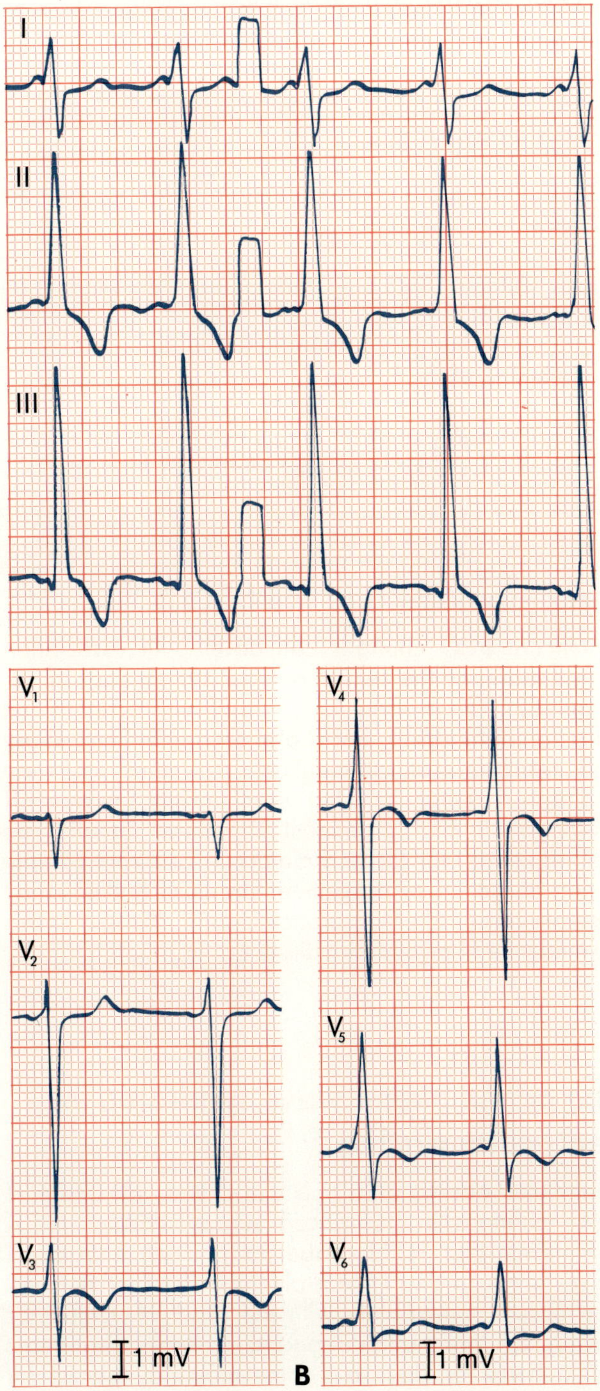

Fig. 14.30
(continued)

Myxoedema and the ECG [34, 35]

The usual ECG changes of myxoedema include (Fig. 14.31):

1 Sinus bradycardia

2 A slightly prolonged PR interval (first degree AV block)

3 Low voltage. (QRS amplitude of less than 5 mm in all limb leads)

4 Flattening of the T wave

5 QT prolongation which in rare cases may be complicated by torsade de pointes ventricular tachycardia.

Brain damage and the ECG [36–38]

Significant ECG changes can develop in association with diseases of the central nervous system (Fig. 14.32, page 352). This is particularly true of subarachnoid and intracranial bleeding, but is also seen with head injury and neurosurgical interventions. The most common findings are deeply inverted or tall upright T waves, QT prolongation and prominent U waves. Torsade de pointes ventricular tachycardia occurs as a rare complication of the QT prolongation. The ECG findings may possibly reflect altered autonomic tone. Autopsy shows no evidence of myocardial disease.

The pacemaker T wave syndrome in ventricular pacing [39, 40]

Ventricular pacing usually is associated with major T wave changes in non-paced supraventricular QRST complexes (Fig. 14.33, page 353). Deep negative T waves are recorded in several leads. The T wave inversion occurs immediately with the onset of ventricular pacing. On termination of pacing, it usually disappears within hours or days but sometimes may persist for weeks.

Pacemaker T wave syndrome should not be misdiagnosed as a non-Q-wave infarction. The differential diagnosis is difficult, particularly as insertion of a pacing lead may be associated with a moderate increase in enzyme levels. Lactate dehydrogenase is often elevated and CKMB may be elevated.

Atrial pacing is not associated with the development of T wave anomalies.

Mitral valve prolapse [41]

The ECG usually is normal in the asymptomatic patient with mitral valve prolapse having typical auscultatory findings (midsystolic click and late systolic murmur) and characteristic echocardiography (systolic sagging of one or both of the mitral valve leaflets). In a minority of patients the ECG shows negative T waves and nonspecific ST changes in leads II, III and aVF or occasionally in the precordial leads.

Other occasional ECG abnormalities include prolongation of the QT interval, prominent U waves and abnormal Q waves. Many reports indicate that patients with mitral valve prolapse have a high incidence of supraventricular and ventricular arrhythmias. Some indicate that these patients may also suffer Stokes-Adams attacks and sudden death related to paroxysms of ventricular tachycardia or AV block (Fig. 6.41, page 178/179). In the patient with mitral valve prolapse and QT prolongation, attacks of torsade de pointes ventricular tachycardia have been observed.

In asymptomatic patients with mitral valve prolapse, a causal relationship between the aforementioned ECG abnormalities and arrhythmias has not been established. Therefore, their simultaneous occurrence may be chance and attributable to the high prevalence of mitral valve prolapse in the general population (2–5 %).

continued page 354

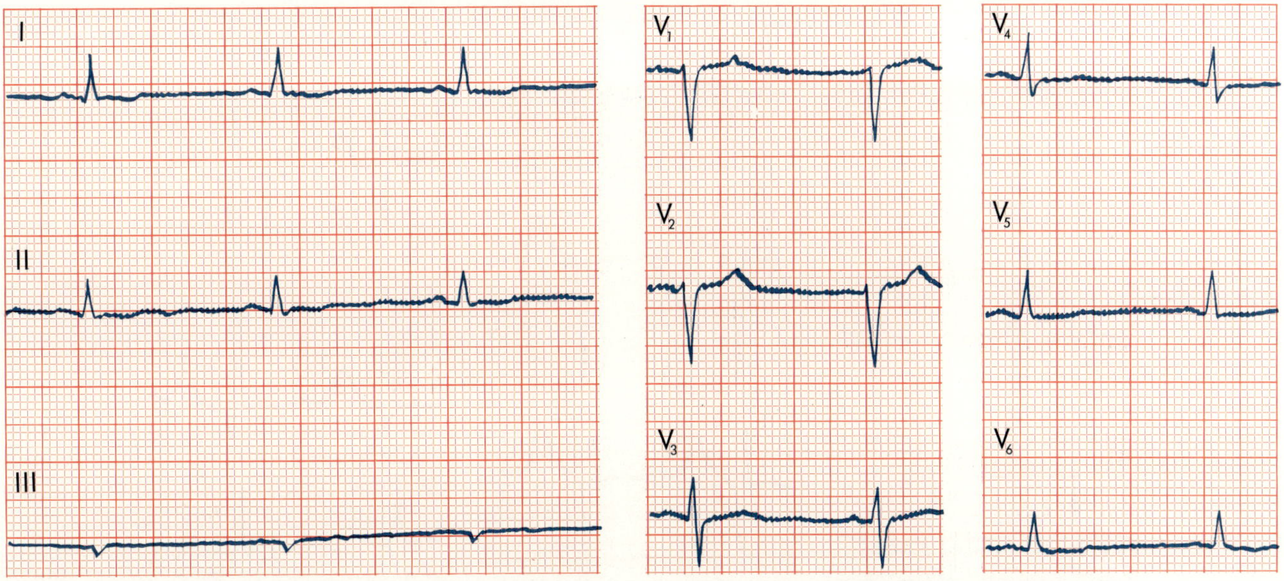

A Low voltage and flattening of the T waves (serum thyroxine 17 nmol/l, triiodothyronine 1.0 nmol/l and TSH 13.2 myU/ml)

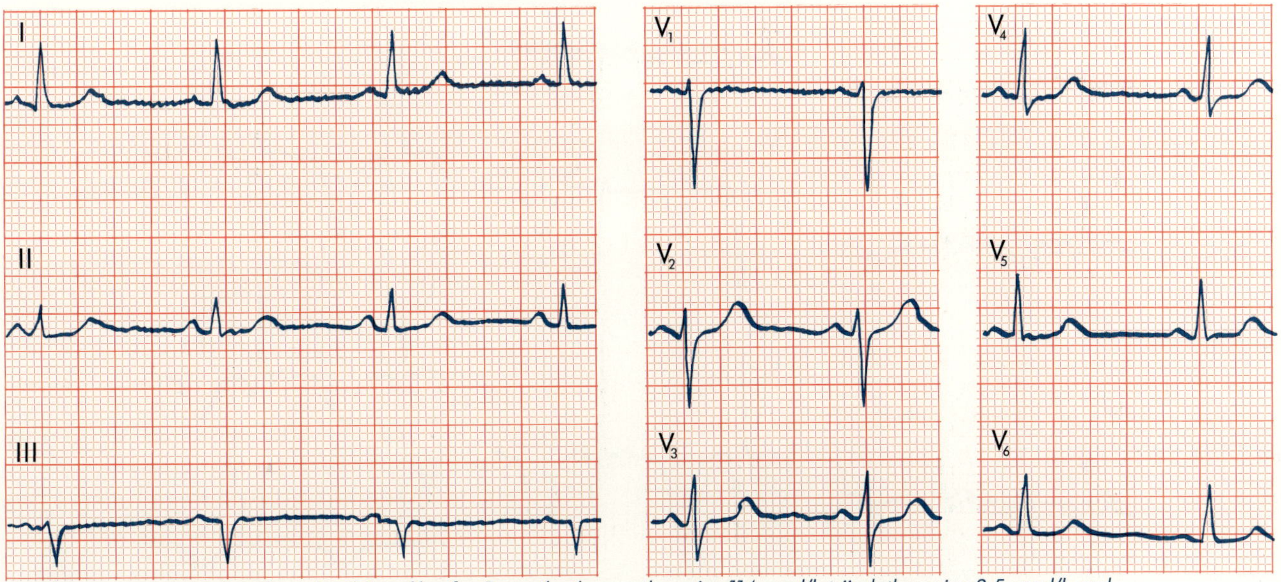

B After treatment with levothyroxine 0.1 mg/day for 8 months (serum thyroxine 114 nmol/l, triiodothyronine 2.5 nmol/l and TSH < 0.2 myU/ml)

Fig. 14.31
Myxoedema. ECG from a 58-year-old woman with hypersensitiviness to cold, increase in weight, hoarseness and fatique for 18 months

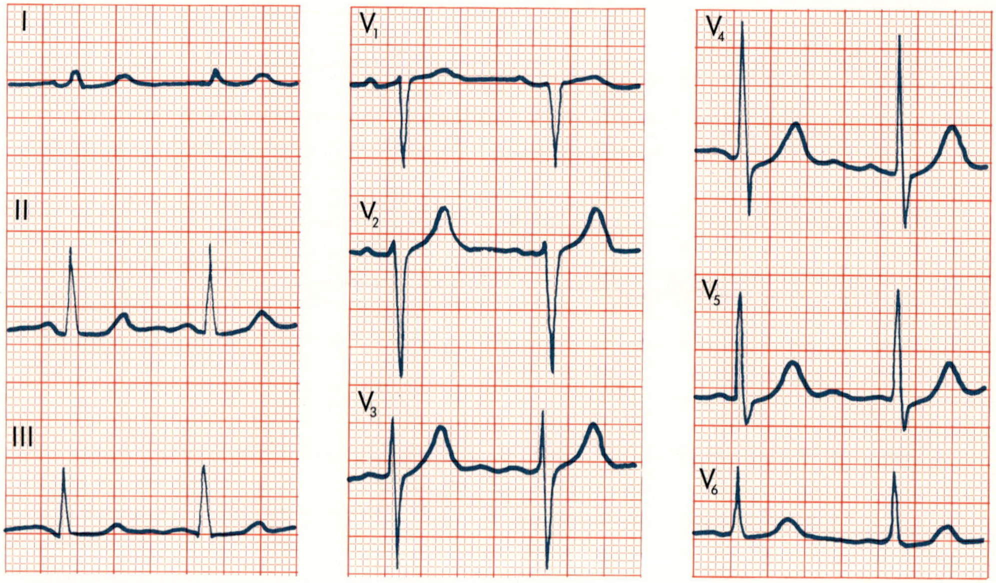

A ECG at admission is normal

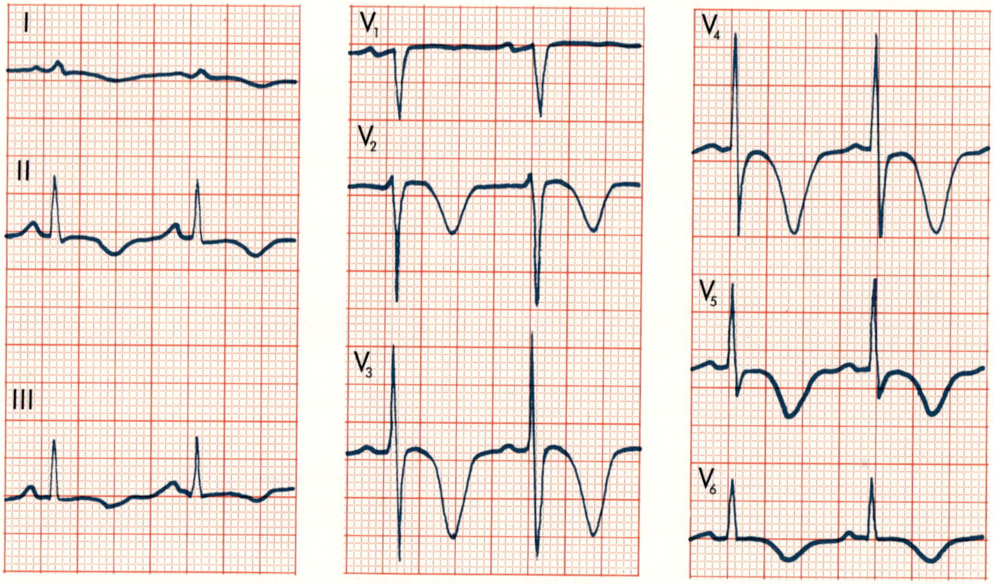

B ECG the day after the development of the hemiparesis. Deep symmetrical negative T waves in V_{1-6} and negative T waves in leads I, II and III

Fig. 14.32
Cerebrovascular accident and T wave changes. ECG from a 73-year-old female who 3 days after admission developed massive left-sided hemiparesis. Blood pressure within normal limits. No history of chest pain and no elevation of serum enzymes

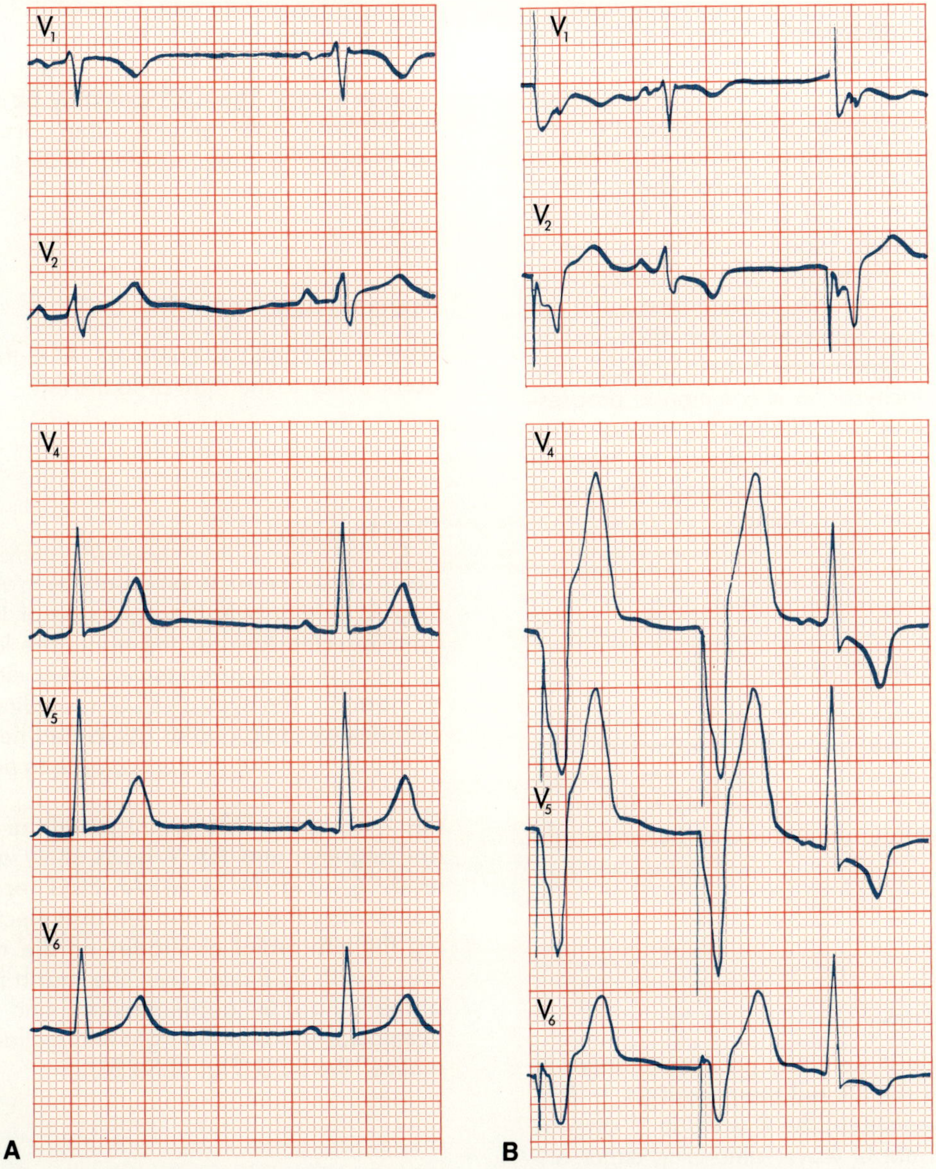

Fig. 14.33
Ventricular (VVI pacing). T wave changes in the non-paced supraventricular QRST complex. ECG from a 69-year-old man with sick sinus syndrome

A Before pacemaker implantation. There is sinus bracycardia (41/min) and there are upright T waves in all precordial leads

B After pacemaker implantation. There is alternation between paced QRS rhythm (rate 74/min) and sinus complexes. The T waves of the sinus complexes are now negative in all precordial leads.

Neuromyopathic disorders [42, 43]

The neuromyopathic disorders: progressive muscular dystrophy of Duchenne's type, Friedreich's ataxia and myotonic dystrophy often are associated with cardiac involvement. ST segment and T wave changes are common in all three conditions. An abnormal Rs pattern in V_1 often is seen in progressive muscular dystrophy of Duchenne's type. Abnormal Q waves simulating the Q waves of a transmural infarction frequently are seen in progressive muscular dystrophy and occasionally in Friedreich's ataxia. Supraventricular and ventricular extrasystoles, paroxysmal supraventricular tachycardia, AV block of varying degrees and bundle branch block are common. Sinus tachycardia is common in progressive muscular dystrophy and Friedreich's ataxia. Sinus bradycardia is common in myotonic dystrophy. Progressive muscular dystrophy may be associated with the development of the sick sinus syndrome.

Connective tissue disease [44–48]

Connective tissue disease e.g. scleroderma and systemic lupus erythematosus can involve the myocardium. The most commonly observed ECG changes are non-specific ST segment and T wave changes. Arrhythmias in the form of extrasystoles, paroxysmal tachycardia and block may occur.

Chest deformities [49, 50]

Deformities of the chest wall may produce changes in the ECG because of the altered heart position. In *funnel chest* (pectus excavatum) the P wave in V_1 often is negative and abnormal Q waves simulating either anterior or inferior transmural myocardial infarction may be observed. T wave inversion is frequent. In the *straight back syndrome* with loss of the normal upper thoracic kyphosis the heart is compressed between the sternum and the vertebral column and T wave changes and sometimes Q wave anomalies are seen.

Obesity [51]

Even in severe obesity ECG changes usually are minor. The R wave may be slightly reduced in height but low voltage is rare. The QRS axis may be shifted slightly to the left but usually remains within normal limits. T wave flattening is the most consistent finding.

Pregnancy [52]

Sinus tachycardia is common. A slight axis shift may occur either to the right or to the left.

Dextrocardia [53]

Dextrocardia refers to all situations in which the heart is located primarily in the right side of the chest with its apex directed towards the right. The lung and the abdominal situs or arrangement may either be reversed or normal. The typical ECG recording in the patient with dextrocardia and/or associated heart disease is an ECG pattern more or less opposite to normal.

The P wave, the QRS complex and the T wave in lead I are negative and the V leads show an RS pattern in leads V_{5-6} (Fig. 14.34 A). An ECG recording made by transposing the right and left arm electrodes and placing the precordial electrodes on the right precordium (V_{1R-6R}) with V_{1R} placed over the fourth intercostal space at the left border of the sternum, and V_{6R} over the fifth intercostal space in the right mid axillary line will "normalize" the ECG (Fig. 14.34 B).

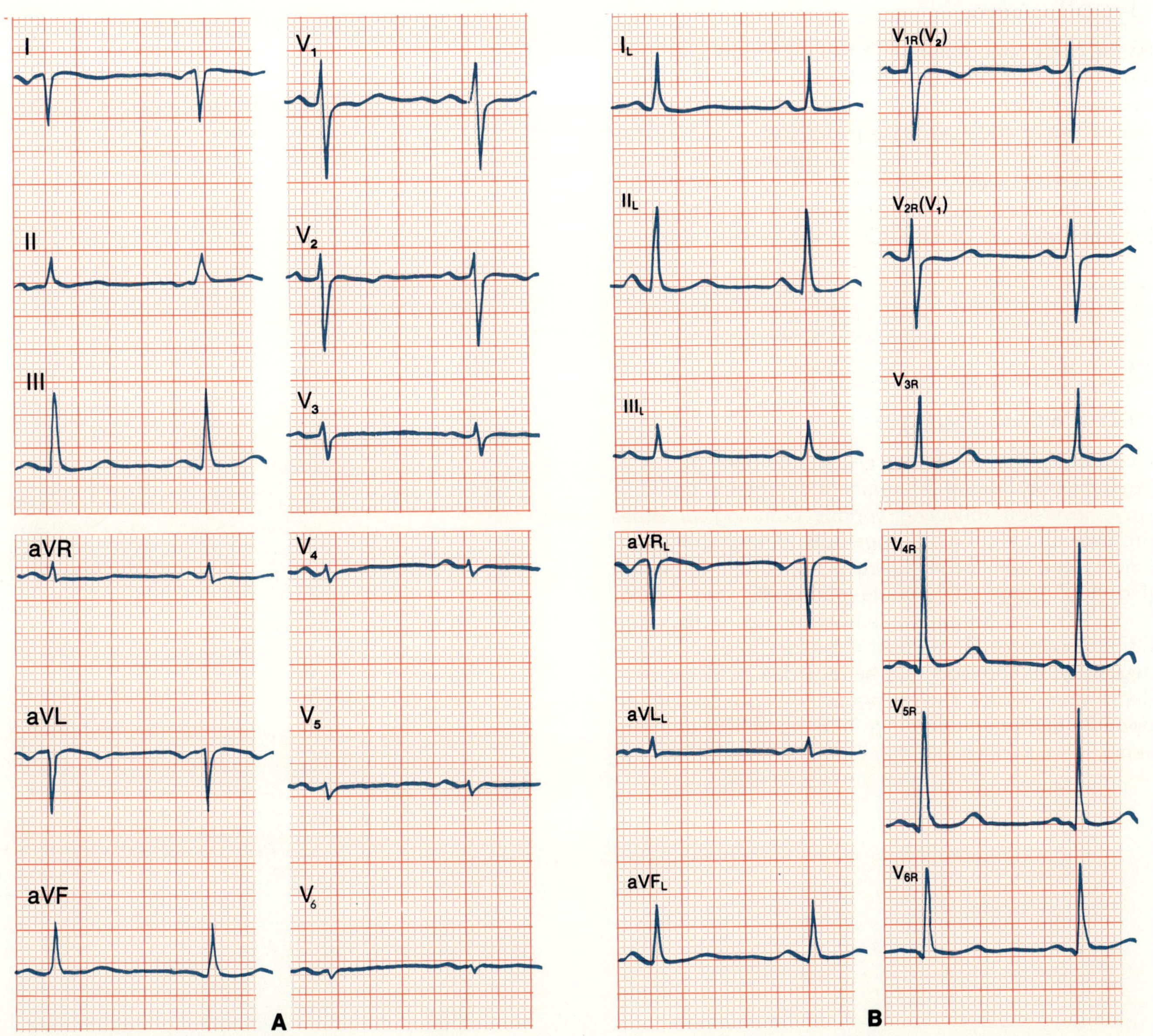

Fig. 14.34
Dextrocardia in healthy boy 15 years of age

A Conventional ECG recording

B ECG recording with transposed left and right arm electrodes and replacement of left precordial leads (V_{1-6}) with right precordial leads (V_{1R-6R}). For explanation see text.

Hypothermia [54, 55]

As the body temperature falls there is progressive slowing of the sinus rate and prolongation of the PR and QT intervals. When the temperature falls below 25° an abnormal wave, the *J wave*, appears early in the ST segment, partly fusing with the QRS complex (Fig. 14.35). Hypothermia often is complicated by atrial fibrillation. Ventricular fibrillation is a major risk at heart temperatures between 27° and 30° C.

Miscellaneous causes of ST segment and T wave changes

There are many conditions which may alter of the ST segment and T wave. ST segment depression and/or T wave inversion reflecting various pathological states are shown in Fig. 14.36, page 358. ST segment elevation is seen with acute Q-wave myocardial infarction (Fig. 14.7, page 317), acute pericarditis (Fig. 14.26, page 343) and transmural ischaemia (Fig. 14.16, page 327). Reciprocal ST segment elevation (and/or T wave negativity) in one lead may be recorded as ST segment depression (and/or T wave positivity) in a lead with an opposite axis orientation (Fig. 14.8, page 319) and vice versa.

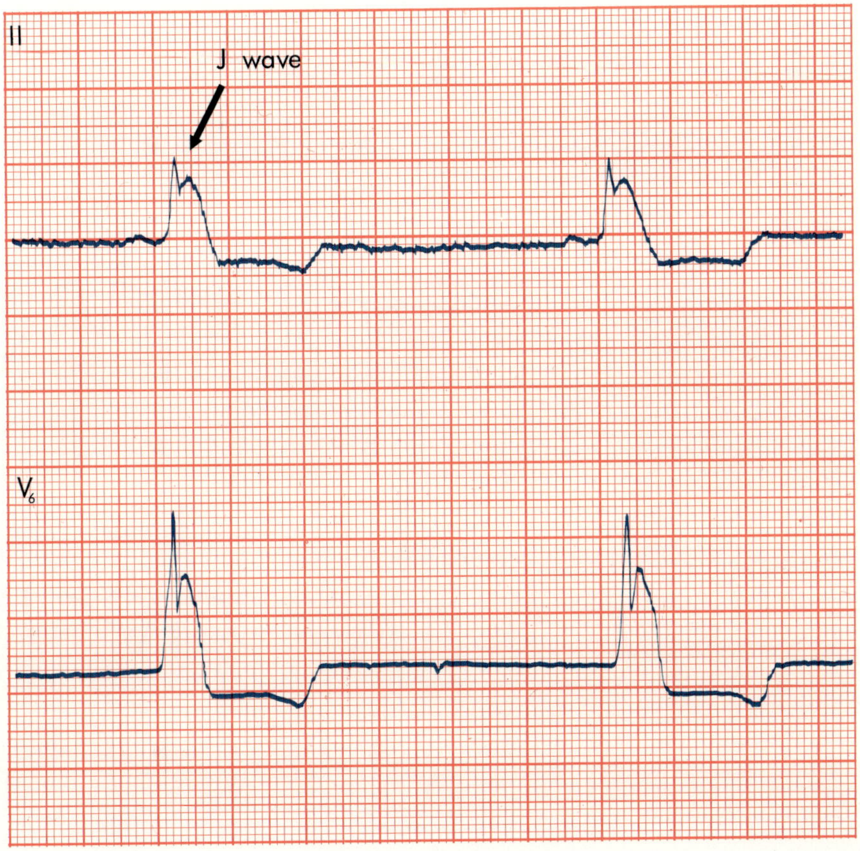

Fig. 14.35
ECG in drowning victim. Rectal temperature 14° of Celsius

A *Left ventricular hypertrophy and strain*

B *Digitalis effect (Cohn effect)*

C *Right ventricular hypertrophy and strain*

D *Acute Q-wave myocardial infarction (days to weeks)*

E *Non-Q-wave infarction*

F *Subendocardial ischaemia*

G *Cerebrovascular accident*

H *After paroxysmal tachycardia*

I *Spontaneous sinus complex in VVI paced patient*

J *Right bundle branch block*

K *Left bundle branch block*

L *WPW pattern*

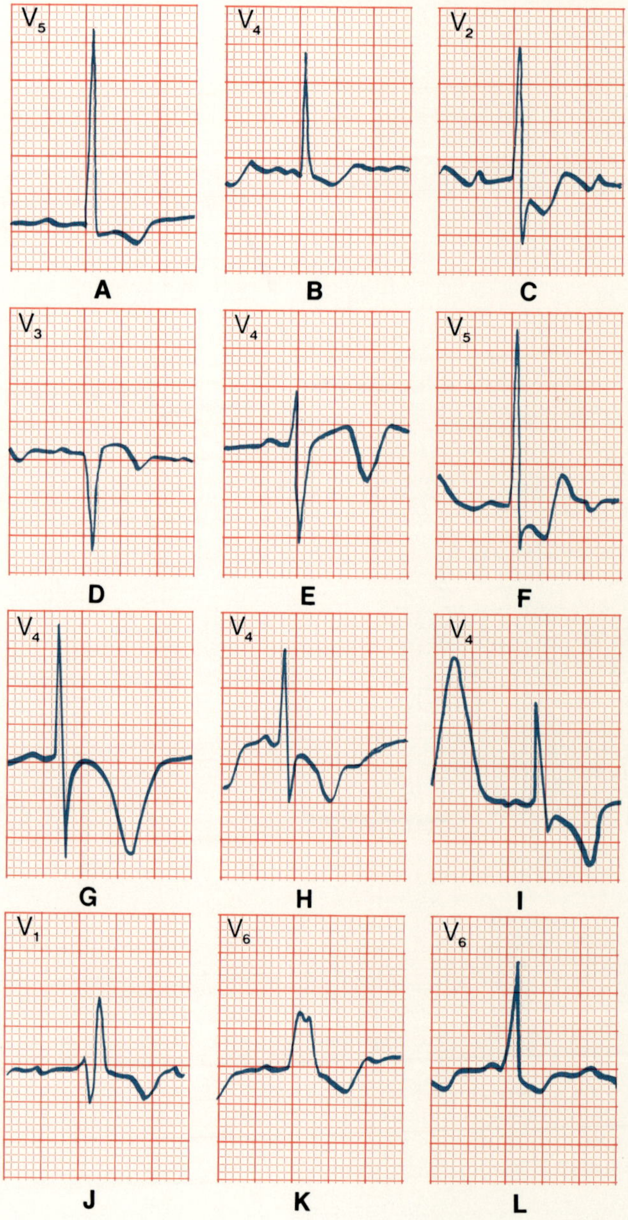

Fig. 14.36
Various causes of ST segment depression and/or T wave negativity

1. The Criteria Committee of the New York Heart Association: Nomenclature and Criteria for Diagnosis of Diseases of the Heart and Great Vessels, 8th edition. Boston: Little, Brown and Co., 1979; 90–119.
2. Schamroth L. An introduction to electrocardiography. Oxford, London: Blackwell Scientific Publications, 1976.
3. Schamroth L. Abnormalities of the P wave. Ingelheim am Rhein: Boehringer Ingelheim Postgraduate Medical Services, 1983; 3–26.
4. Surawicz B. Electrocardiographic diagnosis of chamber en largement. JACC 1986; 711–24.
5. Schamroth L. The electrocardiology of coronary artery disease. 2nd edition. Oxford: Blackwell Scientific Pub lications, 1984.
6. Yasuda T, Ribeiro HG, Holman BL. Accuracy of localization of acute myocardial infarction by 12 lead electrocardiography. J Electrocardiol 1982; 15: 181–88.
7. Phibbs B. "Transmural" versus "subendocardial" myocardial infarction: An electrocardiographic myth. JACC 1983; 1: 561–64.
8. Gibson RS. Non-Q-wave myocardial infarction: Diagnosis, prognosis and management. In: O'Rourke RA, Crawford MH, eds. Current problems in cardiology. Chicago, Illinois: Year Book Medical Publisher, Inc.; 5–72.
9. Mandel WJ, Peter CT, Hoffmann I. Electrocardiographic diagnostic dilemmas in myocardial ischemia and infarction. In: Wellens HJJ, Kulbertus HE, eds. What's new in electrocardiography. The Hague, Boston, London: Martinus Nijhoff Publishers, 1981; 58–78.
10. Christie LG, Conti CR. Systematic approach to evaluation of anginalike chest pain: Pathophysiology and clinical testing with emphasis on objective documentation of myocardial ischemia. Am Heart J 1981; 102: 897–912.
11. Detrano R, Froelicher VF. Exercise testing: Uses and limitations considering recent studies. Prog Cardiovasc Dis 1988; 31: 173–204.
12. Chahine RA. Unstable angina. The problem of definition. Br Heart J 1975; 37: 1246–49.
13. Hugenholtz PG. Unstable angina revisited once more. Europ Heart J 1986; 7: 1010–13.
14. Maseri A, L'Abbate A, Chierchia S, et al. Significance of spasm in the pathogenensis of ischemic heart disease. Am J Cardiol 1979; 44–47.
15. Bertrand ME, Cherrier F. L'Langine de poitrine de Prinz metal: 20 ans après. Arch Mal Coeur 1979; 72: 939–42.
16. Vilhelmsen R, Mortensen SA, Sandøe E. Diagnostic fallacies and drug management in Prinzmetal's variant angina. In: Mason DT, Collins JJ, eds. Myocardial revascularization. Medical and surgical advances in coronary disease. New York: Yorke Medical Books, 1981; 122–37.
17. Egstrup K. The sensitivity of the symptom angina pectoris as a marker of transient myocardial ischaemia in chronic stable angina. Acta med scand 1987; 222: 301–06.
18. Epstein SE, Quyyumi AA, Bonow RO. Myocardial ischemia – silent or symptomatic. New Engl J Med 1988; 318: 1038–43.
19. Amsterdam EA. Relation of silent myocardial ischemia to ventricular arrhythmias and sudden death. Am J Cardiol 1988; 62: 24–27.
20. Pedersen F, Pietersen A, Sandøe E. Silent myocardial ischaemia and life threatening ventricular arrhythmias. Ann Clin Res 1988; 20: 404–09.
21. Sargin O, Demirkol C. Deeply inverted T-waves after supraventricular paroxysmal tachycardia. Dis Chest 1965; 48: 321–23.
22. Campbell M. Inversion of T waves after long paroxysms of tachycardia. Br Heart J 1942; 4: 49–56.
23. Nelson SD, Kou WH, Annesley T, et al. Significance of ST segment depression during paroxysmal supraventricular tachycardia. JACC 1988; 12: 383–87.
24. Brugada P, Gorgeis AP, Wellens HJJ. The electrocardiogram in pulmonary embolism. In: Wellens HJJ, Kulbertus HE, eds. What's new in electrocardiography. The Hague, Boston, London: Martinus Nijhoff Publishers, 1981: 366–80.
25. Spodick DH. Pathogenesis and clinical correlations of the electrocardiographic abnormalities of pericardial disease. Cardiovasc Clin 1977; 8: 201–13.
26. Bruce MA, Spodick DH. Atypical electrocardiogram in acute pericarditis: Characteristics and prevalence. J Electro cardiol 1980; 13: 61–66.
27. Unverferth DV, Williams TE, Fulkerson PK. Electrocardiographic voltage in pericardial effusion. Chest 1979; 75: 157–60.
28. Chesier E, Mitha AS, Matison RE. The ECG of constrictive pericarditis – Pattern resembling right ventricular hypertrophy. Am Heart J 1976; 91: 420–24.
29. Keith JD. Rheumatic fever and rheumatic heart disease. In: Keith JD, Rowe RD, Vlad P, eds. Heart disease in infancy and childhood. New York: Macmillan Publishing Co., 1978; 213–14.
30. Fine I, Bramerd H, Sokolow M. Myocarditits in acute infectious diseases. A clinical and electrocardiographic study. Circulation 1950; 2: 859–71.
31. Oakley CM. Clinical recognition of the cardiomyopathias. Circulation Res 1974; 34,35 (Suppl. II): 152–67.
32. McKenna WJ, Borggrefe M, England D, et al. The natural history of left ventricular hypertrophy in hypertrophic cardiomyopathy: An electrocardiographic study. Circulation 1982; 66: 1233–40.
33. Kuhn H, Breithardt G, Knieriem H-J, et al. Prognosis and possible presymptomatic manifestations of congestive cardiomyopathy (COCM). Postgrad Med J 1978; 54: 451–59.
34. Surawicz B, Mangiardi ML. Electrocardiogram in endocrine and metabolic disorders. In: Rios JC, ed. Clinical-electrocardiographic correlations. Cardiovasc Clin 1977; 8: 243–66.
35. Fredlund B-O, Olsson SB. Long QT interval and ventricular tachycardia of "Torsade de pointe" type in hypothyroidism. Acta med scand 1983; 213: 231–35.
36. Weidler DJ. Myocardial damage and cardiac arrhythmias after intracranial hemorrhage: A critical review. Stroke 1974; 5: 759.
37. Melein J, Fogelholm R. Electrocardiographic findings in subarachnoid hemmorhage. A population study. Acta med scand 1983; 213: 5–8.
38. Nakamura Y, Kaseno K, Kubo T. Transient ST-segment elevation in subarachnoid hemmorrhage. J Electrocardiol 1989; 22: 133–37.
39. Mortensen SA, Meibom J, Nyboe I, et al. Influence on electrocardiogram and cardiac enzymes of permanent pacing simulating myocardial infarction. In: Ferugio GA, ed. Cardiac pacing. Electrophysiology and pacemaker technology. Padova: Piccin Medical Books, 1983; 967–70.
40. Chatterjee K, Harris AM, Davies JG, et al. T-wave changes after artificial pacing. Lnacet 1969; i: 759–62.

41. Ansari A. Syndrome of mitral valve prolapse: Current perspectives. Prog Cardiovasc Dis 1989; 32: 31–72.
42. Waters DD. Cardiovascular manifestations of neuromuscular disease. In: Hurst JW, ed. Update V. The heart. New York: McGraw-Hill Book Co. 1978; 51–79.
43. Olofsson B-O, Forsberg H, Anderson S, et al. Electrocardiographic findings in myotonic dystrophy. Br Heart J 1988; 59: 47–52.
44. Bulkley BH, Ridolfi RL, Salyer WR, et al. Myocardial lesions of progressive systemic sclerosis. A cause of cardiac dysfunction. Circulation 1976; 53: 483–90.
45. Roberts NK, Cabeen WR, Moss J, et al. The prevalence of conduction defects and cardiac arrhythmias in progressive systemic sclerosis. Ann Int Med 1981; 94: 38–40.
46. Bharati S, de la Fuente DJ, Kallen RJ, et al. Conduction system in systemic lupus erythematosus with atrioventricular block. Am J Cardiol 1975; 35: 299–304.
47. Thunen M, Bjerie P, Stjernberg N. ECG abnormalities in patients with sarcoidosis. Acta med scand 1983; 213: 115–18.
48. Eriksson P, Karp K, Bjerie P, et al. Disturbances of cardiac rhythm and conduction in familial amyloidosis with polyneuropathy. Br Heart J 1984; 51: 658–62.
49. Elisberg EI. Electrocardiographic changes associated with pectus excavatum. Ann Int Med 1958; 49: 130–41.
50. De Oliveira JM, Sambhi MP, Zimmermann HA. The electrocardiogram in pectus excavatum. Br Heart J 1958; 20: 495–501.
51. Eisenstein I, Edelstein J, Sarma R, et al. The electrocardiogram in obesity. J Electrocardiol 1982; 15: 115–18.
52. Schwartz DB, Schamroth L. The effect of pregnancy on the frontal plane QRS axis. J Electrocardiol 1979; 12: 279–81.
53. Van Praagh R, Van Praagh S, Vlad P, et al. Diagnosis of the anatomic types of congenital dextrocardia. Am J Cardiol 1965; 15: 234–47.
54. Vandam LD, Burnap TK. Hyopthermia. New Engl J Med 1959; 261: 546–603.
55. Reuler JB. Hypothermia: Pathophysiology, clinical settings and management. Ann Intern Med 1978; 89: 519–27.

Page numbers in *italics* refer to the principal discussion of a subject.

W